# HEALTH PSYCHOLOGY

# HEALTH PSYCHOLOGY

ELEVENTH EDITION

**SHELLEY E. TAYLOR AND ANNETTE L. STANTON**
University of California, Los Angeles

HEALTH PSYCHOLOGY, ELEVENTH EDITION

Published by McGraw Hill LLC, 1325 Avenue of the Americas, New York, NY 10121. Copyright © 2021 by McGraw Hill LLC. All rights reserved. Printed in the United States of America. Previous editions ©2018, 2015, and 2012. No part of this publication may be reproduced or distributed in any form or by any means, or stored in a database or retrieval system, without the prior written consent of McGraw Hill LLC, including, but not limited to, in any network or other electronic storage or transmission, or broadcast for distance learning.

Some ancillaries, including electronic and print components, may not be available to customers outside the United States.

This book is printed on acid-free paper.

2 3 4 5 6 7 8 9 LWI 24 23 22 21 20

ISBN 978-1-260-25390-0 (bound edition)
MHID 1-260-25390-2 (bound edition)
ISBN 978-1-260-83428-4 (loose-leaf edition)
MHID 1-260-83428-X (loose-leaf edition)

Portfolio Manager: *Erika Lo*
Marketing Manager: *Augustine LaFerrera*
Content Project Managers: *Danielle Clement, Katie Reuter*
Buyer: *Laura Fuller*
Design: *Debra Kubiak*
Content Licensing Specialist: *Shawntel Schmitt*
Cover Image: © *Shutterstock/g-stockstudio*
Compositor: *Aptara®, Inc.*

All credits appearing on page or at the end of the book are considered to be an extension of the copyright page.

### Library of Congress Cataloging-in-Publication Data

Names: Taylor, Shelley E., author. | Stanton, Annette L., author.
Title: Health psychology / Shelley E. Taylor and Annette L. Stanton, University of California, Los
    Angeles.
Description: Eleventh edition. | Dubuque : McGraw-Hill Education, [2021] |
    Includes bibliographical references and indexes. | Audience: Ages 18+ |
    Audience: Grades 10–12
Identifiers: LCCN 2019049194 | ISBN 9781260253900 (hardcover) | ISBN
    9781260834284 (spiral bound) | ISBN 9781260834338 (ebook)
Subjects: LCSH: Clinical health psychology. | Medicine, Psychosomatic.
Classification: LCC R726.7 .T39 2021 | DDC 616.001/9—dc23
LC record available at https://lccn.loc.gov/2019049194

mheducation.com/highered

For Everyone Living with
a Chronic Disease Who
So Generously Takes Part
in Our Research

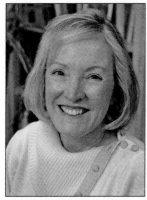

Courtesy of Shelley E. Taylor

**SHELLEY E. TAYLOR** is Distinguished Professor of Psychology at the University of California, Los Angeles. She received her Ph.D. in social psychology from Yale University. After a visiting professorship at Yale and assistant and associate professorships at Harvard University, she joined the faculty of UCLA. Her research interests concern the psychological and social factors that promote or compromise mental and physical health across the life span. Professor Taylor is the recipient of a number of awards—most notably, the American Psychological Association's Distinguished Scientific Contribution to Psychology Award, a 10-year Research Scientist Development Award from the National Institute of Mental Health, and an Outstanding Scientific Contribution Award in Health Psychology. She is the author of more than 350 publications in journals and books and is the author of *Social Cognition*, *Social Psychology*, *Positive Illusions,* and *The Tending Instinct*. She is a member of the National Academy of Sciences and the National Academy of Medicine.

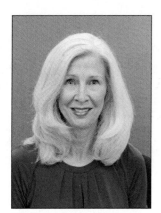

Courtesy of Annette Stanton

**ANNETTE L. STANTON** is Professor of Psychology and Psychiatry/ Biobehavioral Sciences, Senior Research Scientist at the Cousins Center for Psychoneuroimmunology, and Member of the Jonsson Comprehensive Cancer Center at the University of California, Los Angeles. She earned the Ph.D. in clinical psychology at the University of Connecticut. After serving as faculty at Auburn University and the University of Kansas, she joined the faculty of UCLA in 2003. Through her research, Dr. Stanton identifies factors that promote or impede psychological and physical health in adults and couples undergoing chronically stressful experiences, with a focus on the experience of cancer. She translates her findings into action by developing and testing approaches to enhance psychological and physical health in those populations. An author of more than 250 publications in scientific journals and books, she has served as President of the Society for Health Psychology of the American Psychological Association. Her research and professional contributions have been recognized by awards from that society, the International Society of Behavioral Medicine, the American Psychosocial Oncology Society, and the Cancer Support Community. She also is an award-winning teacher and mentor of undergraduate and graduate students.

# CONTENTS

# PART 2

## HEALTH BEHAVIOR AND PRIMARY PREVENTION

PART 3

## STRESS AND COPING

PART 4

# SEEKING AND USING HEALTH CARE SERVICES

CHAPTER 8
## Using Health Services  168

**Recognition and Interpretation of Symptoms  169**

Recognition of Symptoms  169
Interpretation of Symptoms  170
Cognitive Representations of Illness  170
   BOX 8.1 Can Expectations Influence Sensations?
     The Case of Premenstrual Symptoms  171
Lay Referral Network  172
The Internet  172

**Who Uses Health Services?  172**

Age  172
Gender  172
Social Class and Culture  173
Social Psychological Factors  173

**Misusing Health Services  174**

Using Health Services for Emotional
     Disturbances  174
   BOX 8.2 The June Bug Disease: A Case of
     Hysterical Contagion  175
Delay Behavior  175


CHAPTER 9
## Patients, Providers, and Treatments  179

**Health Care Services  180**

Patient Consumerism  180
Structure of the Health Care Delivery System  180
Patient Experiences with Managed Care  181

**The Nature of Patient–Provider Communication  182**

Setting  182
Provider Behaviors That Contribute to Faulty
     Communication  183
   BOX 9.1 What Did You Say?: Language Barriers to
     Effective Communication  184
Patients' Contributions to Faulty Communication  184
Interactive Aspects of the Communication
     Problem  185
Use of Artificial Intelligence  186

**Results of Poor Patient–Provider Communication  186**

Nonadherence to Treatment Regimens  186

   BOX 9.2 What Are Some Ways to Improve
     Adherence to Treatment?  187

**Improving Patient–Provider Communication and Increasing Adherence to Treatment  188**

Teaching Providers How to Communicate  188
   BOX 9.3 What Can Providers Do to Improve
     Adherence?  189

**The Patient in the Hospital Setting  190**

Structure of the Hospital  191
The Impact of Hospitalization
     on the Patient  192
   BOX 9.4 Burnout Among Health Care
     Professionals  193

**Interventions to Increase Information in Hospital Settings  194**

**The Hospitalized Child  194**

   BOX 9.5 Social Support and Distress from
     Surgery  195
Preparing Children for Medical
     Interventions  195

**Complementary and Alternative Medicine  196**

Philosophical Origins of CAM  197

**CAM Treatments  198**

Dietary Supplements and Diets  198
Prayer  199
Acupuncture  199
Yoga  199
Hypnosis  200
Meditation  200
Guided Imagery  200
Chiropractic Medicine  201
Osteopathy  201
Massage  201
Who Uses CAM?  201
Complementary and Alternative Medicine: An Overall
     Evaluation  202

**The Placebo Effect  203**

History of the Placebo  203
   BOX 9.6 Cancer and the Placebo Effect  204
What Is a Placebo?  204
Provider Behavior and Placebo Effects  204
Patient Characteristics and Placebo Effects  205

PART 5

## MANAGEMENT OF CHRONIC AND TERMINAL HEALTH DISORDERS

When I (Dr. Taylor) wrote the first edition of *Health Psychology* over 30 years ago, the task was much simpler than it is now. Health psychology was a new field and was relatively small. In recent decades, the field has grown steadily, and great research advances have been made. Chief among these developments is the use and refinement of the biopsychosocial model: the study of health issues from the standpoint of biological, psychological, and social factors acting together. Increasingly, researchers have identified the biological pathways by which psychosocial factors such as stress may adversely affect health and potentially protective factors such as social support may buffer the impact of stress. With Dr. Stanton joining as an author, our goal in the 11th edition of this text is to convey this increasing sophistication of the field in a manner that makes it accessible, comprehensible, and exciting to undergraduates.

Like any science, health psychology is cumulative, building on past research advances to develop new ones. Accordingly, we have tried to present not only the fundamental contributions to the field but also the current research on these issues. Because health psychology is developing and changing so rapidly, it is essential that a text be up to date. Therefore, we have not only reviewed the recent research in health psychology but also obtained information about research projects that will not be available in the research literature for several years. In so doing, we are presenting a text that is both current and pointed toward the future.

A second goal is to portray health psychology appropriately as being intimately involved with the problems of our times. The aging of the population and the shift in numbers toward the later years have created unprecedented health needs to which health psychology must respond. Such efforts include the need for health promotion with this aging cohort and an understanding of the psychosocial issues that arise in response to aging and its associated chronic disorders. Because AIDS is a leading cause of death worldwide, the need for health measures such as condom use is readily apparent if we are to halt the spread of this disease. Obesity is now one of the world's leading health problems, nowhere more so than in the United States. Reversing this dire trend that threatens to shorten life expectancy worldwide is an important current goal of health psychology. Increasingly, health psychology is an international undertaking, with researchers from around the world providing insights into the problems that affect both developing and developed countries. The 11th edition includes current research that reflects the international focus of both health problems and the health research community.

Health habits lie at the origin of our most prevalent disorders, and this fact underscores more than ever the importance of modifying problematic health behaviors such as smoking and alcohol consumption. Increasingly, research documents the importance of a healthy diet, regular exercise, and weight control among other positive health habits for maintaining good health. The at-risk role has taken on more importance in prevention, as breakthroughs in genetic research have made it possible to identify genetic risks for diseases long before disease is evident. How people cope with being at risk and what interventions are appropriate for them represent important tasks for health psychology research to address.

Health psychology is both an applied field and a basic research field. Accordingly, in highlighting the accomplishments of the field, we present both the scientific progress and its important applications. Chief among these are efforts by clinical psychologists to intervene with people to treat biopsychosocial disorders, such as post traumatic stress disorder; to help people manage health habits that have become life threatening, such as eating disorders; and to develop clinical interventions that help people better manage their chronic illnesses.

Finding the right methods and venues for modifying health continues to be a critical issue. The chapters on health promotion put particular emphasis on the most promising methods for changing health behaviors. The chapters on chronic diseases highlight how knowledge of the psychosocial causes and consequences of these disorders may be used to intervene with people at risk—first, to reduce the likelihood that such disorders will develop, and second, to deal effectively with the psychosocial issues that arise following diagnosis.

The success of any text depends ultimately on its ability to communicate the content clearly to student readers and spark interest in the field. In this 11th edition, we strive to make the material interesting and relevant to the lives of student readers. Many chapters highlight news stories related to health. In addition, the presentation of material has been tied to the needs and interests of young adults. For example, the topic of stress management is tied directly to how students might manage the stresses associated with college life. The topic of problem drinking includes sections on college students' alcohol consumption and its modification. Health habits relevant to this age group—tanning, exercise, and condom use, among others—are highlighted for their relevance to the student population. By learning from anecdotes, case histories, and specific research examples that are relevant to their own lives, students learn how important this body of knowledge is to their lives as young adults.

Health psychology is a science, and consequently, it is important to communicate not only the research itself but also some understanding of how studies were designed and why they were designed that way. The explanations of particular research methods and the theories that have guided research appear throughout the book. Important studies are described in depth so that students have a sense of the methods researchers use to make decisions about how to gather the best data on a problem or how to intervene most effectively.

Throughout the book, we have made an effort to balance general coverage of psychological concepts with coverage of specific health issues. One method of doing so is by presenting groups of chapters, with the initial chapter offering general concepts and subsequent chapters applying those concepts to specific health issues. Thus, Chapter 3 discusses general strategies of health promotion, and Chapters 4 and 5 discuss those issues with specific reference to particular health habits such as exercise, smoking, accident prevention, and weight control. Chapters 11 and 12 discuss broad issues that arise in the context of managing chronic health disorders and terminal illness. In Chapters 13 and 14, these issues are addressed concretely, with reference to specific disorders such as heart disease, cancer, and AIDS.

Rather than adopt a particular theoretical emphasis throughout the book, we have attempted to maintain a flexible orientation. Because health psychology is taught within all areas of psychology (e.g., clinical, social, cognitive, physiological, learning, and developmental), material from each of these areas is included in the text so that it can be accommodated to the orientation of each instructor. Consequently, not all material in the book is relevant for all courses. Successive chapters of the book build on each other but do not depend on each other. Chapter 2, for example, can be used as assigned reading, or it can act as a resource for students wishing to clarify their understanding of biological concepts or learn more about a particular biological system or illness. Thus, each instructor can accommodate the use of the text to his or her needs, giving some chapters more attention than others and omitting some chapters altogether, without undermining the integrity of the presentation.

## ■ NEW TO THIS EDITION

- More than 300 new citations
- Discussion of artificial intelligence and health care (Chapters 1, 9)
- Expanded coverage of web-based interventions (Chapters 1, 3, 11)
- Coverage of the significance of telomeres (Chapters 2, 6)
- Coverage of the gut–brain connection (Chapter 2)
- Discussion of telemedicine (Chapters 2, 8, 15)
- Expanded coverage of dementia (Chapters 2, 11)
- Discussion of socio cultural values and health (Chapters 3, 14)
- Expanded coverage of aging and health (Chapters 3, 4, 11, 14)
- Coverage of just-in-time interventions (Chapters 3, 15)
- Enhanced coverage of marijuana use (Chapter 5)
- New research on positive parenting, stress, and health (Chapter 6)
- Expanded converge on the health effects of prejudice and discrimination (Chapters 6, 13, 14, 15)
- Coverage of the benefits of a sense of purpose and meaning in life (Chapter 7)
- Coverage of research on attempts to cope through actively approaching or avoiding stressful experiences (Chapter 7)
- Enhanced coverage of couples' attempts to cope with shared stressors (Chapter 7)
- Expanded coverage of mindfulness and mindfulness meditation (Chapters 7, 10)
- Enhanced coverage of the health consequences of social support and loneliness (Chapter 7)
- Discussion of the opioid crisis (Chapter 10)
- Expanded coverage of suicide (Chapter 12)
- Coverage of palliative care and end-of-life options (Chapter 12)
- Expanded discussion of bereavement (Chapter 12)
- Enhanced coverage of the prevention and treatment of HIV/AIDS (Chapter 14)
- Expanded coverage of contributors to cancer onset and progression (Chapter 14)
- The changing face of health psychology (Chapter 15)

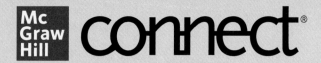

## You're in the driver's seat.

Want to build your own course? No problem. Prefer to use our turnkey, prebuilt course? Easy. Want to make changes throughout the semester? Sure. And you'll save time with Connect's auto-grading too.

# 65%
## Less Time Grading

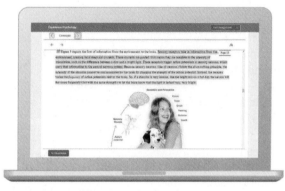

Laptop: McGraw-Hill; Woman/dog: George Doyle/Getty Images

## They'll thank you for it.

Adaptive study resources like SmartBook® 2.0 help your students be better prepared in less time. You can transform your class time from dull definitions to dynamic debates. Find out more about the powerful personalized learning experience available in SmartBook 2.0 at **www.mheducation.com/highered/connect/ smartbook**

## Make it simple, make it affordable.

Connect makes it easy with seamless integration using any of the major Learning Management Systems— Blackboard®, Canvas, and D2L, among others—to let you organize your course in one convenient location. Give your students access to digital materials at a discount with our inclusive access program. Ask your McGraw-Hill representative for more information.

Padlock: Jobalou/Getty Images

## Solutions for your challenges.

A product isn't a solution. Real solutions are affordable, reliable, and come with training and ongoing support when you need it and how you want it. Our Customer Experience Group can also help you troubleshoot tech problems— although Connect's 99% uptime means you might not need to call them. See for yourself at **status. mheducation.com**

Checkmark: Jobalou/Getty Images

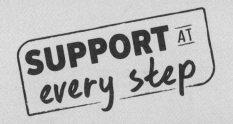

## FOR STUDENTS

## Effective, efficient studying.

Connect helps you be more productive with your study time and get better grades using tools like SmartBook 2.0, which highlights key concepts and creates a personalized study plan. Connect sets you up for success, so you walk into class with confidence and walk out with better grades.

## Study anytime, anywhere.

Download the free ReadAnywhere app and access your online eBook or SmartBook 2.0 assignments when it's convenient, even if you're offline. And since the app automatically syncs with your eBook and SmartBook 2.0 assignments in Connect, all of your work is available every time you open it. Find out more at **www.mheducation.com/readanywhere**

> *"I really liked this app—it made it easy to study when you don't have your textbook in front of you."*
>
> - Jordan Cunningham, Eastern Washington University

Calendar: owattaphotos/Getty Images

## No surprises.

The Connect Calendar and Reports tools keep you on track with the work you need to get done and your assignment scores. Life gets busy; Connect tools help you keep learning through it all.

## Learning for everyone.

McGraw-Hill works directly with Accessibility Services Departments and faculty to meet the learning needs of all students. Please contact your Accessibility Services office and ask them to email accessibility@mheducation.com, or visit **www.mheducation.com/about/accessibility** for more information.

Top: Jenner Images/Getty Images, Left: Hero Images/Getty Images, Right: Hero Images/Getty Images

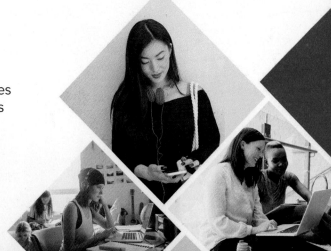

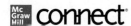

The 11th edition of *Health Psychology* is now available online with Connect, McGraw-Hill's integrated assignment and assessment platform. Connect also offers SmartBook® 2.0 for the new edition, which is an adaptive reading experience proven to improve grades and help students study more effectively. All of the title's ancillary content is also available through Connect, including:

- An Instructor's Manual for each chapter, with student learning objectives and lab exercises.
- A full Test Bank of multiple-choice questions that test students on central concepts and ideas in each chapter.
- Lecture Slides and an Image Bank for instructor use in class.

## ■ ACKNOWLEDGMENTS

Our extensive gratitude goes to Alexandra Jorge and Rachel Caprini for the many hours they put in on the manuscript. We thank our team at McGraw-Hill, Erika Lo and David Patterson, and our development editor Ann Loch, who devoted much time and help to the preparation of the book. We also wish to thank the following reviewers who commented on all or part of the book:

Kaston D. Anderson-Carpenter, *Michigan State University*
Elizabeth Ash, *Morehead State University*
Eric Benotsch, *Virginia Commonwealth University*
David Chun, *Montclair State University*
Len Lecci, *University of North Carolina Wilmington*
Suzanne Morrow, *Old Dominion University*
Ilona Yim, *University of California, Irvine*

**Shelley E. Taylor and Annette L. Stanton**

# PART 1

# Introduction to Health Psychology

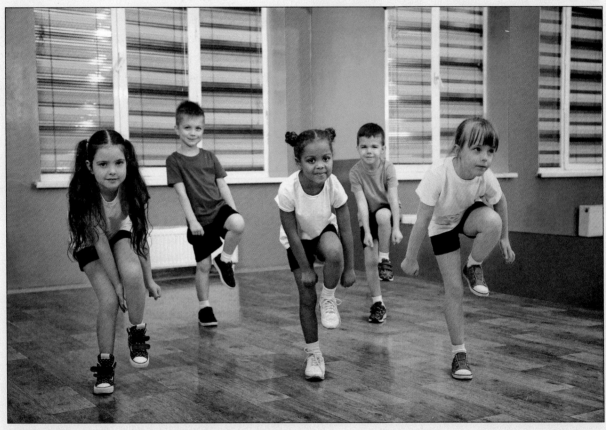

Africa Studio/Shutterstock

CHAPTER 1

# What Is Health Psychology?

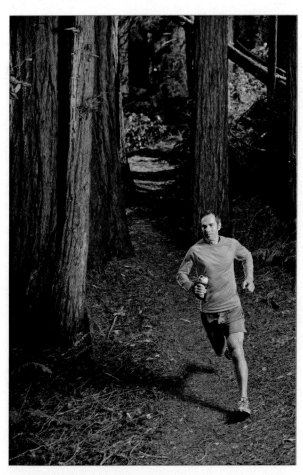

Jacom Stephens/Getty Images

"Government's role in fighting loneliness" (September 12, 2018)

"Vaccination is a social responsibility" (February 4, 2015)

"Risk of concussions from youth sports" (December 25, 2015)

"AI holds promise for improving diagnosis" (September 13, 2018)

"Too little rest is bad for a heart" (January 22, 2019)

"Be kind to your brain—workout" (January 22, 2019)

Every day, we see headlines about health. We are told that smoking is bad for us, that we need to exercise more, and that we've grown obese. We learn about new treatments for diseases about which we are only dimly aware, or we hear that a particular herbal remedy may make us feel better about ourselves. We are told that meditation or optimistic beliefs can keep us healthy or help us get well more quickly. How do we make sense of all these claims? Health psychology addresses important questions like these.

## ■ DEFINITION OF HEALTH PSYCHOLOGY

**Health psychology** is an exciting and relatively new field devoted to understanding psychological influences on how people stay healthy, why they become ill, and how they respond when they do get ill. Health psychologists both study such issues and develop interventions to help people stay well or recover from illness. For example, a health psychology researcher might explore why people continue to smoke even though they know that smoking increases their risk of cancer and heart disease. Understanding this poor health habit leads to interventions to help people stop smoking.

Fundamental to research and practice in health psychology is the definition of health. Decades ago, a forward-looking World Health Organization (1948) defined **health** as "a complete state of physical, mental, and social well-being and not merely the absence of disease or infirmity." This definition is at the core of health psychologists' conception of health. Rather than defining health as the absence of illness, health is recognized to be an achievement involving balance among physical, mental, and social well-being. Many use the term **wellness** to refer to this optimum state of health.

Health psychologists focus on *health promotion and maintenance,* which includes issues such as how to get children to develop good health habits, how to promote regular exercise, and how to design a media campaign to get people to improve their diets.

Health psychologists study the psychological aspects of the *prevention and treatment of illness.* A health psychologist might teach people in a high-stress occupation how to manage stress effectively to avoid health risks. A health psychologist might work with people who are already ill to help them follow their treatment regimen.

Health psychologists also focus on *the etiology and correlates of health, illness, and dysfunction.* **Etiology** refers to the origins or causes of illness. Health psychologists especially address the behavioral and social factors that contribute to health, illness, and dysfunction, such as alcohol consumption, drug use, exercise, the wearing of seat belts, and ways of coping with stress.

Finally, health psychologists analyze and attempt to improve *the health care system and the formulation of health policy.* They study the impact of health institutions and health professionals on people's behavior to develop recommendations for improving health care.

In summary, health psychology examines the psychological and social factors that lead to the enhancement of health, the prevention and treatment of illness, and the evaluation and modification of health policies that influence health care.

### Why Did Health Psychology Develop?

To many people, health is simply a matter of staying well or getting over illnesses quickly. Psychological and social factors might seem to have little to contribute. But consider some of the following puzzles that cannot be understood without the input of health psychology:

- When people are exposed to a cold virus, some get colds whereas others do not.
- Men who are married live longer than men who are not married.
- Throughout the world, life expectancy is increasing. But in countries going through dramatic social upheaval, life expectancy can plummet.
- Women live longer than men in all countries except those in which they are denied access to health care. But women are more disabled, have more illnesses, and use health services more.

- Infectious diseases such as tuberculosis, pneumonia, and influenza used to be the major causes of illness and death in the United States. Now chronic disorders such as heart disease, cancer, and diabetes are the main causes of disability and death.

- Attending a church or synagogue, praying, or otherwise tending to spiritual needs is good for your health.

By the time you have finished this book, you will know why these findings are true.

## ■ THE MIND–BODY RELATIONSHIP: A BRIEF HISTORY

During prehistoric times, most cultures regarded the mind and body as intertwined. Disease was thought to arise when evil spirits entered the body, and treatment consisted primarily of attempts to exorcise these spirits. Some skulls from the Stone Age have small, symmetrical holes that are believed to have been made intentionally with sharp tools to allow the evil spirit to leave the body while the shaman performed the treatment ritual.

The ancient Greeks were among the earliest civilizations to identify the role of bodily factors in health and illness. Rather than ascribing illness to evil spirits, they developed a humoral theory of illness. According to this viewpoint, disease resulted when the four humors or circulating fluids of the body—blood, black bile, yellow bile, and phlegm—were out of balance. The goal of treatment was to restore balance among the humors. The Greeks also believed that the mind was important. They described personality types associated with each of the four humors, with blood being associated with a passionate temperament, black bile with sadness, yellow bile with an angry disposition, and phlegm with a laid-back approach to life. Although these theories are now known not to be true, the emphasis on mind and body in health and illness was a breakthrough for that time.

By the Middle Ages, however, the pendulum had swung to supernatural explanations for illness. Disease was regarded as God's punishment for evildoing, and cure often consisted of driving out the evil forces by torturing the body. Later, this form of "therapy" was replaced by penance through prayer and good works. During this time, the Church was the guardian of medical knowledge, and as a result, medical practice assumed religious overtones. The functions of the physician were typically absorbed by priests, and so healing and the practice of religion became virtually indistinguishable.

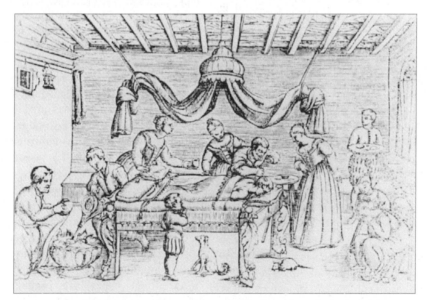

*Sophisticated, though not always successful, techniques for the treatment of illness were developed during the Renaissance. This woodcut from the 1570s depicts a surgeon drilling a hole in a patient's skull, with the patient's family and pets looking on.*
Source: The National Library of Medicine.

Beginning in the Renaissance and continuing into the present day, great strides were made in understanding the technical bases of medicine. These advances include the invention of the microscope in the 1600s and the development of the science of autopsy, which allowed medical practitioners to see the organs that were implicated in different diseases. As the science of cellular pathology progressed, the humoral theory of illness was put to rest. Medical practice drew increasingly on laboratory findings and looked to bodily factors rather than to the mind as bases for health and illness. In an effort to break with the superstitions of the past, practitioners resisted acknowledging any role for the mind in disease processes. Instead, they focused primarily on organic and cellular pathology as a basis for their diagnoses and treatment recommendations.

The resulting **biomedical model,** which has governed the thinking of most health practitioners for the past 300 years, maintains that all illness can be explained on the basis of aberrant somatic bodily processes, such as biochemical imbalances or neurophysiological abnormalities. The biomedical model assumes that psychological and social processes are largely irrelevant to the disease process. The problems with the biomedical model are summarized in Table 1.1.

**TABLE 1.1  |  The Biomedical Model: Why Is It Ill-suited to Understanding Illness?**

- Reduces illness to low-level processes such as disordered cells and chemical imbalances
- Fails to recognize social and psychological processes as powerful influences over bodily states—assumes a mind–body dualism
- Emphasizes illness over health rather than focusing on behaviors that promote health
- Cannot address many puzzles that face practitioners: why, for example, if six people are exposed to a flu virus, do only three develop the flu?

## ■ THE RISE OF THE BIOPSYCHOSOCIAL MODEL

The biomedical viewpoint began to change with the rise of modern psychology, particularly with Sigmund Freud's (1856–1939) early work on **conversion hysteria.** According to Freud, specific unconscious conflicts can produce physical disturbances that symbolize repressed psychological conflicts. Although this viewpoint is no longer central to health psychology, it gave rise to the field of psychosomatic medicine.

## Psychosomatic Medicine

The idea that specific illnesses are produced by people's internal conflicts was perpetuated in the work of Flanders Dunbar in the 1930s (Dunbar, 1943) and Franz Alexander in the 1940s (Alexander, 1950). For example, Alexander developed a profile of the ulcer-prone personality as someone with excessive needs for dependency and love.

Dunbar and Alexander maintained that conflicts produce anxiety, which becomes unconscious and takes a physiological toll on the body via the autonomic nervous system. The continuous physiological changes eventually produce an organic disturbance. In the case of the ulcer patient, for example, repressed emotions resulting from frustrated dependency and love-seeking needs were thought to increase the secretion of acid in the stomach, eventually eroding the stomach lining and producing ulcers (Alexander, 1950).

Dunbar's and Alexander's work helped shape the emerging field of **psychosomatic medicine** by offering profiles of particular disorders believed to be psychosomatic in origin, that is, caused by emotional conflicts. These disorders include ulcers, hyperthyroidism, rheumatoid arthritis, essential hypertension, neurodermatitis (a skin disorder), colitis, and bronchial asthma.

We now know that all illnesses raise psychological issues. Moreover, researchers now believe that a particular conflict or personality type is not sufficient to produce illness. Rather, the onset of disease is usually due to several factors working together, which may include a biological pathogen (such as a viral or bacterial infection) coupled with social and psychological factors, such as high stress, low social support, and low socioeconomic status.

The idea that the mind and the body together determine health and illness logically implies a model for studying these issues. This model is called the **biopsychosocial model.** Its fundamental assumption is that health and illness are consequences of the interplay of biological, psychological, and social factors.

## Advantages of the Biopsychosocial Model

How does the biopsychosocial model of health and illness overcome the disadvantages of the biomedical model? The biopsychosocial model maintains that biological, psychological, and social factors are all important determinants of health and illness. Both macrolevel processes (such as the existence of social support or the presence of depression) and microlevel processes (such as cellular disorders or chemical imbalances) continually interact to influence health and illness and their course.

The biopsychosocial model emphasizes both health and illness. From this viewpoint, health becomes something that one achieves through attention to biological, psychological, and social needs, rather than something that is taken for granted.

## Clinical Implications of the Biopsychosocial Model

The biopsychosocial model is useful for people treating patients as well. First, the process of diagnosis can benefit from understanding the interacting role of biological, psychological, and social factors in assessing a person's health or illness. Treatment can focus on all three sets of factors.

The biopsychosocial model makes explicit the significance of the relationship between patient and practitioner. An effective patient–practitioner relationship can improve a patient's use of services, the efficacy of treatment, and the rapidity with which illness is resolved.

## The Biopsychosocial Model: The Case History of Nightmare Deaths

To see how completely the mind and body are intertwined in health, consider a case study that intrigued medical researchers for nearly 15 years. It involved the bewildering "nightmare deaths" among Southeast Asians.

Following the Vietnam War, in the 1970s, refugees from Southeast Asia, especially Laos, Vietnam, and Cambodia, immigrated to the United States. Around 1977, the Centers for Disease Control and Prevention (CDC) in Atlanta became aware of a strange phenomenon: sudden, unexpected nocturnal deaths among male refugees from these groups. Death often occurred in the first few hours of sleep. Relatives reported that the victim began to gurgle and move about in bed restlessly. Efforts to awaken him were unsuccessful, and shortly thereafter he died. Even more mysteriously, autopsies revealed no specific cause of death.

However, most of the victims appeared to have a rare, genetically based malfunction in the heart's pacemaker. The fact that only men of particular ethnic backgrounds were affected was consistent with the potential role of a genetic factor. Also, the fact that the deaths seemed to cluster within particular families was

consistent with the genetic theory. But how and why would such a defect be triggered during sleep?

As the number of cases increased, it became evident that psychological and cultural, as well as biological, factors were involved. Some family members reported that the victim had experienced a dream foretelling the death. Among the Hmong of Laos, a refugee group that was especially plagued by these nightmare deaths, dreams are taken seriously as portents of the future. Anxiety due to these dreams, then, may have played a role in the deaths (Adler, 1991).

Another vital set of clues came from a few men who were resuscitated by family members. Several of them said that they had been having a severe night terror. One man, for example, said that his room had suddenly grown darker, and a figure like a large black dog had come to his bed and sat on his chest. He had been unable to push the dog off and had become quickly and dangerously short of breath (Tobin & Friedman, 1983). This was also an important clue because night terrors are known to produce abrupt and dramatic physiological changes.

Interviews with the survivors revealed that many of the men had been watching violent TV shows shortly before retiring, and the content of the shows appeared to have made its way into some of the frightening dreams. In other cases, the fatal event occurred immediately after a family argument. Many of the men were said by their families to have been exhausted from combining demanding full-time jobs with a second job or with night school classes to learn English. The pressures to support their families had been taking their toll.

All these clues suggest that the pressures of adjusting to life in the United States played a role in the deaths. The victims may have been overwhelmed by cultural differences, language barriers, and difficulties finding satisfactory jobs. The combination of this chronic strain, a genetic susceptibility, and an immediate trigger provided by a family argument, violent television, or a frightening dream culminated in nightmare death (Lemoine & Mougne, 1983). Clearly, the biopsychosocial model unraveled this puzzle.

## ■ THE NEED FOR HEALTH PSYCHOLOGY

What factors led to the development of health psychology? Since the inception of the field of psychology in the early 20th century, psychologists have made important contributions to health, exploring how and why some people get ill and others do not, how people adjust to their health conditions, and what factors lead people to practice health behaviors. In response to these trends, the American Psychological Association (APA) created a task force in 1973 to focus on psychology's potential role in health research. Participants included counseling, clinical, and rehabilitation psychologists, many of whom were already employed in health settings. Independently, social psychologists, developmental psychologists, and community/environmental psychologists were developing conceptual approaches for exploring health issues (Friedman & Silver, 2007). These groups joined forces, and in 1978, the Division of Health Psychology was formed within the APA. It is safe to say that health psychology is one of the most important developments within the field of psychology in the past 50 years. What other factors have fueled the growing field of health psychology?

## Changing Patterns of Illness

An important factor influencing the rise of health psychology has been the change in illness patterns in the United States and other technologically advanced societies in recent decades. As Table 1.2 shows, until the 20th century, the major causes of illness and death in the United States were **acute disorders.** Acute disorders are short-term illnesses, often a result of a viral or bacterial invader and usually amenable to cure. The prevalence of acute infectious disorders, such as tuberculosis, influenza, measles, and poliomyelitis, has declined because of treatment innovations

and changes in public health standards, such as improvements in waste control and sewage.

Now, **chronic illnesses**—especially heart disease, cancer, and respiratory diseases—are the main contributors to disability and death, particularly in industrialized countries. Chronic illnesses are slowly developing diseases with which people live for many years and that typically cannot be cured but rather are managed by patient and health care providers. Table 1.3 lists the main diseases worldwide at the present time. Note how the causes are projected to change over the next decade or so worldwide.

Why have chronic illnesses helped spawn the field of health psychology? First, these are diseases in which psychological and social factors are implicated as causes. For example, personal health habits, such as diet and smoking, contribute to the development of heart disease and cancer, and sexual activity is critical to the likelihood of developing AIDS (acquired immune deficiency syndrome).

Second, because people may live with chronic diseases for many years, psychological issues arise in their management. Health psychologists help chronically ill people adjust psychologically and socially to their changing health state and treatment regimens, many of which involve self-care. Chronic illnesses affect family functioning, including relationships with a partner or children, and health psychologists help ease the problems in family functioning that may result.

Chronic illnesses may require medication use and self-monitoring of symptoms, as well as changes in

**TABLE 1.2  |  What Are the Leading Causes of Death in the United States? A Comparison of 1900 and 2017, per 100,000 Population**

| 1900 | | 2017 | |
|---|---|---|---|
| Influenza and pneumonia | 202.2 | Heart disease | 165.0 |
| Tuberculosis, all forms | 194.4 | Cancer | 152.5 |
| Gastroenteritis | 142.7 | Unintentional injuries | 49.4 |
| Diseases of the heart | 137.4 | Chronic lower respiratory diseases | 40.9 |
| Vascular lesions of the CNS | 106.9 | Stroke | 37.6 |
| Chronic nephritis | 81.0 | Alzheimer's disease | 31.0 |
| All accidents | 72.3 | Diabetes | 21.5 |
| Malignant neoplasms (cancer) | 64.0 | Influenza and pneumonia | 14.3 |
| Certain diseases of early infancy | 62.6 | Intentional self-harm (suicide) | 14.0 |
| Diphtheria | 40.3 | Nephritis, nephrotic syndrome, and nephrosis | 13.0 |

Note that some accidents and overdoses may be attempts at suicide, so it can be hard to distinguish between those two categories.
*Source:* Xu, Jiaquan, Sherry L. Murphy, Kenneth D. Kochanek, Brigham Bastian, and Elizabeth Arias. "Deaths: Final Data for 2016." *National Vital Statistics Reports* 67, no. 5 (July 2018): 1–76.

**TABLE 1.3 | What Are the Worldwide Causes of Death?**

| | 2016 | | | 2030 |
|---|---|---|---|---|
| Rank | Disease or Injury | Projected Rank | | Disease or Injury |
| 1 | Ischemic heart disease | 1 | | Ischemic heart disease |
| 2 | Stroke | 2 | | Stroke |
| 3 | Chronic obstructive pulmonary disease | 3 | | Chronic obstructive pulmonary disease |
| 4 | Lower respiratory infections | 4 | | Alzheimer's disease and other dementias |
| 5 | Alzheimer's disease and other dementias | 5 | | Lower respiratory infections |
| 6 | Trachea, bronchus, lung cancers | 6 | | Diabetes mellitus |
| 7 | Diabetes mellitus | 7 | | Trachea, bronchus, lung cancers |
| 8 | Road injury | 8 | | Kidney diseases |
| 9 | Diarrheal diseases | 9 | | Cirrhosis of the liver |
| 10 | Tuberculosis | 10 | | Road injury |

*Source:* World Health Organization. "The Top 10 Causes of Death." Accessed June 10, 2019. https://www.who.int/news-room/fact-sheets/detail/the-top-10-causes-of-death.

behavior, such as altering diet and getting exercise. Health psychologists develop interventions to help people learn these regimens and promote adherence to them.

## Advances in Technology and Research

New medical technologies and scientific advances create issues that can be addressed by health psychologists. Just in the past few years, genes have been uncovered that contribute to many diseases including breast cancer. How do we help a college student whose mother has just been diagnosed with breast cancer come to terms with her risk? If she tests positive for a breast cancer gene, how will this change her life? Health psychologists help answer such questions.

Certain treatments that prolong life may severely compromise quality of life. Increasingly, patients are asked their preferences regarding life-sustaining measures, and they may require counseling in these matters. These are just a few examples of how health psychologists respond to scientific developments.

## Expanded Health Care Services

Other factors contributing to the rise of health psychology involve the expansion of health care services. Health care is the largest service industry in the United States, and it is still growing rapidly. Americans spend more than $3.5 trillion annually on health care (National Health Expenditures, 2017). In recent years, the health care industry has come under increasing scrutiny, as substantial increases in health care costs have

not brought improvement in basic indicators of health.

Moreover, huge disparities exist in the United States such that some individuals enjoy the very best health care available in the world while others receive little health care except in emergencies. Prior to the Affordable Care Act (known as Obamacare), 49.9 million Americans had no health insurance at all (U.S. Census Bureau, 2011). Efforts to reform the health care system to provide all Americans with a basic health care package, similar to what already exists in most European countries, have resulted.

Health psychology represents an important perspective on these issues for several reasons:

- Because containing health care costs is so important, health psychology's main emphasis on prevention—namely, modifying people's risky health behaviors before they become ill—can reduce the dollars devoted to the management of illness.

- Health psychologists know what makes people satisfied or dissatisfied with their health care (see Chapters 8 and 9) and can help in the design of a user-friendly health care system.

- The health care industry employs millions of people. Nearly every person in the country has direct contact with the health care system as a recipient of services. Consequently, its impact is enormous.

For all these reasons, then, health care delivery has a substantial social and psychological impact on people, an impact that is addressed by health psychologists.

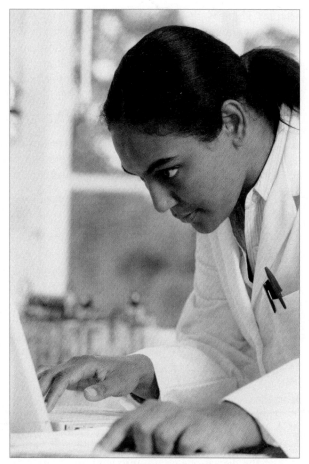

*In the 19th and 20th centuries, great strides were made in the technical basis of medicine. As a result, physicians looked more and more to the medical laboratory and less to the mind as a way of understanding the onset and progression of illness.*
image 100/age fotostock

## Increased Medical Acceptance

There is an increasing acceptance of health psychologists within the medical community. Health psychologists have developed a variety of short-term behavioral interventions to address health-related problems, including managing pain, modifying bad health habits such as smoking, and controlling the side effects of treatments. Techniques that may take a few hours to teach can produce years of benefit. Such interventions, particularly those that target risk factors such as diet or smoking, have contributed to the decline in the incidence of some diseases, especially coronary heart disease.

To take another example, psychologists learned many years ago that informing patients fully about the procedures and sensations involved in unpleasant medical procedures such as surgery improves their adjustment (Janis, 1958; Johnson, 1984). As a consequence of these studies, many hospitals and other treatment centers now routinely prepare patients for such procedures.

Ultimately, if a health-related discipline is to flourish, it must demonstrate a strong track record, not only as a research field but as a basis for interventions as well. Health psychology fulfills both the tasks.

## ■ HEALTH PSYCHOLOGY RESEARCH

Health psychologists make important research contributions to understand health and illness (Riley, 2017). The health psychologist can be a valuable team member by providing the theoretical, methodological, and statistical expertise that is the hallmark of good training in psychology.

### The Role of Theory in Research

Although much research in health psychology is guided by practical problems, such as how to ease the transition from hospital to home care, about one-third of health psychology investigations are guided by theory (Painter, Borba, Hynes, Mays, & Glanz, 2008). A **theory** is a set of analytic statements that explain a set of phenomena, such as why people practice poor health behaviors. The best theories are simple and useful. We will highlight a number of such theories throughout this book.

The advantages of theory for guiding research and treatment are several. Theories provide guidelines for how to do research and interventions (Masters, 2018). For example, the general principles of cognitive–behavioral therapy can tell one investigator what components should go into an intervention with breast cancer patients to help them cope with the aftermath of surgery, and these same principles can help a different investigator develop a weight loss intervention for obese people.

Theories generate specific predictions, so they can be tested and modified as the evidence comes in. For example, testing theories of health behavior change revealed that people need to believe that they can change their behavior, and so the importance of self-efficacy has been incorporated into theories of health behaviors.

Theories help tie together loose ends. Everyone knows that smokers relapse, people go off their diets, and alcoholics have trouble remaining abstinent. A theory of relapse unites these scattered observations into general principles of relapse prevention that can be incorporated into diverse interventions. A wise psychologist once said, "There is nothing so practical as a good theory" (Lewin, 1946), and we will see this wisdom repeatedly borne out.

## Experiments

Much research in health psychology is experimental. In an **experiment,** a researcher creates two or more conditions that differ from each other in exact and predetermined ways. People are then randomly assigned to these different conditions, and their reactions are measured. Experiments to evaluate the effectiveness of treatments or interventions over time are also called **randomized clinical trials,** in which a target treatment is compared against the existing standard of care or a placebo control, that is, an organically inert treatment (Freedland, 2017).

Medical interventions increasingly are based on these methodological principles. **Evidence-based medicine** means that medical and psychological interventions go through rigorous testing and evaluation of their benefits, usually through randomized clinical trials, before they become the standard of care. These criteria for effectiveness are also frequently now applied to psychological interventions.

What kinds of experiments do health psychologists undertake? To determine if social support groups improve adjustment to cancer, cancer patients might be randomly assigned to participate in a support group or to a comparison condition, such as an educational intervention. The patients could be evaluated at a subsequent time to pinpoint how the two groups differed in their adjustment.

Experiments have been the mainstay of science, because they typically provide more definitive answers to problems than other research methods. When we manipulate a variable and see its effects, we can establish a cause–effect relationship definitively. For this reason, experiments and randomized clinical trials are the gold standards of health psychology research. However, sometimes it is impractical to study issues experimentally. People cannot, for example, be randomly assigned to diseases. In this case, other methods, such as correlational methods, may be used.

## Correlational Studies

Much research in health psychology is **correlational research,** in which the health psychologist measures whether changes in one variable correspond with changes in another variable. A correlational study, for example, might reveal that people who are more hostile have a higher risk for cardiovascular disease.

The disadvantage of correlational studies is that it is difficult to determine the direction of causality unambiguously. For example, perhaps cardiovascular risk factors lead people to become more hostile. On the other hand, correlational studies often have advantages over experiments because they are more adaptable, enabling us to study issues when variables cannot be manipulated experimentally.

## Prospective and Retrospective Designs

Some of the problems with correlational studies can be remedied by using a prospective design. **Prospective research** looks forward in time to see how a group of people change, or how a relationship between two variables changes over time. For example, if we were to find that hostility develops relatively early in life, but heart disease develops later, we would be more confident that hostility is a risk factor for heart disease and recognize that the reverse direction of causality—namely, that heart disease causes hostility—is less likely.

Health psychologists conduct many prospective studies in order to understand the risk factors that relate to health conditions. We might, for example, intervene in the diet of one community and not in another and over time look at the difference in rates of heart disease. This would be an experimental prospective study. Alternatively, we might measure the diets that people create for themselves and look at changes in rates of heart disease, based on how good or poor the diet is. This would be an example of a correlational prospective study.

A particular type of prospective study is **longitudinal research,** in which the same people are observed at multiple points in time. For example, to understand what factors are associated with early breast cancer in women at risk, we might follow a group of young women whose mothers developed breast cancer, identify which daughters developed breast cancer, and identify factors reliably associated with that development, such as diet, stress, or alcohol consumption.

Investigators also use **retrospective designs,** which look backward in time in an attempt to reconstruct the conditions that led to a current situation. Retrospective methods, for example, were critical in identifying the risk factors that led to AIDS. Initially, researchers saw an abrupt increase in a rare cancer called Kaposi's sarcoma and observed that the men who developed this cancer often eventually died of general failure of the immune system. By taking extensive histories of the men who developed this disease, researchers were able to determine that the practice of anal-receptive sex without a condom is related to the development of the disorder. Because of retrospective studies, researchers knew some of the risk factors for AIDS even before they had identified the retrovirus.

## The Role of Epidemiology in Health Psychology

Changing patterns of illness have been charted and followed by the field of epidemiology, a discipline closely related to health psychology in its goals and interests (Freeland, 2017). **Epidemiology** is the study of the frequency, distribution, and causes of infectious and noninfectious diseases in a population. For example, epidemiologists study not only who has what kind of cancer but also why some cancers are more prevalent than others in particular geographic areas or among particular groups of people.

Epidemiological studies frequently use two important terms: "morbidity" and "mortality." **Morbidity** refers to the number of cases of a disease that exist at some given point in time. Morbidity may be expressed as the number of new cases (incidence) or as the total number of existing cases (prevalence). Morbidity statistics, then, tell us how many people have what kinds of disorders at any given time. **Mortality** refers to numbers of deaths due to particular causes.

Morbidity and mortality statistics are essential to health psychologists. Charting the major causes of disease can lead to steps to reduce their occurrence. For example, knowing that automobile accidents are a major cause of death among children, adolescents, and young adults has led to safety measures, such as child-safety restraint systems, mandatory seat belt laws, and raising the legal drinking age.

But morbidity is important as well. What is the use of affecting causes of death if people remain ill but simply do not die? Health psychology addresses health-related quality of life. Indeed, some researchers maintain that quality of life and symptom reduction should be more important targets for our interventions than mortality and other biological indicators (Kaplan, 1990). Consequently, health psychologists work to improve quality of life so that people with chronic disorders can live their lives as free from pain, disability, and lifestyle compromise as possible.

## Methodological Tools

This section highlights some of the methodological tools that have proven valuable in health psychology research.

**Tools of Neuroscience**   The field of neuroscience has developed powerful new tools such as functional magnetic resonance imaging (fMRI) that permit glimpses into the brain. This area of research has also produced knowledge about the autonomic, neuroendocrine, and immune systems that have made a variety of breakthrough studies possible. For example, health psychologists can now connect psychosocial conditions, such as social support and positive beliefs, to underlying biology in ways that make believers out of skeptics. The knowledge and methods of neuroscience also shed light on such questions as, how do placebos work? Why are many people felled by functional disorders that seem to have no underlying biological causes? Why is chronic pain so intractable to treatment? What are effective ways to change health behaviors (Hall, Erickson, & Gianaros, 2017)? How does the brain respond to efforts to change health behaviors (Cooper, Tompson, O'Donnell, Vettel, Basset, & Falk, 2018)? We address these issues in later chapters. These and other applications of neuroscience will help address clinical puzzles that have mystified practitioners for decades (Gianaros & Hackman, 2013).

**Web-based Mobile and Wireless Technologies**   Web-based technologies are widely used in health psychology interventions.

Many of these involve efforts to change poor health behaviors, such as insufficient exercise. Others involve providing social support to people in need of more or more helpful social contact. Web-based programs for managing distress in response to illness or treatment now exist for many disorders (Habibovic et al., 2017). Interventions make use of cell phones, pagers, palm pilots, tablets, and other mobile technologies to deliver interventions and assess health-related events in the natural environment. Interventions have included studies of smoking cessation, weight loss, diabetes management, eating disorders, healthy diet, and physical activity (Heron & Smyth, 2010). Telemedicine that provides virtual medical visits is good for treating modest health issues, such as cold, flu, stomachache, and urinary tract infections (Lankford, 2019).

People in these studies typically participate through an apparatus, such as a cell phone, that can provide on-the-spot administration of a treatment or intervention, as well as the collection of data. For example, text messages sent just before meals can remind people about their intentions to consume a healthy diet. Short text messaging has also been used to enhance smoking cessation programs and ensure maintenance of quitting (Berkman, Dickenson, Falk, & Lieberman, 2011). Activity measures and sensors can accurately assess how much exercise a person is getting. Mobile technology can also help people already diagnosed with disorders. People on medications may receive reminders from mobile devices to take their medications. Numerous other applications are possible.

Measuring biological indicators of health has usually required an invasive procedure such as a blood draw. Now, however, mobile health technologies can assess some biological processes. Ambulatory blood pressure monitoring devices help people with high blood pressure identify conditions when their blood pressure goes up. People with diabetes can monitor their blood glucose levels multiple times a day with less invasive technology than was true just a few years ago.

At present, evidence for the success of mobile health-based interventions and assessments is mixed (Kaplan & Stone, 2013), suggesting the need for more research. But these procedures have greatly improved health psychologists' abilities to study health-related phenomena in real time.

Meta-analysis    For some topics in health psychology, enough studies have been done to conduct a meta-analysis. **Meta-analysis** combines results from different studies to identify how strong the evidence is for particular research findings. For example, a meta-analysis might be conducted on 100 studies of dietary interventions to identify which characteristics of these interventions lead to more successful dietary change. Such an analysis might reveal, for example, that only those interventions that enhance self-efficacy, that is, the belief that one will be able to modify one's diet, are successful. Meta-analysis is a particularly powerful methodological tool, because it uses a broad array of diverse evidence to reach conclusions.

## Qualitative Research

In addition to the methods just described, there is an important role for qualitative research in health psychology. Listening to an individual person talk about his or her health needs and experiences is, of course, beneficial for planning an intervention for that person, such as help in losing weight. But more broadly, guided interviews and narratives can provide insights into health processes that summary statistics may not provide. For example, interviews with cancer patients about their chemotherapy experiences may be more helpful in redesigning how chemotherapy is administered than are numerical ratings of how satisfied patients are. Qualitative research can also supplement insights from other research methods. For example, surveys of college students can identify rates of problem drinking, but interviews may be helpful for identifying how to build responsible drinking skills (deVisser et al., 2015). Quantitative and qualitative methods can work hand in hand to develop the research evidence for effective interventions.

## ▧ WHAT IS HEALTH PSYCHOLOGY TRAINING FOR?

Students who are trained in health psychology on the undergraduate level go on to many different occupations. Some students go into medicine, becoming physicians and nurses. Because of their experience in health psychology, some of these health care practitioners conduct research as well. Other health psychology students go into the allied health professional fields, such as social work, occupational therapy, dietetics, physical therapy, or public health. Social workers in medical settings, for example, may assess where patients go after discharge, decisions that are informed by knowledge of their psychosocial needs. Dietetics is important in the dietary management of chronic illnesses, such as cancer, heart disease, and diabetes. Physical therapists help patients regain the use of limbs and functions that may have been compromised by illness and its treatment.

Students who receive either a PhD in health psychology or a PsyD most commonly go into academic research as faculty members or into private practice, where they provide individual and group counseling. Other PhDs in health psychology practice in hospitals and other health care settings. Many are involved in the management of health care, including business and government positions. Others work in medical schools, hospitals and other treatment settings, and industrial or occupational health settings to promote healthy behavior, prevent accidents, and help control health care costs. •

## SUMMARY

1. Health psychology examines psychological influences on how people stay healthy, why they become ill, and how they respond when they do get ill. The field focuses on health promotion and maintenance; prevention and treatment of illness; the etiology and correlates of health, illness, and disability; and improvement of the health care system and the formulation of health policy.

2. The interaction of the mind and the body has concerned philosophers and scientists for centuries. Different models of the relationship have predominated at different times in history.

3. The biomedical model, which has dominated medicine, is a reductionistic, single-factor model of illness that treats the mind and the body as separate entities and emphasizes illness concerns over health.

4. The biomedical model is currently being replaced by the biopsychosocial model, which regards any health disorder as the result of the interplay of biological, psychological, and social factors. The biopsychosocial model recognizes the importance of interacting macrolevel and microlevel processes in producing health and illness. Under this model, health is regarded as an active achievement.

5. The biopsychosocial model guides health psychologists and practitioners in their research efforts to uncover factors that predict states of health and illness and in their clinical interventions with patients.

6. The rise of health psychology can be tied to several factors, including the increase in chronic or lifestyle-related illnesses, the expanding role of health care in the economy, the realization that psychological and social factors contribute to health and illness, the demonstrated importance of psychological interventions to improving people's health, and the rigorous methodological contributions of health psychology researchers.

7. Health psychologists perform a variety of tasks. They develop theories and conduct research on the interaction of biological, psychological, and social factors in producing health and illness. They help treat patients with a variety of disorders and conduct counseling for the psychosocial problems that illness may create. They develop worksite interventions to improve employees' health habits and work in medical settings and other organizations to improve health and health care delivery.

## KEY TERMS

acute disorders
biomedical model
biopsychosocial model
chronic illnesses
conversion hysteria
correlational research
epidemiology
etiology

evidence-based medicine
experiment
health
health psychology
longitudinal research
meta-analysis
morbidity
mortality

prospective research
psychosomatic medicine
randomized clinical trials
retrospective designs
theory
wellness

# CHAPTER 2

# The Systems of the Body

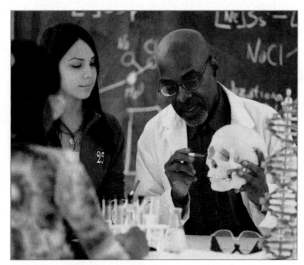

LWA/Dann Tardif/Blend Images/Getty Images

An understanding of health requires a working knowledge of human physiology, namely the study of the body's functioning. Having basic knowledge of physiology clarifies how good health habits make illness less likely, how stress affects the body, how chronic stress can lead to hypertension or coronary artery disease, and how cell growth is radically altered by cancer.

## ■ THE NERVOUS SYSTEM

### Overview

The **nervous system** is a complex network of interconnected nerve fibers. As Figure 2.1 shows, the nervous system is made up of the central nervous system, which consists of the brain and the spinal cord, and the peripheral nervous system, which consists of the rest of the nerves in the body, including those that connect to the brain and the spinal cord. Sensory nerve fibers provide input to the brain and spinal cord by carrying signals from sensory receptors; motor nerve fibers provide output from the brain or spinal cord to muscles and other organs, resulting in voluntary and involuntary movement.

The peripheral nervous system is made up of the somatic nervous system and the autonomic nervous system. The somatic, or voluntary, nervous system connects nerve fibers to voluntary muscles and provides the brain with feedback about voluntary movement, such as a tennis swing. The autonomic, or involuntary, nervous system connects the central nervous system to all internal organs over which people do not customarily have control.

Regulation of the autonomic nervous system occurs via the sympathetic nervous system and the parasympathetic nervous system. The **sympathetic nervous system** prepares the body to respond to emergencies, to strong emotions such as anger or fear, and to strenuous activity. As such, it plays an important role in reaction to stress.

The **parasympathetic nervous system** controls the activities of organs under normal circumstances and acts antagonistically to the sympathetic nervous system. When an emergency has passed, the parasympathetic nervous system helps to restore the body to a normal state.

### The Brain

The brain is the command center of the body. It receives sensory impulses from the peripheral nerve endings and sends motor impulses to the extremities and to internal organs to carry out movement. The parts of the brain are shown in Figure 2.2.

#### The Hindbrain and the Midbrain    The hindbrain has three main parts: the medulla, the pons, and the cerebellum. The **medulla** is responsible for the regulation of heart rate, blood pressure, and respiration. Sensory information about the levels of carbon dioxide and oxygen in the body also comes to the medulla, which, if necessary, sends motor impulses to respiratory muscles to alter the rate of breathing. The **pons** serves as a link between the hindbrain and the midbrain and also helps control respiration.

The **cerebellum** coordinates voluntary muscle movement, the maintenance of balance and equilibrium, and

**FIGURE 2.1 | The Components of the Nervous System**

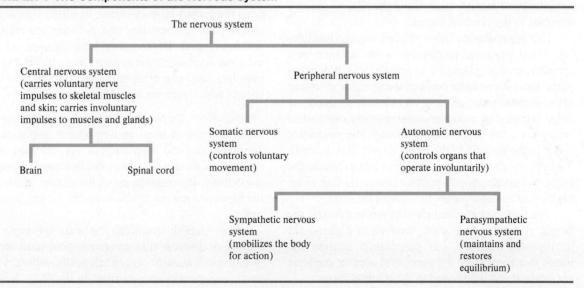

**FIGURE 2.2 | The Brain**    (*Source*: Lankford, T. Randall. *Integrated science for health students*. Virginia: Reston, 1979, p. 232.)

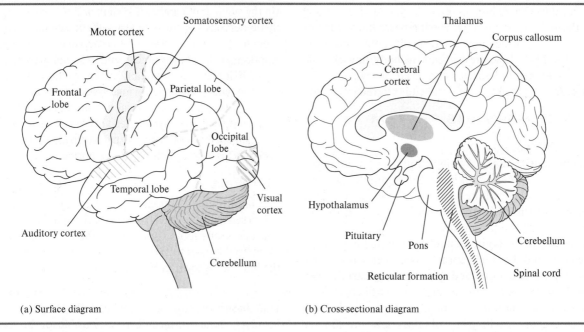

(a) Surface diagram                    (b) Cross-sectional diagram

the maintenance of muscle tone and posture. Damage to this area can produce loss of muscle tone, tremors, and disturbances in posture or gait.

The midbrain is the major pathway for sensory and motor impulses moving between the forebrain and the hindbrain. It is also responsible for the coordination of visual and auditory reflexes.

The Forebrain    The forebrain includes the thalamus and the hypothalamus. The **thalamus** is involved in the recognition of sensory stimuli and the relay of sensory impulses to the cerebral cortex.

The **hypothalamus** helps regulate cardiac functioning, blood pressure, respiration, water balance, and appetites, including hunger and sexual desire. It is an important transition center between the thoughts generated in the cerebral cortex of the brain and their impact on internal organs. For example, embarrassment can lead to blushing via the hypothalamus through the vasomotor center in the medulla to the blood vessels. Together with the pituitary gland, the hypothalamus helps regulate the endocrine system, which releases hormones that affect functioning in target organs throughout the body.

The forebrain also includes the **cerebral cortex,** the largest portion of the brain, involved in higher-order intelligence, memory, and personality. Sensory impulses that come from the peripheral areas of the body are received and interpreted in the cerebral cortex.

The cerebral cortex consists of four lobes: frontal, parietal, temporal, and occipital. Each lobe has its own memory storage area or areas of association. Through these complex networks of associations, the brain is able to relate current sensations to past ones, giving the cerebral cortex its formidable interpretive capabilities.

In addition to its role in associative memory, each lobe is generally associated with particular functions. The frontal lobe contains the motor cortex, which coordinates voluntary movement. The parietal lobe contains the somatosensory cortex, in which sensations of touch, pain, temperature, and pressure are registered and interpreted. The temporal lobe contains the cortical areas responsible for auditory and olfactory (smell) impulses, and the occipital lobe contains the visual cortex, which receives visual impulses.

The Limbic System    The limbic system plays an important role in stress and emotional responses. The amygdala and the hippocampus are involved in the detection of threat and in emotionally charged memories, respectively. The cingulate gyrus, the septum, and areas in the hypothalamus are related to emotional functioning as well.

Many health disorders implicate the brain. One important disorder that was overlooked until recently is chronic traumatic encephalopathy, whose causes and consequences are described in Box 2.1.

A 27-year-old former Marine who had done two tours of Iraq returned home, attempting to resume his family life and college classes. Although he had once had good grades, he found he could not remember small details or focus his attention any longer. He became irritable, snapping at his family, and eventually, his wife initiated divorce proceedings. He developed an alcohol problem, and a car crash caused him to lose his driver's license. When his parents hadn't heard from him, they phoned the police, who found him, a suicide victim of hanging.

Chronic traumatic encephalopathy (CTE) is a degenerative brain disorder that strikes people who have had repeated or serious head injuries. Former boxers and football players, for example, have high rates of CTE. In CTE, an abnormal form of a protein accumulates and eventually destroys cells in the brain, including the frontal and temporal lobes, which are critical for decision making, impulse control, and judgment.

Autopsies suggest that CTE may also be present at high levels among returning veterans, and that blasts from bombs or grenades may have produced these serious effects, including irreversible losses in memory and thinking abilities. More than 27,000 cases of traumatic war injuries were reported by the U.S. military in 2009 alone, and CTE is a likely contributor (Congressional Research Service, 2010). CTE is suspected in some

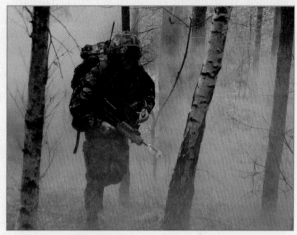

Ingram Publishing/SuperStock

cases that have been diagnosed as post traumatic stress disorder (see Chapter 6). Whether the military will find ways to reduce exposure to its causes or ways to retard the processes CTE sets into effect remains to be seen. Health psychologists can play an important role in addressing the cognitive and social costs of this degenerative disorder.

*Source:* Kristof, Nicholas. "Veterans and Brain Disease." *The New York Times,* April 25, 2012. https://www.nytimes.com/2012/04/26/opinion/kristof-veterans-and-brain-disease.html.

### The Role of Neurotransmitters

The nervous system functions by means of chemicals, called **neurotransmitters,** that regulate nervous system functioning. Stimulation of the sympathetic nervous system prompts the secretion of two neurotransmitters, epinephrine and norepinephrine, together termed the **catecholamines.** These substances are carried through the bloodstream throughout the body, promoting sympathetic activation.

The release of catecholamines prompts important bodily changes. Heart rate increases, the heart's capillaries dilate, and blood vessels constrict, increasing blood pressure. Blood is diverted into muscle tissue. Respiration rate goes up, and the amount of air flowing into the lungs is increased. Digestion and urination are generally decreased. The pupils of the eyes dilate, and sweat glands are stimulated to produce more sweat. These changes are critically important in responses to stressful circumstances. Chronic or recurrent arousal of the sympathetic

nervous system can accelerate the development of several chronic disorders, such as coronary artery disease and hypertension, discussed in greater detail in Chapter 13.

Parasympathetic functioning is a counterregulatory system that helps restore homeostasis following sympathetic arousal. The heart rate decreases, the heart's capillaries constrict, blood vessels dilate, respiration rate decreases, and the metabolic system resumes its activities.

### Disorders of the Nervous System

Approximately 25 million Americans have some disorder of the nervous system. The most common forms of neurological dysfunction are epilepsy and Parkinson's disease. Cerebral palsy, multiple sclerosis, and Huntington's disease also affect substantial numbers of people.

Epilepsy    A disease of the central nervous system affecting 1 in 26 people in the United States (Epilepsy Foundation, 2018), epilepsy is often idiopathic, which means that no specific cause for the symptoms can be identified. Symptomatic epilepsy may be traced to harm during birth, severe injury to the head, infectious disease such as meningitis or encephalitis, or metabolic or nutritional disorders. Risk for epilepsy may also be inherited.

Epilepsy is marked by seizures, which range from barely noticeable to violent convulsions accompanied by irregular breathing and loss of consciousness. Epilepsy cannot be cured, but it can often be controlled through medication and behavioral interventions designed to manage stress (see Chapters 7 and 11).

Parkinson's Disease    People with Parkinson's disease have progressive degeneration of the basal ganglia, a group of nuclei in the brain that control smooth motor coordination. The result of this deterioration is tremors, rigidity, and slowness of movement. As many as 1 million Americans have Parkinson's disease, which primarily strikes people age 50 and older (Parkinson's Disease Foundation, 2018); men are more likely than women to develop the disease. Although the cause of Parkinson's is not fully known, depletion of the neurotransmitter dopamine may be involved. Parkinson's disease may be treated with medication, but large doses, which can cause undesirable side effects, are often required for control of the symptoms.

Cerebral Palsy    Currently, more than 764,000 people in the United States have or experience symptoms of cerebral palsy (CerebralPalsy.org, 2019). Cerebral palsy is a chronic, nonprogressive disorder marked by lack of muscle control. It stems from brain damage caused by an interruption in the brain's oxygen supply, usually during childbirth. In older children, a severe accident or physical abuse can produce the condition. Apart from being unable to control motor functions, those who have the disorder may (but need not) also have seizures, spasms, mental retardation, difficulties with sensation and perception, and problems with sight, hearing, and/or speech.

Multiple Sclerosis    Approximately 2.3 million people worldwide have multiple sclerosis (National Multiple Sclerosis Society, 2016). In the United States, there are nearly 1 million people who have multiple sclerosis (Nelson, Wallin, Marrie, Culpepper, & Langer-Gould, 2019). This degenerative disease can cause paralysis and, occasionally, blindness, deafness, and mental deterioration. Early symptoms include numbness, double vision, dragging of the feet, loss of bladder or bowel control, speech difficulties, and extreme fatigue.

Symptoms may appear and disappear over a period of years; after that, deterioration is continuous.

The effects of multiple sclerosis result from the disintegration of myelin, a fatty membrane that surrounds nerve fibers and facilitates the conduction of nerve impulses. Multiple sclerosis is an autoimmune disorder, so called because the immune system fails to recognize its own tissue and attacks the myelin sheath surrounding nerve fibers.

Huntington's Disease    A hereditary disorder of the central nervous system, Huntington's disease is characterized by chronic physical and mental deterioration. Symptoms include involuntary muscle spasms, loss of motor abilities, personality changes, and other signs of mental disintegration.

The disease affects about 30,000 people directly, and 200,000 more are at risk in the United States (Huntington's Disease Society of America, 2019). The gene for Huntington's has been isolated, and a test is now available that indicates not only if one is a carrier of the gene but also at what age (roughly) one will succumb to the disease. As will be seen later in this chapter, genetic counseling with this group of at-risk people is important.

Polio    Poliomyelitis is a highly infectious viral disease that affects mostly young children. It attacks the spinal nerves and destroys the cell bodies of motor neurons so that motor impulses cannot be carried from the spinal cord outward to the peripheral nerves or muscles. Depending on the degree of damage that is done, the person may be left with difficulties in walking and moving properly, ranging from shrunken and ineffective limbs to full paralysis. Polio cases have decreased substantially worldwide, although polio is still a major health issue in Pakistan and Afghanistan.

Paraplegia and Quadriplegia    Paraplegia is paralysis of the lower extremities of the body; it results from an injury to the lower portion of the spinal cord. Quadriplegia is paralysis of all four extremities and the trunk of the body; it occurs when the upper portion of the spinal cord is severed. People who have these conditions usually lose bladder and bowel control and the muscles below the cut area may lose their tone, becoming weak and flaccid.

Dementia    Dementia (meaning "deprived of mind") is a serious loss of cognitive ability beyond what might be expected from normal aging. A history of brain injuries or a genetically based propensity may be involved in long-term decline. A chronically stressful life, as may result from socioeconomic position, can lead to atrophy in the hippocampus, which can compromise cognitive functioning, often severely (Elbejjani et al., 2017) Although dementia is most common among older adults, it may occur at any stage of adulthood. Memory, attention, language, and problem solving are affected early in the disorder and often lead to diagnosis.

The most common form of dementia is Alzheimer's, accounting for 60 to 70 percent of the cases. In most people, symptoms appear in their mid-60s, and the disease progresses irreversibly, due to plaques and tangles in the progressively shrinking brain. In addition to the early signs of cognitive decline, especially difficulty with short-term memory, social functioning, and use of language, are disrupted as the disease progresses. What leads people to develop Alzheimer's? Lack of physical exercise and intellectual activity are lifestyle factors implicated in its development, and there are also genes that predispose to the disease (Rodriguez et al., 2018). Other contributing factors will be unearthed by the substantial research devoted to this major health issue. About 47 million people worldwide have Alzheimer's (Alzheimer's Association, 2019).

## ■ THE ENDOCRINE SYSTEM

### Overview

The **endocrine system,** diagrammed in Figure 2.3, complements the nervous system in controlling bodily activities. The endocrine system is made up of a number of ductless glands that secrete hormones into the blood, stimulating changes in target organs. The endocrine and nervous systems depend on each other, stimulating and inhibiting each other's activities. The nervous system is chiefly responsible for fast-acting, short-duration responses to changes in the body, whereas the endocrine system mainly governs slow-acting responses of long duration.

The endocrine system is regulated by the hypothalamus and the **pituitary gland.** Located at the base of the brain, the pituitary has two lobes. The posterior pituitary lobe produces oxytocin, which controls contractions during labor and lactation and is also involved in social affiliation, and vasopressin, or antidiuretic hormone (ADH), which controls the water-absorbing ability of the kidneys, among other functions. The anterior pituitary lobe of the pituitary gland secretes hormones responsible for growth: somatotropic hormone (STH), which regulates bone,

**FIGURE 2.3 I The Endocrine System**

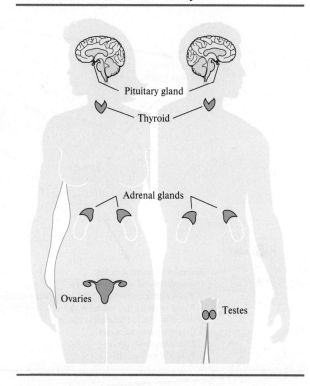

muscle, and other organ development; gonadotropic hormones, which control the growth, development, and secretions of the gonads (testes and ovaries); thyrotropic hormone (TSH), which controls the growth, development, and secretion of the thyroid gland; and adrenocorticotropic hormone (ACTH), which controls the growth and secretions of the cortical region of the adrenal glands.

### The Adrenal Glands

The **adrenal glands** are small glands located on top of each of the kidneys. Each adrenal gland consists of an adrenal medulla and an adrenal cortex. The hormones of the adrenal medulla are epinephrine and norepinephrine, which were described earlier.

As Figure 2.4 implies, the adrenal glands are critically involved in physiological and neuroendocrine reactions to stress. Catecholamines, secreted in conjunction with sympathetic arousal, and corticosteroids are implicated in biological responses to stress. We will consider these stress responses more fully in Chapter 6.

### Disorders Involving the Endocrine System

**Diabetes**    Diabetes is a chronic endocrine disorder in which the body is not able to manufacture or

**FIGURE 2.4 | Adrenal Gland Activity in Response to Stress**

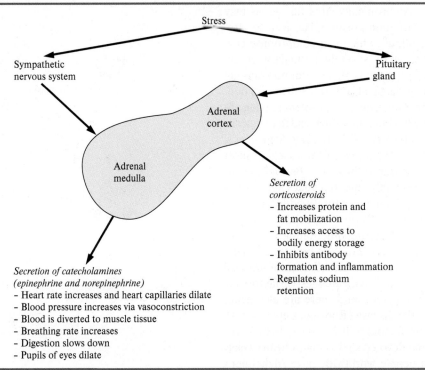

properly use insulin. It is the fourth most common chronic illness in this country and one of the leading causes of death. Diabetes consists of two primary forms. Type I diabetes is a severe disorder that typically arises in late childhood or early adolescence. At least partly genetic in origin, Type I diabetes is an autoimmune disorder, possibly precipitated by an earlier viral infection. The immune system falsely identifies cells in the islets of Langerhans in the pancreas as invaders and destroys those cells, compromising or eliminating their ability to produce insulin.

Type II diabetes, which typically occurs after age 40, is the more common form. In Type II diabetes, insulin may be produced by the body, but there may not be enough of it, or the body may not be sensitive to it. It is heavily a disease of lifestyle, and risk factors include obesity and stress, among other factors.

Diabetic patients have high rates of coronary heart disease, and diabetes is the leading cause of blindness among adults. It accounts for almost 44 percent of all the patients who require renal dialysis for kidney failure (National Institute of Diabetes and Digestive and Kidney Disorders, 2007). Diabetes can also produce nervous system damage, leading to pain and loss

of sensation. In severe cases, amputation of the extremities, such as toes and feet, may be required. As a consequence of these complications, people with diabetes have a considerably shortened life expectancy. In later chapters, we will consider Type I (Chapter 14) and Type II (Chapter 13) diabetes, and the issues associated with their management.

## ■ THE CARDIOVASCULAR SYSTEM

### Overview

The **cardiovascular system** comprises the heart, blood vessels, and blood and acts as the transport system of the body. Blood carries oxygen from the lungs to the tissues and carbon dioxide from the tissues to the lungs. Blood also carries nutrients from the digestive tract to the individual cells so that the cells may extract nutrients for growth and energy. The blood carries waste products from the cells to the kidneys, from which the waste is excreted in the urine. It also carries hormones from the endocrine glands to other organs of the body and transports heat to the surface of the skin to control body temperature.

**FIGURE 2.5 | The Heart**

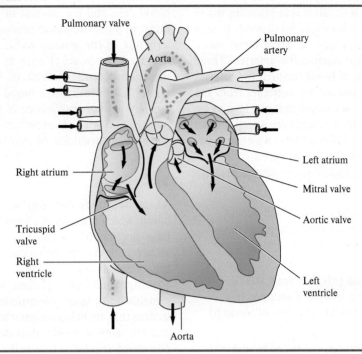

## The Heart

The heart functions as a pump, and its pumping action causes the blood to circulate throughout the body. The left side of the heart, consisting of the left atrium and left ventricle, takes in oxygenated blood from the lungs and pumps it out into the aorta (the major artery leaving the heart), from which the blood passes into the smaller vessels (the arteries, arterioles, and capillaries) to reach cell tissues. The blood exchanges its oxygen and nutrients for the waste materials of the cells and is then returned to the right side of the heart (right atrium and right ventricle), which pumps it back to the lungs via the pulmonary artery. Once oxygenated, the blood returns to the left side of the heart through the pulmonary veins. The anatomy of the heart is pictured in Figure 2.5.

The heart performs these functions through regular rhythmic phases of contraction and relaxation known as the cardiac cycle. There are two phases in the cardiac cycle: systole and diastole. During systole, blood is pumped out of the heart, and blood pressure in the blood vessels increases. As the muscle relaxes during diastole, blood pressure drops, and blood is taken into the heart.

The flow of blood into and out of the heart is controlled by valves at the inlet and outlet of each ventricle. These heart valves ensure that blood flows in one direction only. The sounds that one hears when listening to the heart are the sounds of these valves closing. These heart sounds make it possible to time the cardiac cycle to determine how rapidly or slowly blood is being pumped into and out of the heart.

A number of factors influence the rate at which the heart contracts and relaxes. During exercise, emotional excitement, or stress, for example, the heart speeds up, and the cardiac cycle is completed in a shorter time. A chronically or excessively rapid heart rate can decrease the heart's strength, which may reduce the volume of blood that is pumped. Heart rate variability is a measure of the variability in the time between each heartbeat. It is a measure of cardiac regulation, and is generally viewed as related to cardiovascular fitness and possibly also to psychological well-being (Sloane et al., 2017)

## Disorders of the Cardiovascular System

The cardiovascular system is subject to a number of disorders. Some of these are due to congenital defects—that is, defects present at birth—and others, to infection. By far, however, the major threats to the cardiovascular system are due to lifestyle factors, including stress, poor diet, lack of exercise, and smoking.

**Atherosclerosis**    The major cause of heart disease is atherosclerosis, a problem that becomes worse with age. **Atherosclerosis** is caused by deposits of cholesterol and other substances on the arterial walls, which form plaques that narrow the arteries. These plaques reduce the flow of blood through the arteries and interfere with the passage of nutrients from the capillaries into the cells—a process that can lead to tissue damage. Damaged arterial walls are also potential sites for the formation of blood clots, which can obstruct a vessel and cut off the flow of blood.

Atherosclerosis is associated with several primary clinical manifestations:

- **Angina pectoris,** or chest pain, which occurs when the heart has insufficient supply of oxygen or inadequate removal of carbon dioxide and other waste products.

- **Myocardial infarction (MI),** or heart attack, which results when a clot has developed in a coronary vessel and blocks the flow of blood to the heart.

- **Ischemia,** a condition characterized by lack of blood flow and oxygen to the heart muscle. As many as 3 million to 4 million Americans have silent ischemic episodes without knowing it, and they may consequently have a heart attack with no prior warning.

Other major disorders of the cardiovascular system include the following.

- Congestive heart failure (CHF), which occurs when the heart's delivery of oxygen-rich blood is inadequate to meet the body's needs.

- Arrhythmia, irregular beatings of the heart, which, at its most severe, can lead to loss of consciousness and sudden death.

## Blood Pressure

**Blood pressure** is the force that blood exerts against the blood vessel walls. During systole, the force on the blood vessel walls is greatest; during diastole, it falls to its lowest point. The measurement of blood pressure includes these two indicators.

Blood pressure is influenced by several factors. The first is cardiac output—pressure against the arterial walls is greater as the volume of blood flow increases. A second factor is peripheral resistance, or the resistance to blood flow in the small arteries of the body (arterioles), which is affected by the number of red blood cells and the amount of plasma the blood contains. In addition, blood pressure is influenced by the structure of the arterial walls: If the walls have been damaged, if they are clogged by deposits of waste, or if they have lost their elasticity, blood pressure will be higher. Chronically high blood pressure, called hypertension, is the consequence of too high a cardiac output or too high a peripheral resistance. We will consider hypertension further in Chapter 13.

## The Blood

An adult's body contains approximately 5 liters of blood, which consists of plasma and cells. Plasma, the fluid portion of blood, accounts for approximately 55 percent of the blood volume. The remaining 45 percent of blood volume is made up of cells. The blood cells are suspended in the plasma, which contains plasma proteins and plasma electrolytes (salts) plus the substances that are being transported by the blood (oxygen and nutrients or carbon dioxide and waste materials). The blood also helps to regulate skin temperature.

Blood cells are manufactured in the bone marrow in the hollow cavities of bones. Bone marrow contains five types of blood-forming cells: myeloblasts and monoblasts, both of which produce types of white blood cells; lymphoblasts, which produce lymphocytes; erythroblasts, which produce red blood cells; and megakaryocytes, which produce platelets. Each of these types of blood cells has an important function.

White blood cells play an important role in healing by absorbing and removing foreign substances from the body. They contain granules that secrete digestive enzymes, which engulf and act on bacteria and other foreign particles, turning them into a form conducive to excretion. An elevated white cell count suggests the presence of infection.

Lymphocytes produce antibodies—agents that destroy foreign substances. Together, these groups of cells play an important role in fighting infection and disease. We will consider them more fully in our discussion of the immune system in Chapter 14.

Red blood cells are important mainly because they contain hemoglobin, which is needed to carry oxygen and carbon dioxide throughout the body. Anemia, which involves below-normal numbers of red blood cells, can interfere with this transport function.

**Platelets** serve several important functions. They clump together to block small holes that develop in blood vessels, and they also play an important role in blood clotting.

Clotting Disorders    Clots (or thromboses) can sometimes develop in the blood vessels. This is most likely to occur if arterial or venous walls have been damaged or roughened because of the buildup of cholesterol. Platelets then adhere to the roughened area, leading to the formation of a clot. A clot can have especially serious consequences if it occurs in the blood vessels leading to the heart (coronary thrombosis) or brain (cerebral thrombosis), because it will block the vital flow of blood to these organs. When a clot occurs in a vein, it may become detached and form an embolus, which can become lodged in the blood vessels to the lungs, causing pulmonary obstruction. Death is a common consequence of these conditions.

## ■  THE RESPIRATORY SYSTEM

### Overview

Respiration, or breathing, has three main functions: to take in oxygen, to excrete carbon dioxide, and to regulate the composition of the blood.

The body needs oxygen to metabolize food. During the process of metabolism, oxygen combines with carbon atoms in food, producing carbon dioxide ($CO_2$). The **respiratory system** brings in oxygen through inspiration; it eliminates carbon dioxide through expiration.

## The Structure and Functions of the Respiratory System

Air is inhaled through the nose and mouth and then passes through the pharynx and larynx to the trachea. The trachea, a muscular tube extending downward from the larynx, divides at its lower end into two branches called the primary bronchi. Each bronchus enters a lung, where it then subdivides into secondary bronchi, still-smaller bronchioles, and, finally, microscopic alveolar ducts, which contain many tiny clustered sacs called alveoli. The alveoli and the capillaries are responsible for the exchange of oxygen and carbon dioxide. A diagram of the respiratory system appears in Figure 2.6.

The inspiration of air is an active process, brought about by the contraction of muscles. Inspiration causes the lungs to expand inside the thorax (the chest wall). Expiration, in contrast, is a passive function, brought about by the relaxation of the lungs, which reduces the volume of the lungs within the thorax. The lungs fill most of the space within the thoracic cavity and are very elastic, depending on the thoracic walls for support. If air gets into the space between the thoracic wall and the lungs, one or both lungs will collapse.

Respiratory movements are controlled by a respiratory center in the medulla. The functions of this center depend partly on the chemical composition of the blood. For example, if the blood's carbon dioxide

**FIGURE 2.6 | The Respiratory System**    (*Source:* Lankford, T. Randall. *Integrated science for health students.* Virginia: Reston, 1979, p. 467.)

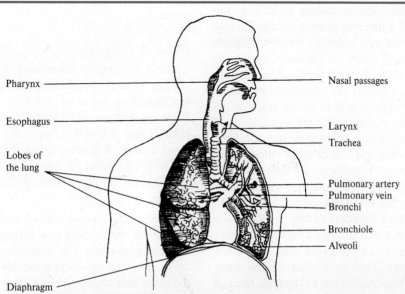

Pharynx

Esophagus

Lobes of the lung

Diaphragm

Nasal passages

Larynx

Trachea

Pulmonary artery
Pulmonary vein
Bronchi

Bronchiole

Alveoli

level rises too high, the respiratory center will be stimulated and respiration will be increased. If the carbon dioxide level falls too low, the respiratory center will slow down until the carbon dioxide level is back to normal.

The respiratory system is also responsible for coughing. Dust and other foreign materials are inhaled with every breath. Some of these substances are trapped in the mucus of the nose and the air passages and are then conducted back toward the throat, where they are swallowed. When a large amount of mucus collects in the large airways, it is removed by coughing (a forced expiratory effort).

## Disorders Associated with the Respiratory System

Asthma    Asthma is a severe allergic reaction typically to a foreign substance, including dust, dog or cat dander, pollens, or fungi. An asthma attack can also be touched off by emotional stress or exercise. These attacks may be so serious that they produce bronchial spasms and hyperventilation.

During an asthma attack, the muscles surrounding air tubes constrict, inflammation and swelling of the lining of the air tubes occur, and increased mucus is produced, clogging the air tubes. The mucus secretion, in turn, may then obstruct the bronchioles, reducing the supply of oxygen and increasing the amount of carbon dioxide.

Statistics show a dramatic increase in the prevalence of allergic disorders, including asthma, in the past 20 to 30 years. Currently, approximately 235 million people worldwide have asthma, 26 million of them in the United States (Centers for Disease Control and Prevention, May 2018; World Health Organization, August 2017). The numbers are increasing, especially in industrialized countries and in urban areas as opposed to rural areas. Asthma rates are especially high in low-income areas, and psychosocial stressors may play a role in aggravating an underlying vulnerability (Vangeepuram, Galvez, Teitelbaum, Brenner, & Wolff, 2012). However, the reasons for the dramatic increase in asthma cases are not yet fully known. Children who have a lot of infectious disorders during childhood are less likely to develop allergies, suggesting that exposure to infectious agents plays a protective role. Thus, paradoxically, the improved hygiene of industrialized countries may actually be contributing to the high rates of allergic disorders currently seen.

Viral Infections    The respiratory system is vulnerable to infections, especially the common cold, a viral infection of the upper and sometimes the lower respiratory tract. The infection that results causes discomfort, congestion, and excessive secretion of mucus. The incubation period for a cold—that is, the time between exposure to the virus and onset of symptoms—is 12 to 72 hours, and the typical duration is a few days. Secondary bacterial infections may complicate the illness. These occur because the primary viral infection causes inflammation of the mucous membranes, reducing their ability to prevent secondary infection.

Bronchitis is an inflammation of the mucosal membrane inside the bronchi of the lungs. Large amounts of mucus are produced in bronchitis, leading to persistent coughing.

A serious viral infection of the respiratory system is influenza, which can occur in an epidemic form. Flu viruses attack the lining of the respiratory tract, killing healthy cells. Fever and inflammation of the respiratory tract may result. A common complication is a secondary bacterial infection, such as pneumonia.

Bacterial Infections    The respiratory system is also vulnerable to bacterial disorders, including strep throat, whooping cough, and diphtheria. Usually, these disorders do not cause permanent damage to the upper respiratory tract. The main danger is the possibility of secondary infection, which results from lowered resistance. However, these bacterial infections can cause permanent damage to other tissues, including heart tissue.

Chronic Obstructive Pulmonary Disease    Chronic obstructive pulmonary disease (COPD), including chronic bronchitis and emphysema, is the fourth-leading cause of death in the United States. Some 16 million Americans have COPD (National Heart, Lung, & Blood Institute, 2017). Although COPD is not curable, it is preventable. Its chief cause is smoking, which accounts for over 80 percent of all cases of COPD (COPD International, 2015).

Pneumonia    There are two main types of pneumonia. Lobar pneumonia is a primary infection of the entire lobe of a lung. The alveoli become inflamed, and the normal oxygen–carbon dioxide exchange between the blood and alveoli can be disrupted. Spread of infection to other organs is also likely.

Bronchial pneumonia, which is confined to the bronchi, is typically a secondary infection that may occur as a complication of other disorders, such as a severe cold or flu. It is not as serious as lobar pneumonia.

### Tuberculosis and Pleurisy

Tuberculosis (TB) is an infectious disease caused by bacteria that invade lung tissue. When the invading bacilli are surrounded by macrophages (a type of white blood cells), they form a clump called a tubercle. Eventually, through a process called caseation, the center of the tubercle turns into a cheesy mass, which can produce cavities in the lung. Such cavities, in turn, can give rise to permanent scar tissue, causing chronic difficulties in oxygen and carbon dioxide exchange between the blood and the alveoli. Once the leading cause of death in the United States, it has been in decline for several decades. However, worldwide, it remains common and deadly, affecting one-fourth of the world's population (Centers for Disease Control and Prevention, 2018).

Pleurisy is an inflammation of the pleura, the membrane that surrounds the organs in the thoracic cavity. The inflammation, which produces a sticky fluid, is usually a consequence of pneumonia or tuberculosis and can be extremely painful.

### Lung Cancer

Lung cancer is a disease of uncontrolled cell growth in tissues of the lung. The affected cells begin to divide in a rapid and unrestricted manner, producing a tumor. Malignant cells grow faster than healthy cells. This growth may lead to metastasis, which is the invasion of adjacent tissue and infiltration beyond the lungs. The most common symptoms are shortness of breath, coughing (including coughing up blood), and weight loss. Smoking is one of the primary causes. There were an estimated 228,150 new lung cancer cases in the United States in 2018 (American Cancer Society, 2019)

### Dealing with Respiratory Disorders

A number of respiratory disorders can be addressed by health psychologists. For example, smoking is implicated in both pulmonary emphysema and lung cancer. Dangerous substances in the workplace and air pollution are also factors that contribute to the incidence of respiratory problems. Both of these causes of disease can be modified.

As we will see in Chapters 3 to 5, health psychologists have conducted research on many of these problems and discussed the clinical issues they raise. Some respiratory disorders are chronic conditions. Consequently, issues of long-term physical, vocational, social, and psychological rehabilitation become important. We cover these issues in Chapters 11, 13, and 14.

## ■ THE DIGESTIVE SYSTEM AND THE METABOLISM OF FOOD

### Overview

Food, essential for survival, is converted through the process of metabolism into heat and energy, and it supplies nutrients for growth and the repair of tissues. But before food can be used by cells, it must be changed into a form suitable for absorption into the blood. This conversion process is called digestion.

### The Functioning of the Digestive System

Food is first lubricated by saliva in the mouth, where it forms a soft, rounded lump called a bolus. It passes through the esophagus by means of peristalsis, a unidirectional muscular movement toward the stomach. The stomach produces various gastric secretions, including pepsin and hydrochloric acid, to further the digestive process. The sight or even the thought of food starts the flow of gastric juices.

As food progresses from the stomach to the duodenum (the intersection of the stomach and lower intestine), the pancreas becomes involved in the digestive process. Pancreatic juices, which are secreted into the duodenum, contain enzymes that break down proteins, carbohydrates, and fats. A critical function of the pancreas is the production of the hormone insulin, which facilitates the entry of glucose into the bodily tissues. The liver also plays an important role in metabolism by producing bile, which enters the duodenum and helps break down fats. Bile is stored in the gallbladder and is secreted into the duodenum as needed.

Most metabolic products are water soluble and can be easily transported in the blood, but some substances, such as lipids, are not soluble in water and so must be transported in the blood plasma. Lipids include fats, cholesterol, and lecithin. An excess of lipids in the blood is called hyperlipidemia, a condition common in diabetes, some kidney diseases, hyperthyroidism, and alcoholism. It is also a causal factor in the development of heart disease (see Chapters 5 and 13).

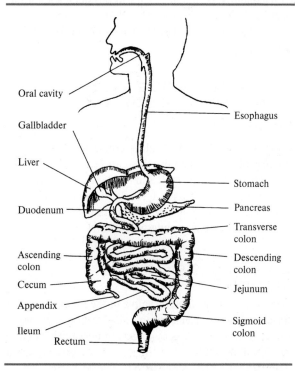

The absorption of food takes place primarily in the small intestine, which produces enzymes that complete the breakdown of proteins to amino acids. The motility of the small intestine is under the control of the sympathetic and parasympathetic nervous systems, such that parasympathetic activity speeds up metabolism, whereas sympathetic nervous system activity reduces it.

Food then passes into the large intestine, which acts largely as a storage organ for the accumulation of food residue and helps in the reabsorption of water. The entry of feces into the rectum leads to the expulsion of solid waste. The organs involved in the metabolism of food are pictured in Figure 2.7.

## Disorders of the Digestive System

The digestive system is susceptible to a number of disorders.

**Gastroesophageal reflux disease**    Gastroesophageal reflux disease (GERD), also known as acid reflux disease, results from an abnormal reflux in the esophagus. This is commonly due to changes in the barrier between the esophagus and the stomach. As much as 60 percent of the U.S. adult population experiences acid reflux at least occasionally (U.S. Healthline, 2012). A systematic review of GERD found that the prevalence in North America was between 18 and 28 percent (El-Serag, Sweet, Winchester, & Dent, 2013).

**Gastroenteritis, Diarrhea, and Dysentery**
Gastroenteritis is an inflammation of the lining of the stomach and small intestine. It may be caused by excessive amounts of food or drink, contaminated food or water, or food poisoning. Symptoms appear approximately 2 to 4 hours after the ingestion of food and include vomiting, diarrhea, abdominal cramps, and nausea.

Diarrhea, characterized by watery and frequent bowel movements, occurs when the lining of the small and large intestines cannot properly absorb water or digested food. Chronic diarrhea may result in serious disturbances of fluid and electrolyte (sodium, potassium, magnesium, calcium) balance.

Dysentery is similar to diarrhea except that mucus, pus, and blood are also excreted. It may be caused by a protozoan that attacks the large intestine (amoebic dysentery) or by a bacterial organism. These conditions are only rarely life threatening in industrialized countries; in developing countries, they are among the most common causes of death.

**Peptic Ulcer**    A peptic ulcer is an open sore in the lining of the stomach or the duodenum. It results from the hypersecretion of hydrochloric acid and occurs when pepsin, a protein-digesting enzyme secreted in the stomach, digests a portion of the stomach wall or duodenum. A bacterium called *Helicobacter pylori* is believed to contribute to the development of many ulcers. Once thought to be primarily psychological in origin, ulcers are now believed to be aggravated by stress, but not caused by it.

**Appendicitis**    Appendicitis is a common condition that occurs when wastes and bacteria accumulate in the appendix. If the small opening of the appendix becomes obstructed, bacteria can easily proliferate. Soon this condition gives rise to pain, increased peristalsis, and nausea. If the appendix ruptures and the bacteria are released into the abdominal cavity or peritoneum, they can cause further infection (peritonitis) or even death.

**Hepatitis**    Hepatitis means "inflammation of the liver," and the disease produces swelling, tenderness, and sometimes permanent damage. When the liver is inflamed, bilirubin, a product of the breakdown of hemoglobin, cannot easily pass into the bile ducts. Consequently, it remains in the blood, causing a yellowing of the skin known as jaundice. Other common symptoms are fatigue, fever, muscle or joint pain, nausea, vomiting, loss of appetite, abdominal pain, and diarrhea.

There are several types of hepatitis, which differ in severity and mode of transmission. Hepatitis A, caused by viruses, is typically transmitted through food and water. It is often spread by poorly cooked seafood or through unsanitary preparation or storage of food. Hepatitis B is more serious. Up to 2.2 million Americans are chronically infected with hepatitis B and thousands will die each year (Hepatitis B Foundation, 2018). Also known as serum hepatitis, it is caused by a virus and is transmitted by the transfusion of infected blood, by improperly sterilized needles, through sexual contact, and through mother-to-infant contact. It is a particular risk among intravenous drug users. Its symptoms are similar to those of hepatitis A but are far more serious.

Hepatitis C, also spread via blood and needles, is most commonly caused by blood transfusions; 130 million to 150 million people worldwide have the disorder, which accounts for half a million deaths annually. Hepatitis D is found mainly in intravenous drug users who are also carriers of hepatitis B, necessary for the hepatitis D virus to spread. Finally, hepatitis E resembles hepatitis A but is caused by a different virus.

## The Gut–Brain Connection

Recent research has focused on how the brain and the gut communicate with each other. The microbial composition of the gut is complex and individualized, making definitive conclusions difficult. However, dysbiosis, the technical term for the microbial imbalance of the gut, has been linked not only to temporary and mild symptoms such as stomach upset but also to potentially more serious conditions such as inflammatory bowel disease, obesity, metabolic syndrome (a frequent precursor to heart disease), and Type II diabetes (Mayer & Hsiao, 2017) as well as to psychiatric disorders and poor mood (Sundin, Ohman, & Simven, 2017). Experiments show that altering the microbial environment through use of probiotics or other dietary interventions may beneficially affect the course of some of these disorders (Dinan & Cryan, 2017) and improve mood and energy. Certain patterns of microbial composition may

represent vulnerabilities for adverse responses to stress, such as post traumatic stress disorder and exposure to extreme stress, such as racism, can alter the gut microbiota adversely (Carson et al., 2018).

The gut sends signals to the brain, which vary with microbial composition, that are then interpreted in the brain leading not only to physical symptoms but to changes in behavior and psychological states. In many important ways, then, the gut and the brain interact to affect physical and psychological health. Moreover, there is some evidence that the benefits of dietary interventions to treat adverse gut–brain interactions may affect not only the target person but subsequent generations (Callaghan, 2017).

## ■ THE RENAL SYSTEM

### Overview

The **renal system** consists of the kidneys, ureters, urinary bladder, and urethra. The kidneys are chiefly responsible for the regulation of bodily fluids; their principal function is to produce urine. The ureters contain smooth muscle tissue, which contracts, causing peristaltic waves to move urine to the bladder, a muscular bag that acts as a reservoir for urine. The urethra then conducts urine from the bladder out of the body. The anatomy of the renal system is pictured in Figure 2.8.

Urine contains surplus water, surplus electrolytes, waste products from the metabolism of food, and

**FIGURE 2.8 | The Renal System**
(*Source:* Lankford, T. Randall. *Integrated science for health students.* Virginia: Reston, 1979, p. 585.)

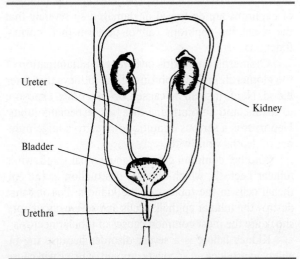

surplus acids or alkalis. By carrying these products out of the body, urine maintains water balance, electrolyte balance, and blood pH. Of the electrolytes, sodium and potassium are especially important because they are involved in muscular contractions and the conduction of nerve impulses, among other vital functions.

One of the chief functions of the kidneys is to control the water balance in the body. For example, on a hot day, when a person has been active and has perspired profusely, relatively little urine will be produced so that the body may retain more water. On the other hand, on a cold day, when a person is relatively inactive or has consumed a good deal of liquid, urine output will be higher so as to prevent overhydration.

Urine can offer important diagnostic clues to many disorders. For example, an excess of glucose may indicate diabetes, and an excess of red blood cells may indicate a kidney disorder. This is one of the reasons that a medical checkup often includes a urinalysis.

To summarize, the urinary system regulates bodily fluids by removing surplus water, surplus electrolytes, and the waste products generated by the metabolism of food.

## Disorders of the Renal System

The renal system is vulnerable to a number of disorders. Among the most common are urinary tract infections, to which women are especially vulnerable and which can result in considerable pain, especially on urination. If untreated, they can lead to more serious infection.

Nephrons are the basic structural and functional units of the kidneys. In many types of kidney disease, such as that associated with hypertension, large numbers of nephrons are destroyed or damaged so severely that the remaining nephrons cannot perform their normal functions.

Glomerular nephritis involves the inflammation of the glomeruli in the nephrons of the kidneys that filter blood. Nephritis can be caused by infections, exposure to toxins, and autoimmune diseases, especially lupus. Nephritis is a serious condition linked to a large number of deaths worldwide.

Another common cause of acute renal shutdown is tubular necrosis, which involves destruction of the epithelial cells in the tubules of the kidneys. Poisons that destroy the tubular epithelial cells and severe circulatory shock are the most common causes of tubular necrosis.

Kidney failure is a severe disorder because the inability to produce an adequate amount of urine will cause the waste products of metabolism, as well as surplus inorganic salts and water, to be retained in the body. An artificial kidney, a kidney transplant, or **kidney dialysis** may be required in order to rid the body of its wastes. Although these technologies can cleanse the blood to remove the excess salts, water, and metabolites, they are highly stressful medical procedures. Kidney transplants carry many health risks, and kidney dialysis can be extremely uncomfortable for patients. Consequently, health psychologists have been involved in addressing these problems.

## ■ THE REPRODUCTIVE SYSTEM

### Overview

The development of the reproductive system is controlled by the pituitary gland. The anterior pituitary lobe produces the gonadotropic hormones, which control the development of the ovaries in females and the testes in males. A diagrammatic representation of the human reproductive system appears in Figure 2.9.

### The Ovaries and Testes

The female has two ovaries located in the pelvis. Each month, one of the ovaries releases an ovum (egg), which is discharged at ovulation into the fallopian tubes. If the ovum is not fertilized (by sperm), it remains in the uterine cavity for about 14 days and is then flushed out of the system with the uterine endometrium and its blood vessels (during menstruation).

The ovaries also produce the hormones estrogen and progesterone. Estrogen leads to the development of secondary sex characteristics in females, including breasts and the distribution of both body fat and body hair. Progesterone, which is produced during the second half of the menstrual cycle to prepare the body for pregnancy, declines if pregnancy does not occur.

In males, testosterone is produced by the interstitial cells of the testes under the control of the anterior pituitary lobe. It brings about the production of sperm and the development of secondary sex characteristics, including growth of the beard, deepening of the voice, distribution of body hair, and both skeletal and muscular growth.

### Fertilization and Gestation

When sexual intercourse takes place and ejaculation occurs, sperm are released into the vagina. These sperm, which have a high degree of motility, proceed upward

**FIGURE 2.9 | The Reproductive System**   (*Sources:* Green, John Herbert. *Basic clinical physiology*. New York: Oxford University Press, 1978; Lankford, T. Randall. *Integrated science for health students*. Virginia: Reston, 1979, p. 688.)

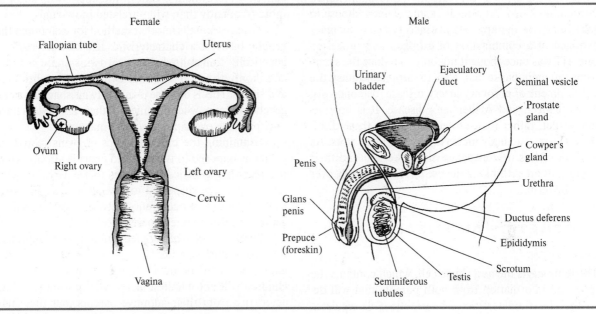

through the uterus into the fallopian tubes, where one sperm may fertilize an ovum. The fertilized ovum then travels down the fallopian tube into the uterine cavity, where it embeds itself in the uterine wall and develops over the next 9 months into a human being.

## Disorders of the Reproductive System

The reproductive system is vulnerable to a number of diseases and disorders. Among the most common and problematic are sexually transmitted diseases (STDs), which occur through sexual intercourse or other forms of sexually intimate activity. STDs include herpes, gonorrhea, syphilis, genital warts, chlamydia, and, most seriously, AIDS.

For women, a risk from several STDs is chronic pelvic inflammatory disease (PID), which may produce severe abdominal pain and infections that may compromise fertility. Other gynecologic disorders to which women are vulnerable include vaginitis, endometriosis (in which pieces of the endometrial lining of the uterus move into the fallopian tubes or abdominal cavity, grow, and spread to other sites), cysts, and fibroids (nonmalignant growths in the uterus that may nonetheless interfere with reproduction). Women are vulnerable to disorders of the menstrual cycle, including amenorrhea, which is the absence of menses, and oligomenorrhea, which is infrequent menstruation.

The reproductive system is also vulnerable to cancer, including testicular cancer in men and gynecologic cancers in women. Every 6 minutes, a woman in the United States is diagnosed with a gynecologic cancer, including cancer of the cervix, uterus, and ovaries (American Cancer Society, 2012a). Endometrial cancer is the most common female pelvic malignancy, and ovarian cancer is the most lethal.

Approximately 12 to 13 percent of U.S. couples may have infertility, defined as the inability to conceive a pregnancy after 1 year of regular sexual intercourse without contraception (U.S. Department of Health & Human Services, 2019). Although physicians once believed that infertility has emotional origins, researchers now believe that distress may complicate but does not cause infertility. Fortunately, over the past few decades, the technology for treating infertility has improved. A variety of drug treatments have been developed, as have more invasive technologies. In vitro fertilization (IVF) is the most widely used method of assistive reproductive technology. The live birth success rate for IVF is 41 to 43 percent per cycle. However, women over age 42 have a 4 percent success rate. (Medline Plus, 2018).

Menopause is not a disorder of the reproductive system; rather, it occurs when a woman's reproductive life ends. A variety of noxious symptoms can occur during the transition into menopause, including sleep disorders, hot flashes, joint pain, forgetfulness, dizziness, and enhanced stress reactivity (Endrighi, Hamer, & Steptoe, 2016). As a result, some women choose to take hormone therapy (HT), which typically includes estrogen or a combination of estrogen and progesterone. HT was once thought not only to reduce the symptoms of menopause but also to protect against the development of coronary artery disease, osteoporosis, breast cancer, and Alzheimer's disease. It is now believed that, rather than protecting against these disorders, HT may actually increase some of these risks. As a result of this new evidence, many women and their physicians are rethinking the use of HT, especially over the long term.

## ■ GENETICS AND HEALTH

### Overview

The fetus starts life as a single cell, which contains the inherited information from both parents that will determine its characteristics. The genetic code regulates such factors as eye and hair color, as well as behavioral factors. Genetic material for inheritance lies in the nucleus of the cell in the form of 46 chromosomes, 23 from the mother and 23 from the father. Two of these 46 are sex chromosomes, which are an X from the mother and either an X or a Y from the father. If the father provides an X chromosome, a female child will result; if he provides a Y chromosome, a male child will result.

### Genetics and Susceptibility to Disorders

Genetic studies have provided valuable information about the inheritance of susceptibility to disease. For example, scientists have bred strains of rats, mice, and other laboratory animals that are sensitive or insensitive to the development of particular diseases and then used these strains to study illness onset and the course of illness. For example, a strain of rats that is susceptible to cancer may shed light on the development of this disease and what other factors contribute to its occurrence. The initial susceptibility of the rats ensures that many of them will develop malignancies when implanted with carcinogenic (cancer-causing) materials.

In humans, several types of research help demonstrate whether a characteristic is genetically based. Studies of families, for example, can reveal whether members of the same family are more likely to develop a disorder, such as heart disease, than are unrelated

individuals in a similar environment. If a factor has genetic determinants, family members will show it more frequently than will unrelated individuals.

Twin research is another method for examining the genetic basis of a characteristic. If a characteristic is genetically transmitted, identical twins share it more commonly than do fraternal twins or other brothers and sisters. This is because identical twins share the same genetic makeup, whereas other brothers and sisters have only partially overlapping genetic makeup.

Examining the characteristics of twins reared together as opposed to twins reared apart is also informative regarding genetics. Attributes that emerge in twins reared apart are suspected to have genetic bases, especially if the rate of occurrence between twins reared together and those reared apart is the same.

Finally, studies of adopted children also help identify which characteristics have genetic origins and which are primarily the product of the environment. Adopted children will not manifest genetically transmitted characteristics from their adoptive parents, but they may manifest environmentally transmitted characteristics.

Consider, for example, obesity, which is a risk factor for a number of disorders, including coronary artery disease and diabetes. If twins reared apart show highly similar body weights, then we would suspect that body weight has a genetic component. If, on the other hand, weight within a family is highly related, and adopted children show the same weight as their parents and any natural offspring, then we would look to the family diet as a potential cause of obesity. For many attributes, including obesity, both environmental and genetic factors are involved.

Research like this has increasingly uncovered the genetic contribution to many health disorders and behavioral factors that may pose risks to health. Such diseases as asthma, Alzheimer's disease, cystic fibrosis, muscular dystrophy, Tay–Sachs disease, and Huntington's disease have a genetic basis. There is also a genetic basis for coronary heart disease and for some forms of cancer, including some breast and colon cancers. This genetic basis does not preclude the important role of the environment, however.

Genetics will continue to be of interest as the contribution of genes to health continues to be uncovered. For example, genetic contributions to obesity and alcoholism have emerged in recent years. Moreover, the contributions of genetics studies to health psychology are broadening. Even some personality characteristics, such as optimism, which is believed to have protective health effects, have genetic underpinnings (Saphire-Bernstein, Way, Kim, Sherman, & Taylor, 2011).

Genetics and Health Psychology   Health psychologists have important roles to play with respect to genetic contributions to health disorders. One question concerns whether people need to be alerted to genetic risks. Many people think that genetic risks are immutable and that any efforts they might undertake to affect their health would be fruitless if genes are implicated (Dar-Nimrod & Heine, 2011). Such erroneous beliefs may deter health behavior change and information seeking about one's risk (Marteau & Weinman, 2006). Genetic risk information may also evoke defensive processes whereby people downplay their risk (Shiloh, Drori, Orr-Urtreger, & Friedman, 2009). Genetic risks may also interact with stress or trauma to increase risks for certain disorders (Zhao, Bremner, Goldberg, Quyyumi, & Vaccarino, 2013). Accordingly, making people aware of genetic risk factors should be accompanied by educational information to offset these potential problems.

Another role for health psychologists involves genetic counseling. Prenatal diagnostic tests permit the detection of some genetically based disorders, including Tay–Sachs disease, cystic fibrosis, muscular dystrophy, Huntington's disease, and breast cancer. Helping people decide whether to be screened and how to cope with genetic vulnerabilities if they test positive represents an important role for health psychologists (Mays et al., 2014). For example, belief in a genetic cause can lead people to take medical actions that may be medically unwarranted (Petrie et al., 2015).

In addition, people who have a family history of genetic disorders, those who have already given birth to a child with a genetic disorder, or those who have recurrent reproductive problems, such as multiple miscarriages, often seek such counseling. In some cases, technological advances have made it possible to treat some of these problems before birth through drugs or surgery. However, if the condition cannot be corrected, the parents often must make the difficult decision of whether to terminate the pregnancy.

Children, adolescents, and young adults sometimes learn of a genetic risk to their health, as research uncovers such causes. Breast cancer, for example, runs in families, and among young women whose mothers, aunts, or sisters have developed breast cancer, vulnerability is higher. Families that share genetic risks may need special attention through family counseling. Some of the genes that contribute to the development

of breast cancer have been identified, and tests are now available to determine whether a genetic susceptibility is present. Although this type of cancer accounts for only 5 percent of breast cancer, women who carry these genetic susceptibilities are more likely to develop the disease at an earlier age; thus, these women are at high risk and need careful monitoring and assistance in making treatment-related decisions. With genetic testing becoming available online to people who submit samples to a genetic testing website, knowledge of genetic risks may increase. However, it is essential to have any genetic risk that is identified independently validated because erroneous results can occur (Kolata, 2018).

Carriers of genetic risks may experience distress (Hamilton, Lobel, & Moyer, 2009). Should people be told about their genetic risks if nothing can be done to treat them? Growing evidence suggests that people at risk for treatable disorders benefit from genetic testing and do not suffer long-term psychological distress (Frieser, Scott, & Vrieze, 2018). Moreover, many people seek to learn their genetic risk factors (Reid et al., 2018). People who are chronically anxious, though, may require special attention and counseling (Rimes, Salkovskis, Jones, & Lucassen, 2006).

In some cases, genetic risks can be offset by behavioral interventions to address the risk factor. For example, one study (Aspinwall, Leaf, Dola, Kohlmann, & Leachman, 2008) found that being informed that one had tested positive for a gene implicated in melanoma (a serious skin cancer) and receiving counseling led to better skin self-examination practices at a 1-month follow-up. Thus health psychologists have an important role to play in research and counseling related to genetic risks, especially if they can help people modify their risk status and manage their distress (Aspinwall, Taber, Leaf, Kohlmann, & Leachman, 2013).

## ■ THE IMMUNE SYSTEM

### Overview

Disease is caused by a variety of factors. In this section, we address the transmission of disease by infection, that is, the invasion of microbes and their growth in the body. The microbes that cause infection are transmitted to people in several ways:

- Direct transmission involves bodily contact, such as handshaking, kissing, and sexual intercourse. For example, genital herpes is typically contracted by direct transmission.

BOX **2.2** Portraits of Two Carriers

Carriers are people who transmit a disease to others without actually contracting that disease themselves. They are especially dangerous because they are not ill and so they can infect dozens, hundreds, or even thousands of people while going about the business of everyday life.

**"TYPHOID MARY"**

Perhaps the most famous carrier in history was "Typhoid Mary," a young Swiss immigrant to the United States who infected thousands of people during her lifetime. During her ocean crossing, Mary was taught how to cook, and eventually, some 100 individuals aboard the ship died of typhoid, including the cook who trained her. Once Mary arrived in New York, she obtained a series of jobs as a cook, continually passing on the disease to those for whom she worked without contracting it herself.

Typhoid is precipitated by a salmonella bacterium, which can be transmitted through water, food, and physical contact. Mary carried a virulent form of the infection in her body but was herself immune to the disease. It is believed that she was unaware she was a carrier for many years. Toward the end of her life, however, she began to realize that she was responsible for the many deaths around her.

Mary's status as a carrier also became known to medical authorities, and she spent the latter part of her life in and out of institutions in a vain attempt to isolate her from others. In 1930, Mary died not of typhoid but of a brain hemorrhage (Federspiel, 1983).

**"HELEN"**

The CBS News program *60 Minutes* profiled an equally terrifying carrier: a prostitute, "Helen," who is a carrier of HIV, the virus that causes AIDS (acquired immune deficiency syndrome). Helen has never had AIDS, but her baby was born with the disease. As a prostitute and heroin addict, Helen is not only at risk for developing the illness herself but also poses a threat to her clients and anyone with whom she shares a needle.

Helen represents a dilemma for medical and criminal authorities. She is a known carrier of AIDS, yet there is no legal basis for preventing her from coming into contact with others. Although she can be arrested for prostitution or drug dealing, such incarcerations are usually short-term and have a negligible impact on her ability to spread the disease to others. For potentially fatal diseases such as AIDS, the carrier represents a nightmare, and medical and legal authorities have been almost powerless to intervene (Moses, 1984).

---

- Indirect transmission (or environmental transmission) occurs when microbes are passed to an individual via airborne particles, dust, water, soil, or food. Influenza is an example of an environmentally transmitted disease.

- Biological transmission occurs when a transmitting agent, such as a mosquito, picks up microbes, changes them into a form conducive to growth in the human body, and passes them on to the human. Yellow fever, for example, is transmitted by this method.

- Mechanical transmission is the passage of a microbe to an individual by means of a carrier that is not directly involved in the disease process. Dirty hands, bad water, rats, mice, and flies can be implicated in mechanical transmission. Box 2.2 tells about two people who were carriers of deadly diseases and transmitted them to others.

### Infection

Once a microbe has reached the body, it penetrates into bodily tissue via any of several routes, including the skin, the throat and respiratory tract, the digestive tract, or the genitourinary system. Whether the invading microbes gain a foothold in the body and produce infection depends on three factors: the number of organisms, the virulence of the organisms, and the body's defensive capacities. The virulence of an organism is determined by its aggressiveness (i.e., its ability to resist the body's defenses) and by its toxigenicity (i.e., its ability to produce poisons, which invade other parts of the body).

### The Course of Infection

Assuming that the invading organism does gain a foothold, the natural history of infection follows a specific course. First, there is an incubation period between the time the infection is contracted and the time the symptoms appear.

Next, there is a period of nonspecific symptoms, such as headaches and general discomfort, which precedes the onset of the disorder. During this time, the microbes are actively colonizing and producing toxins. The next stage is the acute phase, when the illness and its symptoms are at their height. Unless the infection proves fatal, a period of decline follows the acute phase. During this period, the organisms are expelled from the mouth and nose in saliva and respiratory secretions, as well as through the digestive tract and the genitourinary system in feces and urine.

Infections may be localized, focal, or systemic. Localized infections remain at their original site and do not spread throughout the body. Although a local infection is confined to a particular area, it sends toxins to other parts of the body, causing other disruptions. Systemic infections affect a number of areas or body systems.

The primary infection initiated by the microbe may also lead to secondary infections. These occur because the body's resistance is lowered from fighting the primary infection, leaving it susceptible to other invaders. In many cases, secondary infections, such as pneumonia, pose a greater risk than the primary one.

## Immunity

**Immunity** is the body's resistance to invading organisms. It may develop either naturally or artificially. Some natural immunity is passed from the mother to the child at birth and through breast-feeding, although this type of immunity is only temporary. Natural immunity is also acquired through disease. For example, if you have measles once, you are unlikely to develop it a second time; you will have built up an immunity to it.

Artificial immunity is acquired through vaccinations and inoculations. For example, most children and adolescents receive shots for a variety of diseases—among them, diphtheria, whooping cough, smallpox, poliomyelitis, and hepatitis—so that they will not contract these diseases, should they be exposed.

### Natural and Specific Immunity   How does immunity work? The body has a number of responses to invading organisms, some nonspecific and others specific. **Nonspecific immune mechanisms** are a general set of responses to any kind of infection or disorder; **specific immune mechanisms,** which are always acquired after birth, fight particular microorganisms and their toxins.

Natural immunity is involved in defense against pathogens. The cells involved in natural immunity provide defense not against a particular pathogen, but rather against many pathogens. The largest group of cells involved in natural immunity is granulocytes, which include neutrophils and macrophages; both are phagocytic cells that engulf target pathogens. Neutrophils and macrophages congregate at the site of an injury or infection and release toxic substances. Macrophages release cytokines that lead to inflammation and fever, among other side effects, and promote wound healing. Natural killer cells are also involved in natural immunity; they recognize "nonself" material (such as viral infections or cancer cells) and lyse (break up and disintegrate) those cells by releasing toxic substances. Natural killer cells are believed to be important in signaling potential malignancies and in limiting early phases of viral infections.

Natural immunity occurs through four main ways: anatomical barriers, phagocytosis, antimicrobial substances, and inflammatory responses. Anatomical barriers prevent the passage of microbes from one section of the body to another. For example, the skin functions as an effective anatomical barrier to many infections, and the mucous membranes lining the nose and mouth also provide protection.

**Phagocytosis** is the process by which certain white blood cells (called phagocytes) ingest microbes. Phagocytes are usually overproduced when there is a bodily infection, so that large numbers can be sent to the site of infection to ingest the foreign particles.

Antimicrobial substances are chemicals produced by the body that kill invading microorganisms. Interferon, hydrochloric acid, and enzymes such as lysozyme are some antimicrobial substances that help destroy invading microorganisms.

The inflammatory response is a local reaction to infection. At the site of infection, the blood capillaries first enlarge, and a chemical called histamine is released into the area. This chemical causes an increase in capillary permeability, allowing white blood cells and fluids to leave the capillaries and enter the tissues; consequently, the area becomes reddened and fluids accumulate. The white blood cells attack the microbes, resulting in the formation of pus. Temperature increases at the site of inflammation because of the increased flow of blood. Usually, a clot then forms around the inflamed area, isolating the microbes and keeping them from spreading to other parts of the body. Familiar examples of the inflammatory response

**FIGURE 2.10** | **Interaction Between Lymphocytes and Phagocytes**     B lymphocytes release antibodies, which bind to pathogens and their products, aiding recognition by phagocytes. Cytokines released by T cells activate phagocytes to destroy the material they have taken up. In turn, mononuclear phagocytes can present antigen to T cells, thereby activating them.     (*Source:* Roitt, Ivan Maurice, Jonathan Brostoff, and David K. Male. *Immunology.* London: Mosby International, 1998.)

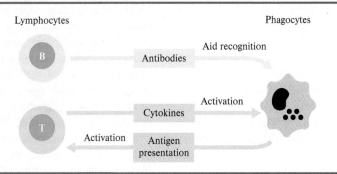

are the reddening, swelling, discharge, and clotting that result when you accidentally cut your skin and the sneezing, runny nose and teary eyes that result from an allergic response to pollen.

Specific immunity is acquired after birth by contracting a disease or through artificial means, such as vaccinations. It operates through the antigen-antibody reaction. Antigens are foreign substances whose presence stimulates the production of antibodies in the cell tissues. Antibodies are proteins produced in response to stimulation by antigens, which combine chemically with the antigens to overcome their toxic effects.

Specific immunity is slower and, as its name implies, more specific than natural immunity. The lymphocytes involved in specific immunity have receptor sites on their cell surfaces that fit with one, and only one, antigen, and thus, they respond to only one kind of invader. When they are activated, these antigen-specific cells divide and create a population of cells called the proliferative response.

Essentially, natural and specific immunity work together, such that natural immunity contains an infection or wound rapidly and early on following the invasion of a pathogen, whereas specific immunity involves a delay of up to several days before a full defense can be mounted. Figure 2.10 illustrates the interaction between lymphocytes and phagocytes.

Humoral and Cell-Mediated Immunity

There are two basic immunologic reactions—humoral and cell mediated. **Humoral immunity** is mediated by B lymphocytes. The functions of B lymphocytes include protecting against bacteria, neutralizing toxins produced

by bacteria, and preventing viral reinfection. B cells confer immunity by the production and secretion of antibodies.

**Cell-mediated immunity,** involving T lymphocytes from the thymus gland, is a slower-acting response. Rather than releasing antibodies into the blood, as humoral immunity does, cell-mediated immunity operates at the cellular level. When stimulated by the appropriate antigen, T cells secrete chemicals that kill invading organisms and infected cells. Components of the immune system are shown in Figure 2.11.

The Lymphatic System's Role in Immunity

The **lymphatic system,** which is a drainage system of the body, is involved in important ways in immune functioning. There is lymphatic tissue throughout the body, consisting of lymphatic capillaries, vessels, and nodes. Lymphatic capillaries drain water, proteins, microbes, and other foreign materials from spaces between the cells into lymph vessels. This material is then conducted in the lymph vessels to the lymph nodes, which filter out microbes and foreign materials for ingestion by lymphocytes. The lymphatic vessels then drain any remaining substances into the blood.

Additional discussion of immunity can be found in Chapter 14, where we consider the rapidly developing field of psychoneuroimmunology and the role of immunity in the development of AIDS.

Disorders Related to the Immune System

The immune system is subject to a number of disorders and diseases. One very important one is AIDS, which

**FIGURE 2.11 | Components of the Immune System**  (*Source:* Roitt, Ivan Maurice, Jonathan Brostoff, and David K. Male. *Immunology.* London: Mosby International, 1998.)

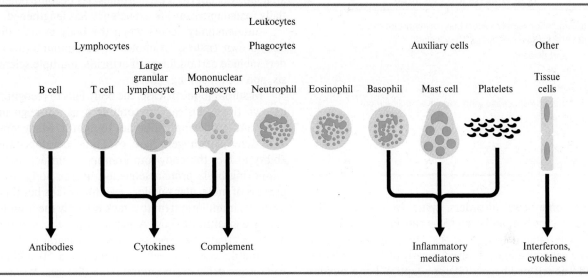

is a progressive impairment of immunity. Another is cancer, which is now believed to depend heavily on immunocompromise. We defer extended discussion of AIDS and cancer to Chapter 14.

**Lupus** affects approximately 1.5 million Americans, most of them women (Lupus Foundation of America, 2016). The disease acquired the name lupus, which means "wolf," because of the skin rash that can appear on the face. It leads to chronic inflammation, producing pain, heat, redness, and swelling, and can be life-threatening when it attacks the connective tissue of the body's internal organs. Depending on the severity of the disease, it may be managed by anti-inflammatory medications or immunosuppressive medications.

A number of infections attack lymphatic tissue. For example, tonsillitis is an inflammation of the tonsils that interferes with their ability to filter out bacteria. Infectious mononucleosis is a viral disorder marked by an unusually large number of monocytes; it can cause enlargement of the spleen and lymph nodes, as well as fever, sore throat, and general lack of energy.

Lymphoma is a tumor of the lymphatic tissue. Hodgkin's disease, a malignant lymphoma, involves the progressive, chronic enlargement of the lymph nodes, spleen, and other lymphatic tissues. As a consequence, the nodes cannot effectively produce antibodies, and the phagocytic properties of the nodes are lost. If untreated, Hodgkin's disease can be fatal.

Infectious disorders were at one time thought to be acute problems that ended when their course had

run. A major problem in developing countries, infectious disorders were thought to be largely under control in developed nations. Now, however, infectious diseases merit closer examination (Morens, Folkers, & Fauci, 2004). First, as noted in the discussion of asthma, the control of at least some infectious disorders through hygiene may have paradoxically increased the rates of allergic disorders. A second development is that some chronic diseases, once thought to be genetic in origin or unknown in origin, are now being traced back to infections. For example, Alzheimer's disease, multiple sclerosis, schizophrenia, and some cancers may have infectious triggers, at least in some cases (Zimmer, 2001). The development of bacterial strains that are resistant to treatment has raised an alarm. The overuse of antibiotics is an active contributor to the development of increasingly lethal strains. Infectious agents have also become an increasing concern in the war on terrorism, with the possibility that smallpox and other infectious agents may be used as weapons.

The inflammatory response that is so protective against provocations ranging from mosquito bites and sunburn to gastritis in response to spoiled food is coming under increasing investigation as a contributor to chronic disease. The destructive potential of inflammation is evident in diseases such as rheumatoid arthritis and multiple sclerosis, but inflammation also underlies many other chronic diseases, including atherosclerosis, diabetes, Alzheimer's disease, asthma, cirrhosis of the

**TABLE 2.1 | Some Consequences of Chronic Low-Level Inflammation**

Inflammation is believed to play an important role in several diseases of aging. They include:
- Heart disease
- Stroke
- Diabetes
- Alzheimer's disease (and cognitive decline more generally)
- Cancer
- Osteoporosis
- Depression

liver, some bowel disorders, cystic fibrosis, heart disease, depression, and even some cancers (Table 2.1).

The inflammatory response, like stress responses more generally, likely evolved in early prehistoric times and was selected because it was adaptive. For example, among hunter-gatherer societies, natural selection would have favored people with vigorous inflammatory responses because life expectancy was fairly short. Few people would have experienced any long-term costs of vigorous or long-lasting inflammatory responses, which now seem to play such an important role in the development of chronic diseases. Essentially, an adaptive pattern of earlier times has become potentially maladaptive, as life expectancy has lengthened.

**Autoimmunity** occurs when the body attacks the body's own tissues. Examples of autoimmune disorders include certain forms of arthritis, multiple sclerosis, and lupus, among others.

In autoimmune disease, the body fails to recognize its own tissue, instead interpreting it as a foreign invader and producing antibodies to fight it. Many viral and bacterial pathogens have, over time, developed the ability to fool the body into granting them access by mimicking basic protein sequences in the body. This process of molecular mimicry eventually fails but then leads the immune system to attack not only the invader but also healthy tissues. A person's genetic makeup may exacerbate this process. Stress can aggravate autoimmune disease. Between 23 million and 50 million Americans suffer from autoimmune diseases. Women are more likely than men to be affected (American Autoimmune Related Diseases Association, 2015; National Institutes of Health, 2018). Although the causes of autoimmune diseases are not fully known, researchers have discovered that a viral or bacterial infection often precedes the onset of an autoimmune disease. •

## SUMMARY

1. The nervous system and the endocrine system act as the control systems of the body, mobilizing it in times of threat and otherwise maintaining equilibrium and normal functioning.

2. The nervous system operates primarily through the exchange of nerve impulses between the peripheral nerve endings and internal organs and the brain, thereby providing the integration necessary for voluntary and involuntary movement.

3. The endocrine system operates chemically via the release of hormones stimulated by centers in the brain. It controls growth and development and augments the functioning of the nervous system.

4. The cardiovascular system is the transport system of the body, carrying oxygen and nutrients to cell tissues and taking carbon dioxide and other wastes away from the tissues for expulsion from the body.

5. The heart acts as a pump to control circulation and is responsive to regulation via the nervous system and the endocrine system.

6. The heart, blood vessels, and blood are vulnerable to a number of problems—most notably, atherosclerosis—which makes diseases of the cardiovascular system the major cause of death in the United States and other developed nations.

7. The respiratory system is responsible for taking in oxygen, expelling carbon dioxide, and controlling the chemical composition of the blood.

8. The digestive system is responsible for producing heat and energy, which—along with essential nutrients—are needed for the growth and repair of cells. Through digestion, food is broken down to be used by the cells for this process.

9. The renal system aids in metabolic processes by regulating water balance, electrolyte balance, and blood acidity-alkalinity. Water-soluble wastes are flushed out of the system in the urine.

10. The reproductive system, under the control of the endocrine system, leads to the development of primary and secondary sex characteristics. Through this system, the species is reproduced, and genetic material is transmitted from parents to their offspring.

11. With advances in genetic technology and the mapping of the genome has come an increased understanding of genetic contributions to disease. Health psychologists play important research and counseling roles with respect to these issues.

12. The immune system is responsible for warding off infection from invasion by foreign substances. It does so through the production of infection-fighting cells and chemicals.

## KEY TERMS

adrenal glands
angina pectoris
atherosclerosis
autoimmunity
blood pressure
cardiovascular system
catecholamines
cell-mediated immunity
cerebellum
cerebral cortex
endocrine system

humoral immunity
hypothalamus
immunity
ischemia
kidney dialysis
lupus
lymphatic system
medulla
myocardial infarction (MI)
nervous system
neurotransmitters

nonspecific immune mechanisms
parasympathetic nervous system
phagocytosis
pituitary gland
platelets
pons
renal system
respiratory system
specific immune mechanisms
sympathetic nervous system
thalamus

# PART 2

# Health Behavior and Primary Prevention

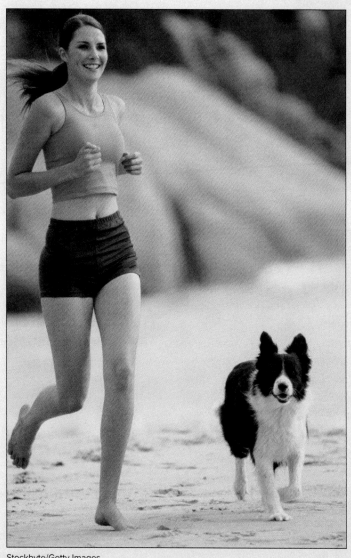

Stockbyte/Getty Images

# Health Behaviors

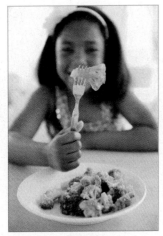

Blend Images/Getty Images

In Chapter 3, we address health behaviors. At the core of this chapter is the idea that good health is achievable through health behaviors that are practiced conscientiously.

## ■ AN INTRODUCTION TO HEALTH BEHAVIORS

### Role of Behavioral Factors in Disease and Disorder

In the past century, patterns of disease in the United States have changed substantially. As noted in Chapter 1, there has been a decline in acute infectious disorders due to changes in public health standards, but there has been an increase in preventable disorders, including lung cancer, cardiovascular disease, alcohol and drug abuse, and vehicular accidents. The role of behavioral factors in the development of these disorders is clear (Table 3.1). Nearly half of the deaths in the United States are caused by preventable factors, with smoking, obesity, drug abuse, and problem drinking being four of the main causes (Centers for Disease Control and Prevention, 2018).

**TABLE 3.1 | Risk Factors for the Leading Causes of Death in the United States**

| Disease | Risk Factors |
| --- | --- |
| Heart disease | Tobacco, high cholesterol, high blood pressure, physical inactivity, obesity and being overweight, diabetes, stress, poor diet, excessive alcohol use |
| Cancer | Smoking, unhealthy diet, environmental factors |
| Unintentional injuries | On the road (failure to wear seat belts), in the home (falls, poison, fire) |
| Chronic lower respiratory diseases | Tobacco, environmental factors (pollution, radon, asbestos) |
| Stroke | High blood pressure, tobacco, diabetes, high cholesterol, physical inactivity, obesity |

*Sources:* American Heart Association. "Coronary Artery Disease - Coronary Heart Disease. Heart Attack and Stroke Symptoms." Last reviewed July 31, 2015. https://www.heart.org/en/health-topics/consumer-healthcare/what-is-cardiovascular-disease/coronary-artery-disease; Xu, Jiaquan, Sherry L. Murphy, Kenneth D. Kochanek, Brigham Bastian, and Elizabeth Arias. "Deaths: Final Data for 2016." *National Vital Statistics Reports* 67, no. 5 (July 2018): 1–76 ; PDQ® Screening and Prevention Editorial Board, 2019.

## ■ HEALTH PROMOTION: AN OVERVIEW

Research on preventable risk factors adopts the perspective of health promotion. **Health promotion** is a philosophy that has at its core the idea that good health, or wellness, is a personal and collective achievement. For the individual, it involves developing a program of good health habits. For the medical practitioner, health promotion involves teaching people how to achieve a healthy lifestyle and helping people **at risk** for particular health problems offset or monitor those risks. For the health psychologist, health promotion involves the development of interventions to help people practice healthy behaviors. For community and national policy makers, health promotion involves emphasizing good health and providing information and resources to help people change poor health habits.

Successful modification of poor health behaviors will have several beneficial effects. First, it will reduce deaths due to lifestyle-related diseases. Second, it may delay the time of death, thereby increasing life expectancy. Third and most important, the practice of good health behaviors may expand the number of years during which a person may enjoy life free from the complications of chronic disease. Finally, modification of health behaviors may begin to make a dent in the more than $3.5 trillion that is spent yearly on health and illness (National Health Expenditures, 2017).

### Health Behaviors and Health Habits

**Health behaviors** are behaviors undertaken by people to enhance or maintain their health. A **health habit** is a health behavior that is firmly established and often performed automatically, without awareness. These habits usually develop in childhood and begin to stabilize around age 11 or 12 years (Cohen, Brownell, & Felix, 1990). Wearing a seat belt, brushing one's teeth, and eating a healthy diet are examples of these behaviors. Although a health habit may develop initially because it is reinforced by positive outcomes, such as parental approval, it eventually becomes independent of the reinforcement process. For example, you may brush your teeth automatically before going to bed. As such, habits can be highly resistant to change. Consequently, it is important to establish good health behaviors and to eliminate poor ones early in life.

An illustration of the importance of good health habits is provided by a classic study of people living in Alameda County, California, conducted by Belloc and

Breslow (1972). These scientists focused on several important health habits:

- Sleeping 7 to 8 hours a night
- Not smoking
- Eating breakfast each day
- Having no more than one or two alcoholic drinks each day
- Getting regular exercise
- Not eating between meals
- Being no more than 10 percent overweight

The scientists asked nearly 7,000 county residents to indicate which of these behaviors they practiced. Residents were also asked about the illnesses they had had, what their energy level had been, and how disabled they had been (e.g., how many days of work they had missed) over the previous 6- to 12-month period. The researchers found that the more good health habits people practiced, the fewer illnesses they had had, the better they had felt, and the less disabled they had been.

A follow-up of these people 9 to 12 years later found that mortality rates were dramatically lower for people practicing the seven health habits. Men following these practices had a mortality rate of only 28 percent and women had a mortality rate of 43 percent, compared to men and women who practiced zero to three of these health habits (Breslow & Enstrom, 1980).

Primary Prevention     Instilling good health habits and changing poor ones is the task of **primary prevention.** This means taking measures to combat risk factors for illness before an illness has a chance to develop. There are two general strategies of primary prevention. The first and most common strategy is to get people to alter their problematic health behaviors, such as helping people lose weight through an intervention. The second, more recent approach is to keep people from developing poor health habits in the first place. Smoking prevention programs with young adolescents are an example of this approach, which we will consider in Chapter 5.

## Practicing and Changing Health Behaviors: An Overview

What factors lead one person to live a healthy life and another to compromise his or her health?

Demographic Factors     Younger, more affluent, better-educated people with low levels of stress and high levels of social support typically practice better health habits than people under higher levels of stress with fewer resources (Hanson & Chen, 2007).

Age     Health habits are typically good in childhood, deteriorate in adolescence and young adulthood, but improve again among older people.

Cultural Values     Values affect the practice of health habits. For example, exercise for women may be considered desirable in one culture but undesirable in another (Guilamo-Ramos, Jaccard, Pena, & Goldberg, 2005). Thus connecting health interventions to cultural values may reduce ethnic health disparities (Sping, Arnat, Handall, & Cameron, 2018).

Personal Control     People who regard their health as under their personal control practice better health habits than people who regard their health as due to chance. The **health locus of control** scale (Wallston, Wallston, & DeVellis, 1978), which includes such items as "I am in control of my health" and "Health professionals control my health," measures the degree to which people perceive their health to be under personal control, control by the health practitioner, or chance.

Social Influence     Social norms that develop in families, among friends, and in communities can have powerful effects on both health-enhancing and health compromising behaviors (Rice & Klein, 2019). Family, friends, and workplace companions all influence health-related behaviors. For example, peer pressure often leads to smoking in adolescence but may influence people to stop smoking in adulthood.

Personal Goals and Values     Health habits are tied to personal goals. If personal fitness is an important goal, a person is more likely to exercise.

Perceived Symptoms     Some health habits are controlled by perceived symptoms. For example, a smoker who wakes up with a smoker's cough and raspy throat may cut back in the belief that he or she is vulnerable to health problems at that time.

Access to the Health Care Delivery System     Access to the health care delivery system affects health behaviors. For example, obtaining a regular Pap smear, getting mammograms, and receiving immunizations for childhood diseases depend on access to health care. Other behaviors such as losing weight and stopping smoking may be indirectly encouraged by the health care system through lifestyle advice.

## Knowledge and Cognition

The practice of health behaviors is tied to cognitive factors, such as knowledge and intelligence (Mõttus et al., 2014). More knowledgeable and smarter people typically take better care of themselves. People who are identified as intelligent in childhood have better health-related biological profiles in adulthood, which may be explained by their practice of better health behaviors in early life (Calvin, Batty, Lowe, & Deary, 2011). Using information like this to develop personalized health behavior change messages, perhaps by computer, shows some promise for optimizing message appeal and efficacy (Nikoloudakis et al., 2018), but the effects of personalized messages are not always strong (French, Cameron, Benton, Deaton, & Harvie, 2017).

## Barriers to Modifying Poor Health Behaviors

There is often little immediate incentive for practicing good health behaviors, however. Health habits develop during childhood and adolescence when most people are healthy. Smoking, a poor diet, and lack of exercise have no apparent effect on health for years, and few children and adolescents are concerned about what their health will be like when they are 40 or 50 years old (Johnson, McCaul, & Klein, 2002). As a result, bad habits have a chance to make inroads.

## Emotional Factors

Emotions may lead to or perpetuate unhealthy behaviors (Conner, McEachan, Taylor, O'Hara, & Lawton, 2015). Poor health behaviors can be pleasurable, automatic, addictive, and resistant to change. Moreover, threatening messages designed to change health behaviors can produce psychological distress and lead people to respond defensively, dismissing risks to their health (Beckjord, Rutten, Arora, Moser, & Hesse, 2008). People may perceive a health threat to be less relevant than it really is, and they may falsely see themselves as less vulnerable than or dissimilar to other people with the same habit (Roberts, Gibbons, Gerrard, & Alert, 2011; Thornton, Gibbons, & Gerrard, 2002). Continuing to practice a risky behavior may itself lead people to minimize their risks and feel a false sense of security (Halpern-Felsher et al., 2001).

## Instability of Health Behaviors

Health habits are only modestly related to each other. The person who exercises faithfully does not necessarily wear a seat belt, for example. Therefore, health behaviors must often be tackled one at a time. Health habits are unstable over time. A person may stop smoking for a year but take it up again during a period of high stress.

Why are health habits relatively independent of each other and unstable? First, different health habits are controlled by different factors. For example, smoking may be related to stress, whereas exercise depends heavily on access to athletic facilities. Second, different factors may control the same health behavior for different people. One person's overeating may be "social," and she may eat primarily in the presence of other people, whereas another person may overeat only when under stress. Even time of day can affect whether people can develop good health habits. Health behaviors completed in the morning have a better chance of becoming automatic than do health habits completed in the evening (Fournier et al., 2017).

Third, factors controlling a health behavior may change over the history of the behavior (Costello, Dierker, Jones, & Rose, 2008). For example, although peer group pressure (social factors) is important in initiating smoking, over time, smoking may be maintained because it reduces feelings of stress.

Fourth, factors controlling a health behavior may change across a person's lifetime. In childhood, regular exercise is practiced because it is built into the school curriculum, but in adulthood, this behavior must be practiced intentionally.

In summary, health behaviors are elicited and maintained by different factors for different people (Nudelman & Shiloh, 2018), and these factors change over the lifetime as well as over the course of the health habit. Consequently, health habit interventions have focused heavily on those who may be helped most—namely, children and adolescents (Patton et al., 2012).

## Intervening with Children and Adolescents

### Socialization

Health habits are strongly affected by early **socialization,** especially the influence of parents as both teachers and role models (Morrongiello, Corbett, & Bellissimo, 2008). Parents instill certain habits in their children (or not) that become automatic, such as brushing teeth regularly and eating breakfast every day. Nonetheless, in many families, even these basic health habits

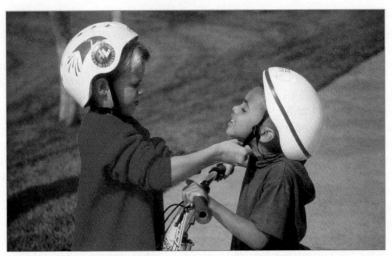

*The foundations for health promotion develop in early childhood, when children are taught to practice good health behaviors.*

Myrleen Ferguson Cate/PhotoEdit

are not taught. Especially in families in which parents are separated or there is chronic family stress, health habits may slip through the cracks (Menning, 2006).

Moreover, as children move into adolescence, they sometimes ignore the early training they received from their parents. In addition, adolescents are exposed to alcohol consumption, smoking, drug use, and sexual risk taking, particularly if their parents aren't monitoring them very closely and their peers practice these behaviors (Andrews, Tildesley, Hops, & Li, 2002).

Using the Teachable Moment    Some times are better than others for modifying health practices. Health promotion efforts capitalize on these **teachable moments.** Many teachable moments arise as early as pregnancy and in early childhood (Martinez et al., 2018). Parents can teach their children basic safety behaviors, such as looking both ways before crossing the street, and basic health habits, such as drinking milk instead of soda with dinner.

Other teachable moments are built into the health care system. For example, many infants in the United States are covered by well-baby care. Pediatricians can make use of these visits to teach motivated new parents the basics of accident prevention and home safety. Many school systems require a physical at the beginning of the school year and immunizations may be available then.

But what can children really learn about health habits? Surprisingly, quite a bit. Interventions with children indicate that choosing healthy foods, brushing teeth regularly, using car seats and seat belts, participating in exercise, crossing the street safely, and behaving appropriately in real or simulated emergencies (such as earthquake drills) are all within the ability of children as young as 3 or 4 years, as long as the behaviors are explained concretely and the children know what to do (Maddux, Roberts, Sledden, & Wright, 1986). Stories or narratives can help make health behavior change especially engaging (O'Malley et al., 2017; Shaffer et al., 2018).

Middle school is an important time for learning several health-related habits. For example, food choices, snacking, and dieting all crystallize around this time (Cohen et al., 1990). There is also a **window of vulnerability** for smoking and drug use during middle school, when students are first exposed to these habits among their peers (D'Amico & Fromme, 1997). Interventions through the schools may reduce these risks.

Teachable moments are not confined to childhood and adolescence. Pregnancy is a teachable moment for stopping smoking and improving diet (Heppner et al., 2011; Levitsky, 2004). The time period immediately after giving birth is also a teachable moment for increasing physical activity and regular exercise, as many new mothers want to get back to their previous level of fitness and appearance, but barriers to physical activity need to be addressed as well, because new mothers may have many new responsibilities, leaving little time for behavior seen as optional, such as exercise (Fjeldsoe, Miller, &

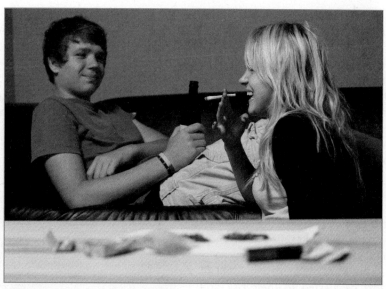

*Adolescence is a window of vulnerability for many poor health habits.*
*Consequently, intervening to prevent health habits from developing is a high priority*
*for children in late elementary and middle school.*
Monkey Business Images/Shutterstock

Marshall, 2013; Rhodes et al., 2014). Adults with newly diagnosed coronary artery disease, another teachable moment, are especially motivated to change contributing health habits such as smoking and poor diet.

### Adolescent Health Behaviors and Adult Health

An important reason for intervening with adolescents is that precautions taken in adolescence may affect disease risk after age 45 more than do adult health behaviors. The health habits a person practices as a teenager or college student may determine which chronic diseases he or she develops and what the person ultimately dies of in adulthood. For adults who make changes in their lifestyle, it may already be too late. This is true for sun exposure and skin cancer and for calcium consumption for the prevention of osteoporosis. Risk factors of other disorders such as coronary heart disease may also be strongly affected by health habits in childhood and adolescence as well.

### Intervening with At-Risk People

> I'm a walking time bomb.
> —37-year-old woman whose female relatives
> had breast cancer.

Another vulnerable group is people who are at risk for particular health problems. For example, people from families with a familial disorder may know that their personal risk is higher (Glenn et al., 2011). For example, a pediatrician may work with obese parents to control the diet of their offspring so that obesity in the children can be avoided.

### Benefits of Focusing on At-Risk People

Working with at-risk populations can be an efficient and effective use of health promotion dollars. First, disease may be prevented altogether. For example, helping men with a family history of heart disease to stop smoking can prevent coronary heart disease. When a risk factor has implications for only some people, it makes sense to target those people for whom the risk factor is relevant. For example, people who have hypertension that implicates salt sensitivity need to be especially vigilant about controlling their salt intake.

Focusing on at-risk people helps to identify other factors that may increase risk. For example, not everyone who has a family history of hypertension will develop hypertension, but by studying people who are at risk, other factors that contribute to its development, such as diet, may be identified.

### Problems of Focusing on At-Risk People

Clearly, however, there are difficulties in working with people at risk. People do not always perceive their risk correctly (Croyle et al., 2006). Most people are unrealistically optimistic and view their poor health behaviors as widely shared but their healthy behaviors as more distinctive. For example, smokers overestimate the number of other people who smoke.

Sometimes testing positive for a risk factor leads people into needless worry or hypervigilant behavior (DiLorenzo et al., 2006). People can become defensive, minimize the significance of their risk factor, and avoid using appropriate services or monitoring their condition.

Ethical Issues   At what point is it appropriate to alarm at-risk people if their personal risk is unknown? Not everyone at risk for a particular disorder will develop the problem and, in many cases, only many years later. For example, should adolescent daughters of breast cancer patients be alerted to their risk and alarmed at a time when they are coming to terms with their emerging sexuality and needs for self-esteem? Psychological distress may be created in exchange for instilling risk reduction behaviors (Croyle, Smith, Botkin, Baty, & Nash, 1997). Some people, such as those predisposed to depression, may react especially poorly to information about their risks. Moreover, in cases involving genetic risk factors, there may not be any effective intervention. For example, alcoholism has a genetic component, particularly among men, and yet exactly how to intervene with the offspring of adult alcoholics is not yet clear.

Emphasizing risks that are inherited can raise complicated issues of family dynamics. For example, daughters of breast cancer patients may suffer stress and exhibit behavior problems, due in part to the enhanced recognition of their risk (Taylor, Lichtman, & Wood, 1984a). Intervening with at-risk populations remains a controversial issue.

## Health Promotion and Older Adults

John Rosenthal, 92, starts each morning with a brisk walk. After a light breakfast of whole wheat toast and orange juice, he gardens for an hour or two. Later, he joins a couple of friends for lunch, and if he can persuade them to join him, they fish during the early afternoon. Reading a daily paper and always having a good book to read keeps John mentally sharp. Asked how he maintains such a busy schedule, John says, "Exercise, friends, and mental challenge" are the keys to his long and healthy life.

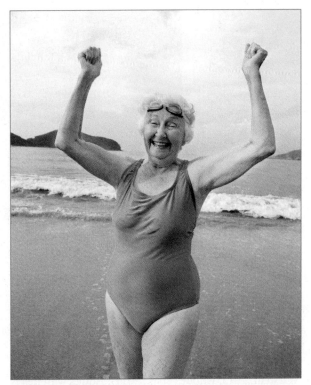

*Among older adults, health habits are a major determinant of whether an individual will have a vigorous or an infirmed old age.*
Marcy Maloy/Getty Images

Rosenthal's lifestyle is right on target. A chief focus of recent health promotion efforts has been older adults. At one time, it was thought that health promotion efforts are wasted in old age. However, policy makers now recognize that a healthy older adult population is essential not only for quality of life but also for controlling health care spending.

Health promotion efforts with older adults focus on several behaviors: maintaining a healthy, balanced diet; maintaining a regular exercise regimen; taking steps to reduce accidents; controlling alcohol consumption; eliminating smoking; reducing the inappropriate use of prescription drugs; obtaining a flu shot; reducing frailty and remaining socially engaged. Often, older adults have multiple issues or health habits that need modification, requiring an integrative biopsychosocial approach to their health care needs (Wild et al., 2014).

Exercise keeps older adults mobile and able to care for themselves, and it does not have to be strenuous (Ku, Fox, Gardiner, & Chen, 2016). Participating in social activities, running errands, and engaging in light housework or gardening reduce the risk of mortality, perhaps by reducing sedentary behavior and fatigue (Park, Thogersen-Houman, vanZarjten, & Ntoumanis, 2018) and by providing social support or a general sense of self-efficacy (Glass, deLeon, Marottoli, & Berkman, 1999). Reducing frailty by targeting activity levels, social functioning, and cognition holds promise (Gwyther et al., 2018). Among the very old, exercise has particularly strong benefits (Kahana et al., 2002), although not for those with chronic pain problems (Park et al., 2018). Group-based exercise programs may be especially successful (Beauchamp et al., 2018).

Controlling alcohol consumption is important for good health among older adults as well. Some older adults develop drinking problems in response to age-related issues, such as loneliness (Brennan & Moos, 1995). Others may try to maintain the drinking habits they had throughout their lives, which become more risky in old age. Metabolic changes related to age may reduce the capacity for alcohol. Moreover, many older people are on medications that may interact dangerously with alcohol, leading to accidents.

Proper medication use is essential to good health. Older adults who are poor may cut back on their medications to save money. Unfortunately, those who do are more likely to experience health problems within the next few years (Reitman, 2004, June 28).

Flu vaccination for older adults is an important health priority. Flu is a major cause of death among older adults, and it increases the risk of heart disease and stroke (Nichol et al., 2003).

Depression and loneliness are problems for older adults. They compromise health habits, leading to accelerated physical decline. Consequently, interventions to increase social engagement can promote this important health behavior (Thomas, 2011). Interventions aimed to increase the level of cognitive functioning and personal self-regulatory skills are also essential, as these skills can be compromised in some older adults (Olson et al., 2017).

The emphasis on health habits among older adults is well placed. By age 80, health habits are the major determinant of whether a person will have a vigorous or an infirmed old age (McClearn et al., 1997). Moreover, the efforts to change older adults' health habits seem to be working: The health of our older adult population is improving (Lubitz, Cai, Kramarow, & Lentzner, 2003), and consequently, so is their well-being (Gana et al., 2013).

## Ethnic and Gender Differences in Health Risks and Habits

Health promotion addresses ethnic and gender differences in vulnerability to health risks. For example, African American and Hispanic women get less exercise than do Anglo women and are more likely to be overweight (Pichon et al., 2007). Anglo and African American women are more likely to smoke than Hispanic women. Alcohol consumption is a greater problem among men than women, and smoking is a somewhat greater problem for Anglo men than for other groups.

Health promotion efforts with different ethnic groups need to take account of culturally different social norms. Culturally appropriate interventions include consideration of health practices in the community, informal networks of communication that can make interventions more successful, and language (Barrera, Toobert, Strycker, & Osuna, 2012; Toobert et al., 2011). Even efficient low-cost interventions such as text messaging and automated telephone messages can be successfully implemented when the messages are culturally adapted to the target group (Migneault et al., 2012).

Health promotion programs for ethnic groups also need to take account of co-occurring risk factors. The combined effects of low socioeconomic status and a biologic predisposition to particular illnesses, for example, put certain groups at great risk. Examples are diabetes among Hispanics and hypertension among African Americans, which we will consider in more detail in Chapter 13.

## ■ CHANGING HEALTH HABITS

> Habit is habit, and not to be flung out of the window by any man, but coaxed downstairs a step at a time.
> —Mark Twain

In the remainder of this chapter, we address how health behaviors can be changed. We especially focus on how theories inform behavior change efforts because theoretically guided interventions: (1) provide specific guidelines for constructing interventions (Masters, Ross, Hookey, & Wooldridge, 2018), (2) provide criteria for evaluating interventions (Michie et al., 2018), and (3) generate conclusions that can have broad applicability to other health behaviors and settings (Masters, 2018).

### Attitude Change and Health Behavior

Educational Appeals  Educational appeals make the assumption that people will change their

**TABLE 3.2 | Educational Appeals**

- Communications should be colorful and vivid rather than steeped in statistics and jargon. If possible, they should also use case histories (Conroy & Hagger, 2018).
- The communicator should be expert, prestigious, trustworthy, likable, and similar to the audience.
- Strong arguments should be presented at the beginning and end of a message, not buried in the middle.
- Messages should be short, clear, and direct.
- Messages should state conclusions explicitly.
- Extreme messages produce more attitude change, but only up to a point. Very extreme messages are discounted. For example, a message that urges people to exercise for half an hour a day will be more effective than one that recommends 3 hours a day.
- For illness detection behaviors (such as HIV testing or obtaining a mammogram), emphasizing problems if the behaviors are not undertaken will be most effective. For health promotion behaviors (such as exercise), emphasizing the benefits may be more effective.
- If the audience is receptive to changing a health habit, then the communication should include only favorable points, but if the audience is not inclined to accept the message, the communication should discuss both sides of the issue.
- Interventions should be sensitive to the cultural norms of the community to which they are directed. For example, family-directed interventions may be especially effective in Latino communities.

health habits if they have good information about their habits. Early and continuing efforts to change health habits have consequently focused heavily on education and changing attitudes. Table 3.2 lists the characteristics that make health communications especially persuasive. More recently, though, the fact that attitude change may not lead to behavior change has prompted research on what additional factors may be involved (Siegel, Navarro, Tan, & Hyde, 2014). Also, the important automatic aspect of health habits has been incorporated into interventions, as unconscious and nonconscious influences on the practice of health habits have become increasingly apparent.

**Affective Aspects of Health Behavior Change**    Attitudinal approaches to changing health habits often make use of **fear appeals.** This approach assumes that if people are afraid that a particular habit is hurting their health, they will change their behavior to reduce their fear. However, this relationship does not always hold (Borland, 2018; Kok, Peters, Kessels, ten Hoor, & Ruiter, 2018).

Persuasive messages that elicit too much fear may actually undermine health behavior change (Becker & Janz, 1987). Moreover, fear alone may not be sufficient to change behavior. Specific action recommendations, such as where and how one can obtain a flu shot, may be needed (Self & Rogers, 1990). Moreover, as already noted, fear can increase defensiveness, which reduces how effective an appeal will be.

People often use affective forecasts, namely their predictions about how a decision will make them feel in the future as a basis for making health decisions (Ellis, Elwyn, Nelson, Scalia, & Kobrin, 2018). For example, the thought "I am going to regret this" might make a person think twice about drinking and driving or staying on the beach all day without sunscreen.

**Message Framing**    A health message can be phrased in positive or negative terms (Gerard & Shepherd, 2016). For example, a reminder card to get a flu immunization can stress the benefits of being immunized or stress the discomfort of the flu itself (Gallagher, Updegraff, Rothman, & Sims, 2011). Which of these methods is more successful? Messages that emphasize problems seem to work better for behaviors that have uncertain outcomes, for health behaviors that need to be practiced only once, such as vaccinations (Gerend, Shepherd, & Monday, 2008), and for issues about which people are fearful (Gerend & Maner, 2011). Messages that stress benefits are more persuasive for behaviors with certain outcomes (Apanovitch, McCarthy, & Salovey, 2003). A meta-analysis of 94 studies indicated that messages stressing benefits are more effective than messages stressing risks for encouraging health behaviors, such as skin cancer prevention, smoking cessation, and physical activity (Gallagher & Updegraff, 2012; Geers et al., 2017).

Which kind of message framing will most affect behavior also depends on people's personal characteristics (Covey, 2014). For example, people who have a promotion or approach orientation that emphasizes maximizing opportunities are more influenced by messages phrased in terms of benefits ("calcium will keep your bones healthy"), whereas people who have a prevention or avoidance orientation that emphasizes minimizing risks are more influenced by messages that stress the risks of not performing a health behavior ("low calcium intake will increase bone loss") (Updegraff, Emanuel, Mintzer, & Sherman, 2015). On the whole, promotion-oriented messages may be somewhat more successful in getting people to initiate

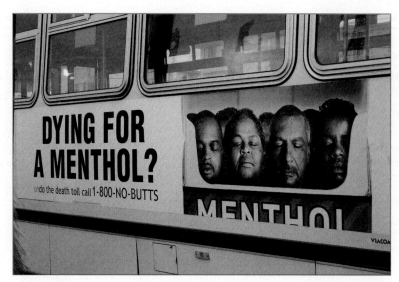

*Fear appeals often alert people to a health problem but do not necessarily change behavior.*

Christopher Kerrigan/McGraw-Hill Education

behavior change, and prevention messages may be more helpful in getting them to maintain behavior change over time (Fuglestad, Rothman, & Jeffery, 2008).

## The Health Belief Model

Attitudinal approaches to health behavior change have been formalized in several specific theories that have guided interventions to change health behaviors. An early influential attitude theory of why people practice health behaviors is the **health belief model** (Hochbaum, 1958; Rosenstock, 1966). According to this model, whether a person practices a health behavior depends on two factors: whether the person perceives a personal health threat, and whether the person believes that a particular health practice will be effective in reducing that threat.

**Perceived Health Threat**   The perception of a personal health threat is influenced by at least three factors: general health values, which include interest in and concern about health; specific beliefs about personal vulnerability to a particular disorder (Dillard, Ferrer, Ubel, & Fagerlin, 2012); and beliefs about the consequences of the disorder, such as whether they are serious. Thus, for example, people may change their diet to include low-cholesterol foods if they value health, feel threatened by the possibility of heart disease, and perceive that the personal threat of heart disease is severe (Brewer et al., 2007).

**Perceived Threat Reduction**   Whether a person believes a health measure will reduce threat has two subcomponents: whether the person thinks the health practice will be effective, and whether the cost of undertaking that measure exceeds its benefits (Rosenstock, 1974). For example, the man who is considering changing his diet to avoid a heart attack may believe that dietary change alone would not reduce his risk of a heart attack and that changing his diet would interfere with his enjoyment of life too much to justify taking the action. So, even if his perceived vulnerability to heart disease is great, he would probably not make any changes. A diagram of the health belief model applied to smoking is presented in Figure 3.1.

**Support for the Health Belief Model**   Many studies have used the health belief model to increase perceived risk and increase perceived effectiveness of steps to modify a broad array of health habits, ranging from health screening programs to smoking (e.g., Goldberg, Halpern-Felsher, & Millstein, 2002). The health belief model does, however, leave out an important component of health behavior change, and that is a sense of **self-efficacy:** the belief that one can control one's practice of a particular behavior (Bandura, 1991). For example, smokers who believe they cannot stop smoking are unlikely to make the effort.

Other theories of health behavior change use a similar conceptual analysis of behavior change. For

**FIGURE 3.1 | The Health Belief Model Applied to the Health Behavior of Stopping Smoking**

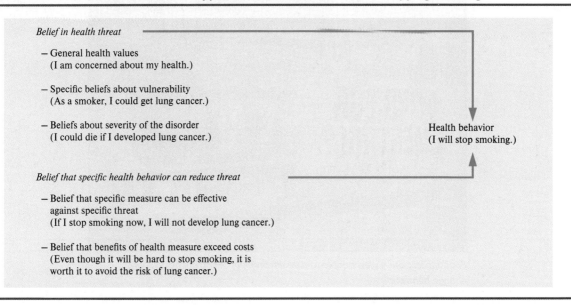

*Belief in health threat*

— General health values
  (I am concerned about my health.)

— Specific beliefs about vulnerability
  (As a smoker, I could get lung cancer.)

— Beliefs about severity of the disorder
  (I could die if I developed lung cancer.)

*Belief that specific health behavior can reduce threat*

— Belief that specific measure can be effective
  against specific threat
  (If I stop smoking now, I will not develop lung cancer.)

— Belief that benefits of health measure exceed costs
  (Even though it will be hard to stop smoking, it is
  worth it to avoid the risk of lung cancer.)

Health behavior
(I will stop smoking.)

example, Protection Motivation Theory (Rogers, 1975) examines how people appraise health threats and how they appraise their abilities to manage threats. This theory, too, has guided many health interventions (Milne, Sheeran, & Orbell, 2000).

## The Theory of Planned Behavior

Health beliefs go some distance in predicting when people will change their health habits. A theory that attempts to link health beliefs directly to behavior is Ajzen's **theory of planned behavior** (Ajzen & Madden, 1986; Fishbein & Ajzen, 1975).

According to this theory, a health behavior is the direct result of a behavioral intention. Behavioral intentions are themselves made up of three components: attitudes toward the specific action, subjective norms regarding the action, and perceived behavioral control (Figure 3.2). Attitudes toward the action center on the likely outcomes of the action and evaluations of those outcomes. Subjective norms are what a person believes *others* think that person should do (normative beliefs) and the motivation to comply with those normative beliefs. Perceived behavioral control is the perception that one can perform the action and that the action will have the intended effect; this component of the model is similar to self-efficacy. These factors combine to produce a behavioral intention and, ultimately, behavior change.

To take a simple example, smokers who believe that smoking causes serious health outcomes, who believe that other people think they should stop smoking, who are motivated to comply with those normative beliefs, who believe that they are capable of stopping smoking, and who form a specific intention to do so will be more likely to stop smoking than people who do not hold these beliefs.

### Evidence for the Theory of Planned Behavior

The theory of planned behavior predicts a broad array of health behaviors and change in health behaviors including risky sexual activity among heterosexuals (Davis et al., 2016; Tyson, Covey, & Rosenthal, 2014), consumption of soft drinks (Kassem & Lee, 2004), and food safety practices (Milton & Mullan, 2012). Moreover, communications targeted to particular parts of the model, such as social norms, have been found to change behaviors (McEachan, Taylor, Harrison, Lawton, & Gardner, 2016). The consideration of future consequences of a health behavior more generally increases its practice (Murphy & Dockray, 2018).

### Criticisms of Attitude Theories

Because health habits are often deeply ingrained and difficult to modify, attitude-change interventions may provide the informational base for altering health habits but not always the impetus to take action. Moreover,

**FIGURE 3.2 | The Theory of Planned Behavior Applied to Adopting a Healthy Diet**   (*Sources:* Ajzen, Icek, Robert Louis Heilbroner, Martin Fishbein, and Lester C. Thurow. *Understanding Attitudes and Predicting Social Behavior.* Englewood Cliffs, NJ: Prentice-Hall, 1980; Ajzen, Icek, and Thomas J. Madden. "Prediction of Goal-Directed Behavior: Attitudes, Intentions, and Perceived Behavioral Control." *Journal of Experimental Social Psychology* 22, no. 5 (September 1986): 453–74. https://doi.org/10.1016/0022-1031(86)90045-4)

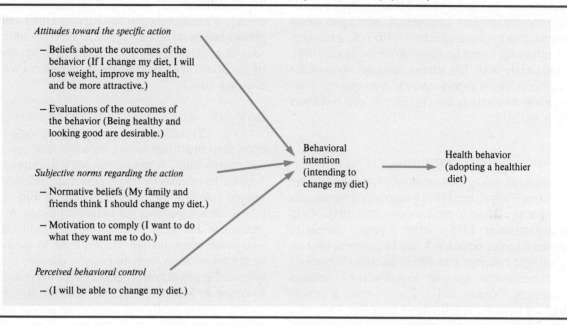

attitude change techniques assume that behavior changes are guided by conscious motivation, and these approaches ignore the fact that some behavior change occurs automatically and is not subject to awareness. That is, a general limitation of health behavior change models is the fact that they heavily emphasize conscious deliberative processes in practicing health behaviors; there is an important role for implicit automatic processes as well. Perhaps the most obvious example concerns health habits that are accomplished automatically in response to a minimal cue, such as putting on a seatbelt when one gets into a car.

## Self-Regulation and Health Behavior

Thus far, we have discussed changing health behaviors primarily through interventions designed to get people to alter their behavior. But people also change on their own. **Self-regulation** refers to the fact that people control their own actions, emotions, and thoughts (Fiske & Taylor, 2013). A lot of self-regulation is automatic, occurring without awareness or thought. But much self-regulation is conscious, designed to meet personal goals and control thoughts, emotions, and behavior in service of those goals. Belief in one's self-regulatory

abilities is essential to their enlistment as well (Jung, Latimer-Cheung, Bourne, & Gunis, 2017). Enhancing health behaviors requires effective self-regulation (Mann, de Ridder, & Fujita, 2013) and the ability to overcome barriers to self-regulation (Millar, 2017), and interventions may need to be aimed at both automatic and conscious, controlled self-regulation processes (Conroy, Maher, Elavsky, Hyde, & Doerksen, 2013).

## Self-Determination Theory

**Self-determination theory (SDT),** a theory that also guides health behavior modification, builds on the idea that people are actively motivated to pursue their goals (Deci & Ryan, 1985; Ryan & Deci, 2000). The theory targets two important components as fundamental to behavior change, namely autonomous motivation and perceived competence. People are autonomously motivated when they experience free will and choice when making decisions. Competence refers to the belief that one is capable of making the health behavior change.

Accordingly, if a woman changes her diet because her physician tells her to, she may not experience a sense of autonomy and instead may experience her actions as under another's control. This may undermine her commitment to behavior change. However, if her dietary change is autonomously chosen, she will be intrinsically motivated to persist. SDT has given rise to interventions that target these beliefs, namely autonomous motivation and competence, and have shown some success in changing behaviors including smoking and adherence to medications (Bruzzese et al., 2014). A meta-analysis of 184 studies indicates support for self-determination theory and the importance of autonomous motivation for changing health behaviors (Ng et al., 2012).

## Implementation Intentions

A theoretical model that emphasizes implementation intentions (Gollwitzer, 1999) integrates conscious processing with automatic behavioral enactment (Gollwitzer & Oettingen, 1998). When a person desires to practice a health behavior, it can be achieved by making a simple coherent plan that links critical situations or environmental cues to goal-directed responses (Sheeren & Conner, 2017). For example, a person might tell herself, "When I finish breakfast, I will take out the dog's leash and walk her." The theory underscores the importance of planning exactly how, when, and where to implement a health behavior. Without these explicit links to action, the good intention might remain at the intention stage.

A second important feature of the theory is the idea that, by forming an implementation intention, a person can delegate the control of goal-directed responses to situational cues (e.g., completing breakfast), which may then elicit the behavior automatically (in this case, taking out the leash to walk the dog). Over time, the link from the implementation to the goal-directed response becomes automatic and need not be brought into conscious awareness to be enacted.

Forming implementation intentions can be a simple but effective way to promote health behaviors (Martin, Sheeran, Slade, Wright, & Dibble, 2009). When a person has a particular health goal, such as remembering to use sunscreen, he or she can strategically engage automatic processes in an effort to make good on that goal. So, for example, a person might say, "Whenever I am going to the beach, I will put on sunscreen first." Having created this implementation intention, she then delegates the control of sunscreen use to anticipated situational cues, in this case, getting ready to go to the beach (Gollwitzer, 1999). Thus, although the original implementation intention is con-

sciously framed, the relation of the health behavior itself to the situation in which it is relevant becomes an automatic process (Sheeran, Gollwitzer, & Bargh, 2013). Adding implementation intentions to attitude models of health behavior has improved their ability to predict behavior (Milne, Orbell, & Sheeran, 2002). Results of a meta-analysis support the idea that changes in intentions lead to changes in behavior (Webb & Sheeran, 2006).

**Self-Affirmation and Self-Transcendent Values**    Self-affirmation occurs when people reflect upon their important values, personal qualities, or social relationships. When people are self-affirmed, they become less defensive about personally relevant risk-related information (Schüz, Schüz, & Eid, 2013), which can set the stage for behavior change. A meta-analysis of 144 studies has shown that inducing self-awareness when people are exposed to persuasive health information leads to positive changes in intentions and in actual health behaviors (Epton et al., 2015; Sweeney & Moyer, 2015). Self-transcendent values such as valuing family and friends can also be invoked to alter health behaviors. In one study, brain reactivity to health threats was reduced among people with strong self-transcendent values (Kanget et al., 2017).

## Health Behavior Change and the Brain

Some successful health behavior change in response to persuasive messages occurs outside of awareness. Despite being inaccessible to conscious awareness, this change may be reflected in patterns of brain activation. Emily Falk and colleagues gave people persuasive messages promoting sunscreen use (Falk, Berkman, Mann, Harrison, & Lieberman, 2010). People who showed significant activation in two particular brain regions, the medial prefrontal cortex (mPFC) and posterior cingulate cortex (pCC), in response to the messages increased their sunscreen use. Most important, attitude change about sunscreen use in response to the persuasive message only weakly predicted people's intentions to use sunscreen, but activity in these two brain regions quite strongly predicted sunscreen use, independent of attitudes and behavioral intentions. In other words, processes apparently not accessible to consciousness nonetheless significantly predicted changes in sunscreen use (Falk, Berkman, Whalen, & Lieberman, 2011).

What this pattern of brain activity means is not yet fully known. One possibility is that activity in mPFC and pCC reflects behavioral intentions at an implicit level that is not consciously accessible (Falk et al., 2010). Alternatively, activity in mPFC may be related to behavior change primarily because participants link the persuasive communication to the self. In any case, health behavior change can occur unconsciously, but the brain may detect these processes nonetheless.

## ◼ COGNITIVE–BEHAVIORAL APPROACHES TO HEALTH BEHAVIOR CHANGE

### Cognitive–Behavioral Therapy (CBT)

Cognitive-behavioral approaches to health habit modification focus on the target behavior itself, the conditions that elicit and maintain it, and the factors that reinforce it (Dobson, 2010). The most effective approach to health habit modification often comes from **cognitive–behavioral therapy (CBT)**. CBT interventions use several complementary methods to intervene in the modification of a target problem and its context. CBT may be implemented individually, through therapy in a group setting, or even on the Internet, and so it is a versatile as well as effective way of intervening to modify poor health habits.

### Self-Monitoring

Many programs of cognitive–behavioral modification use **self-monitoring** as the first step toward behavior change. The rationale is that a person must understand the dimensions of the poor health habit before change can begin. Self-monitoring assesses the frequency of a target behavior and the antecedents and consequences of that behavior.

The first step in self-monitoring is to learn to discriminate the target behavior. For some behaviors, this step is easy. A smoker obviously can tell whether he or she is smoking. However, an urge to smoke may be harder to discriminate; therefore, the person may be trained to monitor internal sensations closely so as to identify the target behavior more readily.

A second stage in self-monitoring is charting the behavior. For example, a smoker may keep a detailed record of smoking-related events, including when a cigarette is smoked, the time of day, the situation in which the smoking occurred, and the presence of other people (if any). She may also record the subjective feelings of craving that existed prior to lighting the cigarette, the emotional responses that preceded the

lighting of the cigarette (such as anxiety or tension), and the feelings that were generated by the actual smoking of the cigarette. In this way, she can begin to get a sense of the conditions under which she is most likely to smoke. Each of these conditions can be a **discriminative stimulus** that is capable of eliciting the target behavior. For example, the sight and smell of food act as discriminative stimuli for eating. The sight of a pack of cigarettes or the smell of coffee may act as discriminative stimuli for smoking. The discriminative stimulus is important because it signals that a positive reinforcement will subsequently occur. CBT aims to eliminate or modify these discriminative stimuli. Although self-monitoring is usually only a beginning step in behavior change, it may itself produce some behavior change (Quinn, Pascoe, Wood, & Neal, 2010). In fact, even being asked questions about a health behavior can launch behavior change (Rodrigues, O'Brien, French, Glidewell, & Sniehotta, 2015).

### Stimulus Control

Once the circumstances surrounding the target behavior are well understood, the factors in the environment that maintain a poor health habit can be modified. **Stimulus-control interventions** involve ridding the environment of discriminative stimuli that evoke the problem behavior, and creating new discriminative stimuli, signaling that a new response will be reinforced.

For example, eating is typically under the control of discriminative stimuli, including the presence of desirable foods and activities (such as watching television). People desiring to lose weight can be encouraged to eliminate these discriminative stimuli for eating, such as ridding their home of rewarding and fattening foods, restricting their eating to a single place in the home, and avoiding eating while engaged in other activities, such as watching television. Other stimuli might be introduced in the environment to indicate that controlled eating will now be followed by reinforcement. For example, people might place signs in strategic locations around the home, reminding them of reinforcements to be obtained after successful behavior change.

### The Self-Control of Behavior

CBT focuses heavily on the beliefs that people hold about their health habits. People often generate internal monologues that interfere with their ability to change their behavior. For example, a person who

BOX **3.1**   Classical Conditioning

First described by Russian physiologist Ivan Pavlov in the early 20th century, **classical conditioning** is the pairing of an unconditioned reflex with a new stimulus, producing a conditioned reflex. Classical conditioning is represented in Figure 3.3.

Classical conditioning was one of the first methods used for health behavior change. For example, consider its use in the treatment of alcoholism. Antabuse (unconditioned stimulus) is a drug that produces extreme nausea, gagging, and vomiting (unconditioned response) when taken in conjunction with alcohol. Over

time, the alcohol becomes associated with the nausea and vomiting caused by the Antabuse and elicits the same nausea, gagging, and vomiting response (conditioned response) without the Antabuse being present.

Classical conditioning approaches to health habit modification do work, but clients know why they work. Alcoholics, for example, know that if they do not take the drug they will not vomit when they consume alcohol. Thus, even if classical conditioning has successfully produced a conditioned response, it is heavily dependent on the client's willing participation.

**FIGURE 3.3 | A Classical Conditioning Approach to the Treatment of Alcoholism**

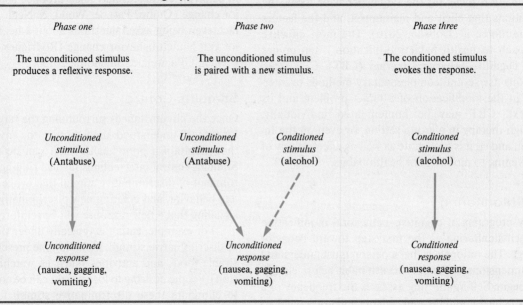

wishes to give up smoking may derail the quitting process by generating self-doubts ("I will never be able to give up smoking"). Unless these internal monologues are modified, the person will be unlikely to change the health habit and maintain that change over time.

Recognition that people's cognitions about their health habits are important in producing behavior change highlights another insight about the behavior change process: the importance of involving the client as co-therapist in the behavior-change intervention. Clients need to actively monitor their own behaviors and apply the techniques of CBT to bring about change. As such, CBT emphasizes **self-control.** The person acts as his or her own therapist and, together

with outside guidance, learns to control the antecedents and consequences of the target behavior.

**Cognitive restructuring** trains people to recognize and modify their internal monologues to promote health behavior change. Sometimes the modified cognitions are antecedents to a target behavior. For example, if a smoker's urge to smoke is preceded by an internal monologue that he is weak and unable to control his smoking urges, these beliefs are targeted for change. The smoker would substitute a monologue that would help him stop smoking (e.g., "I can do this" or "I'll be so much healthier"). Cognitions can also be the consequences of a target behavior. For example, an obese woman trying to lose weight might undermine

In contrast to classical conditioning, which pairs an automatic response with a new stimulus, operant conditioning pairs a voluntary behavior with systematic consequences. The key to **operant conditioning** is reinforcement. When a person performs a behavior and that behavior is followed by positive reinforcement, the behavior is more likely to occur again. Similarly, if an individual performs a behavior and reinforcement is withdrawn or the behavior is punished, the behavior is less likely to be repeated. Over time, these contingencies build up those behaviors paired with positive reinforcement, whereas behaviors that are punished or not rewarded decline.

Many health habits can be thought of as operant responses. For example, drinking may be maintained because mood is improved by alcohol, or smoking may occur because peer companionship is associated with it. In these cases, reinforcement maintains the poor health behavior. Thus, using this principle to change behavior requires altering the reinforcement.

An important feature of operant conditioning is the reinforcement schedule. A continuous reinforcement schedule means that a behavior is reinforced every time it occurs. However, continuous reinforcement is vulnerable to extinction: If the behavior is occasionally not paired with reinforcement, the individual may cease performing the behavior, having come to anticipate reinforcement each time. Psychologists have learned that behavior is often more resistant to extinction if it is maintained by a variable or an intermittent reinforcement schedule than a continuous reinforcement schedule.

her weight-loss program by reacting with hopelessness to every small dieting setback. She might learn, instead, to engage in self-reinforcing cognitions following successful resistance to temptation and constructive self-criticism following setbacks ("Next time, I'll keep those tempting foods out of my refrigerator").

Self-Reinforcement    **Self-reinforcement** involves systematically rewarding oneself to increase or decrease the occurrence of a target behavior. Positive self-reward involves rewarding oneself with something desirable after successful modification of a target behavior, such as going to a movie following successful weight loss. Negative self-reward involves removing an aversive factor in the environment after successful modification of the target behavior. An example of negative self-reward is taking the Miss Piggy poster off the refrigerator once regular controlled eating has been achieved.

For example, suppose Mary smokes 20 cigarettes a day. She might first define a set of reinforcers that can be administered when particular smoking-reduction targets are met—reinforcements such as going out to dinner or seeing a movie. Mary may then set a particular reduction in her smoking as a target (such as 15 cigarettes a day). When that target is reached, she would administer a reinforcement (the movie or dinner out). The next step might be reducing smoking to 10 cigarettes a day, at which time she would receive another reinforcement. The target then might be cut progressively to 5, 4, 3, 2, 1, and none. Through this process, the target behavior of abstinence would eventually be reached.

Like self-reward, self-punishment is of two types. Positive self-punishment involves the administration of an unpleasant stimulus to punish an undesirable behavior. For example, a person might self-administer a mild electric shock each time he or she experiences a desire to smoke. Negative self-punishment consists of withdrawing a positive reinforcer in the environment each time an undesirable behavior is performed. For example, a smoker might rip up money each time he or she has a cigarette that exceeds a predetermined quota. Self-punishment is effective only if people actually perform the punishing activities. If self-punishment becomes too aversive, people often abandon their efforts.

One form of operant conditioning that is effective is **contingency contracting.** In contingency contracting, an individual forms a contract with another person, such as a therapist or friend, detailing what rewards or punishments are contingent on the performance or nonperformance of a behavior. For example, a person who wants to stop drinking might deposit a sum of money with a therapist and arrange to be fined each time he or she has a drink and to be rewarded each day that he or she abstained.

Behavioral Assignments    A technique for increasing client involvement is **behavioral assignments,** home practice activities that support the goals of a

BOX **3.3** | Modeling

**Modeling** is learning that occurs from witnessing another person perform a behavior (Bandura, 1969). Observation and subsequent modeling can be effective approaches to changing health habits. For example, in one study high school students who observed others donating blood were more likely to do so themselves (Sarason, Sarason, Pierce, Shearin, & Sayers, 1991).

Similarity is an important principle in modeling. To the extent that people perceive themselves as similar to the type of person who engages in a risky behavior, they are likely to do so themselves; if people see themselves as similar to the type of person who does not engage in a risky behavior, they may change their behavior (Gibbons & Gerrard, 1995). For example, a swimmer may decline a cigarette from a friend because she perceives that most great swimmers do not smoke.

---

therapeutic intervention. Behavioral assignments are designed to provide continuity in the treatment of a behavior problem. For example, if an early session with an obese client involved training in self-monitoring, the client would be encouraged to keep a log of his eating behavior, including the circumstances in which it occurred. This log could then be used by the therapist and the patient at the next session to plan future behavioral interventions. Figure 3.4 gives an example of the behavioral assignment technique. Note that it includes homework assignments for both client and therapist. This technique can ensure that both parties remain committed to the behavior-change process and that each is aware of the other's commitment.

The chief advantages of behavioral assignments are that (1) the client becomes involved in the treatment process, (2) the client produces an analysis of the behavior that is useful in planning further interventions, (3) the client becomes committed to the treatment process through a contractual agreement to discharge certain responsibilities, (4) responsibility for behavior change is gradually shifted to the client, and (5) the use of homework assignments increases the client's sense of self-control.

**FIGURE 3.4 | Example of a Systematic Behavioral Assignment for an Obese Client**

(*Source:* Shelton, John L., and Rona L. Levy. *Behavioral Assignments and Treatment Compliance: A Handbook of Clinical Strategies.* Champaign, IL: Research Press, 1981., p. 6.)

Homework for Tom [client]

Using the counter, count bites taken.

Record number of bites, time, location, and what you ate.

Record everything eaten for 1 week.

Call for an appointment.

Bring your record.

Homework for John [therapist]

Reread articles on obesity.

## Social Skills and Relaxation Training

Some poor health habits develop in response to the anxiety people experience in social situations. For example, adolescents often begin to smoke to reduce their nervousness in social situations by trying to communicate a cool, sophisticated image. Drinking and overeating may also be responses to social anxiety. Social anxiety can then act as a cue for the maladaptive habit, necessitating an alternative way of coping with the anxiety.

Consequently, many health habit modification programs include either **social skills training** or **assertiveness training,** or both, as part of the intervention package. People are trained in methods that help them deal more effectively with social anxiety.

**Relaxation Training**   Many poor health habits are caused or maintained by stressful circumstances, and so managing stress is important to successful behavior change. A mainstay of stress reduction is **relaxation training** involving deep breathing and progressive muscle relaxation. In deep breathing, a person takes deep, controlled breaths, which decreases heart rate and blood pressure and increases oxygenation of the blood. People typically engage in deep breathing spontaneously when they are relaxed. In progressive muscle relaxation, an individual learns to relax all the muscles in the body progressively to discharge tension or stress.

## Motivational Interviewing

Motivational interviewing (MI) is increasingly used in health promotion interventions. Originally developed to treat addiction, the techniques have been adapted to target smoking, dietary improvements, exercise, cancer screening, and sexual behavior, among other habits (Miller & Rose, 2009). Motivational interviewing is a client-centered counseling style designed to get people to work through any ambivalence they experience about changing their health behaviors. It may be especially effective for people who are initially wary about whether to change their behavior (Resnicow et al., 2002).

In MI, the interviewer adopts a nonjudgmental, nonconfrontational, encouraging, and supportive style. The goal is to help the client express the positive or negative thoughts he or she has regarding the behavior in an atmosphere that is free of negative evaluation (Baldwin, Rothman, Vander Weg, & Christensen, 2013). Typically, clients talk at least as much as counselors during MI sessions.

In MI, there is no effort to dismantle the denial or irrational beliefs that often accompany bad health behaviors or even to persuade a client to stop drinking, quit smoking, or otherwise improve health. Rather, the goal is to get the client to think through and express some of his or her own reasons for and against behavior change. The interviewer listens and provides encouragement in lieu of giving advice (Miller & Rose, 2009). Both the content of the motivational interviewing and the interviewer's style influence its effectiveness (Hardcastle, Forier, Blake, & Hagger, 2017).

## Relapse Prevention

One of the biggest problems faced in health habit modification is the tendency for people to relapse. Following initial successful behavior change, people often return to their old bad habits. Relapse is a particular problem with the addictive disorders of alcoholism, smoking, drug addiction, and overeating (Brownell, Marlatt, Lichtenstein, & Wilson, 1986), but it can be a problem for all behavior change efforts.

What do we mean by "relapse"? A single cigarette smoked at a party or a pint of ice cream consumed on a lonely Saturday night need not lead to full-blown relapse. However, that one cigarette or that single pint of ice cream can produce what is called an **abstinence violation effect**—that is, a feeling of loss of control that results when a person has violated self-imposed rules. The result can be a more serious relapse, as the person's resolve falters. This is especially true for addictive behaviors because the person must also cope with the reinforcing impact of the substance itself.

**Reasons for Relapse**    Why do people relapse? Initially when people change their behaviors, they are vigilant, but over time, vigilance fades and the likelihood of relapse increases. For example, people may find themselves in situations where they used to smoke or drink, such as a party, and relapse at that vulnerable moment. People with low self-efficacy for the behavior change initially are more likely to relapse. Sometimes, people think they have beaten the health problem, and so giving in to a temptation would have few costs (e.g., "a couple drinks would relax me").

A potent catalyst for relapse is negative affect (Witkiewitz & Marlatt, 2004). Relapse is more likely when people are depressed, anxious, or under stress. For example, when people are breaking off a relationship or encountering difficulty at work, they are vulnerable to relapse. Peter Jennings, the national newscaster who died of lung cancer in 2005, had relapsed to smoking after the September 11, 2001, terrorist attacks. Figure 3.5 illustrates the relapse process.

**Relapse prevention** should be integrated into treatment programs from the outset. Enrolling people who are initially committed and motivated to change their behavior reduces the risk of relapse and weeds out people who are not truly committed to behavior change. Although prescreening people for an intervention may seem ethically problematic, including people who are likely to relapse may demoralize other participants in a behavior-change program, demoralize the practitioner, and ultimately make it more difficult for the relapser to change his or her behavior.

Relapse prevention techniques begin by asking people to identify the situations that may lead to relapse so they can develop coping skills that will help them to manage that event. For example, overcoming the temptation to drink at bars might be fostered by scheduling lunches with friends instead. Or, at parties, a person might have a sham drink of club soda, instead of an alcoholic beverage. Mentally rehearsing coping responses in a high-risk situation can promote feelings of self-efficacy. For example, some programs train

**FIGURE 3.5 | A Cognitive–Behavioral Model of the Relapse Process**   This figure shows what happens when a person is trying to change a poor health habit and faces a high-risk situation. With adequate coping responses, the person may be able to resist temptation, leading to a low likelihood of relapse. Without adequate coping responses, however, perceptions of self-efficacy may decline and perceptions of the rewarding effects of the poor health behavior may increase, leading to an increased likelihood of relapse.   (*Source:* Larimer, Mary E., Rebekka S. Palmer, and  G. Alan Marlatt. "Relapse Prevention: An Overview of Marlatt's Cognitive–Behavioral Model." *Alcohol Research and Health* 23, no. 2 (1999): 151–60.)

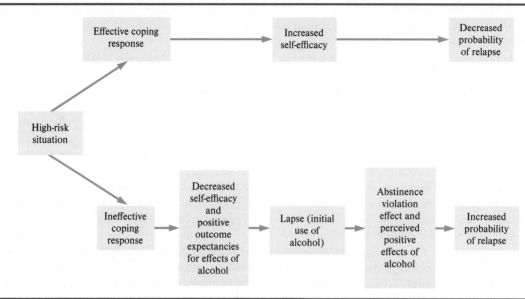

participants to engage in constructive **self-talk** that will help them talk themselves through tempting situations (Brownell et al., 1986).

Cue elimination involves restructuring the environment to avoid situations that evoke the target behavior (Bouton, 2000). For example, the alcoholic who drank exclusively in bars can avoid bars. For other habits, however, cue elimination is impossible. For example, smokers are usually unable to completely eliminate the circumstances in their lives that led them to smoke. Consequently, some relapse prevention programs deliberately expose people to situations that evoke the old behavior to give them practice in using their coping skills (Marlatt, 1990). Making sure that the new habit (such as exercise or alcohol abstinence) is practiced in as many new contexts as possible can ensure that it endures (Bouton, 2000).

Overall, relapse prevention is most successful when people perceive their behavior change to be a long-term goal, develop coping techniques for managing high-risk situations, and integrate their behavior change into a generally healthy lifestyle. In a meta-analysis of 26 studies with more than 9,000 participants treated for alcohol, tobacco, cocaine, and other substance use,

Irvin and colleagues concluded that relapse prevention techniques were effective for reducing substance use and improving psychosocial functioning (Irvin, Bowers, Dunn, & Wang, 1999).

Lifestyle Rebalancing   Long-term maintenance of behavior change can be promoted by leading the person to make other health-oriented lifestyle changes, a technique termed **lifestyle rebalancing**. Lifestyle changes, such as adding an exercise program or using stress management techniques, may promote a healthy lifestyle more generally and help reduce the likelihood of relapse. The role of social support in maintaining behavior change is equivocal. At present, some studies suggest that enlisting the aid of family members in maintaining behavior change is helpful, but other studies suggest not (Brownell et al., 1986). Possibly, research has not yet identified the exact ways in which social support may help maintain behavior change.

### Evaluation of CBT

The advantages of CBT for health behavior change are several. First, a carefully selected set of techniques can deal with all aspects of a problem (van Kessel et al., 2008): Self-observation and self-monitoring define the dimensions of a problem; stimulus control enables a person to modify antecedents of behavior; self-reinforcement controls the consequences of a behavior; and social skills and relaxation training may replace the maladaptive behavior, once it has been brought under some degree of control.

A second advantage is that the therapeutic plan can be tailored to each individual's problem. Each person's faulty health habit and personality are different, so, for example, the particular package identified for one obese client may not be the same as that developed for another obese client (Schwartz & Brownell, 1995). Third, the range of skills imparted by multimodal interventions may enable people to modify several health habits simultaneously, such as diet and exercise, rather than one at a time (Persky, Spring, Vander Wal, Pagoto, & Hedeker, 2005; Prochaska & Sallis, 2004). Overall, CBT interventions have shown considerable success in modifying a broad array of health behaviors.

## ■ THE TRANSTHEORETICAL MODEL OF BEHAVIOR CHANGE

Changing a bad health habit does not take place all at once. People go through stages while they are trying to change their health behaviors (Prochaska, 1994; Rothman, 2000).

### Stages of Change

J. O. Prochaska and colleagues developed the **transtheoretical model of behavior change,** a model that analyzes the stages and processes people go through in bringing about a change in behavior and suggested treatment goals and interventions for each stage (Prochaska, 1994; Prochaska, DiClemente, & Norcross, 1992). Originally developed to treat addictive disorders, such as smoking, drug use, and alcohol addiction, the stage model has now been applied to a broad range of health habits, including exercising and sun protection behaviors (Adams, Norman, Hovell, Sallis, & Patrick, 2009; Hellsten et al., 2008). The transtheoretical model has also been used to modify multiple health behaviors simultaneously (Johnson et al., 2014).

**Precontemplation**   The precontemplation stage occurs when a person has no intention of changing his or her behavior. Many people in this stage are not aware that they have a problem, although families, friends, neighbors, or coworkers may well be. An example is the problem drinker who is largely oblivious to the problems he creates for his family. Sometimes people in the precontemplative phase seek treatment if they have been pressured by others to do so. Not surprisingly, these people often revert to their old behaviors and so make poor targets for intervention.

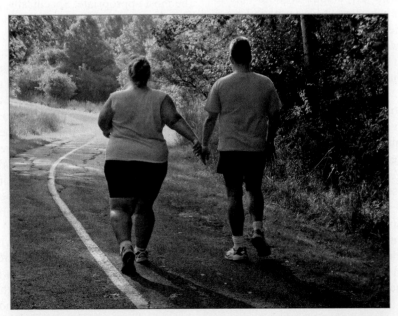

*Readiness to change a health habit is a prerequisite to health habit change.*
Frances L Fruit/Shutterstock

**FIGURE 3.6 | A Spiral Model of the Stages of Change**    (*Source:* Prochaska, James O, Carlo C. DiClemente, and John C. Norcross. "In search of how people change: Applications to addictive behaviors." *American Psychologist* 47, no. 9 (September 1992): 1102–1114.)

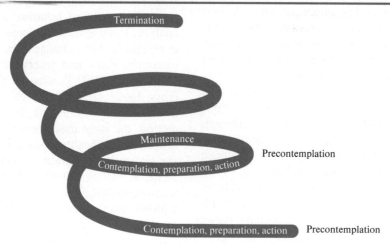

**Contemplation**    Contemplation is the stage in which people are aware that they have a problem and are thinking about it but have not yet made a commitment to take action. Many people remain in the contemplation stage for years. Interventions aimed at increasing receptivity to behavior change can be helpful at this stage (Albarracín, Durantini, Earl, Gunnoe, & Leeper, 2008).

**Preparation**    In the preparation stage, people intend to change their behavior but have not yet done so successfully. In some cases, they have modified the target behavior somewhat, such as smoking fewer cigarettes than usual, but have not yet made the commitment to eliminate the behavior altogether.

**Action**    The action stage occurs when people modify their behavior to overcome the problem. Action requires the commitment of time and energy to making real behavior change. It includes stopping the behavior and modifying one's lifestyle and environment to rid one's life of cues associated with the behavior.

**Maintenance**    In the stage of maintenance, people work to prevent relapse and to consolidate the gains they have made. For example, if a person is able to remain free of an addictive behavior for more than 6 months, he or she is assumed to be in the maintenance stage (Wing, 2000).

Because relapse is the rule rather than the exception with many health behaviors, this stage model is conceptualized as a spiral. As Figure 3.6 indicates, a person may take action, attempt maintenance, relapse, return to the precontemplation phase, cycle through the subsequent stages to action, repeat the cycle again, and do so several times until they have eliminated the behavior (Prochaska et al., 1992).

## Using the Stage Model of Change

At each stage, particular types of interventions may be most appropriate. Specifically, providing people in the precontemplation stage with information about their problem may move them to the contemplation phase. To move people from the contemplation phase into preparation, an appropriate intervention may induce them to assess how they feel and think about the problem and how stopping it will change them. Interventions designed to get people to make explicit commitments as to when and how they will change their behavior may bridge the gap between preparation and action. Interventions that emphasize providing self-reinforcement, social support, stimulus control, and coping skills should be most successful with individuals moving through the action phase into long-term maintenance.

**Perceived Barriers**    **Perceived barriers** are aspects of one's life that interfere with practicing good health behaviors. The person with two jobs may not have enough time to sleep 7 to 8 hours. A woman who wants to exercise may perceive her neighborhood to be too unsafe for walking or running. A family without health insurance may not vaccinate their children.

Perceived barriers are a main reason why people don't practice good health behaviors (Gerend, Shepherd, & Shepherd, 2013), and it can be hard to help people overcome them. In the case of health insurance, social engineering has stepped in, requiring people to have insurance and to vaccinate their children. For the woman who wants to exercise, driving to or getting off a bus where there is a park with other people walking or running may solve the safety issue. Lack of time, stress, competing goals, and inaccessibility of the health care system may be almost inevitable for some people (Gerend et al., 2013; Presseau, Tait, Johnston, Francis, & Sniehotta, 2013). But breaking down perceived barriers is paramount to getting people to practice good health behaviors.

## ■ CHANGING HEALTH BEHAVIORS THROUGH SOCIAL ENGINEERING

Much health behavior change occurs not through programs such as CBT interventions, but through **social engineering.** Social engineering modifies the environment in ways that affect people's abilities to practice a particular health behavior. Often, social engineering solutions are legally mandated. Some examples include requiring vaccinations for school entry, which has led to 90 percent of children in the United States receiving most of the vaccinations they need (Center for the Advancement of Health, December 2002). Others include banning certain drugs, such as heroin and cocaine, and controlling the disposal of toxic wastes. Still others include taxation that may reduce, although not eliminate, poor health habits such as consumption of sugared soft drinks (*The Economist,* November 28, 2015).

Social engineering solutions to health problems can be more successful than individual behavior modification. For example, lowering the speed limit has had more impact on death and disability than interventions to get people to change their driving habits. Raising the legal drinking age and banning smoking in the workplace have had major effects on these health problems. Controlling what is contained in vending machines at school and controlling advertisement of high-fat and high-cholesterol products to children may help to reduce the obesity epidemic.

Still, most health behavior change cannot be legally mandated, and people will continue to engage in bad habits even when their freedoms to do so are limited by social engineering. Consequently, health psychology interventions have a very important role in health behavior change.

## ■ VENUES FOR HEALTH-HABIT MODIFICATION

What is the best venue for changing health habits? There are several possibilities:

### The Practitioner's Office

Many people have regular contact with a physician or other health care professional who knows their medical history and can help them modify their health habits. Physicians are highly credible sources for instituting health habit change, and their recommendations have the force of expertise behind them.

Some health-habit modification is conducted by psychologists and other health practitioners privately on a one-to-one basis, usually using cognitive–behavioral techniques. This approach has two advantages. First, the individual treatment a person receives makes success more likely, and second, the intervention can be tailored to the needs of the particular person. However, only one person's behavior can be changed at a time.

Managed care facilities sometimes run clinics to help people stop smoking, change their diet, and make other healthy lifestyle changes. Advantages are that a number of people can be reached simultaneously, and there is a direct link from knowledge of a person's health risks to the type of intervention that the person receives.

### The Family

Increasingly, health practitioners intervene with families to improve health (Fisher et al., 1998). People from intact families have better health habits than those who live alone or in fractured families. Families typically have more organized, routinized lifestyles than single people do, so family life can be suited to building in healthy behaviors, such as eating three meals a day, sleeping 7 or 8 hours each night, and brushing teeth 2 or 3 times daily.

Children learn their health habits from their parents, so committing the entire family to a healthy lifestyle gives children the best chance at a healthy start in life. Multiple family members are affected by any one member's health habits, and so modifying one family member's behavior, such as diet, is likely to affect other family members.

Finally, and most important, if behavior change is introduced at the family level, all family members are on board, ensuring greater commitment to the behavior-change program and providing social support for the person whose behavior is the target.

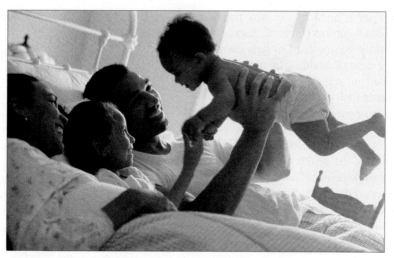

*A stable family life is health promoting, and interventions are increasingly being targeted to families rather than individuals to ensure the greatest likelihood of behavior change.*
Ariel Skelly/Blend Images LLC

Family interventions may be especially helpful in cultures that place a strong emphasis on family. Latinos, Blacks, Asians, and southern Europeans may be especially persuaded by health interventions that emphasize the good of the family (Han & Shavitt, 1994; Klonoff & Landrine, 1999).

## Self-Help Groups

Millions of people in the United States modify their health habits through self-help groups. Self-help groups bring together people with the same health habit problem, and often with the help of a counselor, they attempt to solve their problems together. Some prominent self-help groups include Overeaters Anonymous and TOPS (Take Off Pounds Sensibly) for obesity, Alcoholics Anonymous for alcoholics, and Smokenders for smokers. Many group leaders employ cognitive–behavioral principles in their programs. The social support provided in these groups also contributes to their success. At the present time, self-help groups constitute the major venue for health-habit modification in the United States.

## Schools

Interventions to encourage good health behaviors can be implemented through the school system (Facts of Life, November 2003). The school population is young, and consequently, we may be able to intervene before children have developed poor health habits. Schools have a natural intervention vehicle, namely, classes of

approximately an hour's duration, and many health interventions can fit into this format. Moreover, interventions can change the social climate in a school regarding particular health habits in ways that foster behavior change.

Even in college, social networks continue to be good targets for health interventions. As one or two people change their behavior, their friends may begin to do so as well.

## Workplace Interventions

Approximately 60 percent of the adult population is employed, and consequently, the workplace can reach much of this population (Bureau of Labor Statistics, 2016). Workplace interventions include on-the-job health promotion programs that help employees stop smoking, reduce stress, change their diet, exercise regularly, lose weight, control hypertension, and limit drinking, among other problems. Workplace interventions can be linked to those in other sites; for example, the workplace could free up parents to participate in school interventions with their children (Anderson, Symoniak, & Epstein, 2014). Some workplaces provide health clubs, restaurants that serve healthy foods, and gyms that underscore the importance of good health habits (Figure 3.7). On the whole, workplace interventions have benefits, including higher morale, greater productivity, and reduced health care costs to organizations (Berry, Mirabito, & Baun, 2010).

**FIGURE 3.7 | Percentage of Companies Offering a Particular Wellness Program to Their Employees, by Firm Size, 2011**
(*Source:* Kaiser Family Foundation and Health Research and Education Trust. "Employer Health Benefits: Annual Survey 2011." Accessed June 11, 2019. https://www.kff.org/wp-content/uploads/2013/04/8225.pdf.)
*Note:* "Small firms" are those with 3 to 199 workers; "large firms" are those with 200 or more workers.

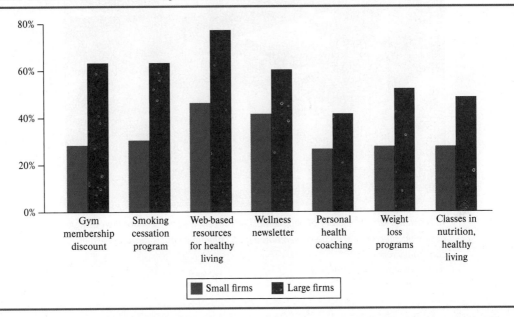

## Community-Based Interventions

There are many kinds of community interventions. A community-based intervention could be a door-to-door campaign about a breast cancer screening program, a media blitz alerting people to the risks of smoking, a grassroots community program to encourage exercise, a dietary modification program that recruits through community institutions, or a mixed intervention involving both media and personal contact.

There are several advantages of community-based interventions. First, such interventions reach more people than individually based interventions or interventions in limited environments, such as a single workplace or classroom. Second, community-based interventions can build on social support for reinforcing adherence to recommended health changes. For example, if all your neighbors have agreed to switch to a low-cholesterol diet, you are more likely to do so as well. Finally, neighborhoods can have profound effects on health practices, especially those of adolescents. Monitoring behavior within neighborhoods has been tied to a lower rate of smoking and alcohol abuse among adolescents, for example (Chuang, Ennett, Bauman, & Foshee, 2005).

But community interventions can be expensive and bring about only modest behavior change (Leventhal, Weinman, Leventhal, & Phillips, 2008). Partnering with existing community organizations such as health maintenance organizations may sustain gains from an initial community intervention and reduce costs.

## The Mass Media

A goal of health promotion is to reach as many people as possible, and consequently, the mass media have great potential. Generally, mass media campaigns bring about modest attitude change but less long-term behavior change. Nonetheless, the mass media can alert people to health risks that they would not otherwise know about.

Recently, health psychologists have studied the effects of health behaviors of characters in soap operas, dramas, and comedies. Characters who smoke, for example, can act as role models, increasing the likelihood that adolescents will begin to smoke (Heatherton & Sargent, 2009). By contrast, characters who engage in healthy activities can encourage healthy behavior change in their viewers.

By presenting a consistent media message over time, the mass media can also have a cumulative effect in changing the values associated with health practices. For example, the cumulative effects of antismoking mass media messages on social norms about smoking have been substantial.

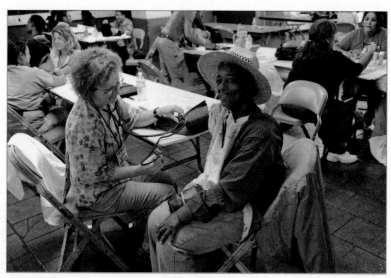

*To reach the largest number of people most effectively, researchers are increasingly designing interventions to be implemented on a community basis through existing community resources.*

Jim Ruymen/UPI/Alamy Stock Photo

### Cellular Phones and Landlines

Venues for low-cost interventions include cell phones and landlines (Eakin, Reeves, Winkler, Lawler, & Owen, 2010). For example, automated phone interventions can prompt people to maintain health behavior change (Kaplan & Stone, 2013; King et al., 2014). Personalized text messages can help smokers quit (Rodgers et al., 2005), and so texting represents another potentially effective low-cost intervention. Programs to contact older adults by telephone each day can make sure their needs are being met, and recent efforts have incorporated lifestyle advice into these volunteer programs, such as recommending physical activity (Castro, Pruitt, Buman, & King, 2011). Moreover, such daily contact can also increase the older adult's experience of social support.

### The Internet

The Internet provides information and low-cost access to health interventions for millions of people (Cohen & Adams, 2011). Websites for smoking cessation (Griffiths et al., 2018) and other health habits have been developed (Linke, Murray, Butler, & Wallace, 2007), and Internet-delivered, computer-tailored lifestyle interventions targeting single or multiple risk factors simultaneously, for example, diet, exercise, handwashing, and smoking, have shown some success (Ainsworth, Steele, Stuart, Joseph, & Miller, 2017; Oenema, Brug, Dijkstra, de Weerdt, & de Vries, 2008). The Internet can also be used to augment the effectiveness of other interventions, such as school-based smoking cessation programs (Norman, Maley, Skinner, & Li, 2008) or interventions with patient groups (Williams, Lynch, & Glasgow, 2007). Tailored e-coaching that provides individualized feedback can supplement standardized interventions for health-related behavior change, such as weight loss (Gabriele, Carpenter, Tate, & Fisher, 2011).

CBT interventions for health habit modification delivered via the Internet can be as effective as face-to-face interventions, and they have advantages of costing less, saving therapists' time, reducing waitlist and travel time, and providing interventions to people who might not seek out a therapist on their own (Cuijpers, van Straten, & Andersson, 2008; Mohr et al., 2010). The Internet also enables researchers to recruit a large number of participants for studies at relatively low cost, thus enabling data collection related to health habits (Lenert & Skoczen, 2002).

The choice of venue for health-habit change is an important issue. Understanding the particular strengths and disadvantages of each venue helps to define interventions that can reach the most people for the least expense.  •

# SUMMARY

1. Health promotion enables people to increase control over and improve their health. It involves the practice of good health behaviors and the avoidance or elimination of health-compromising ones.

2. Health habits are determined by demographic factors (such as age and SES), social factors (such as early socialization in the family), values and cultural background, perceived symptoms, access to medical care, and cognitive factors (such as health beliefs). Health habits are only modestly related to each other and can be unstable over time.

3. Health-promotion efforts target children and adolescents before bad health habits are in place. They also focus on people at risk for disorders to prevent those disorders from occurring. A focus on health promotion among older adults may help contain the soaring costs of health care late in life.

4. Research based on the health belief model and the theory of planned behavior has identified attitudes related to health-habit modification, including the belief that a threat to health is severe, that one is personally vulnerable to the threat, that one is able to perform the response needed to reduce the threat (self-efficacy), that the response will be effective in overcoming the threat (response efficacy), and that social norms support one's practice of the behavior.

5. Attitudinal approaches to health behavior change can instill knowledge and motivation. But by themselves, approaches such as fear appeals and information appeals can have limited effects on behavior change.

6. Cognitive–behavioral approaches to health-habit change use principles of self-monitoring, classical conditioning, operant conditioning, modeling, and stimulus control to modify the antecedents and consequences of a target behavior. CBT brings clients into the treatment process by drawing on principles of self-control and self-reinforcement.

7. Social skills training and relaxation training methods can be incorporated into cognitive–behavioral interventions to deal with the anxiety or social deficits that underlie some health problems.

8. Increasingly, interventions focus on relapse prevention. Practicing coping techniques for managing high-risk-for-relapse situations is a major component of such interventions.

9. Successful modification of health habits does not occur all at once. People go through stages, which they may cycle through several times. When interventions are targeted to the stage an individual is in, they may be more successful.

10. Some health habits are best changed through social engineering, such as mandated childhood immunizations or smoking bans in the workplace.

11. The venue for intervening in health habits is changing. Expensive methods that reach one individual at a time are giving way to group methods that are cheaper, including self-help groups, and school and workplace interventions. The mass media can reinforce health campaigns by alerting people to health risks. Telephone interventions, Internet interventions, and texting all show promise as health behavior change venues.

# KEY TERMS

abstinence violation effect
assertiveness training
at risk
behavioral assignments
classical conditioning
cognitive–behavioral therapy (CBT)
cognitive restructuring
contingency contracting
discriminative stimulus
fear appeals
health behaviors
health belief model
health habit
health locus of control
health promotion
lifestyle rebalancing
modeling
operant conditioning

perceived barriers
primary prevention
relapse prevention
relaxation training
self-control
self-determination theory (SDT)
self-efficacy

self-monitoring
self-regulation
self-reinforcement
self-talk
social engineering
social skills training
socialization

stimulus-control interventions
teachable moment
theory of planned behavior
transtheoretical model of behavior
    change
window of vulnerability

# Health-Promoting Behaviors

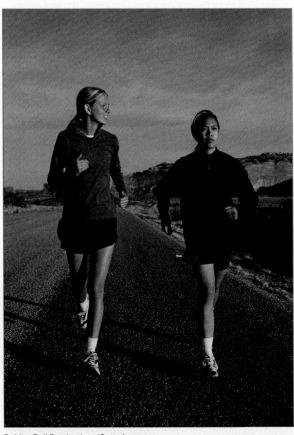

RubberBall Productions/Getty Images

Chapter 4 examines how the principles described in Chapter 3 apply to health-promoting behaviors, including exercise, accident prevention, cancer prevention, healthy diet, and sleep. Each of these important behaviors has been related to at least one major cause of illness and death in industrialized countries. As people in developing countries adopt the lifestyles of industrialized nations, these health habits will assume increasing importance throughout the world.

## ■ EXERCISE

A news headline reads, "Sedentary behavior trumps fat as a killer" (Healy, 2015). In fact, a recent review of 47 studies found that the risk of several chronic diseases and early death increases with long periods of sitting (Alter et al., 2015); even taking breaks from sitting does not fully offset the risk. Adequate physical fitness among adolescents is only 42 percent, with girls worse than boys (Gahche et al., 2014). Consequently, a high level of physical activity is an important health behavior.

Exercise helps to maintain mental and physical health. At one time, scientists believed that only **aerobic exercise** has health benefits, but now evidence suggests that any kind of exercise has benefits, especially for middle-aged and older adults.

### Benefits of Exercise

The health benefits of exercise are substantial. A mere 30 minutes of exercise every day can decrease the risk of several chronic diseases, including heart disease, diabetes, and some cancers. Exercise accelerates wound healing in those with injuries (Emery, Kiecolt-Glaser, Glaser, Malarkey, & Frid, 2005), and can be critical to recovery from disabilities, such as hip fracture (Resnick et al., 2007). Other health benefits are listed in Table 4.1.

However, over two-thirds of American adults do not engage in the recommended levels of physical activity, and about two-thirds of American adults do not engage in any regular leisure-time physical activity (National Center for Health Statistics, 2011). Physical activity is more common among men than women, among Whites than African Americans and Hispanics, among younger than older adults, and among those with higher versus lower incomes (National Center for Health Statistics, 2011b).

### How Much Exercise?

The typical exercise prescription for a normal adult is at least 2½ to 5 hours a

**TABLE 4.1 | Health Benefits of Regular Exercise**

- Helps you control your weight
- Reduces your risk of cardiovascular disease
- Reduces your risk for type 2 diabetes and metabolic syndrome
- Reduces your risk of some cancers
- Strengthens your bones and muscles
- Decreases resting heart rate and blood pressure and increases strength and efficiency of heart
- Improves sleep
- Increases HDL (good) cholesterol
- Improves immune system functioning
- Promotes the growth of new neurons in the brain
- Promotes cognitive functioning

*Sources:* Centers for Disease Control and Prevention. "Physical Activity and Health." Last reviewed April 19, 2019. https://www.cdc.gov/physicalactivity/basics/index.htm?CDC_AA_refVal=https%3A%2F%2Fwww.cdc.gov%2Fphysicalactivity%2Fbasics%2Fpa-health%2Findex.htm; Hamer, Mark, and Andrew Steptoe. "Association between Physical Fitness, Parasympathetic Control, and Proinflmmatory Responses to Mental Stress." *Psychosomatic Medicine* 69, no. 7 (September 2007): 660–66. doi: 10.1097/PSY.0b013e318148c4c0; Heisz, Jennifer, Susan Vandermorris, Johnny Wu, Anthony R. McIntosh, and Jennifer D. Ryan. "Age Differences in the Association of Physical Activity, Sociocognitive Engagement, and TV Viewing on Face Memory." *Health Psychology* 34, no. 1 (January 2014): 83–88. doi: 10.1037/hea0000046.

week of moderate-intensity, or 1¼ to 2½ hours a week of vigorous-intensity aerobic physical activity, or a mixture of both (U.S. Department of Health and Human Services. *Physical Activity Guidelines for Americans*, 2nd edition, 2018). Aerobic exercise is marked by high intensity, long duration, and the need for endurance, and it includes running, bicycling, rope jumping, and swimming. A person with low cardiopulmonary fitness may derive benefits from even less exercise each week. Even short walks or just increasing activity level has physical and psychological benefits for older adults (Ekkekakis, Hall, VanLanduyt, & Petruzzello, 2000; Schechtman, Ory, & the FICSIT group, 2001). In addition, most people simply find exercise to be more intrinsically enjoyable than they expected (Kwan, Stevens, & Bryan, 2017).

### Effects on Psychological Health

Regular exercise improves not only physical health but also mood and emotional well-being (Aggio et al., 2017; Wen et al., 2018). Many people seem to be unaware of these hidden benefits of exercise (Ruby, Dunn, Perrino, Gillis, & Viel, 2011). Some of the positive effects of exercise on

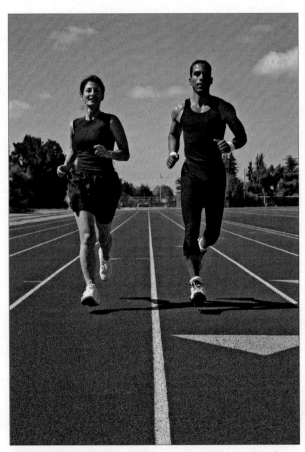

*Regular aerobic exercise produces many physical and emotional benefits, including reduced risk for cardiovascular disease.*

Eliza Snow/Getty Images

mood may stem from factors associated with exercise, such as social activity or being outside (Dunton, Liao, Intille, Huh, & Leventhal, 2015). An improved sense of self-efficacy can also underlie some of the mood effects of exercise (McAuley et al., 2008).

Because of its beneficial effects on mood and self-esteem, exercise has even been used as a treatment for depression (Herman et al., 2002). Several interventions have now shown that exercise can prevent depression in women (Babyak et al., 2000; Wang et al., 2011), and stopping exercise can lead to an increase in symptoms of depression (Berlin, Kop, & Deuster, 2006). Exercise can also reduce stress (Burg et al., 2017) and hasten emotional recovery from stress (Bernstein & McNally, 2017; Puterman, Weiss, Beauchamp, Mogle, & Almeida, 2017).

Health psychologists have also found beneficial effects of exercise on cognitive functioning, especially on executive functioning involved in planning and

higher-order reasoning (Heisz, Vandermorris, Wu, McIntosh, & Ryan, 2015), and consistent with these findings, adherence to an exercise regimen is associated with the volume of several relevant brain regions (Gujral, McAuley, Oberlin, Kramer, & Erickson, 2018). Exercise appears to promote memory and healthy cognitive aging (Erickson et al., 2011; Pereira et al., 2007) and may improve cognitive functioning and executive control in children as well (Arwen, Steele, & Noser, 2018; Heisz et al., 2015). Even modest exercise or increases in activity level can have these beneficial effects on cognitive functioning.

Exercise may offer economic benefits as well. Employee fitness programs can reduce absenteeism, increase job satisfaction, and reduce health care costs, especially among women employees (Rodin & Plante, 1989).

## Determinants of Regular Exercise

Most people's participation in exercise is erratic. Starting young, even in preschool, is important (Gagné & Harnois, 2013) as even very young children start watching TV and using tablets and computers early in life. Currently, only 21 percent of American youths meet the current physical activity guidelines of 60 minutes or more of physical activity each day (Office of Disease Prevention and Health Promotion, 2016). Children get regular exercise through required physical education classes in school, but even these classes have faced budget cutbacks. Moreover, by adolescence, the practice of regular exercise has declined substantially, especially among girls (Davison, Schmalz, & Downs, 2010) and among boys not involved in formal athletics (Crosnoe, 2002). Studying may reduce time for exercise (Kumpulainen et al., 2017). Adults report lack of time, stress, interference with daily activities, and fatigue as barriers to obtaining exercise (Kowal & Fortier, 2007).

**Who Exercises?**   People who come from families in which exercise is practiced, who have positive attitudes toward physical activity, who have a strong sense of self-efficacy for exercising (Goethe, 2018; Peterson, Lawman, Wilson, Fairchild, & Van Horn, 2013), who have energy, who are extroverted and sociable (Kern, Reynolds, & Friedman, 2010), and who are high in well-being (Kim, Kubzansky, Soo, & Boehm, 2017) are more likely to exercise. People who perceive themselves as athletic or as the type of person who exercises (Salmon, Owen, Crawford, Bauman, & Sallis, 2003), who have social support from friends to exercise

(Marquez & McAuley, 2006), who enjoy their form of exercise (Kiviniemi, Voss-Humke, & Seifert, 2007), and who believe that people should take responsibility for their health are also more likely to get exercise than people who do not have these attitudes.

Characteristics of the Setting   Convenient and easily accessible exercise settings promote exercise (Troped et al., 2017). Vigorous walking in your neighborhood can be maintained more easily than participation in an aerobics class in a crowded health club 5 miles from your home. Lack of safe places to do exercise is a particular barrier for people who live in low socioeconomic status (SES) neighborhoods (Estabrooks, Lee, & Gyurcsik, 2003; Feldman & Steptoe, 2004) and for older adults (Thornton, Kerr, Conway, Saelens, & Sallis, 2017).

Improving environmental options for exercise, such as walking trails and recreational facilities, increases rates of exercise (Kärmeniemi, Lankila, Ikäheimo, Koivumaa-Honkanen, & Korpelainen, 2018). When people believe that their neighborhoods are safe, when they are not socially isolated, and when they know what exercise opportunities are available to them in their area, they are more likely to engage in physical activity (Hawkley, Thisted, & Cacioppo, 2009; Sallis, King, Sirard, & Albright, 2007; van Stralen, de Vries, Bolman, Mudde, & Lechner, 2010).

Social support can foster exercise (Berli, Stadler, Shrout, Bolger, & Scholz, 2018; McMahon et al., 2017). Making a commitment to another person to meet for exercise increases the likelihood that it will happen (Prestwich et al., 2012). People who participate in group exercise programs such as jogging or walking say that social support and group cohesion are two of the reasons why they participate (Floyd & Moyer, 2010). This support may be especially important for exercise participation among Hispanics (Marquez & McAuley, 2006). Just seeing others engaging in exercise around one's neighborhood or on a running path can increase how much time a person puts into exercise (Kowal & Fortier, 2007). Even support for exercise from an online social network can increase physical activity (Rovniak et al., 2016).

The best predictor of regular exercise is regular exercise (Phillips & Gardner, 2016). Long-term practice of regular exercise is heavily determined by habit (Kaushal, Rhodes, Spence, & Meldrum, 2017). The first 3 to 6 months appear to be critical, and people who will drop out usually do so in that time period (Dishman, 1982). Developing a regular exercise program, embedding it in regular activities, and doing it regularly means that it begins to become automatic and habitual. However, habit has its limits. Unlike such habitual behaviors as wearing a seat belt or brushing teeth, exercise takes willpower and a belief in personal responsibility in order to be enacted on a regular basis. In summary, if people participate in activities that they like, that are convenient, that they are motivated to pursue, and for which they can develop goals, exercise adherence will be greater (Papandonatos et al., 2012).

## Exercise Interventions

Several types of interventions have shown success in getting people to exercise. Interventions that incorporate principles of self-control (enhancing beliefs in personal efficacy) and that muster motivation can be successful in changing exercise habits (Conroy, Hyde, Doerksen, & Riebeiro, 2010). Helping people to form implementation intentions, and following up with brief text messages can promote activity as well (Prestwich, Perugini, & Hurling, 2010). Several studies confirm the usefulness of the transtheoretical model of behavioral change (that is, the stages of change model) for increasing physical activity. Interventions designed to increase and maintain physical activity that are matched to stage of readiness are more successful than interventions that are not (Blissmer & McAuley, 2002; Dishman, Vandenberg, Motl, & Nigg, 2010; Marshall et al., 2003). When an exercise intervention promotes personal values and social norms, such as the need to be fit, it can be especially successful (Hunt, McCann, Gray, Mutrie, & Wyke, 2013; Kanning & Hansen, 2017; Wally & Cameron, 2017). Affective mental contrasting, a process by which a person contrasts his or her current mental state ("I'm sad to be so out of shape") with the affective state that is imagined once the goal is achieved ("I'll feel great to be in shape") can be an efficient and low-cost way to maintain exercise over time (Ruissen, Rhodes, Crocker, & Beauchamp, 2018).

As is true with other health behaviors, factors that affect the adoption of exercise are not necessarily the same as those that predict long-term maintenance of an exercise program. Believing that physical activity is important predicts initiation of an exercise program, whereas barriers, such as no time or few places to get exercise, predict maintenance (Rhodes, Plotnikoff, & Courneya, 2008). Self-efficacy about one's ability to overcome barriers is a predictor of maintenance (Higgins, Middleton, Winner, & Janelle, 2014).

Family-based interventions designed to induce all family members to be more active have shown some success (Rhodes, Naylor, & McKay, 2010) although if one person is overweight or obese, it may undermine the commitment of others in the family to exercise (Wiseman, Patel, Dwyer, & Nebeling, 2018). Worksite interventions to promote exercise have small but positive effects on increased physical activity (Abraham & Graham-Rowe, 2009). DVD-delivered exercise interventions have shown success and have the potential to reach large numbers of people (Awick et al., 2017). Even minimal interventions such as sending mailers encouraging physical exercise to older adults can increase exercise. Text messaging also shows success in promoting exercise such as brisk walking (Prestwich, Perugini, & Hurling, 2010).The advantages of these interventions, of course, are low cost and ease of implementation.

Relapse prevention techniques increase long-term adherence to exercise programs. For example, helping people figure out how to overcome barriers to obtaining regular exercise, such as stress, fatigue, and a hectic schedule, improves adherence (Blanchard et al., 2007; Fjeldsoe, Miller, & Marshall, 2012).

Incorporating exercise into a more general program of healthy lifestyle change can be beneficial as well (Conroy et al., 2017). Motivation to engage in one health behavior can spill over into another (Mata et al., 2009). For example, among adults at risk for coronary heart disease (CHD), brief behavioral counseling matched to stage of readiness helped them maintain physical activity, as well as reduce smoking and fat intake (Steptoe, Kerry, Rink, & Hilton, 2001). Setting personal goals for exercise can improve commitment (Hall et al., 2010), and forming explicit implementation intentions regarding exactly when and how to exercise facilitates practice as well; planning when to exercise can facilitate the link between intention and actual behavior (Conner, Sandberg, & Norman, 2010).

Exercise interventions may promote more general lifestyle changes. This issue was studied in an intriguing manner with 60 Hispanic and Anglo families, half of whom had participated in a 1-year intervention program of dietary modification and exercise. All the families were taken to the San Diego Zoo as a reward for participating in the program, and while they were there, their food intake and amount of walking were recorded. Families that had participated in the intervention consumed fewer calories, ate less sodium, and walked more than the families in the control condition, suggesting that the intervention had been integrated into their lifestyle (Patterson et al., 1988). The family-based approach of this intervention may have contributed to its success as well (Martinez, Ainsworth, & Elder, 2008).

Physical activity websites would seem to hold promise for inducing people to participate in regular exercise (Napolitano et al., 2003). Of course, if one is on the Internet, one is by definition not exercising. Indeed, thus far, the evidence is mixed that physical activity websites provide the kind of individually tailored recommendations that are needed to get people to exercise on a regular basis (Carr et al., 2012) and initial gains may not be maintained (Carr et al., 2013). However, automated exercise advice can help maintain a physical activity program, once it is initiated (King et al., 2014).

Despite the problems health psychologists have encountered in getting people to exercise and to do so faithfully, the exercise level in the U.S. population has increased substantially in recent decades. A physician's recommendation is one of the factors that lead people to increase their exercise, and trends show that physicians increasingly are advising their patients to begin or continue exercise (Barnes & Schoenborn, 2012). The number of people who participate in regular exercise has increased by more than 50 percent in the past few decades. Increasingly, it is not just sedentary healthy adults who are becoming involved in exercise but also the elderly and chronically ill patients (Courneya & Friedenreich, 2001). These findings suggest that, although the population may be aging, it may be doing so in a healthier way than was true in recent past generations.

## ■ ACCIDENT PREVENTION

No wonder that so many cars collide;
Their drivers are accident prone,
When one hand is holding a coffee cup,
And the other a cellular phone.

—Art Buck

This rhyme captures an important point. Accidents represent one of the major causes of preventable death, both worldwide and in the United States. Moreover, this cause of death is increasing. Worldwide, nearly 1.35 million people die as a result of road traffic injuries, and the estimated economic cost of accidents is $518 billion per year (World Health Organization, 2018).

Nationally, bicycle accidents cause more than 900 deaths per year, prompt more than 494,000 emergency room visits, and constitute the major cause of head injury, making helmet use an important issue (Centers for Disease Control and Prevention, 2015). Over 2,000 people a day are accidentally poisoned in the United States, usually by prescription or illegal drugs, and more than 40,000 people die of poisoning each year (Centers for Disease Control and Prevention, March 2012a; Warner, Chen, Makuc, Anderson, & Miniño, 2011). Occupational accidents and their resulting disability are a particular health risk for working men.

## Home and Workplace Accidents

Accidents in the home, such as accidental poisonings and falls, are the most common causes of death and disability among children under age 5 (Barton & Schwebel, 2007). Interventions to reduce home accidents are typically conducted with parents because they have control over the child's environment. Putting safety catches and gates in the home, placing poisons out of reach, and teaching children safety skills are components of these interventions.

Pediatricians and their staff often incorporate such training into visits with new parents (Roberts & Turner, 1984). Parenting classes help parents to identify the most common poisons in the home and to keep these away from young children. Evaluations of interventions that train parents how to childproof a home (Morrongiello, Sandomierski, Zdzieborski, & McCollam, 2012) show that such interventions can be successful. Even young children can learn about safety in the home. For example, an intervention using a computer game (The Great Escape) improved children's knowledge of fire safety behaviors (Morrongiello, Schwebel, Bell, Stewart, & Davis, 2012). Virtual environmental training on websites can help children learn to cross the street safely (Schwebel, McClure, & Severson, 2014).

At one time, workplace accidents were a primary cause of death and disability. However, statistics suggest that overall, accidents in the workplace have declined since the 1930s. This decline may be due, in part, to better safety precautions by employers. However, accidents at home have actually increased. Social engineering solutions, such as safety caps on medications and required smoke detectors in the home, have mitigated the increase, but the trend is worrisome.

**Accidents and Older Adults**    An estimated 28,000 older adults die each year of fall-related injuries, and many more are disabled. Falls result in more than 2.8 million injuries treated in emergency departments

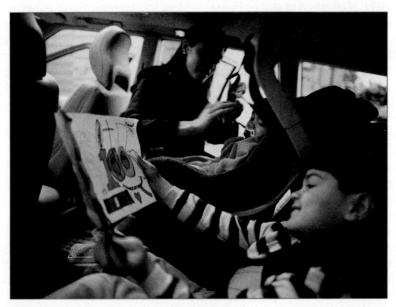

*Automobile accidents represent a major cause of death, especially among the young. Legislation requiring child safety restraint devices has reduced fatalities dramatically.*
Ryan McVay/Photodisc/Getty Images

annually, including over 800,000 hospitalizations (Centers for Disease Control and Prevention, 2017).

Consequently, strategies to reduce accidents among older adults have increasingly been a focus of health psychology research and interventions. Dietary and medication intervention to reduce bone loss can affect risk of fracture. Physical activity training involving balance, mobility, and gait training reduces the risk of falls. Teaching older adults to make small changes in their homes that reduce tripping hazards can help, including nonslip bathmats, shower grab bars, hand rails on both sides of stairs, and better lighting (Facts of Life, March 2006). The evidence suggests that fall prevention programs, often led by health psychologists, can reduce mortality and disability among older adults substantially (Facts of Life, March 2006).

### Motorcycle and Automobile Accidents

> You know what I call a motorcyclist who doesn't wear a helmet? An organ donor.
>
> —Emergency room physician

The single greatest cause of accidental death is motorcycle and automobile accidents (Centers for Disease Control and Prevention, 2009a). Although social engineering solutions such as speed limits and seat belts have major effects on accident rates, psychological interventions can also address factors associated with accidents. These include the way people drive, the speed at which they drive, and the use of preventive measures to increase safety, such as interventions to reduce cell phone usage while driving (Weller, Shackleford, Dieckmann, & Slovic, 2013).

For example, many Americans still do not use seat belts, a problem especially common among adolescents, which accounts, in part, for their high rate of fatal accidents (Facts of Life, May 2004). Community-wide health education programs aimed at increasing seat belt usage and infant restraint devices can be successful. One such program increased the use from 24 to 41 percent, leveling off at 36 percent over a 6-month follow-up period (Gemming, Runyan, Hunter, & Campbell, 1984).

On the whole, though, social engineering solutions may be more effective. Seat belt use is more prevalent in states with laws that mandate their use, and states that enforce helmet laws for motorcycle riders have reduced deaths and lower health care costs related to disability due to motorcycle accidents (*Wall Street Journal,* 2005, August 9).

### ■ VACCINATIONS AND SCREENING

Vaccinations and screening represent two ways of avoiding or detecting early some of the main causes of death in the United States. Yet many people fail to use these health resources, which makes behavior change important for health psychologists.

### Vaccinations

Parents are urged to get their children vaccinated against measles, polio, diphtheria, whooping cough, and tetanus, among other childhood diseases. Most do, because school registration typically requires these vaccines. However, some do not and instead are freeriders; that is, if most children are vaccinated, the minority that is not are protected by those who are (Korn, Betsch, Böhm, & Meier, 2018). In some cases, refusing to get vaccinations for one's children comes from the mistaken beliefs that a vaccine actually causes the disease or that the vaccine causes another disorder, such as autism (Martin & Petrie, 2017). Interventions have attempted to correct the incorrect beliefs that can undermine vaccination and stressed the social benefits of vaccination in the hopes of keeping rates high (Betsch et al., 2013).

Vaccinations of girls and boys against HPV (human papillomavirus) by age 13 is now recommended by the National Institutes of Health. HPV is a sexually transmitted virus tied to cervical as well as other cancers. The Centers for Disease Control and Prevention report, however, that as of 2016, only 40 percent of girls and 21 percent of boys had received it. This rate compares very unfavorably to many other countries, including Australia (75 percent), the United Kingdom (about 88 percent), and Rwanda (93 percent) (Winslow, 2016). Family-focused messages aimed at parents and adolescents have been suggested as one focus of public health interventions to increase vaccination rates (Alexander et al., 2014), and direct payments to adolescents in the United Kingdom have been tried (Mantzari, Vogt, & Marteau, 2015). As yet, the most effective way to encourage this behavior has not been found.

### Screenings

The two most common cancers in the United States are breast cancer in women and prostate cancer in men. Until recently, routine screening was the frontline against these cancers. At present, however, routine screening through mammography for women and the PSA (prostate-specific antigen) test for men is no longer recommended for all adults; false positives (when the test falsely suggests the presence of cancer) has led to unnecessary treatment, including surgeries. Moreover, although diagnosed cases from both tests increased, there has been little to no impact on mortality from these causes.

At present, men who are symptomatic or at high risk (who have a family history of prostate cancer; Watts et al., 2014) and women who are symptomatic or at high risk (having a family history of breast cancer; having genes implicated in breast cancer) should be monitored. Otherwise, routine PSA screening is not recommended and a mammogram is recommended every year between ages 45 and 55 and every other year for women between the ages of 55 and 74. In older women, the value of the test is less clear.

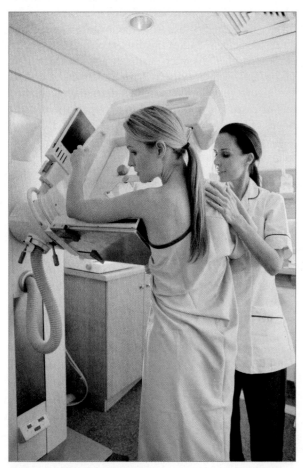

*Mammograms are an important way of detecting breast cancer in women over 50. Finding ways to reach older women to ensure that they obtain mammograms is a high priority for health scientists.*
Cultura/Getty Images

Why is screening through mammography important for high-risk women? The reasons are several:

- One in every eight women in the United States develops breast cancer.

- The majority of breast cancers are detected in women over age 40, and so screening this age group is cost-effective.

- Early detection, as through mammograms, can improve survival rates.

Unfortunately, compliance with mammography recommendations is low. Fear of radiation, embarrassment over the procedure, anticipated pain, anxiety, fear of cancer (Gurevich et al., 2004; Schwartz, Taylor, & Willard, 2003), and most importantly, especially among poorer women, concern over costs act as deterrents to getting regular mammograms (Lantz, Weigers, & House, 1997). Lack of awareness of the importance of mammograms, little time, and lack of available services also contribute to low screening rates.

Changing attitudes toward mammography can increase the likelihood of obtaining a mammogram. For example, the theory of planned behavior predicts the likelihood of obtaining regular mammograms: Women who have positive attitudes regarding mammography and who perceive social norms as favoring their obtaining a mammogram are more likely to participate in a mammography program (Montano & Taplin, 1991). Social support predicts the use of mammograms and may be especially important for low-income and older women (Messina et al., 2004). If your friends are getting mammograms, you are more likely to do so as well. Interventions are more successful if they are geared to the stage of readiness of prospective participants (Champion & Springston, 1999; Lauver, Henriques, Settersten, & Bumann, 2003).

## Colorectal Cancer Screening

In Western countries, colorectal cancer is the second-leading cause of cancer deaths. Medical guidelines have recommended routine colorectal screening for older adults (Wardle, Williamson, McCaffery et al., 2003) beginning at age 50 and every 3 to 5 years after that.

Factors that predict the practice of other health behaviors also predict participation in colorectal cancer screening, including SES, self-efficacy, perceived benefits of the procedure, a physician's recommendation to participate, social norms favoring participation, messages that stress personal risk (Brumbach, Birmingham,

Boonyasiriwat, Walters, & Kinney, 2017), and few barriers to taking advantage of a screening program (Manne et al., 2002; Sieverding, Matterne, & Ciccarello, 2010; Orbell, Szczepura, Weller, Gumber, & Hagger, 2017). As is true of many health behaviors, beliefs predict the intention to participate in colorectal screening, whereas life difficulties (low SES, poor health status) interfere with actually getting screened (Kiviniemi, Klasko-Foster, Erwin, & Jandorf, 2018).

Community-based programs that use the mass media, community-based education, interventions through social networks such as churches, health care provider recommendations, and reminder notices promote participation in cancer screening programs and can attract older adults (Curbow et al., 2004; Kerrison et al., 2018). Telephone-based interventions tailored to people's resistance to colorectal screening can increase the likelihood of obtaining screening as well (Menon et al., 2011). Hispanics are at particular risk for colorectal cancer, and so it is especially important to reach them (Gorin, 2005).

## ■ SUN SAFETY PRACTICES

The past 30 years have seen a nearly fourfold increase in the incidence of skin cancer in the United States. Although basal cell and squamous cell carcinomas do not typically kill, malignant melanoma takes over

9,000 lives each year (American Cancer Society, 2018). In the past two decades, melanoma incidence has risen by 155 percent. Moreover, these cancers are among the most preventable. The chief risk factor for skin cancer is well known: excessive exposure to ultraviolet (UV) radiation. Living or vacationing in southern latitudes, participating in outdoor activities, and using tanning salons all contribute to dangerous sun exposure. Less than one-third of American children adequately protect themselves against the sun, and more than three-quarters of American teens get at least one sunburn each summer (Facts of Life, July 2002).

As a result, health psychologists have developed interventions to promote safe sun practices. Typically, these efforts begin with educational interventions to alert people to the risks of skin cancer and to the effectiveness of sunscreen use for reducing risk (Stapleton, Turrisi, Hillhouse, Robinson, & Abar, 2010). However, education alone is not entirely successful (Jones & Leary, 1994). Tans are still perceived to be attractive (Blashill, Williams, Grogan, & Clark-Carter, 2015), and many people are oblivious to the long-term consequences of tanning (Orbell & Kyriakaki, 2008). Many people use sunscreens with an inadequate sun protection factor (SPF), and few people apply sunscreen often enough during outdoor activities (Wichstrom, 1994). Effective sunscreen use requires knowledge about skin cancer, perceived need for sunscreen, perceived

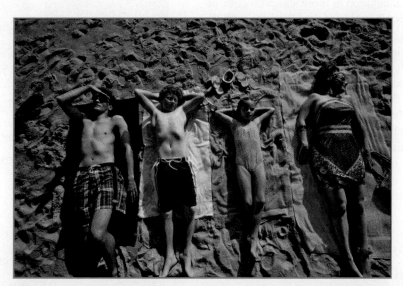

*Despite the risks of exposure to the sun, millions of people each year continue to sunbathe.*

Ingram Publishing/Superstock

efficacy of sunscreen as protection against skin cancer, and social norms that favor sunscreen use (Gonzales & Blashill, 2018; Turrisi, Hillhouse, Gebert, & Grimes, 1999). All of these factors change only grudgingly.

Parents play an important role in ensuring that children reduce sun exposure (Hamilton, Kirkpatrick, Rebar, & Hagger, 2017). Parents' own sun protection habits influence how attentive they are to their children's practices and what their children do when they are on their own (Turner & Mermelstein, 2005).

Communications to adolescents and young adults that stress the gains that sunscreen use will bring them, such as freedom from concern about skin cancers or improvements in appearance, may be more successful than those that emphasize the risks (Detweiler, Bedell, Salovey, Pronin, & Rothman, 1999; Jackson & Aiken, 2006). When risks are emphasized, it is important to stress the immediate adverse effects of rather than the long-term risks of chronic illness, because adolescents and young adults are especially influenced by immediate concerns.

In one clever investigation, one group of beachgoers was exposed to a photo-aging intervention that showed premature wrinkling and age spots; a second group received a photo intervention that made the negative appearance-related consequences of UV exposure very salient; a third group received both interventions; and a fourth group was assigned to a control condition. Those beachgoers who received the UV photo information engaged in more sun protective behaviors, and the combination of the UV photo with the photo-aging information led to substantially less sunbathing over the long-term (Mahler, Kulik, Gerrard, & Gibbons, 2007; Mahler, Kulik, Gibbons, Gerrard, & Harrell, 2003). Similar interventions appear to be effective in reducing the use of tanning salons (Gibbons, Gerrard, Lane, Mahler, & Kulik, 2005).

Health psychologists have explored Internet-based strategies as a vehicle for distributing sun safety materials. Even brief interventions directed to sun safety practices can be effective, especially for people at risk (Heckman, Handorf, Darlow, Ritterband, & Manne, 2017).

# ■ DEVELOPING A HEALTHY DIET

Diet is an important and controllable risk factor for many of the leading causes of death and disease. For example, diet is related to serum cholesterol level and to lipid profiles. The dramatic rise in obesity in the

United States has added urgency to this issue. However, only about 13 percent of adults get the recommended servings of fruit and only about 9 percent get the recommended servings of vegetables each day (Centers for Disease Control and Prevention, July 2015; Table 4.2). Experts estimate that unhealthful eating contributes to more than 678,000 deaths per year (U.S. Burden of Disease Collaborators, 2013).

**TABLE 4.2 | Current USDA Recommendations for a Balanced Diet**

The U.S. Agriculture Department currently recommends a 2,000-calorie-a-day diet made up of the following components:

–Dairy (3 cups)

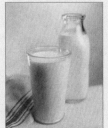

Mitch Hrdlicka/ Getty Images

–Fruits (2 cups)

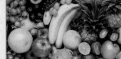

Lex van Lieshout/Image shop/Alamy Stock Photo

–Vegetables (2.5 cups)

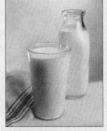

Lex van Lieshout/Image shop/Alamy Stock Photo

–Grain (3 oz)

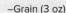

Comstock/Getty Images

–Meat (6 oz)

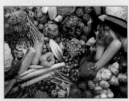

IT Stock/Getty Images

–Oil (6 tsp)

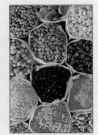

Ken Karp/McGraw-Hill Education

Much eating is pleasure-driven, called hedonic eating; this eating is not to satisfy hunger or obtain needed calories, but rather driven by the sheer delight of eating (Bejarano & Cushing, 2018).

As such, it is hard to modify. Because adolescence is an important time when young people's food preferences form and can drive their behavior, interventions need to focus on building the intrinsic motivation to eat well and enlisting the influence of social groups, both family and peers, to increase adolescents' consumption of healthy foods (Smit et al., 2018). Dietary change is critical, especially for people at risk for or already diagnosed with chronic diseases such as coronary artery disease, hypertension, diabetes, and cancer (Center for the Advancement of Health, 2000f). These are diseases for which people low in SES are more at risk, and diet may explain some of the relation between low SES and these disorders. For example, supermarkets in high-SES neighborhoods carry more health-oriented food products than do supermarkets in low-income areas. Thus, even if the motivation to change one's diet is there, the food products may not be (Conis, 2003, August 4).

## Changing Diet

The human diet evolved thousands of years ago, and to meet energy demands required foods high in fat, sugar, and calories. Humans still have a preference for such foods, although they are no longer essential and can compromise health (Ahlstrom, Dinh, Haselton, & Tomiyama, 2017). The good news is that changing one's diet can improve health. A diet high in fruits, vegetables, with some whole grains, peas and beans, poultry, and fish and low in refined grains, potatoes, and red and processed meats lowers the risk of coronary heart disease (Fung, Willett, Stampfer, Manson, & Hu, 2001). Switching from trans fats (as are used for fried and fast foods) and saturated fats (from meat and dairy products) to polyunsaturated fats and monounsaturated fats is a healthful change as well (Marsh, 2002, September 10). Current U.S. government guidelines for a balanced diet are described in Table 4.2.

Several specific diets, in addition to low-fat diets, have health benefits. Healthy "Mediterranean" diets are rich in vegetables, nuts, fruits, and fish and low in red meat. Low-carbohydrate diets with vegetarian sources of fat and protein and little bread and other high-carbohydrate foods can have healthful effects. Many people like these diets, and so they can be fairly easily adopted and adhered to over time.

## Resistance to Modifying Diet

It is difficult to get people to modify their diet, however, even when they are at high risk for CHD or when their physician recommends it. The typical reason that people switch to a diet low in cholesterol, fats, calories, and additives and high in fiber, fruits, and vegetables is to improve appearance, not to improve health. Even so, fewer than half of U.S. adults meet the dietary recommendations for reducing fat levels and for increasing fiber, fruit, and vegetable consumption (Kumanyika et al., 2000).

Rates of adherence to a new diet may be high at first but fall off over time. Some diets are restrictive, monotonous, expensive, and hard to implement. Changes in shopping, meal planning, cooking methods, and eating habits may be required. Snacking at times when resolve is low can undermine healthy eating, as many snacks are unhealthy (Inauen, Shrout, Bolger, Stadler, & Scholz, 2016). Tastes are hard to alter. Foods that are high in fat and sugars help turn off stress hormones, such as cortisol, but they contribute to an unhealthy diet. A preference for meat, a lack of health consciousness, a limited interest in exploring new foods, and low awareness of the link between eating habits and illness are all tied to poor dietary habits.

**Stress and Diet**    Stress has a direct and negative effect on diet. People under stress eat more fatty foods, fewer fruits and vegetables, and are more likely to snack and skip breakfast (O'Connor, Jones, Ferguson, Conner, & McMillan, 2008). People with low-status jobs, high workloads, and little control at work also have less healthy diets. When people are under stress, they are distracted, may fail to practice self-control, and may not pay much attention to what they are eating (Devine, Connors, Sobal, & Bisogni, 2003). Thus, the sheer cognitive burden of daily life can interfere with the ability to control food consumption by preventing people from monitoring their eating (Ward & Mann, 2000).

**Who Controls Their Diet?**    People who are high in conscientiousness and intelligence do a better job of adhering to a healthy diet. People who have high self-control are better able to manage a healthy diet than people without executive control skills (Powell, McMinn, & Allan, 2017). A strong sense of self-efficacy, well-being, interest in health, knowledge about dietary issues, family support, and the perception that dietary change has important health benefits are also critical to developing a healthy diet (Boehm et al., 2018; Steptoe, Doherty, Kerry, Rink, & Hilton, 2000; van Rijn, Wegman, Aarts, de Graaf, & Smeets, 2017; Wu, Fisher-Hoch, Reininger, & McCormick, 2018).

When people are informed about social norms regarding diet, they are more likely to make a change toward those norms (Robinson, Fleming, & Higgs, 2014). For example, if the people around you have stopped drinking soda because they think it is unhealthy, you are more likely to do so as well. Associating healthy food choices with the self can change attitudes in a healthy direction (Mattavelli, Avishai, Perugini, Richetin, & Sheeran, 2017).

Interventions to Modify Diet    Recent efforts to induce dietary change have focused heavily on reducing portion size, snacking, and sugary drink consumption. Portion size has increased greatly over the past decades, contributing to obesity. Snacking has also been tied to obesity. Sugary drinks have been tied to higher heart disease risk (de Koning et al., 2012) and are suspected of contributing to the rising rates of type 2 diabetes. Accordingly, interventions have been directed to these issues, as well as to reducing fat and increasing vegetable and fruit consumption. Specific health risks such as obesity, diabetes, or CHD often lead people to change their diets, and physicians, nurses, dieticians, and health psychologists work with patients to develop an appropriate diet.

Most diet change is implemented through cognitive–behavioral interventions. Efforts to change diet begin with education and training in self-monitoring: Most people are poorly informed about what a healthy diet is and do not pay sufficient attention to what they actually eat (O'Brien, Fries, & Bowen, 2000). Additional components are stimulus control and contingency contracting, coupled with relapse prevention techniques for high-risk-for-relapse situations, such as parties. Drawing on social support for making a dietary change and increasing one's sense of self-efficacy are two critical factors for improving diet (Steptoe, Perkins-Porras, Rink, Hilton, & Cappuccio, 2004). Self-affirmation and motivational interviewing have shown to be helpful in getting people to increase their fruit and vegetable intake and otherwise improve their diets (Ahluwalia et al., 2007; Harris et al., 2014). Training in self-regulation, including planning skills and formation of explicit behavioral intentions (Stadler, Oettingen, & Gollwitzer, 2010) can improve dietary adherence.

Implementation intentions regarding exactly when, where, and what food will be consumed can also help people bring snacking under intentional control (Harris et al., 2014). However, much eating and snacking occurs mindlessly, when people are exerting little self-control. For example, just seeing other people snacking can increase a person's likelihood of also doing so (Schüz, Papadakis, & Ferguson, 2018). In such cases, simple environmental interventions, such as a sign in a cafe promoting healthy eating, can help people make good choices (Allan, Johnston, & Campbell, 2015).

Recent efforts to change the dietary habits of high-risk people have focused on the family (Gorin et al., 2013). Eating meals together promotes better eating habits. In family interventions, family members typically meet with a dietary counselor to discuss ways to change the family diet. When all family members are committed to and participate in dietary change, it is easier for a target family member (such as a cardiac patient) to do so as well (Wilson & Ampey-Thornhill, 2001). Children who are involved in these interventions may practice better dietary habits into adolescence and adulthood. An intervention with Latina mothers with type 2 diabetes and their overweight daughters made use of this strong social tie to promote weight loss and healthy eating (Sorkin et al., 2014).

Community interventions aimed at dietary change have been undertaken. For example, nutrition education campaigns in supermarkets have shown some success. In one study, a computerized, interactive nutritional information system placed in supermarkets significantly decreased high-fat purchases and somewhat increased high-fiber purchases (Jeffery, Pirie, Rosenthal, Gerber, & Murray, 1982; Winett et al., 1991). A workplace restaurant intervention posted a message stating "Most people here choose to eat vegetables with their lunches" which increased the purchase of vegetables (Thomas et al., 2017). Restaurants often describe the nutritious menu options in unappealing terms, which can undermine healthy meal choices (Turnwald, Jurafsky, Conner, & Crumm, 2017).

Tailoring dietary interventions to ethnic identity and making them culturally and linguistically appropriate may achieve particularly high rates of success (Eakin et al., 2007; Martinez et al., 2008; Resnicow, Davis, et al., 2008). In Latino populations, face-to-face contact with a health adviser who goes through the steps for successful diet modification may be especially important, due to the emphasis on personal contact in Latino culture and communities (Elder et al., 2005).

Researchers are moving toward interventions that are cost-effective to alter behavior related to diet and exercise, rather than large-scale CBT interventions. For example, computer-tailored dietary fat intake interventions can be effective both with adults and with adolescents (Haerens et al., 2007). Telephone counseling can achieve beneficial effects (Madlensky et al., 2008). Such interventions can reach many people at relatively low cost.

Change is likely to come from social engineering as well. When children have access to school snack bars that include sodas, candy, and other unhealthy foods, it undermines their consumption of healthier foods (Cullen & Zakeri, 2004).

Some of these interventions may seem heavy-handed. After all, most people eat what they want based on their preferences or what is available. Nudging people in the right direction through subtle messages may work as well as, or better than, explicit warnings (van der Laan, Papies, Hooge, & Smeets, 2017; Wagner, Howland, & Mann, 2015). Eliminating snack foods from schools, making school lunch programs more nutritious, making snack foods more expensive and healthy foods less so, and taxing products high in sugar or fats (Brownell & Frieden, 2009) will make some inroads into promoting healthy food choices.

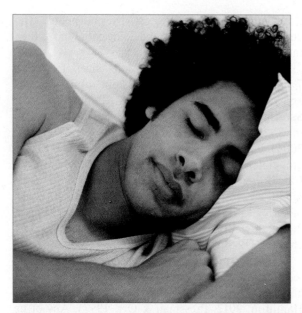

*Scientists have begun to identify the health risks associated with little or poor-quality sleep.*
Stockbyte/Getty Images

■ **SLEEP**

Michael Foster, a trucker who carried produce, was behind in his truck payments. To catch up, he needed to make more runs each week. To do so, he began cutting back from 6 hours of sleep a night to 3 or 4, stretches that he grabbed in his truck between jobs. On an early-morning run between Fresno and Los Angeles, he fell asleep at the wheel and his truck went out of control, hitting a car and killing a family.

## What Is Sleep?

Sleep is a vital health habit. It has a powerful effect on risk of infectious disease, risk of depression, poor responses to vaccines, and the occurrence and progression of several chronic disorders, including cardiovascular disease and cancer (Hall, Brindle, & Buysse, 2018). But sleep is often abused.

There are two broad types of sleep: non–rapid eye movement (NREM) and rapid eye movement (REM). NREM sleep consists of four stages. Stage 1, the lightest

and earliest stage of sleep, is marked by theta waves, when we begin to tune out the sounds around us, although we are easily awakened by any loud sound. In stage 2, breathing and heart rates even out, body temperature drops, and brain waves alternate between short bursts called sleep spindles and large K-complex waves. Stages 3 and 4, deep sleep, are marked by delta waves. These are the phases most important for restoring energy, strengthening the immune system, and prompting the body to release growth hormone (Brindle et al., 2018b). During REM sleep, eyes dart back and forth, breathing and heart rates flutter, and we often dream vividly. This stage of sleep is marked by beta waves and is important for consolidating memories, solving problems from the previous day, and turning knowledge into long-term memories (Irwin, 2015). All of these phases of sleep are essential.

## Sleep and Health

An estimated 70 million Americans suffer from chronic sleep disorders—most commonly, insomnia (Centers for Disease Control and Prevention, June 2017). Many other people, such as college students, choose to deprive themselves of sleep in order to keep up with all the demands on their time. But sleep is an important restorative activity, and people who deny themselves sleep may be doing more harm than they realize.

Roughly 40 percent of adults sleep less than 7 hours a night on weeknights, one-third of adults experience sleep problems (Stein, Belik, Jacobi, & Sareen, 2008), and 54 percent of people over age 55 report insomnia at least once a week (Weintraub, 2004). For women, sleep disorders may be tied to hormonal levels related to menopause (Manber, Kuo, Cataldo, & Colrain, 2003). Even children who sleep too little or too much incur health risks, including risk of early death (Duggan, Reynolds, Kern, & Friedman, 2014); low SES contributes to poor sleep among children (El-Sheikh et al., 2013).

Insufficient sleep (less than 7 hours a night) affects cognitive functioning, mood, job performance, and quality of life (Karlson, Gallagher, Olson, & Hamilton, 2012; Pressman & Orr, 1997). Any of us who has spent a sleepless night tossing and turning over some problem knows how unpleasant the following day can be. Insomnia compromises well-being on the short term and quality of life on the long-term (Karlson, Gallagher, Olson, & Hamilton, 2013). Poor sleep can be a particular problem in certain high-risk occupations, such as police work, in which officers are exposed to traumatic events (Irish, Dougall, Delahanty, & Hall, 2013).

As noted, there are health risks of inadequate and poor quality sleep (Patterson, Malone, Lozano, Grandner, & Hanlon, 2016). Chronic insomnia can compromise the ability to secrete and respond to insulin (suggesting a link between sleep and diabetes); it increases the risk of coronary heart disease (Ekstedt, Åkerstedt, & Söderström, 2004); it can alter the structure and functioning of the heart (Lee et al., 2018) and it augments cardiovascular reactivity to stress (Brindle et al., 2018); it increases blood pressure and dysregulates stress physiology (Franzen et al., 2011); it can affect weight gain (Motivala, Tomiyama, Ziegler, Khandrika, & Irwin, 2009); it exacerbates pain and emotional responses to it (Gerhart, Burns, Post, Smith, & Porter, 2017), including lower back pain (Pinheiro et al., 2018); it can reduce the efficacy of flu shots; and it is tied to adverse immune changes including chronic inflammation (Park et al., 2016). More than 70,000 of the nation's annual automobile crashes are accounted for by sleepy drivers, and 1,550 of these are fatal each year. In one study of healthy older adults, sleep disturbances predicted all-cause mortality over the next 4 to 19 years

of follow-up (Dew et al., 2003). Children who do not get enough sleep may show behavioral problems (Pesonen et al., 2009). By contrast, good sleep quality can act as a stress buffer (Hamilton, Catley, & Karlson, 2007).

Who can't sleep? People who are going through or who have been through major stressful life events or traumas (Brindle et al., 2018a), who are suffering from depression (Bouwmans, Conradi, Bos, Oldehinkel, & de Jonge, 2017), who are experiencing stress at work (Burgard & Ailshire, 2009), who are experiencing socioeconomic adversity (Jarrin, McGrath, & Quon, 2014), who have high levels of hostility or arousal (Fernández-Mendoza et al., 2010; Granö, Vahtera, Virtanen, Keltikangas-Järvinen, & Kivimäki, 2008), who use maladaptive coping strategies to cope with stress (Fernández-Mendoza et al., 2010), and who ruminate on the causes of their stress (Zawadzki, Graham, & Gerin, 2012) have poor sleep quality and report sleep disturbances. Stressful events regarded as uncontrollable can produce insomnia (Morin, Rodrigue, & Ivers, 2003). People who deal with stressful events by ruminating or focusing on them are more prone to insomnia than are those who deal with stressful events by blunting their impact or distracting themselves (Fernández-Mendoza et al., 2010; Voss, Kolling, & Heidenreich, 2006; Zoccola, Dickerson, & Lam, 2009). Sleep may have particular significance for people low in SES, as low SES is linked to poor subjective and objective sleep quality (Friedman et al., 2007; Mezick et al., 2008). Abuse of alcohol is also related to poor sleep quality (Irwin, Cole, & Nicassio, 2006). People with good social support sleep well (de Grey, Uchino, Trettevik, Cronan, & Hogan, 2018).

Although the health risks of insufficient sleep are now well known, less well known is the fact that people who habitually sleep more than 7 hours every night also incur health risks (van den Berg et al., 2008a). Long sleepers, like short sleepers, also have more symptoms of psychopathology, including chronic worrying (Grandner & Kripke, 2004).

Behavioral interventions have been undertaken for the treatment of insomnia, including mindfulness-based interventions (Britton, Haynes, Fridel, & Bootzin, 2010), relaxation therapy, control of sleep-related behaviors (such as the routine a person engages in before going to sleep), and cognitive–behavioral interventions. All these treatments show some success in treating insomnia (Irwin et al., 2006). Other health-related outcomes can improve as well, such as increased heart

**TABLE 4.3 | A Good Night's Sleep**

- Get regular exercise, at least three times a week.
- Keep the bedroom cool at night.
- Sleep in a comfortable bed that is big enough.
- Establish a regular schedule for awakening and going to bed.
- Develop nightly rituals that can get you ready for bed, such as taking a shower.
- Use a fan or other noise generator to mask background sound.
- Don't consume too much alcohol and don't smoke.
- Don't eat too much or too little at night.
- Don't have strong smells in the room, such as from incense, candles, or lotions.
- Don't nap after 3 PM
- Cut back on caffeine, especially in the afternoon or evening.
- If awakened, get up and read quietly in another place, so that bed is associated with sleep, not sleeplessness.

*Sources:* Gorman, Christine. "Get Some Sleep." *Time,* March 29, 1999. http://content.time.com/time/magazine/article/0,9171,990567,00.html; Murphy, S. L. "Deaths: Final Data for 1998." *National Vital Statistics Reports* 28, no. 11 (July 24): 1–105.

rate variability and quality of life. Table 4.3 lists some of the recommendations used in interventions to promote better sleep.

# ■ REST, RENEWAL, SAVORING

An important set of health behaviors that is only beginning to be understood involves relaxation and renewal, the restorative activities that help people savor the positive aspects of life, reduce stress, and restore emotional balance (Pressman et al., 2009). For example, simply not taking a vacation is a risk factor for heart attack among people with heart disease (Gump & Matthews, 1998; Steptoe, Roy, & Evans, 1996). Participating in enjoyable leisure time activities, such as hobbies, sports, socializing, or spending time in nature, has been tied to lower blood pressure, lower cortisol, lower weight, and better physical functioning. Satisfaction with leisure activities can improve cognitive functioning among the elderly (Singh-Manoux, Richards, & Marmot, 2003; Steinberg, Christy, Batch, Askew, & Moore, 2017) and promote good health behaviors such as good sleep (Kim, Kubzansky, & Smith, 2015; Sin, Almeida, Crain, Kossek, & Berkman, 2017).

Unfortunately, little other than intuition currently guides our thinking about restorative processes. Nonetheless, health psychologists suspect that rest, renewal, and savoring—involving activities such as going home for the holidays, relaxing after exams, and enjoying a walk or a sunset—have health benefits. •

## SUMMARY

1. Health-enhancing behaviors are practiced by people to improve their current and future health. Such behaviors include exercise, accident prevention measures, cancer detection processes, consumption of a healthy diet, 7 to 8 hours of sleep each night, and opportunities for rest and renewal.

2. Exercise reduces risk for heart attack and improves other aspects of bodily functioning. Exercise also improves mood and reduces stress.

3. Few people adhere regularly to the standard exercise prescription of at least 30 minutes at least three times a week. People are more likely to exercise when the form of exercise is convenient and they like it, if their attitudes favor exercise, and if they come from families in which exercise is practiced.

4. Cognitive–behavioral interventions, including relapse prevention components, have been moderately successful in helping people adhere to regular exercise programs.

5. Accidents are a major cause of preventable death, especially among children and adolescents. Publicity in the mass media, legislation promoting accident prevention measures, training of parents by health practitioners, and interventions to promote safety measures for children have reduced these risks.

6. Mammograms are recommended for women over age 50, yet not enough women, especially minority and older women, undergo them because of lack of information, unrealistic fears, and the high cost and lack of availability of mammograms. Colorectal screening is also an important cancer-related health behavior.

7. Dietary interventions involving reductions in cholesterol, fats, calories, and additives and increases in fiber, fruits, and vegetables are widely recommended. Yet long-term adherence to such diets is limited for many reasons: Recommended diets are sometimes boring; tastes are hard to change; and behavior change often falls off over time.

8. Dietary interventions through the mass media and community resources have promise. Intervening with the family is also helpful in promoting and maintaining dietary change. Cognitive–behavioral therapeutic interventions have been successfully employed to alter diet, although recent interventions have moved to less costly formats, such as telephone interventions.

9. Sufficient sleep, rest renewal, and relaxation are also important health behaviors. Many people abuse their sleep intentionally or suffer from insomnia. A variety of behavioral methods that promote relaxation can offset these risks. In addition, setting aside time to savor the pleasant aspects of life and simply taking a vacation may have health benefits.

## KEY TERM

aerobic exercise

CHAPTER 5

# Health-Compromising Behaviors

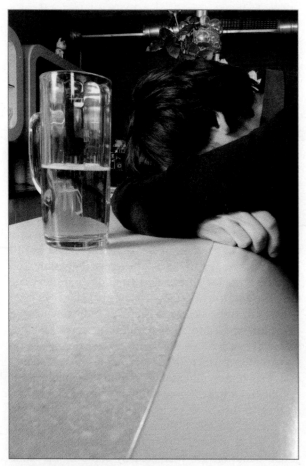

Clandestini/Getty Images

CHAPTER OUTLINE

**Characteristics of Health-Compromising Behaviors**
**Marijuana Use**

**Obesity**
   *What Is Obesity?*
   *Obesity in Childhood*
   *SES, Culture, and Obesity*
   *Obesity and Dieting as Risk Factors for Obesity*
   *Stress and Eating*
   *Interventions*
   *Cognitive–Behavioral Therapy (CBT)*
   *Evaluation of Cognitive–Behavioral Weight-Loss Techniques*
   *Taking a Public Health Approach*
**Eating Disorders**
   *Anorexia Nervosa*
   *Bulimia*
   *Binge Eating Disorder*
**Alcoholism and Problem Drinking**
   *The Scope of the Problem*
   *What Is Substance Dependence?*
   *Alcoholism and Problem Drinking*
   *Origins of Alcoholism and Problem Drinking*
   *Treatment of Alcohol Abuse*
   *Treatment Programs*
   *Evaluation of Alcohol Treatment Programs*
   *Preventive Approaches to Alcohol Abuse*
   *Drinking and Driving*
   *Is Modest Alcohol Consumption a Health Behavior?*
**Smoking**
   *Synergistic Effects of Smoking*
   *A Brief History of the Smoking Problem*
   *Why Do People Smoke?*
   *Nicotine Addiction and Smoking*
   *Interventions to Reduce Smoking*
   *Smoking Prevention Programs*

83

Some years back, my (S.E.T.) father went for his annual physical examination, and his doctor told him, as the doctor did each year, that he had to stop smoking. As usual, my father told his doctor that he would stop when he was ready. He had already tried several times and had been unsuccessful. My father had begun smoking at age 14, long before the health risks of smoking were known, and it was now an integrated part of his lifestyle, which included a couple of cocktails before a dinner high in fat and cholesterol and a hectic life with few opportunities for regular exercise. Smoking was part of who he was. His doctor then said, "Let me put it this way. If you expect to see your daughter graduate from college, stop smoking *now.*"

That warning did the trick. My father threw his cigarettes in the wastebasket and never had another one. Over the years, as he read more about health, he began to change his lifestyle in other ways. He began to swim regularly for exercise, and he pared down his diet to one of mostly fish, chicken, vegetables, fruit, and cereal. Despite the fact that he once had many of the risk factors for early heart disease, he lived to age 83.

## ■ CHARACTERISTICS OF HEALTH-COMPROMISING BEHAVIORS

In this chapter, we address health-compromising behaviors—behaviors practiced by people that undermine or harm their current or future health. My father's problems with stopping smoking illustrate several important points about these behaviors. Many health-compromising behaviors are habitual, and several, including smoking, are addictive, making them very difficult habits to break. On the other hand, with proper interventions, even the most intractable health habit can be modified. When a person succeeds in changing a poor health behavior, often he or she will make other healthy lifestyle changes. The end result is that risk declines, and a disease-free middle and old age becomes a possibility.

Many health-compromising behaviors share several additional important characteristics. First, there is a window of vulnerability in adolescence. Behaviors such as drinking to excess, smoking, using illicit drugs, practicing unsafe sex, and taking risks that can lead to accidents or early death all begin in early adolescence and sometimes cluster together as part of a problem behavior syndrome (Donovan & Jessor, 1985; Lam,

Stewart, & Ho, 2001). In the past, adolescent boys were more at risk of falling into these patterns, but girls are catching up (Mahalik et al., 2013). Not all health-compromising behaviors develop during adolescence; obesity, for example, can begin early in childhood. Nonetheless, there is an unnerving similarity in the factors that elicit and maintain many health-compromising behaviors.

Many of these behaviors are tied to the peer culture, as children learn from and imitate their peers, especially the male peers they like and admire (Long, Barrett, & Lockhart, 2017). Wanting to be attractive to others becomes very important in adolescence, and this factor is significant in the development of eating disorders, alcohol consumption, tobacco and drug use, tanning, unsafe sexual encounters, and vulnerability to injury (Shadel, Niaura, & Abrams, 2004). Exposure to peers' risky behavior, such as unsafe driving, increases risk-taking (Simons-Morton et al., 2014).

Many of these behaviors are pleasurable, enhancing the adolescent's ability to cope with stressful situations, and some represent thrill seeking, which can be rewarding in its own right. However, each of these behaviors is also dangerous. Each has been tied to at least one major cause of death, and several, especially smoking and obesity, are risk factors for more than one major chronic disease. Adolescents who slip into these patterns are less likely to practice good health habits and use leisure time for exercise in midlife, setting the stage for an unhealthy middle and older age (Wichstrøm, von Soest, & Kvalem, 2013).

Third, these behaviors develop gradually, as the person is exposed to the behavior, experiments with it, and later engages in it regularly. As such, many health-compromising behaviors are acquired through a process that makes different interventions important at the different stages of vulnerability, experimentation, and regular use.

Fourth, substance abuse of all kinds, whether cigarettes, food, alcohol, drugs, or health-compromising sexual behavior, are predicted by some of the same factors (Peltzer, 2010). Adolescents who get involved in risky behaviors often have conflict with their parents (Cooper, Wood, Orcutt, & Albino, 2003). Adolescents with a penchant for deviant behavior and with low self-esteem also show these behaviors (Duncan, Duncan, Strycker, & Chaumeton, 2002). Adolescents who try to combine long hours of employment with school have an increased risk of alcohol, cigarette, and marijuana abuse (Johnson, 2004). Adolescents who abuse substances typically do poorly in school; family problems, deviance, and low self-esteem appear to explain this relationship (Andrews & Duncan, 1997). Reaching puberty early (van Jaarsveld, Fidler, Simon, & Wardle, 2007) and having a low IQ, a difficult temperament, and deviance-tolerant attitudes predict poor health behaviors (Repetti, Taylor, & Seeman, 2002). Good self-control diminishes and poor self-regulation facilitates vulnerability to illicit substance use (Wills et al., 2013). But co-occurring mental health disorders, such as depression or anxiety, may fuel these problem behaviors and make them harder to treat (Vannucci et al., 2014).

A particular dilemma is that many of these behaviors—drinking or cigarette smoking, for example—may start out as experiments but smoking, drugs, excessive alcohol consumption, and compulsive eating can become addictions. There may be common underlying brain pathways for all these seemingly different behaviors, especially the circuitry that controls reward and pleasure/pain (Salamone & Correa, 2013; Smith & Robbins, 2013; Stice, Yokum, & Burger, 2013).

Finally, problem behaviors, including obesity, smoking, and alcoholism, are more common in the lower social classes (Fradklin et al., 2015). Lower-class children and adolescents are exposed more to problem behaviors and may use these behaviors to cope with the stressors of low social class (Novak, Ahlgren, & Hammarstrom, 2007). Practice of these health-compromising behaviors are one reason that social class is so strongly related to most causes of disease and death (Adler & Stewart, 2010).

## ■ MARIJUANA USE

Is marijuana use a health-compromising behavior (National Institute on Drug Abuse, 2018)?

Drug use is a major issue in the United States. Heroin (and other opioids) and cocaine, for example, can all lead to overdoses and death.

Marijuana is the most popular recreational drug, with over 94 million people admitting to using it at least once, and 22 million of them in the past month. Adolescent and young adult men are particularly likely to have used it.

Euphoria, relaxation, heightened sensory perceptions, altered time perception, and increased appetite are among the common effects, but other experiences are less positive including anxiety, fear, paranoia, or panic; these negative side effects are especially likely if the marijuana is high in potency or the person using it is inexperienced.

Is marijuana addictive? Some users develop a dependency even though it interferes with daily activities. About 4 million users fall into this category and are adversely affected over the long term.

Among men in their 20s from low-income backgrounds, frequent, escalating use of marijuana has been linked to changes in brain neural circuitry; specifically changes in communication between key brain regions that affect motivation and mood have been found, as well as poorer cognitive functioning, lower educational achievement and higher risk for depression (Sarlin, 2018). Whether these changes are permanent is still under investigation.

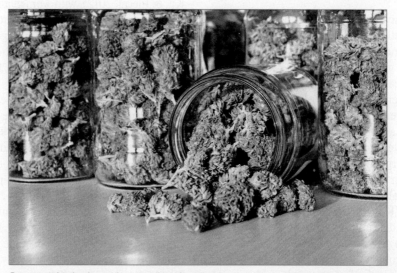

*Dry cannabis buds can be stored in glass jars.*
Soru Epotok/Shutterstock

**TABLE 5.1 | Body Mass Index Table**

| | Normal | | | | | | Overweight | | | | | Obese | | | | | |
|---|---|---|---|---|---|---|---|---|---|---|---|---|---|---|---|---|---|
| BMI | 19 | 20 | 21 | 22 | 23 | 24 | 25 | 26 | 27 | 28 | 29 | 30 | 31 | 32 | 33 | 34 | 35 |
| Height (inches) | Body Weight (pounds) | | | | | | | | | | | | | | | | |
| 58 | 91 | 96 | 100 | 105 | 110 | 115 | 119 | 124 | 129 | 134 | 138 | 143 | 148 | 153 | 158 | 162 | 167 |
| 59 | 94 | 99 | 104 | 109 | 114 | 119 | 124 | 128 | 133 | 138 | 143 | 148 | 153 | 158 | 163 | 168 | 173 |
| 60 | 97 | 102 | 107 | 112 | 118 | 123 | 128 | 133 | 138 | 143 | 148 | 153 | 158 | 163 | 168 | 174 | 179 |
| 61 | 100 | 106 | 111 | 116 | 122 | 127 | 132 | 137 | 143 | 148 | 153 | 158 | 164 | 169 | 174 | 180 | 185 |
| 62 | 104 | 109 | 115 | 120 | 126 | 131 | 136 | 142 | 147 | 153 | 158 | 164 | 169 | 175 | 180 | 186 | 191 |
| 63 | 107 | 113 | 118 | 124 | 130 | 135 | 141 | 146 | 152 | 158 | 163 | 169 | 175 | 180 | 186 | 191 | 197 |
| 64 | 110 | 116 | 122 | 128 | 134 | 140 | 145 | 151 | 157 | 163 | 169 | 174 | 180 | 186 | 192 | 197 | 204 |
| 65 | 114 | 120 | 126 | 132 | 138 | 144 | 150 | 156 | 162 | 168 | 174 | 180 | 186 | 192 | 198 | 204 | 210 |
| 66 | 118 | 124 | 130 | 136 | 142 | 148 | 155 | 161 | 167 | 173 | 179 | 186 | 192 | 198 | 204 | 210 | 216 |
| 67 | 121 | 127 | 134 | 140 | 146 | 153 | 159 | 166 | 172 | 178 | 185 | 191 | 198 | 204 | 211 | 217 | 223 |
| 68 | 125 | 131 | 138 | 144 | 151 | 158 | 164 | 171 | 177 | 184 | 190 | 197 | 203 | 210 | 216 | 223 | 230 |
| 69 | 128 | 135 | 142 | 149 | 155 | 162 | 169 | 176 | 182 | 189 | 196 | 203 | 209 | 216 | 223 | 230 | 236 |
| 70 | 132 | 139 | 146 | 153 | 160 | 167 | 174 | 181 | 188 | 195 | 202 | 209 | 216 | 222 | 229 | 236 | 243 |
| 71 | 136 | 143 | 150 | 157 | 165 | 172 | 179 | 186 | 193 | 200 | 208 | 215 | 222 | 229 | 236 | 243 | 250 |
| 72 | 140 | 147 | 154 | 162 | 169 | 177 | 184 | 191 | 199 | 206 | 213 | 221 | 228 | 235 | 242 | 250 | 258 |
| 73 | 144 | 151 | 159 | 166 | 174 | 182 | 189 | 197 | 204 | 212 | 219 | 227 | 235 | 242 | 250 | 257 | 265 |
| 74 | 148 | 155 | 163 | 171 | 179 | 186 | 194 | 202 | 210 | 218 | 225 | 233 | 241 | 249 | 256 | 264 | 272 |
| 75 | 152 | 160 | 168 | 176 | 184 | 192 | 200 | 208 | 216 | 224 | 232 | 240 | 248 | 256 | 264 | 272 | 279 |
| 76 | 156 | 164 | 172 | 180 | 189 | 197 | 205 | 213 | 221 | 230 | 238 | 246 | 254 | 263 | 271 | 279 | 287 |

*Source:* U.S. Department of Health & Human Services and National Heart, Lung, and Blood Institute. "Aim for a Healthy Weight. Body Mass Index Table 1." Accessed June 27, 2019. https://www.nhlbi.nih.gov/health/educational/lose_wt/BMI/bmi_tbl.htm.

# ■ OBESITY

## What Is Obesity?

**Obesity** is an excessive accumulation of body fat. Generally, fat should constitute about 20 to 27 percent of body tissue in women and about 15 to 22 percent in men. Table 5.1 presents guidelines from the National Institutes of Health for calculating your body mass index and determining whether you are overweight or obese.

The World Health Organization estimates that 650 million people worldwide are obese and 1.9 billion are overweight, including 41 million children under age 5 (World Health Organization, January 2018). Obesity is now so common that it has replaced malnutrition as the most prevalent dietary contributor to poor health worldwide (Kopelman, 2000), and it will soon account for more diseases and deaths in the United States than smoking.

The obesity problem is most severe in the United States. Americans are the fattest people in the world. At present, 68 percent of the adult U.S. population is overweight, and about 40 percent is obese (Centers for Disease Control and Prevention, 2017; Ogden, Carroll, Kit, & Flegal, 2012), with women and older adults somewhat more likely to be overweight or obese than men and younger adults (Fakhouri, Ogden, Carroll, Kit, & Flegal, 2012) (Figure 5.1). Although obesity levels have begun to level off, the trend has not yet reversed (Kaplan, 2014).

There is no mystery why people in the United States have become so heavy. The average American's food intake rose from 1,826 calories a day in the 1970s to more than 2,000 by the mid-1990s (O'Connor, 2004, February 6). Soda consumption has skyrocketed from 22.2 gallons to 56 gallons per person per year (Ervin, Kit, Carroll, & Ogden, 2012). Portion sizes at meals have increased substantially over the past 20 years (Nielsen & Popkin, 2003). Muffins that weighed 1.5 ounces in 1957 now average half a pound each (Raeburn, Forster, Foust, & Brady, 2002, October 21). Snacking has increased more than 60 percent over the last three decades (Critser, 2003), and easy access to

| Obese | | | | Extreme Obesity | | | | | | | | | | | | | | |
| 36 | 37 | 38 | 39 | 40 | 41 | 42 | 43 | 44 | 45 | 46 | 47 | 48 | 49 | 50 | 51 | 52 | 53 | 54 |
|---|---|---|---|---|---|---|---|---|---|---|---|---|---|---|---|---|---|---|
| Body Weight (pounds) | | | | | | | | | | | | | | | | | | |
| 172 | 177 | 181 | 186 | 191 | 196 | 201 | 205 | 210 | 215 | 220 | 224 | 229 | 234 | 239 | 244 | 248 | 253 | 258 |
| 178 | 183 | 188 | 193 | 198 | 203 | 208 | 212 | 217 | 222 | 227 | 232 | 237 | 242 | 247 | 252 | 257 | 262 | 267 |
| 184 | 189 | 194 | 199 | 204 | 209 | 215 | 220 | 225 | 230 | 235 | 240 | 245 | 250 | 255 | 261 | 266 | 271 | 276 |
| 190 | 195 | 201 | 206 | 211 | 217 | 222 | 227 | 232 | 238 | 243 | 248 | 254 | 259 | 264 | 269 | 275 | 280 | 285 |
| 196 | 202 | 207 | 213 | 218 | 224 | 229 | 235 | 240 | 246 | 251 | 256 | 262 | 267 | 273 | 278 | 284 | 289 | 295 |
| 203 | 208 | 214 | 220 | 225 | 231 | 237 | 242 | 248 | 254 | 259 | 265 | 270 | 278 | 282 | 287 | 293 | 299 | 304 |
| 209 | 215 | 221 | 227 | 232 | 238 | 244 | 250 | 256 | 262 | 267 | 273 | 279 | 285 | 291 | 296 | 302 | 308 | 314 |
| 216 | 222 | 228 | 234 | 240 | 246 | 252 | 258 | 264 | 270 | 276 | 282 | 288 | 294 | 300 | 306 | 312 | 318 | 324 |
| 223 | 229 | 235 | 241 | 247 | 253 | 260 | 266 | 272 | 278 | 284 | 291 | 297 | 303 | 309 | 315 | 322 | 328 | 334 |
| 230 | 236 | 242 | 249 | 255 | 261 | 268 | 274 | 280 | 287 | 293 | 299 | 306 | 312 | 319 | 325 | 331 | 338 | 344 |
| 236 | 243 | 249 | 256 | 262 | 269 | 276 | 282 | 289 | 295 | 302 | 308 | 315 | 322 | 328 | 335 | 341 | 348 | 354 |
| 243 | 250 | 257 | 263 | 270 | 277 | 284 | 291 | 297 | 304 | 311 | 318 | 324 | 331 | 338 | 345 | 351 | 358 | 365 |
| 250 | 257 | 264 | 271 | 278 | 285 | 292 | 299 | 306 | 313 | 320 | 327 | 334 | 341 | 348 | 355 | 362 | 369 | 376 |
| 257 | 265 | 272 | 279 | 286 | 293 | 301 | 308 | 315 | 322 | 329 | 338 | 343 | 351 | 358 | 365 | 372 | 379 | 386 |
| 265 | 272 | 279 | 287 | 294 | 302 | 309 | 316 | 324 | 331 | 338 | 346 | 353 | 361 | 368 | 375 | 383 | 390 | 397 |
| 272 | 280 | 288 | 295 | 302 | 310 | 318 | 325 | 333 | 340 | 348 | 355 | 363 | 371 | 378 | 386 | 393 | 401 | 408 |
| 280 | 287 | 295 | 303 | 311 | 319 | 326 | 334 | 342 | 350 | 358 | 365 | 373 | 381 | 389 | 396 | 404 | 412 | 420 |
| 287 | 295 | 303 | 311 | 319 | 327 | 335 | 343 | 351 | 359 | 367 | 375 | 383 | 391 | 399 | 407 | 415 | 423 | 431 |
| 295 | 304 | 312 | 320 | 328 | 336 | 344 | 353 | 361 | 369 | 377 | 385 | 394 | 402 | 410 | 418 | 426 | 435 | 443 |

food through microwave ovens and fast-food restaurants contributes to the increase. The average American weight gain over the past 20 years is the caloric equivalent of only three Oreo cookies or one can of soda a day (Critser, 2003), so it does not take vast quantities of food or sugary drinks to gain weight.

Risks of Obesity   Obesity is a risk factor for many disorders. It contributes to death rates for all cancers and for the specific cancers of the colon, rectum, liver, gallbladder, pancreas, kidney, and esophagus, as well as non-Hodgkin's lymphoma and multiple myeloma. Estimates are that excess weight may account for 14 percent of all deaths from cancer in men and 20 percent of all deaths from cancer in women (Calle, Rodriguez, Walker-Thurmond, & Thun, 2003). Obesity also contributes substantially to deaths from cardiovascular disease (Flegal, Graubard, Williamson, & Gail, 2007), and it is tied to atherosclerosis, hypertension, type 2 diabetes, and heart failure (Kerns, Rosenberg, & Otis, 2002). Obesity increases risks in surgery, anesthesia administration, and childbearing (Brownell & Wadden, 1992). It has been tied to poorer cognitive skills as early as adolescence, well in advance of any diagnosable chronic health condition (Hawkins, Gunstad, Calvo, & Spitznagel, 2016).

Obesity is a chief cause of disability. The number of people age 30 to 49 who are too heavy to care for themselves or perform routine household tasks has jumped by 50 percent. This increase bodes poorly for the future. People who are disabled in their 30s and 40s are more likely to have health care expenses and to need nursing home care in older age, if they live that long (Richardson, 2004, January 9). Being obese also reduces the likelihood that a person will exercise, and lack of exercise increases obesity, yet obesity and lack of exercise appear to exert independent adverse effects on health, leading to greater risks than either risk factor alone (Hu et al., 2004). One in four people over 50 is obese, and as the population ages, the numbers of people who will have difficulty performing the basic tasks of daily living, such as bathing, dressing,

**FIGURE 5.1** | **Percentage of Obese Adults**    Obese adults have a BMI greater than or equal to 30.

Source. U.S. Department of Health & Human Services and Centers for Disease Control and Prevention. "Prevalence of Obesity among Adults and Youth: United States, 2015–2016." Accessed June 27, 2019. https://www.cdc.gov/nchs/data/databriefs/db288.pdf.

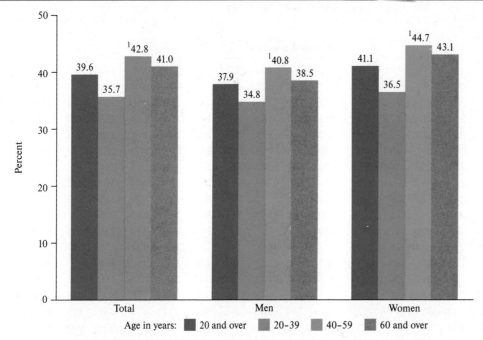

[1]Significantly different from those aged 20–39.
NOTES: Estimates for adults aged 20 and over were age adjusted by the direct method to the 2000 U.S. census population using the age groups 20–39, 40–59, and 60 and over. Crude estimates are 39.8% for total, 38.0% for men, and 41.5% for women.
Access data table for Figure 1 at: https://www.cdc.gov/nchs/data/databriefs/db288_table.pdf#1.
SOURCE: NCHS, National Health and Nutrition Examination Survey, 2015-2016.

or even walking, will be substantial (Facts of Life, December, 2004).

Obesity is associated with early mortality (Adams et al., 2006). People who are overweight at age 40 die, on average, 3 years earlier than people who are thin (Peeters et al., 2003). Abdominally localized fat, as opposed to excessive fat in the hips, buttocks, or thighs, is an especially potent risk factor for cardiovascular disease, diabetes, hypertension, cancer, and decline in cognitive function (Dore, Elias, Robbins, Budge, & Elias, 2008). People with excessive abdominal weight (sometimes called "apples," in contrast to "pears," who carry their weight on their hips) are more psychologically and physiologically reactive to stress (Epel et al., 2000). Fat tissue produces proinflammatory cytokines, which may exacerbate diseases related to inflammatory processes (see Chapter 2). Box 5.1 explores the biological regulation more fully.

Often ignored among the risks of obesity is the psychological distress that can result. Although there

is a robust stereotype of overweight people as "jolly," studies suggest that the obese are prone to neuroticism and psychiatric conditions, especially depression (Sutin et al., 2013; Toups et al., 2013), perhaps in part because other stereotypes of the obese are negative and unkind.

There are social and economic consequences of obesity as well. An obese person may have to pay for two seats on an airplane, have difficulty finding clothes, endure derision and rude comments, and experience other reminders that the obese, quite literally, do not fit. Obesity is stigmatized as a disability whose fault lies squarely with the obese person (Mata & Hertwig, 2018). Even health care providers may hold these stereotypes. One woman reported that her physician told her she was too fat for a proper exam and to come back when she'd lost 50 pounds (Center for the Advancement of Health, 2008). Obese people are perceived to be unattractive and insecure, and so people keep their distance. **Weight stigma** may actually undermine

All animals, including humans, have sensitive and complex systems for regulating food. Taste has been called the chemical gatekeeper of eating. It is an ancient sensory system and plays a role in selecting certain foods and rejecting others.

An important player in weight control is the protein leptin, which is secreted by fat cells. Leptin signals the neurons of the hypothalamus whether the body has sufficient energy stores of fat or whether it needs additional energy. The brain's eating control center reacts to the signals sent from the hypothalamus to increase or decrease appetite. Leptin inhibits the neurons that stimulate appetite and activates those that suppress appetite. As such, it holds promise as a target for interventions (Morton, Cummings, Baskin, Barsh, & Schwartz, 2006).

Ghrelin may play a role in why dieters who lose weight often gain it back so quickly. Ghrelin is secreted by specialized cells in the stomach, spiking just before meals and dropping afterward. When people are given ghrelin injections, they feel extremely hungry. Therefore, blocking ghrelin levels or the action of ghrelin may help people lose weight and keep it off (Grady, 2002, May 23).

weight loss efforts (Puhl, Quinn, Weisz, & Suh, 2017). The resulting effect of repeated exposure to others' judgments about their weight can be heightened biological responses to stress (Tomiyama et al., 2014), social alienation, and low self-esteem (Himmelstein, Puhl, & Quinn, 2018). The perception of weight stigma and weight discrimination can contribute to mental and physical health risks over time (Rodriguez et al., 2017). As a result, obese people sometimes become reclusive, and one consequence is that diabetes, heart disease, and other complications of obesity may be far advanced by the time they seek a physician. Positive media portrayals of overweight and obese people can go some distance to mitigate the stigma (Brochu, Pearl, Puhl, & Brownell, 2014). Imagining contact with a counter-stereotype obese person, namely one who is attractive, confident, and appealing may help counter the stereotypes that can plague interactions between obese and nonobese people (Dunaev, Brochu, & Markey, 2018).

## Obesity in Childhood

In the United States, approximately 42 million children under 5 are overweight or obese (World Health Organization, 2016). Nearly two-thirds of overweight and obese children already have risk factors for cardiovascular disease, such as elevated blood pressure, elevated lipid levels, or hyperinsulemia (Sinha et al., 2002). African American and Hispanic children and adolescents are at particular risk. For the first time in over 200 years, the current generation of children has a shorter life expectancy than their parents due to high rates of obesity (Belluck, 2005, March 17).

What causes the high rates of obesity in childhood? There are genetic contributors to obesity, the knowledge of which may eventually contribute to treatment (McCaffery, 2018). Genetic risks may combine with risks conferred by low socioeconomic status (SES), increasing overall risk to be obese (Dinescu, Horn, Duncan, & Turkheimer, 2016). The impact of genetics on weight may be exerted in part by a vigorous feeding style that is evident early in life. There are also genetically based tendencies to store energy as fat rather than lean tissue. Another important factor is sedentary lifestyles, involving television, video games, and the Internet. Consumption of snacks and sugary drinks during the sedentary activities greatly increases the risks associated with obesity (Ervin & Ogden, 2013). Sugary drinks alone have been tied to 25,000 deaths per year in the United States and 180,000 worldwide in adulthood, due to a practice that typically begins in childhood (Healy, July 15, 2015).

Adverse social relationships in childhood, including being bullied, are related to higher body mass index into adulthood (Baldwin et al., 2016; Elsenburg et al., 2017). These long-term changes appear to result from patterns of gene activation (Loucks et al., 2016).

Children are less likely to be obese if they participate in organized sports or physical activity, but obese children may come from families that do not value or do not have access to exercise facilities (Kozo et al., 2012; Veitch et al., 2011). Too much television time can also contribute to obesity (Grummon, Vaughn, Jones, & Ward, 2017). Children who take in too many

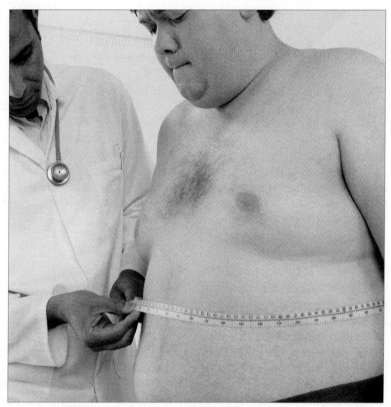

*More than one-third of the adult population in the United States is overweight, putting them at risk for heart disease, kidney disease, hypertension, diabetes, and other health problems.*

Adam Gault/Science Source

calories in infancy and childhood are more likely to become obese adults (Kuhl et al., 2014). Even the family dog is more likely to be overweight in families that have large portion sizes and low activity levels. By contrast, positive parenting can mitigate poorly controlled eating in children (Connell & Francis, 2014). Figure 5.2 illustrates the high rates of obesity among children.

Obesity depends on both the number and the size of an individual's fat cells. Among moderately obese people, fat cells are typically large, but there is not an unusually large number of them. Among the severely obese, there are a large number of fat cells, and the fat cells themselves are exceptionally large (Brownell, 1982). Childhood constitutes a window of vulnerability for obesity because the number of fat cells a person has is typically determined in the first few years of life, by genetic factors and by early eating habits (Wilfley, Hayes, Balantekin, Van Buren, & Epstein, 2018).

## SES, Culture, and Obesity

Additional risk factors for obesity include social class and culture (Gallo et al., 2012). In the United States, women of low SES are heavier than high-SES women, and African American women, in particular, are more likely to be obese (Ogden, Lamb, Carroll, & Flegal, 2010). For reasons that remain unclear, the prevalence of obesity among men is not related to SES. Obesity, thus, may be part of the accumulating disadvantage that women of low SES experience over the lifespan (Zajacova & Burgard, 2010). Values are implicated in obesity. Thinness is valued in women from high-SES levels in developed countries, which in turn leads to a cultural emphasis on weight control and physical activity (Wardle et al., 2004). Weight stigma targeted at obese people can lead to rude comments and mistreatment, adding to the anxiety and depression that obese people can feel.

**FIGURE 5.2 | Percentage of Obese Youth**   Obesity in youth is a BMI of greater than or equal to the age- and sex-specific 95th percentile growth chart.

Source: U.S. Department of Health & Human Services and Centers for Disease Control and Prevention. "Prevalence of Obesity among Adults and Youth: United States, 2015–2016." Accessed June 27, 2019. https://www.cdc.gov/nchs/data/databriefs/db288.pdf.

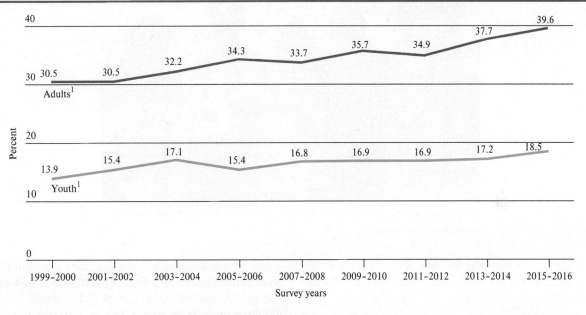

[1]Significant increasing linear trend from 1999-2000 through 2015-2016.
NOTES: All estimates for adults are age adjusted by the direct method to the 2000 U.S. census population using the age groups 20-39, 40-59, and 60 and over. Access data table for Figure 5 at: https://www.cdc.gov/nchs/data/databriefs/db288_table.pdf#5.
SOURCE: NCHS, National Health and Nutrition Examination Survey, 1999-2016.

Depression, stress (Mason et al., 2019), and weight gain are linked (Olive, Telford, Byrne, Abhayaratna, & Telford, 2017). Depression in mothers has been tied to a higher likelihood of obesity in their teenage children (Marmorstein & Iacono, 2016). People who are depressed are more likely to gain weight, and people who are obese or overweight are more likely to be depressed (Kubzansky, Gilthorpe, & Goodman, 2012; van Reedt Dortland, Giltay, van Veen, Zitman, & Penninx, 2013). Anxiety can also play a role, especially in adolescence (Roberts & Duong, 2016). Perceived discrimination against obese people may partly explain this relationship (Robinson, Sutin, & Daly, 2017). People who are high in neuroticism, extraversion, and impulsivity and low in conscientiousness are more likely to be obese (Sutin, Ferrucci, Zonderman, & Terracciano, 2011).

Obesity spreads through social networks, almost like an epidemic. A person's chances of becoming obese increase substantially when he or she has a friend, sibling, or partner who has become obese. It may be that obesity changes the social norms associated with obesity, making it more acceptable to become obese (Christakis & Fowler, 2007). Most people seem unaware of the social influences on their eating (Spanos, Vartanian, Herman, & Polivy, 2014).

## Obesity and Dieting as Risk Factors for Obesity

Obesity is a risk factor for becoming even more so. Many obese people have a high basal insulin level, which promotes overeating due to increased hunger. Moreover, the obese have large fat cells, which have a greater capacity for producing and storing fat than do small fat cells.

Dieting contributes to the propensity for obesity. Successive cycles of dieting and weight gain, so-called **yo-yo dieting,** enhance the efficiency of food use and lower the metabolic rate (Robinson, Sutin, & Daly, 2018). When dieters begin to eat normally again, their

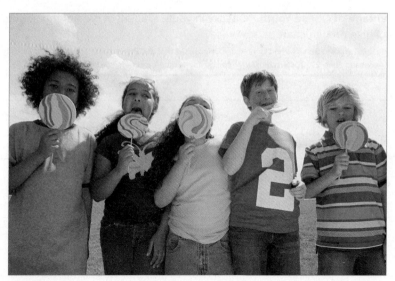

*Obesity in childhood is one of the fastest growing health concerns in the United States.*
Image Source/Getty Images

metabolic rate may stay low, and it can become easier for them to put on weight again even though they eat less food.

Set Point Theory of Weight    Evidence has accumulated for a **set point theory of weight:** the idea that each individual has an ideal biological weight, which cannot be greatly modified (Garner & Wooley, 1991). According to the theory, the set point acts like a thermostat regulating heat in a home. A person eats if his or her weight gets too low and stops eating as the weight reaches its ideal point. Some people have a higher set point than others, leading to a risk for obesity (Brownell, 1982). The theory argues that efforts to lose weight may be compensated for by adjustments in energy expenditure, as the body actively attempts to return to its original weight. This theory applies to obese people too. Once obesity is established, it is often stamped in, and the body will defend against efforts to lose weight (Healy, 2015).

Stress and Eating

Stress affects eating (Cotter & Kelly, 2018), although in different ways for different people. About half of people eat more when they are under stress, and half eat less (Willenbring, Levine, & Morley, 1986). For non-dieting and nonobese normal eaters, stress or anxiety may suppress physiological cues of hunger, leading to lower consumption of food. For overweight and obese people, however, stress and anxiety can disinhibit food consumption, removing the self-control that usually guards against eating (Sinha & Jastreboff, 2013). Whereas men tend to eat less in stressful circumstances, many women eat more (Grunberg & Straub, 1992). Stress also influences what food is consumed. People who eat in response to stress usually consume more low-calorie and salty foods, although when not under stress, stress eaters show a preference for high-calorie foods (Willenbring et al., 1986).

Anxiety and depression figure into **stress eating** as well. One study found that stress eaters experience greater fluctuations in anxiety and depression than do nonstress eaters. Overweight people also have greater fluctuations in anxiety, hostility, and depression than do normal-weight individuals (Lingsweiler, Crowther, & Stephens, 1987), and this pattern predicts variability in weight (Pacanowski et al., 2018). People who eat in response to negative emotions show a preference for sweet and high-fat foods (Oliver, Wardle, & Gibson, 2000). These "comfort foods," however, do not actually lift moods (Wagner, Ahlstrom, Redden, Vickers, & Mann, 2014).

Interventions

More people are treated for obesity in the United States than for all other health habits or conditions combined. More than half a million people attend weight-loss clinics, and Amazon.com lists more than

Nearly half of all adults in the United States are trying to lose weight at any given time, and the most popular way is through dieting. Although dieting (or caloric restriction) leads to weight loss on the short term, over the long term, most people gain back at least as much or more weight that they lost when they were dieting. Why would dieting have exactly the opposite of its intended effects?

Health psychologist Janet Tomiyama and her colleagues set out to answer this question (Tomiyama et al., 2010). Their hypothesis was that diets fail because they increase stress and levels of the stress hormone cortisol. Both of these factors can cause weight gain. Tomiyama reasoned that the stress of monitoring one's caloric intake and restricting food consumption enhances stress and cortisol production, leading to the unexpected and paradoxical effect that dieting leads to more weight gain.

In their study, 121 young women who wanted to lose weight were assigned to one of four dieting interventions for 3 weeks. They were told either to monitor their diet (or not) and/or to restrict their calories (or not). Tomiyama provided all of the dieters with prepared food, so that everybody consumed the same number of calories.

The results showed that the women who restricted their calories (the dieters) had higher cortisol levels, and monitoring calories increased perceived stress. Thus, dieting seems to harm both psychological well-being and

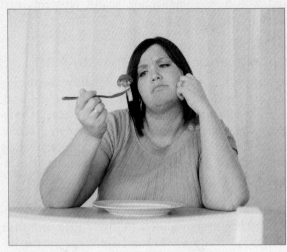

Vstock/UpperCut Images/Getty Images

biological functioning. The stress of dieting may be one reason why diets usually fail.

If dieting does not work, what will? The answer is lifestyle change. Rather than restricting calories, changing one's diet permanently in a way that involves more fruits and vegetables, less starch (white bread, dinner rolls), and smaller portions, coupled with regular exercise will lead to sustainable weight loss. Adding exercise also helps people take off extra weight and keep it off.

---

150,000 book titles that refer to diet or dieting. However, obesity is a very difficult condition to treat. Even initially successful weight-loss programs show high rates of relapse.

Dieting    Most weight-loss programs begin with dietary treatment. People are trained to restrict their caloric and/or carbohydrate intake. Knowledge of the nutritional qualities of food, termed nutritional literacy, is important in this stage (Rosenbaum, Clark, Convertino, Call, & Forman, 2018). In some cases, food may be provided to the dieters to ensure that the appropriate foods are being consumed. Generally, weight loss produced through dietary methods is small and rarely maintained for long (Agras et al., 1996). In fact, as Box 5.2 shows, dieting has risks. Very low-carbohydrate or low-fat diets do the best job in helping people lose weight initially, but these diets are the hardest to maintain, and people commonly revert to their old habits. Reducing caloric intake,

increasing exercise, and sticking with an eating plan over the long term are the only factors reliably related to staying slim. Beginning as early as preschool, these are the best ways to tackle obesity (Kuhl et al., 2014).

Surgery    Surgical procedures represent a radical way of controlling extreme obesity. In one common surgical procedure, the stomach is literally stapled up to reduce its capacity to hold food, so that the overweight individual must restrict his or her intake. Psychiatric problems may also decline along with weight (Kalarchian et al., 2016). In another approach known as lap band surgery, an adjustable gastric band is inserted surgically around the top of the stomach to create a small pouch in the upper stomach to reduce the stomach's capacity to take in food. As with all surgeries, there are potential side effects such as gastric and intestinal distress. Consequently, this procedure is usually reserved for people who are at least 100 percent overweight, who have failed repeatedly to lose weight through other methods, and who have complicating health problems that make weight loss urgent.

## Cognitive–Behavioral Therapy (CBT)

Researchers now believe that compulsive overeating that can lead to obesity shares the same brain circuitry as other addictive disorders, making it a difficult problem to treat, like smoking or drug addiction (Volkow, Wang, Tomasi & Baler, 2013). Many interventions with obese people use CBT to combat maladaptive eating behavior.

**Screening**    Some programs begin by screening applicants for their readiness to lose weight and their motivation to do so. Unsuccessful prior dieting attempts, weight lost and regained, high body dissatisfaction, and low self-esteem can all undermine weight-loss efforts (Teixeira et al., 2002).

**Self-Monitoring**    Obese clients are trained in self-monitoring, to keep careful records of what they eat, when they eat it, how much they eat, and where they eat it. This record keeping simultaneously defines the behavior, makes clients more aware of their eating patterns, and can lead to beginning efforts to lose weight (Baker & Kirschenbaum, 1998). Even online self-monitoring has been tied to weight loss (Krukowski, Harvey-Berino, Bursac, Ashikaga, & West, 2013). Many clients are surprised to discover what, when, and how much they actually eat. Monitoring is always important for weight loss. Even daily self-weighing seems to be a safe self-monitoring technique (Gorin et al., 2019), but it becomes especially so at high-risk times, such as during the holidays, when weight gain reliably occurs (Boutelle, Kirschenbaum, Baker, & Mitchell, 1999). Most eating occurs in social situations, and social cues such as how much other people are eating affect food consumption; yet many people are unaware of the social influences on their eating (Vartanian, Spanos, Herman, & Polivy, 2017).

**Attentional Retraining**    People who are battling a health issue such as obesity or smoking will often show an attentional bias in favor of cues related to the issue. For example, an obese person may orient to food cues, such as appealing high-calorie foods, or a store window with rich foods (Kemps, Tiggemann, & Hollitt, 2014). Obese children whose attention goes to food

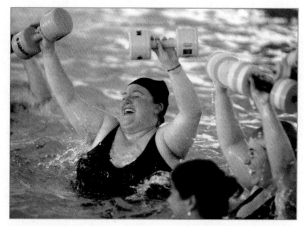

*Approximately 500,000 Americans participate in organized weight-reduction programs. Many of these programs include exercise.*
Natacha Pisarenko/AP Images

may also gain weight (Werthmann et al., 2015). Attentional retraining involves breaking or at least moderating this automatic attentional bias by distracting one's self, focusing on other aspects of the environment, or engaging in physical activity.

**Stimulus Control**    The immediate food environment has powerful effects on eating (Elliston, Ferguson, Schüz, & Schüz, 2017). For this reason, clients are trained to modify the stimuli in their environment that have previously elicited and maintained their eating and to take steps to modify their food consumption. Such steps include purchasing low-calorie foods (such as raw vegetables) and limiting the high-calorie foods kept in the house. Clients are taught to confine eating to one place at particular times of day, and to develop new discriminative stimuli that will be associated with eating, for example, using a particular place setting, such as a special placemat or napkin, and to eat only when those stimuli are present. Keeping portion size modest is also important (Kerameas, Vartanian, Herman, & Polivy, 2015). Creating and increasing non-food-related novel and enjoyable activities in one's life can also help in controlling obesity (Carr & Epstein, 2018; Xu et al., 2017).

**Controlling Eating**    The next step is to gain control over the eating process itself. For example, clients may be urged to count each mouthful of food. They may be told to put down eating utensils after every few mouthfuls until the food in their mouths is chewed and swallowed. Longer and longer delays are introduced between mouthfuls so as to encourage slow eating (which tends to reduce intake). Finally, clients are urged to savor their food—to make a conscious effort to appreciate it while they are eating. The goal is to teach the obese person to eat less and enjoy it more. This mindful eating also helps reduce impulsive snacking and food choices (Hendrickson & Rasmussen, 2017).

Self-Reinforcement   Success in modifying eating habits can be supported by a positive reinforcement, such as going to a movie or posting a facebook message. Developing a sense of self-control over eating is an important part of behavioral treatment of obesity and can help people overcome temptations. Succeeding in losing weight is tied to greater vitality and psychological well-being (Swencionis et al., 2013), and this can act as another source of self-reinforcement.

Controlling Self-Talk   Cognitive restructuring is an important part of weight-reduction programs. As noted in Chapter 3, poor health habits can be maintained through dysfunctional monologues ("I'll never lose weight—I've tried before and failed so many times"). Participants in weight-loss programs are urged to identify the maladaptive thoughts they have regarding weight loss and to substitute positive self-instruction. As with other health behavior changes, self-efficacy is important for success, and may be especially so for men (Crane, Ward, Lutes, Bowling, & Tate, 2016).

The formation of explicit implementation intentions (Luszczynska, Sobczyk, & Abraham, 2007) and a strong sense of self-efficacy—that is, the belief that one will be able to lose weight—also predicts weight loss (Warziski, Sereika, Styn, Music, & Burke, 2008). The goal of these aspects of interventions is to increase a sense of self-determination, which can enhance intrinsic motivation to continue diet modification and weight loss (Mata et al., 2009).

Exercise   Exercise is a critical component of any weight-loss program. As people age, increasing physical activity is essential just to maintain weight, let alone avoid gaining it (Jameson, 2004). It can even change the underlying propensity to gain weight; that is, exercise can help reprogram genes that influence how fat is stored, making obesity less likely (*The Economist,* July 13, 2013). Maintaining an exercise program requires strong self-regulation skills as well as attitudes and intentions that favor exercise (Chevance,

Stephan, Héraud, & Boiché, 2018). Positive parenting about exercise can help foster the behavior in adolescents (Huffman, Wilson, Van Horn, & Pate, 2018).

Stress Management   Efforts to lose weight can be stressful (Tomiyama et al., 2010), and so reducing life stress can be helpful. Among the techniques that have been used are mindfulness training and acceptance and commitment theory (ACT).

Social Support   Social support is important for losing weight (Cornelius, Gettens, & Gorin, 2016). Consequently, most CBT programs include training in eliciting effective support from families, friends, and coworkers. Even supportive messages from a behavioral therapist over the Internet seem to help people lose weight (Oleck, 2001). Autonomy support, that is, social support that conveys the belief that the person is an autonomous, responsible agent of his/her own behavior appears to foster self-regulation that can lead to more weight loss better than more directive support (Gorin, Powers, Koestner, Wing, & Raynor, 2014). Family support or negativity strongly influences weight gain or loss, especially among Latinas (Jewell, Letham-Hamlett, Ibrahim, Leucken, & MacKinnon, 2017).

The family environment is critical for weight loss, especially for children and adolescents. Families typically eat together, and so meals, which are usually planned by one person, are consumed by all (Lytle et al., 2011; Samuel-Hodge et al., 2010). Family-based interventions have shown particular promise for modifying obesity-related health behaviors (Crespo et al., 2012; Gorin et al., 2013) especially among Latinas (Marquez, Norman, Fowler, Gans, & Marcus, 2018). When support from family becomes prescriptive with pressure to lose weight, however, it may undermine weight loss efforts (Cornelius et al., 2018).

Relapse Prevention   Relapse prevention techniques are incorporated into treatment programs, including matching treatments to the eating problems of particular clients, restructuring the environment to remove temptation, rehearsing high-risk situations for relapse (such as parties and holidays), and developing coping strategies to deal with high-risk situations.

Moreover, weight-loss efforts can fail and lapses are likely, and so people need to be protected against their self-recrimination and tendency to let a lapse turn into a full-blown loss of control. (Forman, Schumacher, Crosby, Manasse, & Goldstein, 2017; Schumacher et al., 2018). Maintenance of weight loss is an ongoing

**TABLE 5.2 | Weight-Management Tips**

| Increasing Awareness | Exercise |
|---|---|
| Keep track of what you eat.<br>Keep track of your weight.<br>Write down when you eat and why. | Track your exercise progress: What do you enjoy doing?<br>Incorporate exercise into your lifestyle—become more active in all areas of life. |
| **While You're Eating** | **Attitudes** |
| Pace yourself—eat slowly.<br>Pay attention to your eating process.<br>Pay attention to how full you are.<br>Eat at the same place and at the same time.<br>Eat one portion, and serve yourself before beginning the meal. | Think about your weight-loss goals—make them realistic.<br>Remember that any progress is beneficial and that not reaching your goal does not mean you failed.<br>Think about your desire for foods—manage and work through cravings. |
| **Shopping for Food** | **Working with Others** |
| Structure your shopping so that you know what you are buying beforehand.<br>Limit the number of already prepared items.<br>Don't shop when you are hungry. | Incorporate friends and family into your goals and your new lifestyle, including meal preparation and exercise routines.<br>Communicate to them what they can do to help you reach your goals. |
| **The Eating Environment** | **Nutrition** |
| Make healthy foods more available than unhealthy ones.<br>Do your best to stick to your eating routine when dining out.<br>Think about the limitations and possible adjustments to your eating routine before dining out or eating with other people. | Be informed about nutrition.<br>Know your recommended daily intake of calories, vitamins, and minerals.<br>Know which foods are good sources of vitamins, minerals, proteins, carbohydrates, and healthy fats.<br>Eat a balanced diet.<br>Prepare foods that are both healthy and taste good. |

process (Greaves, Poltawski, Garside, & Briscoe, 2017). Motivation and implementation of intentions must be maintained for both eating and exercise (Elsborg & Elbe, 2018).

Weight-loss programs such as these can be implemented successfully, over the Internet (Krukowski, Harvey-Berino, Bursac, Ashikaga, & West, 2013), through workplace weight-loss interventions, and through commercial weight-loss programs. Indeed, more than 500,000 people each week are exposed to behavioral methods to control obesity through commercial programs such as Weight Watchers and Jenny Craig.

## Evaluation of Cognitive–Behavioral Weight-Loss Techniques

Cognitive–behavioral programs typically produce modest success, with weight loss of nearly 2 pounds a week for up to 20 weeks and long-term maintenance over at least 2 years (Brownell & Kramer, 1989). Programs that emphasize diet modification self-direction and ex-

ercise and include relapse prevention techniques are particularly successful (Jeffery, Hennrikus, Lando, Murray, & Liu, 2000). Interventions with children and adolescents show particularly good results when parents are involved (Kitzmann et al., 2010). A meta-analysis showed that these interventions also can reduce emotional eating and increase cognitive restraint (Jacob et al., 2018). A meta-analysis of online interventions showed similar effects, although they were not as strong (Podina & Fodor, 2018). Long-term maintenance of weight loss can be improved by daily weighing (Crain, Sherwood, Martinson, & Jeffery, 2018).

Table 5.2 describes some of the promising leads that current research suggests for enhancing long-term weight loss in cognitive–behavioral programs.

## Taking a Public Health Approach

The increasing prevalence of obesity makes it evident that prevention is essential for combating this problem (National Academy of Medicine, 2011d).

Health psychologists have criticized the media and the products they popularize for perpetuating false images of feminine beauty. The Barbie doll has come under particular criticism because its popularity with young girls may contribute to excessive dieting and the development of eating disorders. Using hip measurement as a constant, researchers have calculated that for a young, healthy woman to attain the same body proportions as the Barbie doll, she would have to increase her bust by 5 inches, her neck length by more than 3 inches, and her height by more than 2 feet while decreasing her waist by 6 inches (Brownell & Napolitano, 1995). This clearly unattainable standard may contribute to the false expectations that girls and women develop for their bodies. Consequently, Mattel, who makes Barbie dolls, has now added diverse Barbies including curvy ones with proportions more similar to those of many adolescent girls (Li, 2016).

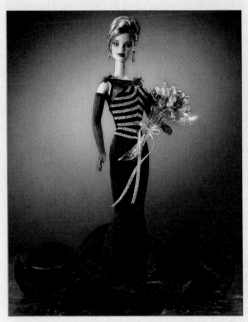

AP Images

Prevention with families at risk for having obese children is an important strategy. Parents should be trained early to adopt sensible meal-planning and eating habits that they can convey to their children. Although obesity has proven to be very difficult to modify with adults, it is easier to teach children healthy eating and activity habits. Obese children can benefit from lifestyle interventions involving reinforcements for giving up sedentary activities like television watching, inducements to engage in sports and other physical activities, and steps to encourage healthier eating practices including avoiding or eliminating snacking (Wilfley et al., 2007). School-based interventions directed to making healthy foods available and modifying sedentary behavior help (Dietz & Gortmaker, 2001).

The World Health Organization has argued for several changes, including food labels that contain more nutrition and serving size information, a special tax on foods that are high in sugar and fat (the so-called junk food tax), and restriction of advertising to children or required health warnings (Arnst, 2004). Some states now control the availability of junk food and sugary drinks in schools, products that have been linked directly to weight in children (Taber, Chriqui, Perna, Powell, & Chaloupka, 2012). Some of these real or proposed changes in food and drink availability have led to bitter battles between food and beverage companies and state, local, and even the Federal government.

## EATING DISORDERS

In pursuit of the elusive perfect body (Box 5.3), many women and an increasing number of men chronically restrict their diet and engage in other weight-loss efforts, such as laxative use, cigarette smoking, and chronic use of diet pills (Facts of Life, November 2002). Women ages 15 to 24 are most likely to practice these behaviors, but cases of eating disorders have been documented in people as young as 7 years and as old as their mid-80s (Facts of Life, November 2002).

The epidemic of eating disorders suggests that, like obesity, the pursuit of thinness is a major public health threat. Recent years have seen an increase in the incidence of eating disorders, especially among adolescent girls. Chief among these are anorexia nervosa and bulimia. Eating disorders have some of the highest disability and mortality rates of all behavioral disorders (Park, 2007). Eating disorders result in death for about 6 percent of those who have them (Facts of Life, November 2002). Suicide attempts are not uncommon (Bulik et al., 2008). Women with eating disorders or tendencies toward them are also more likely to be depressed, anxious, and low in self-esteem and to have a poor sense of mastery.

## Anorexia Nervosa

One of my most jarring memories is of driving down a street on my university campus during Christmas vacation and seeing a young woman clearly suffering from anorexia nervosa about to cross the street. She had obviously just been exercising. The wind blew her sweatpants around the thin sticks that had once been normal legs. The skin on her face was stretched so tight that the bones showed through, and I could make out her skeleton under what passed for flesh. I realized that I was face-to-face with someone who was shortly going to die. I looked for a place to pull over, but by the time I had found a parking space, she had disappeared into one of the dormitories, and I could not see which one. Nor do I know what I would have said if I had caught up with her.

**Anorexia nervosa** is an obsessive disorder amounting to self-starvation, in which a person diets and exercises to the point that body weight is grossly below optimum level, threatening health and potentially leading to death (Kask et al., 2016). Most sufferers are young women, but gay and bisexual men and transgender people are also at risk (Blashill, Goshe, Robbins, Mayer, & Safren, 2014; Haug & Balsam, 2017).

Developing Anorexia Nervosa    Genetic factors are clearly implicated, especially genes involving the serotonin, dopamine, and estrogen systems. These systems have been implicated in both anxiety and food intake. Interactions between genetic factors and risks in the environment, such as early exposure to stress, may also play a role (Striegel-Moore & Bulik, 2007), and dysregulated biological stress systems may be involved (Zucker et al., 2017).

Personality characteristics and family interaction patterns may be causal factors in anorexia. People with anorexia may experience a lack of control coupled with a need for approval and exhibit conscientious, perfectionistic behavior. Body image distortions are also common among anorexic girls, although it is not clear whether this distortion is a consequence or a cause of the disorder. For example, these girls still see themselves as overweight when they have long since dropped below their ideal weight (Hewig et al., 2008).

Anorexic girls can come from families with psychopathology or alcoholism or from families that are extremely close but have poor skills for communicating emotion or dealing with conflict (Garfinkel & Garner, 1983; Rakoff, 1983). Mothers of daughters with eating disorders appear to be more dissatisfied with their families, more dissatisfied with their daughters' appearance, and more vulnerable to eating disorders themselves (Pike & Rodin, 1991). Mothers who are preoccupied with their own weight and eating behaviors place their daughters at risk for developing eating problems (Francis & Birch, 2005). More generally, eating disorders have been tied to insecure attachment in relationships, that is, to the expectation of criticism or rejection from others (Troisi et al., 2006). By the time a young woman or man goes into treatment for anorexia, the behavior may have become a habit that is, consequently, much harder to treat (Goode, 2015).

Treating Anorexia    Initially, the chief target of therapy is to bring the patient's weight back up to a safe level, a goal that often must be undertaken in a residential treatment setting, such as a hospital. To achieve weight gain, most therapies use cognitive–behavioral approaches (Brown & Keel, 2012). However, the standard principles of cognitive–behavioral therapy do not always work well with anorexia (Brown & Keel, 2012). Motivational issues are especially important, as inducing the anorexic person to want to change her behavior is essential (Wilson, Grilo, & Vitousek, 2007).

Family therapy may help families learn positive methods of communicating emotion and conflict. During the early phases of treatment, parents are urged to assume control over the anorexic family member's eating, but as the anorexic family member begins to gain weight and comply with parental authority, she or he begins to assume more control over eating (Wilson, Grilo, & Vitousek, 2007).

Because of the health risks and difficulties in treating anorexia nervosa, research has increasingly moved toward prevention. Some interventions address social norms regarding thinness directly (Neumark-Sztainer, Wall, Story, & Perry, 2003). For example, one study gave women information about other women's weight and body type, on the grounds that women who develop eating disorders often wrongly believe that other women are smaller and thinner than they actually are (Sanderson, Darley, & Messinger, 2002). The intervention succeeded in changing women's estimates of their actual and ideal weight (Mutterperl & Sanderson, 2002). Drawing on the concept of dissonance, some studies have found that writing essays denouncing the thinness ideal can help women at risk for anorexia and can reduce their symptoms (Green et al., 2017).

But the factors that may prevent new cases from arising may be quite different from those that lead students who already have symptoms to seek out treatment (Mann et al., 1997). One eating disorder prevention program had college freshmen meet classmates who had recovered from an eating disorder; they described their experience and provided information about the disorder. To the researchers' dismay, following the intervention, the participants had slightly more symptoms of eating disorders than those who had not participated. The program may have inadvertently normalized the problem. Consequently, ideal strategies for prevention may require stressing the health risks of eating disorders, whereas the strategies for inducing symptomatic women to seek treatment may involve normalizing the behavior and urging them to accept treatment (Mann et al., 1997).

## Bulimia

**Bulimia** is characterized by alternating cycles of binge eating and purging through such techniques as vomiting, laxative abuse, extreme dieting or fasting, and drug or alcohol abuse. **Bingeing** appears to be caused at least in part by dieting. About half of the people diagnosed with anorexia are also bulimic. Bulimia affects 1 to 3 percent of women (Wisniewski, Epstein, Marcus, & Kaye, 1997) and an increasing number of men (Striegel, Bedrosian, Wang, & Schwartz, 2012), and up to 10 percent of people with bulimia may also have bingeing episodes.

### Developing Bulimia
Whereas many people with anorexia are thin, people with bulimia are typically of normal weight or overweight, especially through the hips. The binge phase is regarded as an out-of-control reaction of the body to restore weight, and the purge phase as an effort to regain control over weight.

Women prone to bulimia, especially binge eating, appear to have altered stress responses, especially an atypical hypothalamic–pituitary-adrenal diurnal pattern (Ludescher et al., 2009). Cortisol levels, especially in response to stress, may be elevated, promoting eating (Gluck et al., 2004). Food can become a constant thought (Blechert, Feige, Joos, Zeeck, & Tuschen-Caffier, 2011). Restrained eating, then, can set the stage for a binge.

Bulimia may have a genetic basis, inasmuch as eating disorders cluster in families, and twin studies show a high concordance rate for binge eating (Wade, Bulik, Sullivan, Neale, & Kendler, 2000). Families that place a high value on thinness and appearance are also likely to have bulimic daughters (Boskind-White & White, 1983).

Physiological theories of bulimia focus on hormonal dysfunctions (Monteleone et al., 2001), low leptin functioning (Jimerson, Mantzoros, Wolfe, & Metzger, 2000), hypothalamic dysfunction, food allergies, or disordered taste responsivity (Wisniewski et al., 1997), disorder of the endogenous opioid system (Mitchell, Laine, Morley, & Levine, 1986), neurological disorder, and a combination of these. In other words, bulimia appears to have or create underlying physiological disruptions but exactly what they are and if they are causal is not yet clear.

### Treating Bulimia
A barrier to treating bulimia is that many women do not believe either that their problem is a serious one, or that a medical intervention will overcome it. Accordingly, one of the first steps in treatment is to convince bulimics that the disorder threatens their health and that interventions can help them overcome the disorder (Smalec & Klingle, 2000). When bulimia becomes compulsive, outright prevention of the behavior may be required, with the patient placed in a treatment facility. CBT has been moderately successful in treating bulimia (Mitchell, Agras, & Wonderlich, 2007), in either an individual or group setting (Katzman et al., 2010). Internet interventions may also be somewhat successful in modifying disordered eating and weight gain prevention (Stice, Durant, Rohde, & Shaw, 2014).

A combination of medication and cognitive-behavioral therapy appears to be the most effective therapy (Brown & Keel, 2012; Wilson et al., 2007). Typically, this treatment begins with self-monitoring, keeping a diary of eating habits, including time, place, type of food consumed, and emotions experienced. Simple self-monitoring can produce decreases in binge-purge behavior.

Specific techniques are then added and include inducing the client to increase the regularity of meals, eat a greater variety of foods, delay the impulse to purge as long as possible, and eat favorite foods in new settings not previously associated with binges. Perceptions of self-efficacy facilitate the success of cognitive–behavioral interventions.

Relapse prevention techniques are often added to therapeutic programs. These include learning to identify situations that trigger binge eating and developing coping skills to avoid them. Relaxation and stress management skills are often added to these programs as well.

### Binge Eating Disorder

**Binge eating** usually occurs when the individual is alone; it may be triggered by negative emotions produced by stressful experiences (Telch & Agras, 1996). The dieter begins to eat and then cannot stop, and although the bingeing is unpleasant, the binger feels out of control, unable to stop eating. Low self-esteem is implicated in binge eating and may be a good target for prevention and treatment (Goldschmidt, Wall, Loth, Bucchianeri, & Neumark-Sztainer, 2014). Many people with binge eating disorder also have a mental health disorder, such as anxiety or depression (Kessler et al., 2013), and child abuse may be implicated in some cases (Caslini et al., 2016).

A related eating disorder, termed binge eating disorder, characterizes the many people who engage in recurrent binge eating but do not engage in the compensatory purging behavior to avoid weight gain (Spitzer et al., 1993).

Binge eating disorder is a health problem at least on a scale with bulimia. However, many people with the disorder do not seek or obtain treatment (Kessler et al., 2014). Binge eating increases in response to stress, and a rise in ghrelin, which controls the urge to eat, may be responsible (Gluck, Yahav, Hashim, & Geliebter, 2014). People with binge eating disorders are characterized by an excessive concern with body image and weight; a preoccupation with dieting; a history of depression, psychopathology, and alcohol or drug abuse; and difficulties with managing work and social situations (Spitzer et al., 1993). Overvaluing body appearance, a larger body mass than is desired, dieting, and symptoms of depression are implicated in triggering binge episodes (Stice, Presnell, & Spangler, 2002).

## ■ ALCOHOLISM AND PROBLEM DRINKING

### The Scope of the Problem

Alcohol is responsible for approximately 88,000 deaths each year, making it the third-leading cause of preventable death after tobacco and improper diet and exercise (Centers for Disease Control and Prevention, 2013). More than 20 percent of Americans drink at levels that exceed government recommendations (Centers for Disease Control and Prevention, September 2008). About 15.1 million American adults meet criteria for alcohol use disorder (Substance Abuse and Mental Health Services Administration, 2015).

As a health issue, alcohol consumption has been linked to high blood pressure, stroke, cirrhosis of the liver, and some forms of cancer. Excessive alcohol consumption has also been tied to brain atrophy and consequent deteriorating cognitive function (Anstey et al., 2006). Alcoholics can have sleep disorders, which, in turn, may contribute to immune alterations that elevate risk for infection (Redwine, Dang, Hall, & Irwin, 2003). Every day, nearly 30 people die of drunk-driving crashes in the United States—that's one person every 48 minutes in 2017 (National Highway Traffic Safety Administration, 2019).

An estimated 15 percent of the national health bill goes to the treatment of alcoholism (Dorgan & Editue, 1995). Economically, the costs of alcohol abuse and alcoholism are estimated to be approximately $249 billion per year and include the following:

- Most of the costs, 73 percent of the total cost, resulted from losses in the workplace
- 11 percent went to health care expenses to treat problems due to excessive drinking
- 10 percent was spent on law enforcement and criminal justice expenses
- 5 percent of the costs went to losses from motor vehicle crashes (Centers for Disease Control and Prevention, January 2016).

In addition to the direct costs of alcoholism through illness, accidents, and economic costs, alcohol abuse contributes to social problems. Alcohol disinhibits aggression, so homicides, suicides, and assaults occur under the influence of alcohol. Alcohol can also facilitate other risky behaviors. For example, among sexually active adults, alcohol leads to more impulsive sexuality (Weinhardt, Carey, Carey, Maisto, & Gordon, 2001) and poorer skills for negotiating condom use (Gordon, Carey, & Carey, 1997).

Overall, though, it has been difficult to define the scope of alcoholism. Many problem drinkers keep their problem successfully hidden, at least for a time. By drinking at particular times of day or at particular places, and by restricting contacts with other people during these times, the alcoholic may be able to drink without noticeable disruption in his or her daily activities.

## What Is Substance Dependence?

A person is said to be dependent on a substance when he or she has repeatedly self-administered it, resulting in tolerance, withdrawal, and compulsive behavior (American Psychiatric Association, 2000). Substance dependence can include **physical dependence,** when the body has adjusted to the substance and incorporates the use of that substance into the normal functioning of the body's tissues. Physical dependence often involves **tolerance,** the process by which the body increasingly adapts to the use of a substance, requiring larger and larger doses of it to obtain the same effects, and eventually reaching a plateau. **Craving** is a strong desire to engage in a behavior or consume a substance. It results from physical dependence and from a conditioning process: As the substance is paired with environmental cues, the presence of those cues triggers an intense desire for the substance. **Addiction** occurs when a person has become physically or psychologically dependent on a substance following repeated use over time. **Withdrawal** refers to the unpleasant symptoms, both physical and psychological, that people experience when they stop using a substance on which they have become dependent. Although the symptoms vary, they include anxiety, irritability, intense cravings for the substance, nausea, headaches, tremors, and hallucinations.

## Alcoholism and Problem Drinking

**Problem drinking** and **alcoholism** are substance dependence disorders that are defined by several specific behaviors. These patterns include the need for daily use of alcohol, the inability to cut down on drinking, repeated efforts to control drinking through temporary abstinence or restriction of alcohol to certain times of the day, binge drinking, occasional consumption of large quantities of alcohol, loss of memory while intoxicated, continued drinking despite known health problems, and drinking of nonbeverage alcohol, such as cough syrup.

The term *alcoholic* is usually reserved for someone who is physically addicted to alcohol. Alcoholics show withdrawal symptoms when they stop drinking, they have a high tolerance for alcohol, and they have little ability to control their drinking. Problem drinkers may not have these symptoms, but they may have

social, psychological, and medical problems resulting from alcohol.

Physiological dependence can be manifested in stereotypic drinking patterns (particular types of alcohol in particular quantities at particular times of day), drinking that maintains blood alcohol at a particular level, the ability to function at a level that would incapacitate less tolerant drinkers, increased frequency and severity of withdrawal, early-in-the-day and middle-of-the-night drinking, a sense of loss of control over drinking, and a subjective craving for alcohol (Straus, 1988).

## Origins of Alcoholism and Problem Drinking

The origins of alcoholism and problem drinking are complex. Based on twin studies and on the frequency of alcoholism in sons of alcoholic fathers, genetic factors appear to be implicated (Hutchison, McGeary, Smolen, Bryan, & Swift, 2002). Modeling a parent's drinking is also implicated (van der Zwaluw et al., 2008). Men have traditionally been at greater risk for alcoholism than women (Robbins & Martin, 1993), although younger women and women employed outside the home are catching up (Christie-Mizell & Peralta, 2009; Williams, 2002). Sociodemographic factors, such as low income, also predict alcoholism.

**Drinking and Stress**   Drinking occurs, in part, as an effort to buffer the impact of stress. People who have a lot of negative life events, experience chronic stressors, and have little social support are more likely to become problem drinkers than people without these problems (Brennan & Moos, 1990; Sadava & Pak, 1994). For example, alcohol abuse rises among people who have been laid off from their jobs (Catalano, Dooley, Wilson, & Hough, 1993). Alienation from work, low job autonomy, the sense that one's abilities are not being used, and lack of participation in decision making at work are associated with heavy drinking (Greenberg & Grunberg, 1995). Financial strain, especially if it produces depression, leads to drinking (Peirce, Frone, Russell, & Cooper, 1994), and a sense of powerlessness in one's life has also been related to alcohol use and abuse (Seeman, Seeman, & Budros, 1988).

Many people begin drinking to enhance positive emotions and reduce negative ones (Repetto, Caldwell, & Zimmerman, 2005), and alcohol does reliably lower anxiety and depression and improve self-esteem, at least temporarily (Steele & Josephs, 1990). For many people, drinking is associated with pleasant social occasions (Collins et al., 2017), and people may develop a social life centered on drinking, such as going to bars or attending parties (Emslie, Hunt, & Lyons, 2013). Thus, there can be psychological rewards to drinking.

There are two windows of vulnerability for alcohol use and abuse. The first, when chemical dependence generally starts, is between the ages of 12 and 21 (DuPont, 1988). The other is in late middle age, in which problem drinking may act as a coping method for managing stress (Brennan & Moos, 1990). Late-onset problem drinkers are more likely to control their drinking on their own or be successfully treated, compared with people who have more long-term drinking problems (Moos, Brennan, & Moos, 1991).

Depression and alcoholism are linked. Alcoholism may represent untreated symptoms of depression, or depression may act as an impetus for drinking in an effort to improve mood. Accordingly, in some cases, symptoms of both disorders must be treated simultaneously (Oslin et al., 2003).

## Treatment of Alcohol Abuse

As many as half of all alcoholics stop or reduce their drinking on their own (Cunningham, Lin, Ross, & Walsh, 2000). This "maturing out" of alcoholism is especially likely in the later years of life (Stall & Biernacki, 1986). Cutting back can also be a result of learning just how much they drink, relative to other people (Taylor, Vlaev, Maltby, Brown, & Wood, 2015). In addition, alcoholism can be successfully treated. Nonetheless, as many as 60 percent of the people treated through such programs may return to alcohol abuse (Finney & Moos, 1995).

Alcoholics who are of higher SES and who are in highly socially stable environments (i.e., who have regular jobs, intact families, and a circle of friends) do very well in treatment programs, achieving success rates as high as 68 percent. In contrast, alcoholics of low SES often have success rates of 18 percent or less. Without employment and social support, the prospects for recovery are dim. Box 5.4 presents an example of these problems.

## Treatment Programs

For hard-core alcoholics, the first phase of treatment is **detoxification.** Because this process can produce severe symptoms and health problems, detoxification is typically conducted in a carefully supervised and monitored medical setting. Once the alcoholic has at least partly dried out, therapy is initiated. The typical program begins with a short-term, intensive inpatient treatment followed by a period of continuing treatment on an outpatient basis (NIAAA, 2000a).

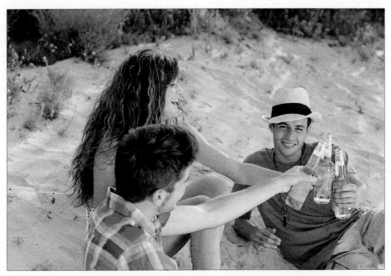

*Adolescence and young adulthood represent a window of vulnerability to problem drinking and alcoholism. Successful intervention with this age group may reduce the scope of the alcoholism problem.*
Frank Herholdt/Image Source

When the Berlin Wall came down in 1989, there were celebrations worldwide. In the midst of the jubilation, few fully anticipated the problems that might arise in its wake. Hundreds of thousands of East Germans, who had lived for decades under a totalitarian regime with a relatively poor standard of living, were now free to stream across the border into West Germany, which enjoyed prosperity, high employment rates, and a high standard of living. But for many people, the promise of new opportunities failed to materialize. Employment was less plentiful than had been assumed, and the East Germans were less qualified for the jobs that did exist. East Germans experienced more discrimination and hostility than they expected, and many migrating East Germans found themselves unemployed.

Two German researchers, Mittag and Schwarzer (1993), examined alcohol consumption among men who had found employment in West Germany and those who had remained unemployed. In addition, they measured self-efficacy with respect to coping with life's problems through such items as "When I am in trouble, I can rely on my ability to deal with the problem effectively."

The researchers found that the men with a high sense of self-efficacy were less likely to consume high levels of alcohol. The men who were unemployed and also had a low sense of self-efficacy drank more than any other group. Thus, being male, being unemployed for a long time, and not having a sense of personal agency led to heavy drinking.

Although health psychologists cannot provide jobs to the unemployed, perhaps they can empower people to develop a sense of self-efficacy. If one believes that one can control one's behavior, cope effectively with life, and solve one's problems, one may be better able to deal effectively with setbacks (Mittag & Schwarzer, 1993).

Approximately 745,200 people in the United States received treatment for alcoholism in 2008 (National Institute on Drug Abuse, 2011). A self-help group, especially Alcoholics Anonymous (AA), is the most commonly sought source of help for alcohol-related problems (NIAAA, 2000a) (Box 5.5).

Cognitive–Behavioral Treatments    Treatment programs for alcoholism and problem drinking typically use cognitive–behavioral therapy (CBT) to treat the biological and environmental factors involved in alcoholism simultaneously (NIAAA, 2000b). The goals of CBT are to decrease the reinforcing properties of alcohol, to teach people new behaviors inconsistent with alcohol abuse, and to modify the environment to include reinforcements for activities that do not involve alcohol. Learning coping techniques for dealing with stress and relapse prevention skills enhance the prospects for long-term maintenance.

Many CBT programs begin with a self-monitoring phase, in which the alcoholic or problem drinker charts situations that give rise to drinking. Motivational enhancement procedures are often included because the responsibility and the capacity to change rely entirely on the client (NIAAA, 2000a). Some programs also include medications for blocking the alcohol–brain interactions that may contribute to alcoholism (Demody, Wardell, Stoner, & Hendershot, 2018).

Many treatment programs include stress management techniques that can be substituted for drinking. Drink refusal skills and the substitution of nonalcoholic beverages in high-risk social situations are also important components of CBT interventions. In some cases, family therapy and group counseling are added. The advantage of family counseling is that it eases the alcoholic's or problem drinker's transition back into his or her family (NIAAA, 2000a).

Relapse Prevention    A meta-analysis of alcohol treatment outcome studies estimates that more than 50 percent of treated patients relapse within the first 3 months after treatment (NIAAA, 2000a). Accordingly, relapse prevention techniques are essential. Practicing coping skills or social skills for high-risk-for-relapse situations is a mainstay of relapse prevention interventions. In addition, the recognition that people often stop and restart an addictive behavior several times before they are successful has led to the development of techniques for managing relapses. Understanding that an occasional relapse is normal helps the problem drinker realize that any given lapse does not signify failure. Overall, the evidence shows that cognitive–behavioral treatments to treat alcohol disorders are

BOX **5.5**    A Profile of Alcoholics Anonymous

No one knows exactly when Alcoholics Anonymous (AA) began, but it is believed that the organization was formed around 1935 in Akron, Ohio. The first meetings were attended by a few acquaintances who discovered that they could remain sober by attending the services of a local religious group and sharing their problems and efforts to remain sober with other alcoholics. By 1936, weekly AA meetings were taking place around the country.

Currently, AA's membership is estimated to be more than 2 million individuals worldwide (Alcoholics Anonymous, 2018). The sole requirement for participation in AA is a desire to stop drinking. Members come from all walks of life, including all socioeconomic levels, races, cultures, sexual preferences, and ages.

Members are encouraged to immerse themselves in the culture of AA—to attend "90 meetings in 90 days." At these meetings, AA members speak about the drinking experiences that prompted them to seek out AA and what sobriety has meant to them. Time is set aside for prospective new members to talk informally with long-time members so that they can learn and imitate the coping techniques that recovered alcoholics have used.

AA has a firm policy regarding alcohol consumption. It maintains that alcoholism is a disease that can be managed but never cured. Recovery means that an individual must acknowledge that he or she has a disease, that it is incurable, and that alcohol can play no part in future life. Recovery depends completely on staying sober.

Is AA successful in getting people to stop drinking? AA's dropout rate is unknown, and success over the long term has not been measured. Moreover, because the organization keeps no membership lists (it is anonymous), it is difficult to evaluate its success. However, AA itself maintains that two out of three people have been able to stop drinking through its program, and one authorized study reported a 75 percent success rate for a New York AA chapter.

AA programs are effective for several reasons. Participation in AA is like a religious conversion experience in which a person adopts a new way of life; such experiences can be powerful in bringing about behavior change. Also, the member who shares his or her experiences develops a commitment to other members. The process of giving up alcohol contributes to a sense of emotional maturity and responsibility, helping the alcoholic accept responsibility for his or her life. AA may also provide a sense of meaning and purpose in a person's life—most chapters have a strong spiritual or religious bent and urge members to commit themselves to a power greater than themselves. In addition, the group can provide satisfying personal relationships that help people overcome the isolation that many alcoholics experience. Too, the members provide social reinforcement for each other's abstinence.

AA was one of the earliest self-help programs for people suffering from a health problem and therefore, has provided a model for self-help organizations. Moreover, in having successfully treated alcoholics for decades, AA has demonstrated that the problem of alcoholism is not intractable.

successful across a broad range of people and situations (Magill & Ray, 2009). Interventions with heavy-drinking college students have made use of these approaches (Box 5.6).

## Evaluation of Alcohol Treatment Programs

Several factors are associated with successful alcohol treatment programs: a focus on factors in the environment that elicit drinking and modifying those factors or instilling coping skills to manage them; a moderate length of participation (about 6 to 8 weeks) and involving relatives and employers in the treatment process. Interventions that include these components can produce up to a 40 percent treatment success rate (Center for the Advancement of Health, 2000d).

Even minimal interventions administered by a computer can make a dent in drinking-related problems (Freyer-Adam et al., 2018). Online interventions from a credible source that emphasize problem-solving skills and substituting other behaviors for drinking may be especially effective (Garrett et al., 2018). For example, a few sessions devoted to a discussion of problem drinking and telephone interventions have shown some success in reducing drinking (Oslin et al., 2003). Most alcoholics, though, approximately 85 percent, do not receive formal treatment. As a result, social engineering approaches such as banning alcohol advertising, raising the drinking age, and enforcing

Most U.S. college students drink alcohol, and as many as 40 percent of them are heavy drinkers (O'Malley & Johnston, 2002). Moreover, if you are a college student who drinks, the odds are 7 in 10 that you have engaged in binge drinking (Wechsler, Seibring, Liu, & Ahl, 2004) (Table 5.3).

Many colleges have tried to deal with the heavy-drinking problem by providing educational materials about the harmful effects of alcohol. However, dogmatic alcohol prevention messages may actually increase drinking (Bensley & Wu, 1991). Moreover, the information conflicts markedly with the personal experiences of many college students who find drinking in a party situation to be enjoyable. Consequently, motivating students even to attend alcohol abuse programs, much less to follow their recommendations, is difficult.

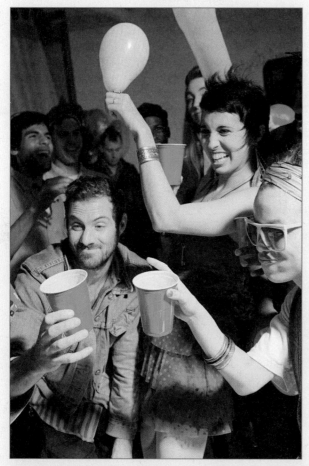

Craig Wetherby Photography/Image Source/age fotostock

Some of the more successful efforts to modify college students' drinking have encouraged them to gain self-control over drinking rather than trying to get them to eliminate alcohol consumption altogether. Interventions that include self-affirmation (Fox, Harris, & Jessop, 2017) or that couple self-affirmation with implementation intentions have been successful (Ehret & Sherman, 2018). Cognitive–behavioral interventions help college students gain such control. These programs begin by getting students to monitor their drinking and learn what blood alcohol levels mean and what their effects are. Often, merely monitoring drinking leads to a reduction in drinking. The program includes information about the risks of alcohol consumption, the acquisition of skills to moderate alcohol consumption, relaxation training and lifestyle rebalancing, nutritional information, aerobic exercise, relapse prevention skills designed to help students cope with high-risk situations, assertiveness training, and drink-refusal training. Changing perceptions of the drinker from a fun party guy to a loser can foster alcohol reduction and prevention programs with students (Teunissen et al., 2012). Moreover, if the student can alter his or her identity away from the prototype of the drinker, it may reduce alcohol consumption.

Many intervention programs include social skills training designed to get students to find alternative ways to relax and have fun in social situations without abusing alcohol. To gain personal control over drinking, students are taught **controlled drinking** skills. For example, one technique involves **placebo drinking,** namely consuming nonalcoholic beverages or alternating an alcoholic with a nonalcoholic beverage.

**TABLE 5.3 | Patterns of College Student Binge Drinking**

|  | 1999 | 2001 |
|---|---|---|
| All students | 44.5% | 44.4% |
| Men | 50.2 | 48.6 |
| Women | 39.4 | 40.9 |
| Live in dormitory | 44.5 | 45.3 |
| Live in fraternity/sorority house | 80.3 | 75.4 |

*Source:* Wechsler, H., J. E. Lee, M. Kuo, M. Seibring, T. F. Nelson, and H. Lee. "Trends in College Binge Drinking During a Period of Increased Prevention Efforts: Findings from 4 Harvard School of Public Health College Alcohol Study Surveys: 1993–2001." *Journal of American College Health* 50, no. 5 (2002): 203–17.

*(continued)*

BOX **5.6** The Drinking College Student (*continued*)

An evaluation of an 8-week training program with college students involving these components showed moderate success. Students reported significant reductions in their drinking compared with a group that received only educational materials about the adverse effects of excessive drinking. Moreover, these gains persisted over a year long follow-up period (Marlatt & George, 1988).

Lengthy interventions such as this one are expensive and time consuming, and consequently, as is the case with other health habits, efforts have gone into finding briefer interventions that may be successful (Fried & Dunn, 2012). For example, many college students are now required to attend brief alcohol interventions incorporated into freshman orientation (e.g., DiFulvio, Linowski, Mazziotti, & Puleo, 2012).

Even online interventions have been created. AlcoholEdu® is an online alcohol prevention program used by more than 500 college and university campuses nationwide. This program is designed to challenge students' expectations about alcohol while enabling them to make healthy and safe decisions about their personal alcohol consumption.

Efforts have also focused on preventing students from getting into a heavy drinking lifestyle in the first place. For example, one intervention (Marlatt et al., 1998) employed motivational interviewing to induce students to question their drinking practices and develop goals for changing their behavior, as drinking to excess has been tied to severe behavioral consequences (see Tables 5.4 and 5.5). Over a 2-year follow-up, students in the intervention drank significantly less and experienced fewer consequences of heavy drinking.

**TABLE 5.4 | Alcohol-Related Problems of College Students Who Had a Drink in the Past Year**

| Alcohol-Related Problem | Drinkers Who Reported Problems |
|---|---|
| Had a hangover | 51.7% |
| Missed class | 27.3 |
| Did something you regret | 32.7 |
| Forgot where you were or what you did | 24.8 |
| Engaged in unplanned sexual activity | 19.5 |
| Got hurt or injured | 9.3 |

*Source:* Wechsler, H., J. E. Lee, M. Kuo, M. Seibring, T. F. Nelson, and H. Lee. "Trends in College Binge Drinking During a Period of Increased Prevention Efforts: Findings From 4 Harvard School of Public Health College Alcohol Study Surveys: 1993–2001." *Journal of American College Health* 50, no. 5 (2002): 203–17.

**TABLE 5.5 | Alcohol Use by U.S. College Students Age 18 to 24**

| Alcohol-Related Incidents per Year |
|---|
| Deaths: 1,825 |
| Injuries: 599,000 |
| Assaults: 690,000 students assaulted by student who had been drinking |
| Sexual abuses: 97,000 victims of alcohol-related sexual assault or date-rape |
| Academic problems: about 25% of students report academic consequences of their drinking (missing class, falling behind, doing poorly on exams or papers, receiving lower grades overall) |
| Health problems: 150,000 students develop an alcohol-related health problem |
| Suicide attempts: about 1.2 to 1.5 percent of students indicate that they tried to commit suicide within the past year due to drinking or drug use |

*Source:* U.S. Department of Health & Human Services and National Institute on Alcohol Abuse and Alcoholism. "Alcohol Facts and Statistics." Accessed June 27, 2019. https://www.niaaa.nih.gov/alcohol-health/overview-alcohol-consumption/alcohol-facts-and-statistics.

penalties for drunk driving can complement formal intervention efforts.

## Preventive Approaches to Alcohol Abuse

Many researchers believe that a prudent approach to alcohol-related problems is prevention: inducing adolescents to avoid drinking altogether or to control their drinking before the problems of alcohol abuse set in. Social influence programs in middle schools are typically designed to teach young adolescents drink-refusal techniques and coping methods for dealing with high-risk situations.

Research suggests some success with these programs. First, such programs enhance adolescents' self-efficacy, which, in turn, may enable them to resist the passive social pressure that comes from seeing peers drink (Donaldson, Graham, Piccinin, & Hansen, 1995). Second, these programs can change social norms that typically foster adolescents' motivation to begin using alcohol, replacing them with norms stressing abstinence or controlled alcohol consumption (Donaldson, Graham, & Hansen, 1994). Third, these programs can be low-cost options for low-income areas, which have traditionally been the most difficult to reach. Ultimately, taxes on alcohol may be one way to improve public health (*The Economist,* July 28, 2018).

## Drinking and Driving

Thousands of vehicular fatalities result from drunk driving each year. Programs such as MADD (Mothers Against Drunk Driving), founded and staffed by the families and friends of those killed by drunk drivers, put pressure on state and local governments for tougher alcohol control measures and stiffer penalties for convicted drunk drivers. Moreover, hosts and hostesses are now pressured to assume responsibility for the alcohol consumption of their guests.

With increased media attention to the problem of drunk driving, drinkers seem to be developing self-regulatory techniques to avoid driving while drunk. However, in some cases drinking and driving warnings may actually lead to an increase in the behavior (Johnson & Kopetz, 2017). Self-regulatory skills are, thus, essential and include limiting drinks to a prescribed number, arranging for a designated driver, getting a taxi, or delaying or avoiding driving after consuming alcohol. Although eliminating drinking altogether is unlikely to occur, the rising popularity of self-regulation to avoid drunk driving may help reduce this serious problem.

## Is Modest Alcohol Consumption a Healthy Behavior?

Paradoxically, modest alcohol intake may contribute to a longer life. Approximately one to two drinks a day (less for women) reduces risk of a heart attack, lowers risk factors associated with coronary heart disease, and reduces risk of stroke (Britton & Marmot, 2004; Facts of Life, December 2003). These benefits may be especially true for older adults and senior citizens. Although many health care practitioners fall short of recommending that people have a drink or two each day, the evidence is mounting that modest drinking may actually reduce the risk for some major causes of death. Nonetheless, this remains an area of controversy.

## ■ SMOKING

Smoking is one of the greatest causes of preventable death. By itself and in interaction with other risk factors, it remains a chief cause of death in developed countries. In the United States, smoking accounts for at least 480,000 deaths each year—smoking is known to be the cause of 9 out of 10 lung cancer deaths in men and women (Centers for Disease Control and Prevention, February 2016) (Table 5.6). Nearly 17 percent of people in the United States still smoke (Tavernise, 2015), about 38 million people overall. Smoking is related to a fourfold increase in women's risk of developing breast cancer after menopause (Ambrosone et al., 1996). Smoking also increases the risk for chronic bronchitis, emphysema, respiratory disorders, damage and injuries due to fires and accidents, lower birth weight in offspring, and retarded fetal development (Center for the Advancement of Health, 2000h; Waller, McCaffery, Forrest, & Wardle, 2004). Smoking also increases risk of erectile dysfunction by 50 percent (Bacon et al., 2006).

The dangers of smoking are not confined to the smoker. Studies of secondhand smoke reveal that spouses, family members, and coworkers are at risk for a variety of health disorders (Marshall, 1986). Parental cigarette smoking can lower cognitive performance in adolescents by reducing blood oxygen capacity and increasing carbon monoxide levels (Bauman, Koch, & Fisher, 1989).

## Synergistic Effects of Smoking

Smoking enhances the detrimental effects of other risk factors. For example, smoking and cholesterol interact to produce higher rates of heart disease than would be

**TABLE 5.6 | U.S. Cigarette Smoking-Related Mortality**

| Disease | Deaths |
|---|---|
| Lung cancer | 127,700 |
| Chronic obstructive pulmonary disease (COPD) | 100,600 |
| Heart disease | 99,300 |
| Other cancers | 36,000 |
| Other heart disease | 25,500 |

*Source:* U.S. Department of Health & Human Services and Centers for Disease Control and Prevention. "Tobacco-Related Mortality." Accessed June 27, 2019. https://www.cdc.gov/tobacco/data_statistics/fact_sheets/health_effects/tobacco_related_mortality/index.htm.

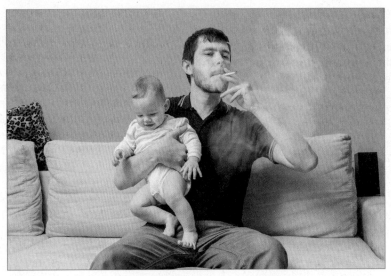

*The risks of smoking are not confined to the smoker. Coworkers, spouses, and other family members of smokers are at risk for many smoking-related disorders.*
vchal/Shutterstock

expected from simply adding together their individual risks (Perkins, 1985). Stress and smoking can also interact in dangerous ways. For men, nicotine can increase heart rate reactivity to stress. For women, smoking can reduce heart rate but increase blood pressure responses to stress (Girdler, Jamner, Jarvik, Soles, & Shapiro, 1997). Trauma exposure and post-traumatic stress disorder increase the health risks of smoking (Read et al., 2013). Smoking acts synergistically with low SES as well: Smoking inflicts greater harm among disadvantaged groups than among more advantaged groups (Pampel & Rogers, 2004).

Weight and smoking can interact to increase mortality. Cigarette smokers who are thin are at increased risk of mortality, compared with average-weight smokers (Sidney, Friedman, & Siegelaub, 1987). Thinness is not associated with increased mortality in people who have never smoked or among former smokers. Smokers engage in less physical activity than nonsmokers, which represents an indirect contribution of smoking to ill health.

Smoking is more likely among people who are depressed (Pratt & Brody, 2010; Prinstein & La Greca, 2009), and smoking interacts synergistically with depression to increase risk for cancer and heart disease (Carroll et al., 2017). Smoking may also be a cause of depression, especially in young people (Goodman & Capitman, 2000), which makes the concern about the synergistic effects of smoking and depression on health more alarming. Smoking is related to anxiety in

adolescence; whether smoking and anxiety have a synergistic effect on health disorders is not yet known, but the chances of panic attacks and other anxiety disorders are increased (Johnson et al., 2000).

The synergistic health risks of smoking are very important and may be responsible for a substantial percentage of smoking-related deaths; however, research suggests that the public is largely unaware of the synergistic adverse effects of smoking (Hermand, Mullet, & Lavieville, 1997).

## A Brief History of the Smoking Problem

For years, smoking was considered to be a sophisticated and manly habit. Characterizations of 19th- and 20th-century gentry, for example, often depicted men retiring to the drawing room after dinner for cigars and brandy. Cigarette advertisements of the early 20th century built on this image, and by 1955, 53 percent of the adult male population in the United States smoked. Women did not begin to smoke in large numbers until the 1940s, but once they did, advertisers began to tie cigarette smoking to feminine sophistication as well (Pampel, 2001).

In 1964, the first surgeon general's report on smoking came out (U.S. Department of Health, Education, and Welfare and U.S. Public Health Service, 1964), accompanied by an extensive publicity campaign to highlight the dangers of smoking. The good news is that, in the United States, the number of adults who smoke has fallen dramatically to 15.5 percent. It continues to be a major health problem, however.

Critics argue that the tobacco industry has disproportionately targeted smoking appeals to minority group members and teens, and indeed, the rates among certain low-SES minority groups, such as non-Hispanic American Indians/Alaska Natives, are especially high (Centers for Disease Control and Prevention, 2017). These differences may be due in part to differences in cultural attitudes regarding smoking (Johnsen, Spring, Pingitore, Sommerfeld, & MacKirnan, 2002). At present, 27 percent of high school students use tobacco products, with electronic cigarettes most commonly used in 2018 (Centers for Disease Control and Prevention, 2019). Table 5.7 presents current figures on the prevalence of smoking, Figure 5.3 shows the relation of smoking prevalence to smoking-related historical events, and Figure 5.4 shows the prevalence of smoking by black, white, and Hispanic teens.

**TABLE 5.7 | Smoking Prevalence by Age and Sex**

| Age (years) | Percentage of Population | |
|---|---|---|
| | Males | Females |
| 18–24 | 18.5 | 14.8 |
| 25–44 | 22.9 | 17.2 |
| 45–64 | 19.4 | 16.8 |
| 65+ | 9.8 | 7.5 |

*Source:* Centers for Disease Control and Prevention. "Current Cigarette Smoking Among Adults — United States, 2005–2014." Accessed June 27, 2019. https://www.cdc.gov/mmwr/preview/mmwrhtml/mm6444a2.htm.

As pressures to reduce smoking among children and adolescents have mounted, tobacco companies have turned their marketing efforts overseas. In developing countries, smoking represents a growing health problem. For example, smoking is reaching epidemic proportions in China.

**FIGURE 5.3 | Adult per Capita Cigarette Consumption (Thousands per Year) and Major Smoking and Health Events, United States**    *Source:* Adapted from Warner (1985) with permission from Massachusetts Medical Society, 1985; U.S. Department of Health and Human Services, 1989; Creek et al., 1994; U.S. Department of Agriculture, 2000; U.S. Census Bureau, 2013; and U.S. Department of the Treasury, 2013.

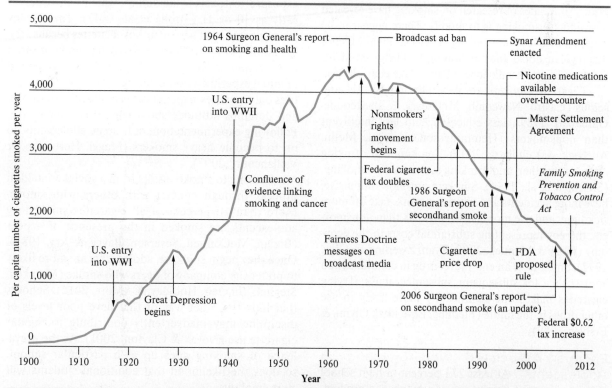

**FIGURE 5.4 | Percentage of High School Students Who Smoke**  *Source:* Centers for Disease Control and Prevention. "Cigarette Use Among High School Students — United States, 1991–2009." Accessed June 27, 2019. https://www.cdc.gov/mmwr/preview/mmwrhtml/mm5926a1.html.

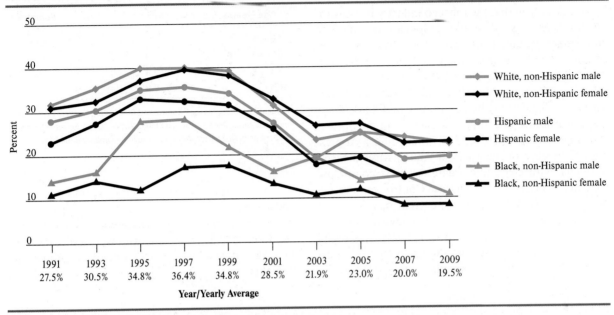

## Why Do People Smoke?

Nearly 3 decades of research on smoking have revealed how difficult smoking is to modify. There appear to be genetic influences on smoking (Piasecki, 2006). Genes that regulate dopamine functioning are likely candidates for these heritable influences (Timberlake et al., 2006).

Cigarette smokers are generally less health conscious (Castro, Newcomb, McCreary, & Baezconde-Garbanati, 1989), less educated, and less intelligent than nonsmokers (Hemmingsson, Kriebel, Melin, Allebeck, & Lundberg, 2008). Smoking and drinking often go together, and drinking seems to cue smoking, (Shiffman et al., 1994). Smokers are more impulsive, have more accidents and injuries at work, take off more sick time, and use more health benefits than nonsmokers, thereby representing substantial costs to the economy (Flory & Manuck, 2009; Ryan, Zwerling, & Orav, 1992). Smoking is an entry-level drug in childhood and adolescence for subsequent substance abuse: Trying cigarettes makes one significantly more likely to use other drugs in the future (Fleming, Leventhal, Glynn, & Ershler, 1989).

**Factors Associated with Smoking in Adolescents**    At least 27.1 percent of high school students reported current use of any tobacco product.

But smoking does not start all at once. A first step is exposure to tobacco marketing, which can occur as early as 10 or 11 (Strong et al., 2017). Then, many young people start with menthol cigarettes because the irritation and harsh flavor of smoking can be masked (*The Economist,* November 24, 2018). There is a period of initial experimentation, during which the adolescent tries out cigarettes, experiences peer pressure to smoke, and develops attitudes about what a smoker is like. Following experimentation, only some adolescents go on to become heavy smokers (Maggi, Hertzman, & Vaillancourt, 2007).

Starting to smoke results from a social contagion process through contact with others who smoke. More than 70 percent of all cigarettes smoked by adolescents are smoked in the presence of a peer (Biglan, McConnell, Severson, Bavry, & Ary, 1984). Once they begin smoking, adolescents are more likely to prefer the company of peers who smoke (Mercken, Steglich, Sinclair, Holliday, & Moore, 2012). Schools that look the other way or that have poor levels of discipline may inadvertently contribute to regular cigarette use (Novak & Clayton, 2001). As the prevalence of smoking goes up at a particular school, so does the likelihood that additional students will start smoking.

Smoking runs in families. Adolescents are more likely to start smoking if their parents smoke, and if their parents smoked early and often (Jester et al., 2019). If their parents stopped smoking before the child turned approximately 8, smoking cessation actually reduces the risk of smoking, presumably because of the family's anti-smoking attitudes (Wyszynski, Bricker, & Comstock, 2011). Adolescents are more likely to start smoking if they are from a lower social class, if they feel social pressure to smoke, and if there has been a major stressor in the family, such as parental separation or job loss (Swaim, Oetting, & Casas, 1996; Unger, Hamilton, & Sussman, 2004). These effects are partly due to the increase in stress and depression that may result (Kirby, 2002; Unger et al., 2004). Even watching people smoke in movies and on television contributes to high rates of adolescent smoking (Sargent & Heatherton, 2009) (Figure 5.4). Once adolescents begin to smoke, the risks they perceive from smoking decline, and so smoking itself reduces perceptions of risk (Morrell, Song, & Halpern-Felsher, 2010).

Smoking clusters in social networks, almost as an infectious disease might (Christakis & Fowler, 2008). Although smoking has declined overall, clusters of smokers who know each other increase the likelihood that a friend or relative will continue to smoke. The good news is that these geographic clusters also appear to spread quitting: The likelihood that someone will stop smoking increases by two-thirds if their spouse has stopped smoking, by 25 percent if a sibling has quit, and by 36 percent if a friend has quit. Even smoking cessation by a coworker decreases the likelihood that one will continue to smoke by 34 percent. Smoking, like so many other risky behaviors, spreads through social ties (Christakis & Fowler, 2008).

Self-Identity and Smoking   The image of one's self is a significant factor in beginning smoking (Tombor et al., 2015). Low self-esteem, dependency, feelings of powerlessness, and social isolation all increase the tendency to imitate others' behavior, and smoking is no exception. Feelings of being hassled, angry, or sad increase the likelihood of smoking (Whalen, Jamner, Henker, & Delfino, 2001; Wills, Sandy, & Yaeger, 2002). For example, sexual and gender minority (SGM) young adults are more likely to smoke than non-SGM young adults, and the experience of discrimination may contribute to their higher rate (Vogel, Thrul, Humfleet, Delucchi, & Ramo, 2018). Feelings of self-efficacy and good self-control

skills help adolescents resist temptations to smoke (Wills et al., 2010). Self-identity is also important for stopping smoking. Identifying oneself as a smoker impedes the ability to quit smoking, whereas identifying oneself as a quitter can promote it (Van den Putte, Yzer, Willemson, & de Bruijn, 2009).

## Nicotine Addiction and Smoking

Smoking is an addiction, reported to be harder to stop than heroin addiction or alcoholism (see Table 5.8). Only so-called chippers are able to smoke casually without showing signs of addiction. However, the exact mechanisms underlying nicotine addiction are unknown.

People smoke to maintain blood levels of nicotine and to prevent withdrawal symptoms. In essence, smoking regulates the level of nicotine in the body, and when plasma levels of nicotine depart from the ideal levels, smoking occurs. Nicotine alters levels of neuroregulators, including acetylcholine, norepinephrine, dopamine, endogenous opioids, and vasopressin. Nicotine may be used by smokers to engage these neuroregulators because they produce temporary improvements in performance or affect. Acetylcholine, norepinephrine,

**TABLE 5.8 | Why Is Smoking So Hard to Change?**

Relapse rates among smoking quitters are very high. Why is smoking such a hard habit to change?

- Tobacco addiction typically begins in adolescence, when smoking is associated with pleasurable activities.
- Smoking patterns are highly individualized, and group interventions may not address all the motives underlying any particular smoker's smoking.
- Stopping smoking leads to short-term unpleasant withdrawal symptoms such as distractibility, nausea, headaches, constipation, drowsiness, fatigue, insomnia, anxiety, irritability, and hostility.
- Smoking is mood elevating and helps to keep anxiety, irritability, and hostility at bay.
- Smoking keeps weight down, a particularly significant factor for adolescent girls and adult women.
- Smokers are unaware of the benefits of remaining abstinent over the long term, such as improved psychological well-being, higher energy, better sleep, higher self-esteem, and a sense of mastery.

*Sources:* Hertel, A. W., Emily A. Finch, Kristina Kelly, and Christie King. "The Impact of Expectations and Satisfaction on the Initiation and Maintenance of Smoking Cessation: An Experimental Test." *Health Psychology* 27, no. 3 (2008): 197–206; Stewart, A. L., A. C. King, J. D. Killen, and P. L. Ritter. "Does Smoking Cessation Improve Health-Related Quality-of-Life?." *Annals of Behavioral Medicine* 17, no. 4 (2017): 331–38.

and vasopressin appear to enhance memory, and acetylcholine and beta endorphins can reduce anxiety and tension. Alterations in dopamine, norepinephrine, and opioids improve mood. Smoking among habitual smokers improves concentration, recall, alertness, arousal, psychomotor performance, and the ability to screen out irrelevant stimuli, and consequently smoking can improve performance. Habitual smokers who stop smoking report that their concentration is reduced; their attention becomes unfocused; their memory suffers; and they experience increases in anxiety, tension, irritability, craving, and moodiness.

However, this is not a complete picture. In studies that alter nicotine level in the bloodstream, smokers do not alter their smoking behavior enough to compensate for these changes. Moreover, smoking is responsive to rapidly changing forces in the environment long before such forces can affect blood plasma levels of nicotine. High rates of relapse are found among smokers long after plasma nicotine levels are at zero. Thus, the role of nicotine in addiction may be more complex.

## Interventions to Reduce Smoking

**Changing Attitudes Toward Smoking**    The mass media have been effective in providing the educational base for anti smoking attitudes. Effective messages must be clear and based on facts (Hoover et al., 2008); this is particularly important for smokers who are knowledgeable about health issues (Hoover et al., 2008). Emotional appeals may work better for people whose knowledge of health issues is low. Pictures that evoke negative emotions have been particularly effective (Romer et al., 2018). Most people now view smoking as an addiction with negative social consequences. Antismoking media messages have also been effective in discouraging adults and adolescents from beginning to smoke (Hersey et al., 2005). However, education provides only a base and by itself may nudge people closer to the desire to quit but not to quitting itself. Moreover, many smokers do not want to stop (Borrelli et al., 2018).

**Nicotine Replacement Therapy**    Many therapies begin with some form of nicotine replacement, such as nicotine patches, which release nicotine in steady doses into the bloodstream. Nicotine replacement therapy significantly increases initial smoking cessation (Cepeda-Benito, 1993; Hughes, 1993). E-cigarettes, which work by turning a nicotine-infused liquid into a vapor, are based on this principle. Whether e-cigarettes are safe, however, is unclear (Bold, Krishnan-Sarin, & Stoney, 2018). Finding the answer to this question is important, because more youngsters now smoke e-cigarettes than traditional ones.

**The Therapeutic Approach to the Smoking Problem**    Accordingly, health psychologists have moved to a therapeutic approach to the smoking problem.

Attentional retraining involves helping smokers reorient their attention away from smoking-related cues, both internal and in the environment. It can be a first step in a stopping smoking intervention to help reduce craving and orienting toward smoking-related cues (Kerst & Waters, 2014). Exercise also helps reduce attentional bias toward smoking-related cues (Oh & Taylor, 2014).

Many smoking intervention programs have used the stages of change model as a basis for intervening. Interventions to move people from the precontemplation to the contemplation stage center on changing attitudes, emphasizing the adverse health consequences of smoking and the negative social attitudes that most people hold about smoking. Motivating a readiness to quit may, in turn, increase a sense of self-efficacy that one will be able to do so, contributing further to readiness to quit.

Moving people from contemplation to action requires that the smoker develop implementation intentions to quit, including a timetable for quitting, a program for how to quit, and an awareness of the difficulties associated with quitting (Armitage, 2008). Moving people to the action phase employs many of the cognitive–behavioral techniques that have been used to modify other health habits.

As this account suggests, smoking would seem to be a good example of how the stage model might be applied. However, interventions matched to the stage of smoking are inconsistent in their effects (Quinlan & McCaul, 2000; Segan, Borland, & Greenwood, 2004; Stotts, DiClemente, Carbonari, & Mullen, 2000).

**Social Support and Stress Management**    As is true for other health habit interventions, would-be ex-smokers are more likely to be successful over the short term if they have a supportive partner and nonsmoking supportive friends. The presence of smokers in one's social network is a hindrance to maintenance and predicts relapse (Mermelstein, Cohen, Lichtenstein, Baer,

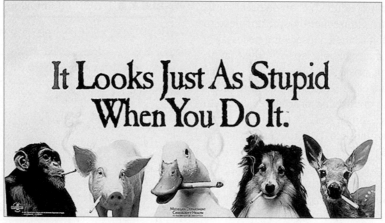

It Looks Just As Stupid
When You Do It.

*Smoking has been represented by the tobacco industry as a glamorous habit, and
one task of interventions has been to undermine that image.*
Courtesy State of Health Products. www.buttout.com 888-428-8868.

& Kamarck, 1986). Consequently, couple-based interventions have been developed that seem to be especially effective (Khaddouma et al., 2015).

Stress management training is helpful for successful quitting (Yong & Borland, 2008). Because smoking is relaxing for so many people, teaching smokers how to relax in situations in which they might be tempted to smoke provides an alternative method for coping with stress or anxiety (Manning, Catley, Harris, Mayo, & Ahluwalia, 2005). Lifestyle rebalancing through changes in diet and exercise also helps people cut down on smoking or maintain abstinence after quitting (Prapavessis et al., 2016; Zvolensky et al., 2018).

Image is also important in helping people stop. People who have a strong sense of themselves as nonsmokers do better in treatment than those who have a strong sense of themselves as smokers (Gibbons & Eggleston, 1996; Shadel & Mermelstein, 1996). Interventions with young women who smoke must take into account appearance-related issues, as young women often fear that if they stop smoking, they will put on weight (Grogan et al., 2011).

Interventions with Adolescents   Earlier, we noted how important the image of the cool, sophisticated smoker is in getting teenagers to start smoking. Several interventions to induce adolescents to stop smoking have made use of self-determination theory. Because adolescents often begin smoking to shore up their self-image with a sense of autonomy and control, self-determination theory targets those same cognitions—

namely, autonomy and self-control—but from the opposite vantage point; that is, they target the behavior of stopping smoking instead (Williams et al., 2006).

Relapse Prevention   Relapse prevention techniques are typically incorporated into smoking cessation programs (Piasecki, 2006). Relapse prevention is important because the ability to remain abstinent shows a steady month-by-month decline, such that, within 2 years after smoking cessation, even the best programs do not exceed a 50 percent abstinence rate (Piasecki, 2006).

Relapse prevention techniques begin by preparing people for withdrawal, including cardiovascular changes, increases in appetite, variations in the urge to smoke, increases in coughing and discharge of phlegm, and increases in irritability. These problems occur intermittently during the first 7 to 11 days. Relapse prevention also focuses on the ability to manage high-risk situations that lead to a craving for cigarettes, such as drinking coffee or alcohol (Piasecki, 2006) and on coping techniques for dealing with stressful interpersonal situations. Some relapse prevention approaches include contingency contracting, in which the smoker pays a sum of money that is returned only on the condition of cutting down or abstaining.

Like most addictive health habits, smoking shows an abstinence violation effect, whereby a single lapse reduces perceptions of self-efficacy, increases negative mood, and reduces beliefs that one will be successful in stopping smoking (Shadel et al., 2011). Stress-triggered lapses lead to relapse more quickly than do other kinds (Shiffman et al., 1996). Consequently, smokers need to remind themselves that a single lapse is not necessarily worrisome, because many people lapse on the road to quitting. Focusing on positive emotions may reduce the risk of lapse (Vinci et al., 2017). Sometimes, buddy systems or telephone counseling procedures can help quitters avoid turning a single lapse or temptation into a full-blown relapse (Lichtenstein, Glasgow, Lando, Ossip-Klein, & Boles, 1996).

Evaluation of Interventions   How successful have smoking interventions been? Adult smokers are well served by cognitive–behavioral interventions that include self-monitoring, modification of the stimuli that elicit and maintain smoking, reinforcing successful smoking cessation, and relapse prevention techniques such as rehearsing alternative coping techniques in high-risk situations. This is especially true if the health care professional has strong behavioral counseling skills (Hagimoto, Nakamura, Masui, Bai, & Oshima, 2018; Lorencatto, West, Bruguera, Brose, & Michie, 2016). However, these approaches may be less successful with adolescents. What may be needed instead are inexpensive, efficient, short-term interventions (McVea, 2006). Programs that include a motivation enhancement component, a focus on self-efficacy, stress management, and social skills training can be successful and can be delivered in school clinics and classrooms (Sussman, Sun, & Dent, 2006; Van Zundert, Ferguson, Shiffman, & Engels, 2010).

Virtually every imaginable combination of therapies for getting people to stop has been tested. Typically, these programs show high initial success rates for quitting, followed by high rates of return to smoking, sometimes as high as 90 percent. Those who relapse are more likely to be depressed, young and dependent on nicotine (Stepankova et al., 2017). Those who relapse often have a low sense of self-efficacy, concerns about gaining weight after stopping smoking, more previous quit attempts, and more slips (occasions when they used one or more cigarettes) (Lopez, Drobes, Thompson, & Brandon, 2008; Ockene et al., 2000).

Although the rates of relapse suggest some pessimism, it is important to consider the cumulative effects of smoking cessation programs. Any single effort to stop smoking yields only a 20 percent success rate, but with multiple efforts to quit, eventually the smoker may become an ex-smoker (Lichtenstein & Cohen, 1990). In fact, hundreds of thousands of smokers have

**TABLE 5.9 | Quitting Smoking**

**Here are some steps to help you prepare for your Quit Day:**

- Pick the date and mark it on your calendar.
- Tell friends and family about your Quit Day.
- Stock up on oral substitutes—sugarless gum, carrot sticks, and/or hard candy.
- Decide on a plan. Will you use nicotine replacement therapy? Will you attend a class? If so, sign up now.
- Set up a support system. This could be a group class, Nicotine Anonymous, or a friend who has successfully quit and is willing to help you.

**On your Quit Day, follow these suggestions:**

- Do not smoke.
- Get rid of all cigarettes, lighters, ashtrays, and any other items related to smoking.
- Keep active—try walking, exercising, or doing other activities or hobbies.
- Drink lots of water and juice.
- Begin using nicotine replacement if that is your choice.
- Attend a stop-smoking class or follow a self-help plan.
- Avoid situations where the urge to smoke is strong.
- Reduce or avoid alcohol.
- Use the four "A's" (avoid, alter, alternatives, activities) to deal with tough situations.

*Source:* American Cancer Society, Inc. "Deciding to Quit Smoking and Making a Plan." Accessed June 27, 2019. https://www.cancer.org/healthy/stay-away-from-tobacco/guide-quitting-smoking/deciding-to-quit-smoking-and-making-a-plan.html.

quit, albeit not necessarily the first time they tried. Over time, people may amass enough techniques and the motivation to persist.

People who quit on their own are typically well-educated and have good self-control skills, self-confidence in their ability to stop, and a perception that the health benefits of stopping are substantial (McBride et al., 2001). Stopping on one's own is easier if one has a supportive social network that does not smoke and if one is able to distance oneself from the typical smoker and identify with nonsmokers instead (Gerrard, Gibbons, Lane, & Stock, 2005). Stopping is also more successful following an acute or chronic health threat, such as a diagnosis of heart disease, especially among middle-aged smokers (Falba, 2005). Stopping smoking can lead spontaneously to other beneficial changes in health behaviors (Noonan et al., 2016). A list of guidelines for people who wish to stop on their own appears in Table 5.9.

Brief Interventions   Brief interventions by physicians and other health care practitioners can bring about smoking cessation and control relapse (Vogt, Hall, Hankins, & Marteau, 2009). Providing smoking cessation guidelines during medical visits may improve the quit rate (Williams, Gagne, Ryan, & Deci, 2002). One health maintenance organization targeted the adult smokers in their program with telephone counseling and newsletters that offered quitting guidelines; the program achieved its goal of reducing smoking, and, most notably, it reached smokers who otherwise would not have participated in cessation programs (Glasgow et al., 2008). The state of Massachusetts began offering free stop-smoking treatment to poor residents in 2006 and achieved a remarkable decline in smoking from 38 to 28 percent, suggesting that incorporating brief interventions into Medicaid programs can be successful (Goodnough, 2009, December 17).

Workplace   Initially, workplace interventions were thought to hold promise in smoking cessation efforts. To date, however, workplace interventions are not more effective than other intervention programs (Facts of Life, July 2005). However, when workplace environments are entirely smoke-free, employees smoke much less (Facts of Life, July 2005).

Commercial Programs and Self-Help   A variety of **self-help aids** and programs have been developed for smokers to quit on their own. These include nicotine patches, as well as more intensive self-help programs. Cable television programs designed to help people stop initially and to maintain their resolution have been broadcast in some cities. Although it is difficult to evaluate self-help programs formally, studies suggest that initial quit rates are lower but that long-term maintenance rates are just as high as with more intensive behavioral interventions. Because self-help programs are inexpensive, they represent an important attack on the smoking problem for both adults and adolescents (Lipkus et al., 2004).

Quitlines provide telephone counseling to help people stop smoking and are quite successful (Lichtenstein, Zhu, & Tedeschi, 2010). People can call in when they want to get help for quitting or if they are worried about relapse. Most such programs are based on principles derived from CBT. Both adults and younger smokers can benefit from this kind of telephone counseling (Rabius, McAlister, Geiger, Huang, & Todd, 2004).

Internet interventions are a recent approach to the smoking problem (Graham, Papandonatos, Cha, Erar, & Amato, 2018) that has several advantages: People can seek them out when they are ready to and without regard to location. They can deal with urges to smoke by getting instant feedback from an Internet service. In a randomized control trial sponsored by the American Cancer Society, an Internet program for smoking cessation was significantly more helpful to smokers trying to quit than a control condition. Moreover, the effects lasted longer than a year, suggesting the long-term efficacy of Internet interventions for smoking cessation (Seidman et al., 2010).

Public health approaches to reducing smoking begin with warning labels on cigarette packs, billboards, and other places where they are likely to be noticed. These warnings help raise concerns, which can lead to quit attempts (Yong et al., 2014). More broad-based approaches initially focused on community interventions combining media blitzes with behavioral interventions directed especially at high-risk people, such as people with other risk factors for CHD. However, such interventions are often expensive, and long-term follow-ups suggest limited long-term effects (Facts of Life, July 2005). Ultimately, banning cigarette smoking from workplaces and public settings and raising cigarette taxes have been most successful in reducing smoking (Orbell et al., 2009; *The Economist,* July 28, 2018).

## Smoking Prevention Programs

The war on smoking also focuses on keeping potential smokers from starting. These **smoking prevention programs** aim to catch potential smokers early and attack the underlying motivations that lead people to smoke. Typically, these programs are implemented through the school system. They are inexpensive and efficient because little class time is needed and no training of school personnel is required.

The central components of social influence interventions are:

* Information about the negative effects of smoking is carefully constructed to appeal to adolescents.

* Materials are developed to convey a positive image of the nonsmoker (rather than the smoker) as an independent, self-reliant individual.

* The peer group is used to foster not smoking rather than smoking.

BOX **5.7** The Perils of Secondhand Smoke

Norma Broyne was a flight attendant with American Airlines for 21 years. She had never smoked a cigarette, and yet, in 1989, she was diagnosed with lung cancer, and part of a lung had to be removed. Broyne became the center of a class-action suit brought against the tobacco industry, seeking $5 billion on behalf of 60,000 current and former nonsmoking flight attendants for the adverse health effects of the smoke they inhaled while performing their job responsibilities prior to 1990, when smoking was legal on most flights (Collins, 1997, May 30). Norma Broyne finally saw her day in court. The tobacco companies that she and other flight attendants sued agreed to pay $300 million to set up a research foundation on cancer.

**Passive smoking,** or **secondhand smoke,** is the third-leading cause of preventable death in the United States, killing more than 41,000 nonsmokers every year (Table 5.10). It causes about 3,000 cases of lung cancer annually, as many as 62,000 heart disease deaths, and exacerbation of asthma in 1 million children (California Environmental Protection Agency, 2005; Endrighi, McQuaid, Bartlett, Clawson, & Borrelli, 2018).

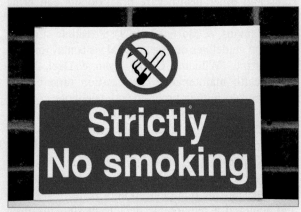

Trevor Benbrook/123RF

**TABLE 5.10 | The Toll of Secondhand Smoke**

| Disease | Annual Consequences |
| --- | --- |
| Lung cancer | 7,330 deaths |
| Heart disease | 33,950 deaths |
| Sudden infant death syndrome | 430 deaths |
| Buildup of fluid in the middle ear | 790,000 doctor's office visits |
| Asthma in children | 202,000 asthma flare-ups |
| Lower respiratory infection | 150,000–300,000 |

*Source:* American Lung Association. "Health Effects of Secondhand Smoke." Accessed June 27, 2019. https://www.lung.org/stop-smoking/smoking-facts/health-effects-of-secondhand-smoke.html.

Babies with prenatal exposure to secondhand smoke have a 7 percent lower birth weight (Environmental Health Perspectives, 2004). Exposure to secondhand smoke also increases the risk of depression (Bandiera et al., 2010).

In a dramatic confirmation of the problems associated with workplace smoking, the state of Montana imposed a ban on public and workplace smoking in June 2002 and then overturned it 6 months later. Two physicians charted the number of heart attacks that occurred before the ban, during it, and afterward. Heart attack admissions dropped 40 percent when the workplace ban on smoking was in place but immediately bounced back when smoking resumed. What is remarkable about the Montana study is its demonstration of its immediate impact on a major health outcome—heart attacks—in such a short time (Glantz, 2004).

Overall, the best way to reduce smoking is to tax tobacco products, restrict where people can smoke, and deliver cost-effective cognitive–behavioral interventions with relapse prevention techniques to people who are already smokers (Federal Tax Increase, 2009).

**Evaluation of Social Influence Programs** Do these programs work? Overall, social influence programs can reduce smoking rates (Resnicow et al., 2008) for as long as 4 years (Murray, Davis-Hearn, Goldman, Pirie, & Luepker, 1988). However, experimental smoking may be affected more than regular smoking, and experimental smokers may stop on their own anyway (Flay et al., 1992). What is needed are programs that will reach the child destined to become a regular smoker, and as yet, we know less about what helps to keep these youngsters from starting to smoke. •

## SUMMARY

1. Health-compromising behaviors are those that threaten or undermine good health. Many of these behaviors cluster and first emerge in adolescence.

2. Obesity has been linked to cardiovascular disease, kidney disease, diabetes, some cancers, and other chronic conditions.

3. Causes of obesity include genetic predisposition, early diet, a family history of obesity, low SES, little exercise, and consumption of large portions of high-calorie food and drinks. Ironically, dieting may contribute to the propensity for obesity.

4. Obesity has been treated through diets, surgical procedures, drugs, and CBT. CBT includes monitoring eating behavior, modifying the environmental stimuli that control eating, gaining control over the eating process, and reinforcing new eating habits. Relapse prevention skills help in long-term maintenance.

5. Cognitive–behavioral techniques can produce weight losses of 2 pounds a week for up to 20 weeks, maintained over a 2-year period.

6. Increasingly, interventions are focusing on weight-gain prevention with children in obese families and with high-risk adults.

7. Eating disorders, especially anorexia nervosa, bulimia, and bingeing are major health problems, especially among adolescents and young adults, and health problems, including death, commonly result.

8. Alcoholism accounts for thousands of deaths each year through cirrhosis, cancer, fetal alcohol syndrome, and accidents connected with drunk driving.

9. Alcoholism has a genetic component and is tied to sociodemographic factors such as low SES. Drinking also arises in an effort to buffer the impact of stress and appears to peak between ages 18 and 25.

10. Residential treatment programs for alcoholism begin with an inpatient "drying out" period, followed by the use of cognitive–behavioral change methods including relapse prevention. However, most programs are outpatient and use principles of CBT.

11. The best predictor of success is the patient. Alcoholics with mild drinking problems, little abuse of other drugs, and a supportive, financially secure environment do better than those without such supports.

12. Smoking accounts for more than 480,000 deaths annually in the United States due to heart disease, cancer, and lung disorders.

13. Theories of the addictive nature of smoking focus on nicotine and nicotine's role as a neuroregulator.

14. Attitudes toward smoking have changed dramatically for the negative, largely due to the mass media. Attitude change has kept some people from beginning smoking, motivated many to try to stop, and kept some former smokers from relapsing.

15. Many programs for stopping smoking begin with some form of nicotine replacement, and use CBT to help people stop smoking. Interventions also include social skills training programs and relaxation therapies. Relapse prevention is an important component of these programs.

16. Smoking is highly resistant to change. Even after successfully stopping for a short time, most people relapse. Factors that contribute to relapse include addiction, lack of effective coping techniques for dealing with social situations, and weight gain.

17. Smoking prevention programs are designed to keep youngsters from beginning to smoke. Many of these programs use a social influence approach and teach youngsters how to resist peer pressure to smoke and help adolescents improve their coping skills and self-image.

18. Social engineering approaches to control smoking have also been used, in part, because secondhand smoke harms others in the smoker's environment.

## KEY TERMS

addiction
alcoholism
anorexia nervosa
binge eating disorder
bingeing
bulimia
controlled drinking
craving

detoxification
obesity
passive smoking
physical dependence
placebo drinking
problem drinking
secondhand smoke
self-help aids

set point theory of weight
smoking prevention programs
stress eating
tolerance
withdrawal
weight stigma
yo-yo dieting

# PART 3

# Stress and Coping

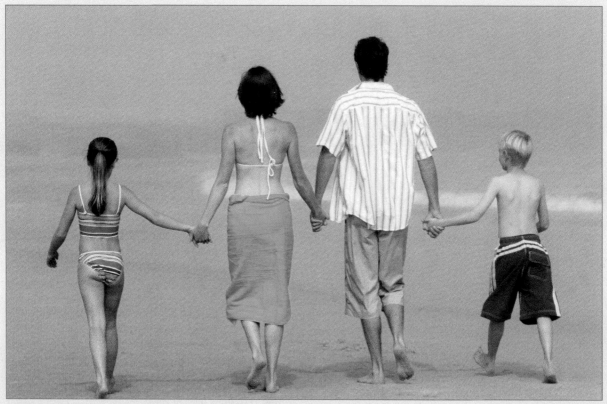

Stockbyte/Getty Images

CHAPTER 6

# Stress

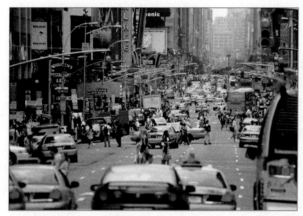

Grant V Faint/Photodisc/Getty Images

# ■ WHAT IS STRESS?

Most of us have more first-hand experience with stress than we care to remember. Stress is being stopped by a police officer after accidentally running a red light. It is waiting to take a test when you are not sure that you have studied enough or studied the right material. It is missing a bus on a rainy day full of important appointments.

**Stress** is a negative emotional experience accompanied by predictable biochemical, physiological, cognitive, and behavioral changes that are directed either toward altering the stressful event or accommodating to its effects.

## What Is a Stressor?

Initially, researchers focused on stressful events themselves, called **stressors.** In the United States, for example, people report that money, the economy, work, family health problems, and family responsibilities are their top five stressors (American Psychological Association, 2008).

But an experience may be stressful to some people but not to others. If "noise" is the latest rock music playing on your radio, then it will probably not be stressful to you, although it may be to your neighbor.

## Appraisal of Stressors

Stress is the consequence of a person's appraisal processes (Lazarus & Launier, 1978): **primary appraisal** occurs as a person is trying to understand what the event is and what it will mean. Events may be appraised for their harm, threat, or challenge. Harm is the assessment of the damage that has already been done, as for example being fired from a job. Threat is the assessment of possible future damage, as a person anticipates the problems that loss of income will create for him and his family. But events may also be appraised in terms of their challenge, that is, the potential to overcome or even profit from the event. For example, a woman who lost her job may regard her unemployment as an opportunity to try something new. Challenge assessments lead to more confident expectations that one can cope with the stressful event, more favorable emotional reactions to the event, and lower blood pressure, among other benefits (Blascovich, 2008).

**Secondary appraisals** assess whether personal resources are sufficient to meet the demands of the environment. When a person's resources are more than adequate to deal with a difficult situation, he or she may feel little stress and experience a sense of challenge instead. When the person perceives that his or her resources will probably be sufficient to deal with the event but only with a lot of effort, he or she may feel a moderate amount of stress. When the person perceives that his or her resources will probably not be sufficient to overcome the stressor, he or she may experience a great deal of stress.

Stress, then, is determined by **person-environment fit** (Lazarus & Folkman, 1984; Lazarus & Launier, 1978). It results from the process of appraising events (as harmful, threatening, or challenging), of assessing potential resources, and of responding to the events. To see how stress researchers have arrived at this current understanding, we examine the origins of stress research.

# ■ ORIGINS OF THE STUDY OF STRESS

## Fight or Flight

The earliest contribution to stress research was Walter Cannon's (1932) description of the **fight-or-flight response.** Cannon proposed that when an organism perceives a threat, the body is rapidly aroused and motivated via the sympathetic nervous system and the endocrine system. This concerted physiological response mobilizes the organism to attack the threat or to flee; hence, it is called the fight-or-flight response.

At one time, fight or flight literally referred to fighting or fleeing in response to stressful events such as attack by a predator. Now, more commonly, *fight* refers to aggressive responses to stress, such as getting angry or taking action, whereas *flight* is reflected in social withdrawal or withdrawal through substance use or distracting activities. On the one hand, the fight-or-flight response is adaptive because it enables the organism to respond quickly to threat. On the other hand, it can be harmful because stress disrupts emotional and physiological functioning, and when stress continues unabated, it lays the groundwork for health problems.

## Selye's General Adaptation Syndrome

Another important early contribution to stress was Hans Selye's (1956, 1976) work on the **general adaptation syndrome.** Selye exposed rats to a variety of stressors, such as extreme cold and fatigue, and observed

**FIGURE 6.1 | The Three Phases of Selye's General Adaptation Syndrome**
Hans Selye, a pioneering stress researcher, formulated the General Adaptation Syndrome. He proposed that people go through three phases in response to stress. The first is the alarm phase, in which the body reacts to a stressor with diminished resistance. In the second stage, the stage of resistance that follows continued exposure to a stressor, stress responses rise above normal. The third phase, exhaustion, results from long-term exposure to the stressor, and at this point, resistance will fall below normal.

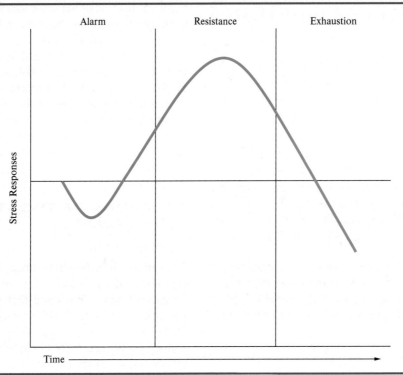

their physiological responses. To his surprise, all stress-ors, regardless of type, produced essentially the same pattern of physiological changes. They all led to an enlarged adrenal cortex, shrinking of the thymus and lymph glands, and ulceration of the stomach and duodenum.

From these observations, Selye (1956) developed the general adaptation syndrome. He argued that when a person confronts a stressor, it mobilizes itself for ac-tion. The response itself is nonspecific with respect to the stressor; that is, regardless of the cause of the threat, the person will respond with the same physiological pattern of reactions. (As will be seen, this particular conclusion has now been challenged.) Over time, with repeated or prolonged exposure to stress, there will be wear and tear on the system.

The general adaptation syndrome consists of three phases. In the first phase, *alarm,* the person be-comes mobilized to meet the threat. In the second

phase, *resistance,* the person makes efforts to cope with the threat, as through confrontation. The third phase, *exhaustion,* occurs if the person fails to over-come the threat and depletes physiological resources in the process of trying. These phases are pictured in Figure 6.1.

Criticisms of the General Adaptation Syn-drome    Selye's model has been criticized on several grounds. First, it assigns a very limited role to psycho-logical factors, and researchers now believe that the psychological appraisal of events is critical to experi-encing stress (Lazarus & Folkman, 1984). A second criticism concerns the fact that not all stressors pro-duce the same biological responses (Kemeny, 2003). How people respond to stress is influenced by their personalities, emotions, and biological constitutions (e.g., Moons, Eisenberger, & Taylor, 2010). A third criticism concerns whether exhaustion of physiological resources or their chronic activation is most implicated in stress; research suggests that continued activation (the second phase) may be most important for accumulating damage to physiological systems, rather than exhaustion. Finally, Selye assessed stress as an outcome, that is, the endpoint of the general adaptation syndrome. In fact, people experience many debilitating effects of stress after an event has ended and even in anticipation of its occurrence. Despite these limitations and reservations, Selye's model remains a cornerstone in the field.

## Tend-and-Befriend

In response to stress, people (and animals) do not merely fight, flee, and grow exhausted. They also affiliate with each other, whether it is the herding behavior of antelope in response to a predator or the coordinated responses to a stressor that a community shows when it is under the threat of a hurricane. Taylor et al. (2000) developed a theory of responses to stress termed **tend-and-befriend.** The theory maintains that, in addition to fight or flight, people and animals respond to stress with social affiliation and nurturant behavior toward offspring. These responses to stress may be especially true of women.

During the time that responses to stress evolved, men and women faced somewhat different adaptive challenges. Whereas men were responsible for hunting and protection, women were responsible for foraging and child care. These activities were largely sex segregated, with the result that women's responses to stress would have evolved so as to protect not only the self but offspring as well. These responses are not distinctive to humans. The offspring of most species are immature and would be unable to survive, were it not for the attention of adults. In most species, that attention is provided by the mother.

Tend-and-befriend has an underlying biological mechanism, in particular, the hormone oxytocin. Oxytocin is a stress hormone, rapidly released in response to some stressful events, and its effects are especially influenced by estrogen, suggesting a particularly important role in the responses of women to stress. Oxytocin acts as an impetus for affiliation in both animals and humans, and oxytocin increases affiliative behaviors of all kinds, especially mothering (Taylor, 2002). In addition, animals and humans with high levels of oxytocin are calmer and more relaxed, which may contribute to their social and nurturant behavior.

Research supports some key components of the theory. Women are indeed more likely than men to respond to stress by turning to others (Luckow, Reifman, & McIntosh, 1998; Tamres, Janicki, & Helgeson, 2002). Mothers' responses to offspring during times of stress also appear to be different from those of fathers in ways encompassed by the tend-and-befriend theory. Nonetheless, men, too, show social responses to stress, and so elements of the theory apply to men as well.

## How Does Stress Contribute to Illness?

These early contributions to the study of stress have helped researchers identify the pathways by which stress leads to poor health. The first set of pathways involves direct effects on physiology. As both Cannon and Selye showed, stress alters biological functioning. The ways in which it does so and how it interacts with existing risks or genetic predispositions to illness determine what illnesses a person will develop. Direct physiological effects include such processes as elevated blood pressure, a decreased ability of the immune system to fight off infection, and changes in lipid levels and cholesterol, among other changes. We explore these more fully in the next sections.

A second set of pathways concerns health behaviors (Chapters 3 to 5). People who live with chronic stress have poorer health habits than people who do not, and acute stress, even when it is short-term, often compromises health habits. These poor health habits can include smoking, poor nutrition, little sleep, little exercise, and use of substances such as drugs and alcohol. Over the long term, each of these poor health habits contributes to specific illnesses. For example, smoking can cause lung disease. Even in the short term, changes in these health habits may increase the risk for illness and set the stage for longer-term adverse health outcomes.

Third, stress affects psychosocial resources in ways that can adversely affect health (Chapter 7). Supportive social contacts are protective of health, but stress can make a person avoid these social contacts or, worse, behave in ways that drive others away. Optimism, self-esteem, and a sense of personal control also contribute to good health, yet many stressors undermine these beneficial resources. To the extent that time, money, and energy must be put into combating the stressor, these external resources are compromised as well, falling especially hard on people who have very little of those resources.

**FIGURE 6.2 | Stress and Mental and Physical Health**
Stress contributes to mental and physical health disorders. This figure shows some of the routes by which these effects may occur.    *Source.* Cohen, Sheldon, Ronald C. Kessler, and Lynn Underwood Gordon. *Measuring Stress: A Guide for Health and Social Scientists*. Michigan: Oxford University Press, 1965.

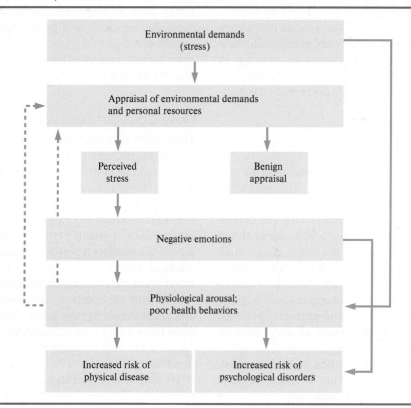

A fourth set of pathways by which stress adversely affects health involves the use of health services and adherence to treatment recommendations. People are less likely to adhere to a treatment regimen when they are under stress, and they are more likely to delay seeking care for disorders that should be treated. Alternatively, they may not seek care at all. These pathways are addressed primarily in Chapters 8 and 9.

These four routes—physiology, health behaviors, psychosocial resources, and use of health services—represent the most important pathways by which stress affects health (see Figure 6.2).

## ■ THE PHYSIOLOGY OF STRESS

Stress engages psychological distress and leads to changes in the body that may have short- and long-term consequences for health. Two interrelated systems are heavily involved in the stress response. They are the sympathetic adrenomedullary (SAM) system and the hypothalamic–pituitary–adrenocortical (HPA) axis.

Sympathetic Activation    When events are perceived as harmful or threatening, they are identified as such by the cerebral cortex in the brain, which, in turn, sets off a chain of reactions mediated by these appraisals. Information from the cortex is transmitted to the hypothalamus, which initiates one of the earliest responses to stress—namely, sympathetic nervous system arousal. Sympathetic arousal stimulates the medulla of the adrenal glands, which, in turn, secrete the catecholamines epinephrine (EP) and norepinephrine (NE). These effects result in the cranked-up feeling we usually experience in response to stress: increased blood pressure, increased heart rate, increased sweating, and constriction of peripheral blood vessels, among other changes. The catecholamines modulate the immune system as well.

Parasympathetic functioning may also become dysregulated in response to stress. For example, stress can affect heart rate variability. Parasympathetic modulation is an important restorative aspect of rest and sleep, and so, changes in heart rate variability may both represent a pathway to disturbed sleep and help to explain the relation of stress to illness and increased risk for mortality.

**HPA Activation**    The HPA axis is also activated in response to stress. The hypothalamus releases corticotrophin-releasing hormone (CRH), which stimulates the pituitary gland to secrete adrenocorticotropic hormone (ACTH), which, in turn, stimulates the adrenal cortex to release glucocorticoids. Of these, cortisol is especially significant. It acts to conserve stores of carbohydrates and helps reduce inflammation in the case of an injury. It also helps the body return to its steady state following stress. When its functioning is compromised, as happens, for example, in people of low SES under chronic stress, it may contribute to the chronic disease burden carried by low SES populations (Le-Scherban et al., 2018).

Repeated activation of the HPA axis in response to chronic or recurring stress can ultimately compromise its functioning. Daily cortisol patterns may be altered. Normally, cortisol levels are high upon waking in the morning, but decrease during the day (although peaking following lunch) until they flatten out at low levels in the afternoon. People under chronic stress, however, can show any of several deviant patterns: elevated cortisol levels long into the afternoon or evening, a general flattening of the daily rhythm, an exaggerated cortisol response to a challenge, a protracted cortisol response following a stressor, or, alternatively, no response at all (McEwen, 1998). Any of these patterns is suggestive of compromised ability of the HPA axis to respond to and recover from stress with concomitant health effects (Piazza, Dmitrieva, Charles, Almeida, & Orona, 2018). (Figure 6.3). For example, a blunted cortisol response that implies physiological dysregulation has been tied to risk for cardiovascular disease, enhanced pain sensitivity, and exacerbation of symptoms of withdrawal in addictive disorders (al'Absi, 2018). Even preschoolers with flat cortisol rhythms show compromised sleep over time (Saridjan et al., 2019).

## Effects of Long-Term Stress

Although physiological mobilization prepared humans to fight or flee in prehistoric times, only rarely do our current stressful events require these kinds of adjustments. That is, job strain, commuting, family quarrels, and money worries are not the sorts of stressors that demand this dramatic mobilization of physical resources. Nonetheless, people still experience sudden elevations of circulating stress hormones in response to current-day stressors, and this process, in certain respects, does not serve the purpose for which it originally developed.

Over the long term, excessive discharge of epinephrine and norepinephrine can lead to suppression of immune function; produce adverse changes such as increased blood pressure and heart rate; provoke variations in normal heart rhythms, such as ventricular arrhythmias, which can be a precursor to sudden death; and produce neurochemical imbalances that may contribute to the development of psychiatric disorders. The catecholamines may also have effects on lipid levels and free fatty acids, which contribute to the development of atherosclerosis, as was seen in Chapter 2.

Corticosteroids have immunosuppressive effects, which can compromise the functioning of the immune system. Prolonged cortisol secretion has also been related to the destruction of neurons in the hippocampus, which can lead to problems with verbal functioning, memory, and concentration (Starkman, Giordani, Brenent, Schork, & Schteingart, 2001) and may be one of the mechanisms leading to senility. Pronounced HPA activation is common in depression, with episodes of cortisol secretion being more frequent and longer among depressed than nondepressed people. Storage of fat in central visceral areas (i.e., belly fat), rather than in the hips, is another consequence of prolonged HPA activation. This accumulation leads to a high waist-to-hip ratio, which is used by some researchers as a marker for chronic stress (Bjorntorp, 1996).

Which of these responses to stress have implications for disease? The health consequences of HPA axis activation may be more significant than those of sympathetic activation (Blascovich, 1992; Dientsbier, 1989; Jamieson, Mendes, & Nock, 2013). Sympathetic arousal in response to stress by itself may not be a pathway for disease; HPA activation may be required as well. This reasoning may explain why exercise, which produces sympathetic arousal but not HPA activation, is protective for health rather than health compromising. However, unlike exercise, stressors can be experienced long after a stressful event has terminated, and cardiovascular activation may persist for hours, days,

**FIGURE 6.3 | How Does Stress Cause Illness?**
Direct physiological effects result from sympathetic nervous system and/or HPA activation. In addition, as this figure shows, stress may affect health via behaviors, first, by influencing health behavior, second, by affecting the use of psychosocial resources and, third, by interfering with treatment and the use of health services.

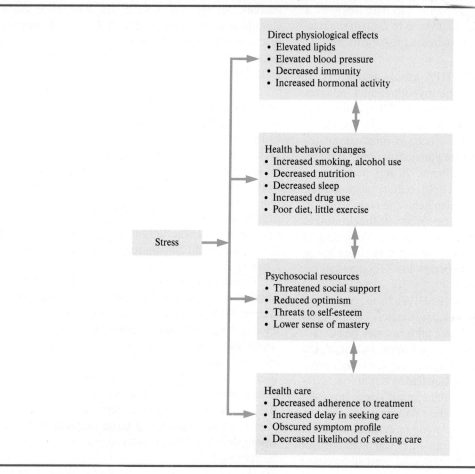

Stress

Direct physiological effects
• Elevated lipids
• Elevated blood pressure
• Decreased immunity
• Increased hormonal activity

Health behavior changes
• Increased smoking, alcohol use
• Decreased nutrition
• Decreased sleep
• Increased drug use
• Poor diet, little exercise

Psychosocial resources
• Threatened social support
• Reduced optimism
• Threats to self-esteem
• Lower sense of mastery

Health care
• Decreased adherence to treatment
• Increased delay in seeking care
• Obscured symptom profile
• Decreased likelihood of seeking care

weeks, or even years after an initial stressful event has occurred, even without awareness (Pieper, Brosschot, van der Leeden, & Thayer, 2010). Such wear and tear on the cardiovascular system may foster illness.

Stress may also compromise immune functioning (Chapter 14). Among these changes is impairment of the immune system's ability to terminate inflammation, which is an early response to stress. Chronic inflammation, even low-level chronic inflammation, is implicated in many diseases including coronary artery disease (Rohleder, 2014) (see Chapter 2), and so the impaired ability to terminate inflammation may be an important pathway by which stress affects illness outcomes. Slow wound healing, for example, may be one consequence (Walburn et al., 2017).

Poor sleep can be a consequence of chronic stress. Because sleep represents a vital restorative activity, this mechanism, too, represents a pathway to disease.

## Individual Differences in Stress Reactivity

People vary in their reactivity to stress. **Reactivity** is the degree of change that occurs in autonomic, neuroendocrine, and/or immune responses as a result of stress. Some people are predisposed by their genetic makeup, prenatal experiences, and/or early life experiences to be more biologically reactive to stress than others and, consequently, they may be especially vulnerable to adverse health consequences due to stress (Boyce et al., 1995; Jacobs et al., 2006).

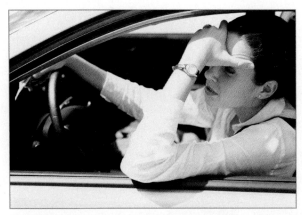

*Stressful events such as being stuck in traffic produce agitation and physiological arousal.*

Stockbyte/Getty Images

**TABLE 6.1 | Indicators of Allostatic Load**

- Decreases in cell-mediated immunity
- The inability to shut off cortisol in response to stress
- Lowered heart rate variability
- Elevated epinephrine levels
- A high waist-to-hip ratio (reflecting abdominal fat)
- Hippocampal volume (which can decrease with repeated stimulation of the HPA)
- Problems with memory (an indirect measure of hippocampal functioning)
- Elevated blood pressure

*Source:* "Seeman, Teresa E., Burton Singer, John W. Rowe, and Ralph Horwitz. "Price of Adaptation - Allostatic Load and Its Health Consequences." *Archives of Internal Medicine 157* (November 1997): 2259–2268."

For example, S. Cohen and colleagues (2002) found that people who reacted to laboratory stressors with high cortisol responses and who also had a high level of negative life events were especially vulnerable to upper respiratory infections when exposed to a virus. People who reacted to laboratory stressors with low immune responses were especially vulnerable to upper respiratory infection only if they were also under high stress. High immune reactors, in contrast, did not show differences in upper respiratory illness as a function of the stress they experienced, perhaps because their immune systems were quick to respond to the threat that a potential infection posed.

Studies like these suggest that psychobiological reactivity to stress is an important factor that influences the stress–illness relationship (McCubbin et al., 2018). As will be seen in Chapter 13, differences in reactivity are believed to contribute to the development of hypertension and coronary artery disease.

### Physiological Recovery

Recovery following stress is also important in the physiology of the stress response. The inability to recover quickly from a stressful event may be a marker for the cumulative damage that stress has caused. Researchers have paid special attention to the cortisol response, particularly, prolonged cortisol responses that occur under conditions of high stress.

In one intriguing study (Perna & McDowell, 1995), elite athletes were divided into those who were experiencing a high versus a low amount of stress in their lives, and their cortisol response was measured following vigorous training. Those athletes under more stress had a protracted cortisol response. Stress may, accordingly, widen the window of susceptibility for illness and injury among competitive athletes by virtue of its impact on cortisol recovery.

### Allostatic Load

Multiple physiological systems within the body fluctuate to meet demands from stress, as we have seen. The concept of **allostatic load** has been developed to refer to the physiological costs of chronic exposure to the physiological changes that result from repeated or chronic stress (McEwen, 1998). Allostatic load can begin to accumulate in childhood, affecting multiple disease risks across the lifespan (Wiley, Gruenewald, Karlamangla, & Seeman, 2016). The buildup of allostatic load can be assessed by a number of indicators, including increasing weight and higher blood pressure (Seeman, Singer, Horwitz, & McEwen, 1997). Telomeres, a sequence of DNA at the ends of chromosomes, protect DNA and regulate aging at the cellular level. Shorter telomeres have accordingly been regarded as a sign of accelerated aging. Many experiences of stress, such as discrimination, have been tied to shorter telomeres and other signs of accelerated aging (Lee, Kim, & Neblett, 2017). More of these indicators are listed in Table 6.1. Allostatic load is tied not only to multisystem adverse changes prognostic for poor health, but also with personality changes, such as increases in neuroticism and decreases in extroversion and conscientiousness. These adverse personality changes may be another route by which allostatic load increases health risks (Yannick, Sutin, Luchetti, & Terracciano, 2016).

BOX **6.1** | Can Stress Affect Pregnancy?

Common wisdom has long held that pregnant women should be treated especially well and avoid major stressors in their lives. Research now supports that wisdom by showing that stress can actually endanger the course of pregnancy and childbirth.

Stress affects the immune and endocrine systems in ways that directly affect the growing fetus. These changes are potentially dangerous because they can lead to spontaneous abortion (Wainstock, Lerner-Geva, Glasser, Shoham-Vardi, & Anteby, 2013), and preterm birth and low birth weight, among other adverse outcomes (Glynn, Dunkel-Schetter, Hobel, & Sandman, 2008; Tegethoff, Greene, Olsen, Meyer, & Meinlschmidt, 2010). African American women and acculturated Mexican American women appear to be especially vulnerable, due in large part to the stress they experience (D'Anna-Hernandez et al., 2012; Hilmert et al., 2008) even stress experienced in childhood (Mitchell, Porter, & Christian, 2018). The mother's elevated cortisol levels in response to stress act as a signal to the fetus that it is time to be born, leading to preterm birth (Mancuso, Dunkel-Schetter, Rini, Roesch, & Hobel, 2004).

Are there any factors that can protect against adverse birth outcomes due to stress? Social support, especially from a partner, protects against adverse birth outcomes (Feldman, Dunkel-Schetter, Sandman, & Wadhwa, 2000). Psychosocial resources such as mastery, self-esteem, and optimism may also help guard against adverse birth outcomes (Rini, Dunkel-Schetter,

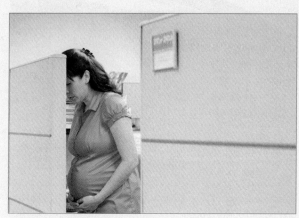

Terry Vine Photography/Blend Images LLC

Wadhwa, & Sandman, 1999). Pregnancy-specific stress can elevate birth risks as well (Cole-Lewis et al., 2014) and affect the child's characteristics years later (Wu et al., 2018). The anxiety that can accompany stress and the prenatal period exacerbates cortisol levels and increases the likelihood of an adverse birth outcome, and so interventions to reduce anxiety may be helpful as well (Mancuso et al., 2004).

But the old adage about taking it easy during pregnancy and the more dire warnings about the high risks for adverse birth outcomes in disadvantaged groups make it clear that pregnancy is an especially important time to avoid stress and to draw on one's psychological and social resources.

Many of these changes occur normally with age, so to the extent that they occur early, accumulating allostatic load may be thought of as accelerated aging in response to stress. Over time, this kind of wear and tear can lead to illness and increased risk of death (Gallo, Fortmann, & Mattei, 2014). The damage due to chronic stress is made worse if people also cope with stress via a high-fat diet, infrequent exercise, alcohol abuse, and smoking, all of which stress can encourage (Doan et al., 2014). Bisexual men appear to be especially at risk for accumulation of allostatic load (Mays et al., 2018).

The relationship of stress to both acute disorders, such as infection, and chronic disorders, such as heart disease, is now well known. We explore these processes more fully with heart disease and hypertension in Chapter 13

and cancer and arthritis in Chapter 14. Stress can even affect the course of pregnancy, as Box 6.1 shows.

### ■ WHAT MAKES EVENTS STRESSFUL?

#### Dimensions of Stressful Events

Although events are not necessarily inherently stressful, some characteristics of events make them more likely to be appraised as stressful.

Negative Events Negative events produce more stress than do positive events. Shopping for the holidays, coping with an unexpected job promotion, and getting married are all positive events that draw off time and energy. Nonetheless, these positive experiences are less stressful than negative or undesirable events, such as getting a traffic ticket, trying to find a job, coping with a death in the family, getting divorced or experiencing daily conflict (Tobin et al., 2015). Rejection targeted at you specifically by another person or group is particularly toxic (Murphy, Slavich, Chen, & Miller, 2015). Negative events produce more psychological distress and physical symptoms than positive ones do (Sarason, Johnson, & Siegel, 1978). Both rumination and psychological distress can have adverse effects on health (Chiang, Turiano, Mroczek, & Miller, 2018; Zawadzki, Sliwinski, & Smyth, 2018). A positive stress mindset toward a potentially stressful event, such as rethinking it as a challenge and proactively meeting its demands, can beneficially affect health outcomes (Keech, Hagger, O'Callaghan-Hamilton, 2018).

**Uncontrollable Events**   Uncontrollable or unpredictable events are more stressful than controllable or predictable ones especially if they are also unexpected (Cankaya, Chapman, Talbot, Moynihan, & Duberstein, 2009). When people feel that they can predict, modify, or terminate an aversive event or feel they have access to someone who can influence it, they experience less stress, even if they actually can do nothing about it (Thompson, 1981). Feelings of control not only mute the subjective experience of stress but also influence biochemical reactions to it, including catecholamine levels and immune responses (Brosschot et al., 1998).

**Ambiguous Events**   Ambiguous events are more stressful than clear-cut events. When a potential stressor is ambiguous, a person cannot take action, but must instead devote energy to trying to understand the stressor, which can be a time-consuming, resource-sapping task. Clear-cut stressors, on the other hand, let the person get on with finding solutions and do not leave him or her stuck at the problem definition stage. The ability to take confrontative action is usually associated with less distress and better coping (Billings & Moos, 1984).

**Overload**   Overloaded people experience more stress than people with fewer tasks to perform (Cohen & Williamson, 1988). For example, one of the main sources of work-related stress is job overload, the perception that one is responsible for doing too much in too short a time.

**Which Stressors?**   People are more vulnerable to stress in central life domains than in peripheral ones, because important aspects of the self are heavily invested in central life domains (Swindle & Moos, 1992). For example, one study of working women for whom parental identity was very important found that strains associated with the parent role, such as feeling that their children did not get the attention they needed, took a toll (Simon, 1992).

To summarize, then, events that are negative, uncontrollable, ambiguous, or overwhelming or that involve central life goals are experienced as more stressful than

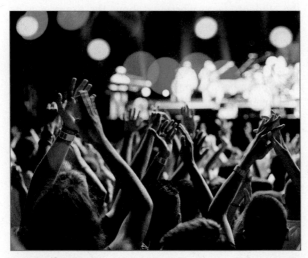

momcilog/Getty Images

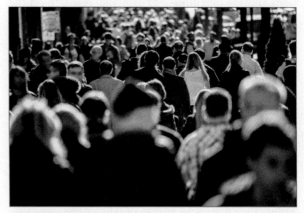

blvdone/Shutterstock

*Events such as crowding are experienced as stressful to the extent that they are appraised that way. Some situations of crowding make people feel happy, whereas other crowding situations are experienced as aversive.*

events that are positive, controllable, clear-cut, or manageable or that involve peripheral life tasks.

## Must Stress Be Perceived as Such to Be Stressful?

The discussion of stress thus far has emphasized the importance of perception, that is, the subjective experience of stress. However, objective stressors can have effects independent of the perceived stress they cause. For example, in a study of air traffic controllers, Repetti (1993b) assessed their subjective perceptions of stress on various days and also gathered objective measures of daily stress, including the weather conditions and the amount of air traffic. She found that both subjective and objective measures of stress independently predicted psychological distress and health complaints. Even when the air traffic controllers reported that they were not under stress, if air traffic was heavy and weather conditions poor, they were more likely to show evidence of stress, both physiologically and behaviorally.

## Can People Adapt to Stress?

If a stressful event becomes a permanent or chronic part of the environment, will people eventually habituate to it, or will they develop **chronic strain?** The answer to this question depends on the type of stressor, the subjective experience of stress, and the indicator of stress.

Most people are able to adapt psychologically to moderate or predictable stressors. At first, any novel or threatening situation can produce stress, but such reactions subside over time. For example, research on the effects of environmental noise (Nivison & Endresen, 1993) and crowding (Cohen, Glass, & Phillip, 1978) indicates few or no long-term adverse physiological or psychological effects, suggesting that most people simply adapt to these chronic stressors.

However, vulnerable populations, such as children, the elderly, and the poor, show little adaptation to chronic stressors (Cohen et al., 1978). One reason is that these groups already experience little control over their environments and, accordingly, may already be at high levels of stress; the addition of an environmental stressor may push their resources to the limits. For example, the cumulative effects of daily stress can compromise older adults' cognitive functioning (Stawski, Cerino, Witzel, & MacDonald, 2019).

Most people, then, can adapt to mildly stressful events; however, it may be difficult or impossible to adapt to highly stressful events, and already-stressed people may be unable to adapt to even moderate stressors. Moreover, even when psychological adaptation may have occurred, physiological changes in response to stress may persist. Chronic stress can impair cardiovascular, neuroendocrine, and immune system recovery from stressors and, through such effects, contribute to an increased risk for diseases such as cardiovascular disorders (Matthews, Gump, & Owens, 2001).

## Must a Stressor Be Ongoing to Be Stressful?

One of the wonders and curses of human beings' symbolic capacities is the ability to anticipate things before they materialize. We owe our abilities to plan, invent, and reason abstractly to this skill, but we also get from it our ability to worry. We do not have to be exposed to a stressor to suffer stress.

**Anticipating Stress**    The anticipation of a stressor can be as stressful as its actual occurrence, and sometimes more so (Wirtz et al., 2006). Consider the strain of anticipating a confrontation with one's partner or worrying about an upcoming test. Sleepless nights and days of distracting anxiety attest to the human being's capacity for anticipatory distress.

In one study that illustrates this point, medical students' blood pressure was assessed on an unstressful lecture day, on the day before an important examination, and during the examination itself. Although the students had stable blood pressure on the lecture day, blood pressure on the preexamination day, when the students were worrying about the exam, was as high as that seen during the examination (Sausen, Lovallo, Pincomb, & Wilson, 1992).

**Aftereffects of Stress**    Adverse **aftereffects of stress** often persist long after the stressful event itself is no longer present. These aftereffects include a shortened attention span and poor performance on intellectual tasks as well as ongoing psychological distress and physiological arousal. Cognitive disruptions such as difficulty concentrating are common, and social behavior is affected as well; people seem to be less willing to help others when they are suffering from the aftereffects of stress. Worry or rumination, even when one is not aware that one is doing it, can keep heart rate, blood pressure, and immune markers at high levels (Zoccola, Figueroa, Rabideau, Woody, & Benencia, 2014). Box 6.2 profiles a particular kind of aftereffect of stress, post traumatic stress disorder.

**TABLE 6.2 | The Social Readjustment Rating Scale**

Here are some examples of items from the Social Readjustment Rating Scale, including some that are viewed as very taxing and others, much less so.

| Rank | Life Event | Mean Value |
|---|---|---|
| 1 | Death of a spouse | 100 |
| 2 | Divorce | 73 |
| 4 | Detention in jail or other institution | 63 |
| 5 | Death of a close family member | 63 |
| 6 | Major personal injury or illness | 53 |
| 8 | Being fired at work | 47 |

Here are some of the smaller stressful events that nonetheless can aggravate accumulating stress as well.

| Rank | Life Event | Mean Value |
|---|---|---|
| 41 | Vacation | 13 |
| 42 | Christmas | 12 |
| 43 | Minor violations of the law (e.g., traffic tickets, jaywalking, and disturbing the peace) | 11 |

*Source*: Acuna, Laura, and Diana Alejandra González-García. "The Social Readjustment Rating Scale of Holmes and Rahe in Mexico: A Rescaling after 16 Years." *Journal of Psychosomatic Research 11* (January 2012): 213–218.

## ■ HOW HAS STRESS BEEN STUDIED?

Health psychologists have used several different methods for studying stress and assessing its effects on psychological and physical health.

### Studying Stress in the Laboratory

A common way to study stress is to bring people into the laboratory, expose them to short-term stressful events, and observe the impact of that stress on their physiological, neuroendocrine, and psychological responses. This **acute stress paradigm** consistently finds that when people perform stressful tasks (such as counting backward quickly by 7s or delivering an impromptu speech to an unresponsive audience), they become psychologically distressed and show physiological arousal (Kirschbaum, Klauer, Filipp, & Hellhammer, 1995; Ritz & Steptoe, 2000).

The acute stress paradigm has been helpful for identifying who is most vulnerable to stress (Pike et al., 1997). For example, people who are chronically stressed react more strongly during these laboratory stressors as do people who are high in hostility (Davis, Matthews, & McGrath, 2000). Box 6.3 provides an example of how an acutely stressful event can lead to dramatic health consequences. These methods have also shown that when people experience stress in the presence of a supportive partner or even a stranger, their stress responses can be reduced (Ditzen et al., 2007).

### Inducing Disease

Another way of studying the effects of stress has involved intentionally exposing people to viruses and then assessing whether they get ill and how ill they get. For example, S. Cohen and colleagues (1999) measured levels of stress in a group of adults, infected them with an influenza virus by swabbing their nose with cotton soaked in a viral culture, and measured their respiratory symptoms, the amount of mucus they produced, and immune responses to stress. They found that people experiencing more stress are more likely to get sick and mount a stronger immune response than people exposed to the virus whose lives were less stressful. This approach has also been used to study factors that protect against stress, such as social support (e.g., Cohen et al., 2008).

### Stressful Life Events

Another line of stress research assesses **stressful life events.** Two pioneers in stress research, Holmes and Rahe (1967), maintained that when a person must adjust to a changing environment, the likelihood of stress increases. They created an inventory of stressful life events (Table 6.2) by developing ratings of stressful

Post traumatic stress disorder (PTSD) affects 8 percent of veterans, according to the Veteran's Administration but the adverse effects may go unrecognized. As a 71-year-old veteran of the Vietnam War put it, "It only took me 47 years to seek treatment. I had no joy in my life" (*Los Angeles Times,* December 29, 2018, p. A9).

When a person has experienced intense stress, symptoms of the stress experience may persist long after the event is over and affect health long afterward as well (Litcher-Kelly et al., 2014; Lowe, Willis, & Rhodes, 2014). In the case of major traumas, these stressful after-effects may go on intermittently for months or years. Among people also exposed to early life trauma, the adverse health affects are worse (Franz et al., 2019). Such long-term reactions are especially likely following combat exposure, as occurred in Iraq and Afghanistan (McNally, 2012). But they may also occur in response to assault, rape, domestic abuse, a violent encounter with nature (such as an earthquake or flood), a disaster (such as 9/11) (Fagan, Galea, Ahern, Bonner, & Vlahov, 2003), being a hostage (Vila, Porche, & Mouren-Simeoni, 1999), or having a child with a life-threatening disease (Cabizuca, Marques-Portella, Mendlowicz, Coutinho, & Figueria, 2009). Particular occupations such as being a police officer in a high-crime city (Mohr et al., 2003) or having responsibility for clearing up remains following war, disaster, or mass death (McCarroll, Ursano, Fullerton, Liu, & Lundy, 2002) increase the risk of trauma. PTSD can be the result.

Symptoms of PTSD include psychic numbing, reduced interest in once-enjoyable activities, detachment from friends, or constriction in emotions. The person

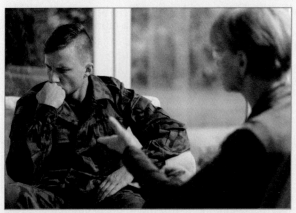

Photographee.eu/Shutterstock

may relive aspects of the trauma, as the Iraq War veteran did. Other symptoms include excessive vigilance, sleep disturbances, headaches (Arcaya et al., 2017) and poor respiratory health (Waszczuk et al., 2017), feelings of guilt, impaired memory and concentration, an exaggerated startle response to loud noise (Lewis, Troxel, Kravitz, Bromberger, Matthews, & Hall, 2013), and even suicidal behavior. Sometimes the onset of symptoms is delayed, necessitating following people at risk over time (O'Donnell et al., 2013). PTSD can lead to severe conflict in couples and with other family members and friends (Caska et al., 2014). PTSS (post-traumatic stress symptoms) are experienced by a broader swath of people who go through a traumatic event, which can include hospitalization, injury, a workplace accident, and the illness or hospitalization of one's child (Egberts, van de Schoot, Geenen, & Van Loey, 2017; Thompson et al., 2017). Reactions may include avoidant coping, anxiety, and extreme appraisals of the event, a pattern that can be at least partly offset by early intervention (Marsac et al., 2017). Confronting rather than avoiding the stressor is a therapeutic target.

PTSD/PTSS can produce temporary and permanent changes in cardiovascular functioning, especially in response to distressing situations (Dennis et al., 2016). People with PTSD show cortisol dysregulation (Mason et al., 2002), alterations in immune functioning (Boscarino & Chang, 1999), chronically higher levels of norepinephrine, epinephrine, and testosterone (Lindauer et al., 2006; O'Donnell, Creamer, Elliott, & Bryant, 2007), and higher blood pressure (Edmondson et al., 2018).

PTSD leads to poor health, especially cardiovascular and lung disorders (Ahmadi et al., 2018; Pietrzak, Goldstein, Southwick, & Grant, 2011), vulnerability to chronic pain (Tsur, Defrin, & Ginzburg, 2017), and early mortality, especially from heart disease (Dedert, Calhoun, Watkins, Sherwood, & Beckham, 2010). It also is tied to poor health issues such as obesity, problem drinking and smoking, lack of exercise and poor eating which contribute to poor health (Lee & Park, 2018; Mason et al., 2017; van den Berk-Clark et al., 2018), and to worsening symptoms of already existing disorders such as asthma (Fagan et al., 2003).

Nearly half of adults in the United States experience at least one traumatic event in their lifetime, but only 10 percent of women and 5 percent of men develop

PTSD (Ozer & Weiss, 2004). Who is most likely to develop PTSD? People who have poor cognitive skills (Gilbertson et al., 2006) or catastrophic thinking about stress (Bryant & Guthrie, 2005), and people who have a preexisting emotional disorder such as anxiety (Dohrenwend, Yager, Wall, & Adams, 2013) are vulnerable. People who use avoidant coping, have low levels of social support, have a history of chronic stress, have preexisting heightened reactivity to trauma-related stimuli (Suendermann, Ehlers, Boellinghaus, Gamer, & Glucksman, 2010), and are generally negative all have increased risk of developing PTSD in the wake of a traumatic stressor (Gil & Caspi, 2006; Widows, Jacobsen, & Fields, 2000). African Americans and Latinx have higher rates of PTSD than do whites (Sibrava et al. 2019).

Characteristics of the trauma matter, too. Soldiers who had combat experience, who observed atrocities, and who participated in atrocities are most likely to experience PTSD (Dohrenwend et al., 2013). The more traumas one is exposed to, the greater the risk of PTSD, and the greater the health risk that may result (Sledjeski, Speisman, & Dierker, 2008).

Can PTSD be alleviated? Cognitive–behavioral therapies are used to treat PTSD (Harvey, Bryant, & Tarrier, 2003; Nemeroff et al., 2006). Reducing negative affect-related autonomic arousal is one important interventions focus, as this arousal can enhance cardiovascular risk (Dennis et al., 2017). Perhaps counterintuitively, repeated exposure to the trauma through imagined exposure and discussion of thoughts and feelings related to the trauma can reduce symptoms of PTSD and enhance emotional processing of the traumatic event (Reger et al., 2011). This exposure therapy early after the trauma may be best (Rothbaum et al., 2012). Virtual reality exposure therapy after or even before exposure to wartime trauma has been used (Rizzo et al., 2009). The goals of repeated exposure involve isolating the trauma as a discrete event, habituating to it and reducing overwhelming distress. In turn, this repeated exposure can foster new interpretations of the event and its implications, reduce anxiety, and build a sense of mastery (Harvey et al., 2003). Once habituation is achieved, cognitive restructuring is added to integrate the trauma into the client's self-view and worldview. Anxiety management training is often included so that the patient can recognize and deal with intrusive traumatic memories (Harvey et al., 2003). Interventions such as these have been successfully used with military veterans (Monson et al., 2006) and women who were sexually abused as children (McDonagh et al., 2005) among other groups. People who have both PTSD and a concomitant medical condition, such as cardiovascular disease or epilepsy, will need treatment that sensitively addresses the needs dictated by both conditions (Chen et al., 2017).

events based on the amount of change those events cause. Thus, for example, if one's spouse dies, virtually every aspect of life is disrupted. On the other hand, getting a traffic ticket may be annoying but is unlikely to produce much change in one's life. Although all people experience at least some stressful events, some people will experience a lot, and it is this group, according to Holmes and Rahe, that is most vulnerable to illness.

Although scores on life event inventories predict illness, the relation is quite modest. Why is this the case? First, some of the items on the list are vague; for example, "personal injury or illness" could mean anything from the flu to a heart attack. Second, because events have preassigned point values, individual differences in how events are experienced are not taken into account. For example, a divorce may mean welcome freedom to one partner but a collapse in living standard or self-esteem to the other.

Third, inventories include both positive and negative events, as well as events that people choose, such as getting married, and events that simply happen, such as the death of a close friend. As noted, sudden, negative, unexpected, and uncontrollable events are reliably more stressful. Fourth, researchers typically do not assess whether stressful events have been successfully resolved, which mutes adverse effects (Thoits, 1994; Turner & Avison, 1992).

Life event inventories may pick up chronic strains and also personality factors that influence how intensely a person experiences an event. Many people believe that stress causes illness, and so if they have been ill, they may remember more events in their lives as having been stressful.

Everyone knows that fans get worked up during excit- ing sports matches. Near misses by one's own team, questionable calls by referees, and dirty plays can all rouse fans to fever pitch. But do these events actually have health effects? To examine this question, Wilbert- Lampen and colleagues (2008) studied acute cardio- vascular events in 4,279 Germans when the German national team played in World Cup soccer events. On days with matches involving the German team, cardiac emergencies were nearly three times as likely as on days when they did not play. Nearly half of these peo- ple, mostly men, had previously been diagnosed with coronary heart disease.

The study concluded that viewing a stressful soc- cer match, or indeed any other exciting sports event, may more than double the risk of a heart attack or stroke. This increased risk falls especially hard on people who have already been diagnosed with heart

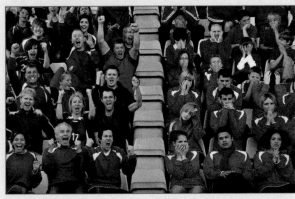

Cultural Limited/SuperStock

disease. So if someone you care about has a cardiovas- cular disorder and is a sports fan, that person may want to rethink whether exciting matches are worth the risk.

A final difficulty concerns the time between stress and illness. Usually, in these studies, stress over a 1-year period is related to the most recent 6 months of illness bouts. Yet, January's crisis is unlikely to have caused June's cold and April's financial problems are unlikely to have produced a malignancy detected in May. Obviously, these cases are extreme, but they illustrate some of the problems in studying the stress–illness relationship over time. For all these reasons, life event inventories are no longer used as much and some researchers have turned instead to perceived stress (Box 6.4).

### Daily Stress

In addition to major stressful life events, researchers have studied minor stressful events, or **daily hassles,** and their cumulative impact on health and illness. Such hassles include being stuck in traffic, waiting in a line, doing household chores, having difficulty making small decisions, and daily conflict (Tobin et al., 2015). Daily minor problems produce psychological distress, adverse physiological changes, physical symptoms, and use of health care services (Gouin, Glaser, Malarkey, Beversdorf, & Kiecolt-Glaser, 2012; Sin, Graham- Engeland, Ong, & Almeida, 2015). An example of how daily hassles can be measured is shown in Box 6.5.

Minor hassles affect physical and psychological health in several ways. First, the cumulative impact of small stressors may wear a person down, leading to ill- ness. Second, such events may aggravate reactions to major life events or chronic stress to produce distress or illness (Marin, Martin, Blackwell, Stetler, & Miller, 2007; Serido, Almeida, & Wethington, 2004).

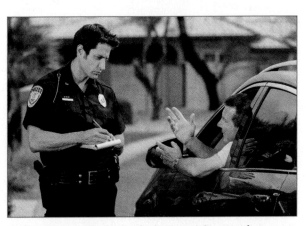

*Traffic enforcement agents who have social support from coworkers are better able to deal with these stressful working conditions (Karlan, Brondolo, & Schwartz, 2003).*

Jacom Stephens/Avid Creative, Inc./iStockphoto.com

Because people vary so much in what they consider to be stressful, many researchers measure perceived stress instead. S. Cohen and his colleagues (1983) developed a measure of perceived stress, some items of which follow. Perceived stress predicts a broad array of health outcomes (Kojima et al., 2005; Young et al., 2004).

**ITEMS ON THE PERCEIVED STRESS SCALE**

For each question, choose from the following alternatives:

0   Never
1   Almost never
2   Sometimes
3   Fairly often
4   Very often

1. In the last month, how often have you been upset because of something that happened unexpectedly?
2. In the last month, how often have you felt nervous and stressed?
3. In the last month, how often have you found that you could not cope with all the things that you had to do?
4. In the last month, how often have you been angered because of things that happened that were outside your control?
5. In the last month, how often have you found yourself thinking about things that you had to accomplish?
6. In the last month, how often have you felt difficulties were piling up so high that you could not overcome them?

If your score is high, you may want to try to reduce the stress in your life.

---

Although useful for identifying the smaller hassles of life, measurement of daily strain has some of the same problems as the measurement of major stressful life events. For example, people who report a lot of hassles may be anxious or neurotic.

### ■ SOURCES OF CHRONIC STRESS

Earlier, we posed the question of whether people can adapt to chronically stressful events. The answer is that people can adapt to a degree but continue to show signs of stress in response to severe chronic strains in their lives. Indeed, chronic stress may be more important than major life events for developing illness.

#### Effects of Early Stressful Life Experiences

Early life adversity in childhood can affect not only health in childhood, but also health across the lifespan into adulthood and old age (Gebreab et al., 2018; Llabre et al., 2017). Offspring can even experience health consequences of their parent's childhood exposure to mistreatment (Tomfohr-Madsen, Bayrampour, & Tough, 2016). Some of this work grew out of the

allostatic load view of stress, which argues that major, chronic, or recurrent stress dysregulates stress systems, which, over time, produce accumulating risk for disease (Slatcher & Robles, 2012). These early risks include low socioeconomic status, exposure to violence, acculturative stress (namely the stress of adapting to a new culture), living in poverty-stricken neighborhoods,

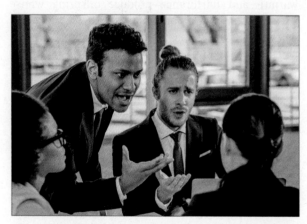

*Work strains, like the argument between these coworkers, are common sources of stress that compromise well-being and physical health.*

LightFieldStudios/iStock/Getty Images

BOX **6.5** The Measurement of Daily Strain

## INSTRUCTIONS

Each day, we experience minor annoyances as well as major problems or difficulties. Indicate how much of a strain each of these annoyances has been for you in the past month.

### Severity

0   Did not occur

1   Mild strain

2   Somewhat of a strain

3   Moderate strain

4   Extreme strain

### Hassles

| | | | | | | |
|---|---|---|---|---|---|---|
| 1. A quarrel or problems with a neighbor | 0 | 1 | 2 | 3 | 4 |
| 2. Traffic congestion | 0 | 1 | 2 | 3 | 4 |
| 3. Thoughts of poor health | 0 | 1 | 2 | 3 | 4 |
| 4. An argument with a romantic partner | 0 | 1 | 2 | 3 | 4 |
| 5. Concerns about money | 0 | 1 | 2 | 3 | 4 |
| 6. A parking ticket | 0 | 1 | 2 | 3 | 4 |
| 7. Preparation of meals | 0 | 1 | 2 | 3 | 4 |

and other community level stressors (Blair & Raver, 2012; Garcia, Wilborn, & Mangold, 2017; McLaughlin et al., 2016).

Physical or sexual abuse in childhood increases health risks (Midei, Matthews, Chang, & Bromberger, 2013) because abuse can result in intense, chronic stress that taxes physiological systems (Wegman & Stetler, 2009) and difficulties regulating emotions (Broody et al., 2014). Biological aging may be affected, with children who go through traumas reaching puberty very early; early puberty can lead to later early health risks (Lei, Beach, & Simons, 2018). Even more modest family stress can increase risk for disease. Repetti and colleagues (2002) found that "risky families"—that is, families that are high in conflict or criticism and low in warmth and nurturance—produce offspring whose stress responses are compromised. These difficulties include problems with emotion regulation, social skills, and health habits (Schrepf, Markon, & Lutgendorf, 2014). Children who grow up in harsh families do not learn how to recognize other people's emotions and respond to them appropriately or regulate their own emotional responses to situations. As a result, they may overreact to mild stressors (Hanson & Chen, 2010). These adverse reactions can be compounded by low socioeconomic status (Appleton et al., 2012) and by exposure to trauma (Schrepf et al., 2014).

Children who grow up in risky families also have difficulty forming good social relationships. These deficits in emotion regulation and social skills can persist across the lifespan long into adulthood, compromising the ways in which people from risky families cope with stress (Raposa, Hammen, Brennan, O'Callaghan, &

Najman, 2014; Taylor, Eisenberger, Saxbe, Lehman, & Lieberman, 2006). Physiological systems are affected as well (Miller, Chen, & Parker, 2011). Children from risky families can develop heightened sympathetic reactivity to stress, enhanced pain sensitivity (You & Meagher, 2016), exaggerated cortisol responses leading to health risks, an immune profile marked by chronic inflammation (Miller & Chen, 2010; Schreier & Chen, 2012), and shorter telomere length (Brody, Yu, & Shalev, 2017).

For example, in a retrospective study, Felitti et al. (1998) asked adults to complete a questionnaire regarding their early family environment that inquired, among other things, how warm and supportive the environment was versus how cold, critical, hostile, or conflictridden it was. The more negative characteristics these adults reported from their childhood, the more vulnerable they were in adulthood to many disorders, including depression, lung disease, cancer, heart disease, and diabetes (Loucks, Almeida, Taylor, & Matthews, 2011). Because children from risky families often have poor health habits, some enhanced risk for disease may come from smoking, poor diet, and lack of exercise.

Stress in adolescence also affects health both during adolescence (Schreier, Roy, Frimer, & Chen, 2014) and into adulthood (Quon & McGrath, 2014). For example, social disadvantage in adolescence is linked to increased body weight, to inflammation (Pietras & Goodman, 2013), and to high-blood pressure and poor blood pressure recovery from stress (Evans, Exner-Cortens, Kim & Bartholomew, 2013). Perceived financial stress is especially strongly related to multiple health markers and outcomes, attesting again to the adverse health effects of low SES (Quon & McGrath, 2014).

Good parenting can mitigate these effects (Manczak et al., 2017; Farrell, Simpson, Carlson, Englund, & Sung, 2017). In one study, adolescents who were positively parented had lower inflammation several years later (Byrne et al., 2017). Parental warmth may help reduce biological responses to stress (Nelson et al., 2017), can better the effects of parental divorce (Luecken, Hagan, Wolchik, Sandler, & Tein, 2016), and can mitigate the adverse effects of low SES on health (Boylan, Cundiff, Jakubowski, Pardini, & Matthews, 2018). Overall, it appears that parental warmth moderates the biological and psychological fallout that can result from stress during adolescence (Levine, Hoffer, & Chen, 2017).

Are these effects reversible? At present it is unknown whether early life stress permanently programs stress systems or whether some of these effects are reversible. However, some factors, such as maternal nurturance in a high poverty environment, can be protective against the health risks usually found in high-stress areas (Miller et al., 2011). Interventions undertaken early in childhood may have health payoffs across the life span (Puig, Englund, Simpson, & Collins, 2012).

## Chronic Stressful Conditions

Sometimes, chronic stress is long-term and grinding, such as living in poverty, being in a bad relationship, remaining in a high-stress job, and experiencing sexual harassment. Chronic stress is also an important contributor to psychological distress and physical illness. Uncontrollable stressors may be particularly virulent (McGonagle & Kessler, 1990). Even something as mundane as commuting can affect daily cortisol levels and perceived stress, affecting the over 100 million Americans who commute to work every weekday (Evans & Wener, 2006).

Research relating chronic stress to health outcomes is difficult to conduct, though, because it is hard to show that a particular chronic stressor is the factor that caused illness. Second, unlike life events, which can often be assessed objectively, chronic stress can be more difficult to measure objectively. Third, as in the measurement of life events, inventories that assess chronic strain may also tap psychological distress and neuroticism. Nonetheless, the evidence indicates that chronic stress is related to illness (Matthews, Gallo, & Taylor, 2010).

Box 6.6 focuses on a particular type of chronic stress, namely, prejudice, and its relation to poor health.

Research showing social class differences in death from all causes, including cancers and cardiovascular disease, also attests to the relationship between chronic stress and health (Grzywacz, Almeida, Neupert, & Ettner, 2004). Socioeconomic disadvantage, including poverty, exposure to crime, neighborhood stress, and other chronic stressors, vary with SES and are all tied to poor health outcomes and at early ages (Fuller-Rowell, Curtis, Chae, & Ryff, 2018). People who are low in SES typically have low-prestige occupations, which may expose them to greater interpersonal conflict and stress at work. Chronic SES-related stress has also been related to alterations in cortisol patterns, catecholamines, and inflammation (Friedman & Herd, 2010; Kumari et al., 2010). A meta-analysis showed that even subjective measures of SES or rank, that is, how people perceive their SES level in comparison to others, show robust relations to biological markers of compromised health (Murray, Haselton, Fales, & Cole, 2019), to perceived health (Cundiff & Matthews, 2017) and to health outcomes (Zell, Strickhouser, & Krizan, 2018). Children in low SES circumstances suffer health risks, including sleep problems (El-Sheikh et al., 2013), weight gain (Puterman et al., 2016), and increases in allostatic load (Doan, Dich, & Evans, 2014). Some of these risks tied to low SES may be lessened in families marked by warm parenting (Hagan, Roubinov, Adler, Boyce, & Bush, 2016) and reversible if circumstances improve (Cundiff, Boylan, Pardini, & Matthews, 2017). Living in a good neighborhood can offset some of the disadvantages of low SES as well (Roubinov, Hagan, Boyce, Adler, & Bush, 2018).

## Stress in the Workplace

Workplace stress is estimated to cost $300 billion a year (American Institute of Stress, n.d.). Studies of stress in the workplace are important for several additional reasons:

- They help identify some of the most common stressors of everyday life.
- They provide evidence for the stress–illness relationship.
- Work stress may be one of our preventable stressors and so provide possibilities for intervention.
- Stress-related physical and mental health disorders account for a growing percentage of disability and social security payments to workers.

BOX **6.6** Can Prejudice Harm Your Health?

A young African American father pulled up in front of a house in a largely white neighborhood to pick up his daughter from a birthday party. Because he was early and the party had not ended, he sat waiting in the car. Within 8 minutes, a security car had pulled up behind him; two officers approached him and asked him to exit his vehicle. Neighbors had reported seeing a suspicious-looking African American man casing their neighborhood.

Prejudice and racism adversely affect health (Klonoff, 2014). It has long been known that African Americans experience greater health risks than the rest of the population. Life expectancy for African American men is about 5 years less than that for white men, and life expectancy for African American women is 3 years less than that for white women (National Vital Statistics Reports, 2016). For example, African American men and women die of cardiovascular disease at nearly one and a half times the rate for white men and women. A meta-analytic review showed that minority adolescents who perceive discrimination have higher risk of poor health habits, poor emotional functioning, and lower academic achievement, among other adverse outcomes (Benner et al., 2018).

Many of these differences can be traced to differences in SES and social status (Major, Mendes, & Dovidio, 2013; Myers, 2009). Poverty, lower educational attainment, imprisonment, and unemployment are more prevalent among blacks than among whites (Browning & Cagney, 2003). The day-in, day-out grinding strain associated with poor housing, little available employment, poor schools, and poor neighborhoods also contributes to stress through chronic exposure to violence and an enduring sense of danger (Ross & Mirowsky, 2011). Discrimination can erode personal resources, such as social support, the ability to regulate emotions effectively (Gibbons et al., 2014) and even sleep (Peterson et al., 2017). Medical services in minority areas are often inadequate. African Americans are less likely to receive preventive services and more likely to experience delayed medical attention (National Academy of Medicine, 2002).

Racism and racial discrimination also contribute to disease risk, especially risk of cardiovascular disease (Brondolo, ver Halen, Pencille, Beatty, & Contrada, 2009; Williams & Mohammed, 2009) and insulin resistance (Brody, Yu, Chen, Ehrlich, & Miller, 2018).

One may be treated badly by a store clerk or stopped by the police for no reason (driving while black). The adverse effects of prejudice and discrimination on health are explained in part by the higher anxiety, depression, and hostility that people develop in response to their experiences of prejudice and discrimination (Brondolo et al., 2011). Experiences of discrimination have been related to shorter telomere length, an indicator of aging and susceptibility to aging-related diseases (Lee, Kim, & Neblett, 2017).

There are physiological and health effects of racism as well. Perceived racism coupled with inhibited angry responses to it are related to high blood pressure, contributing to the high incidence of hypertension among African Americans (Smart Richman, Pek, Pascoe, & Bauer, 2010). Risk of kidney disease may also increase (Beydoun et al., 2017). Racism may also help to explain the high levels of depression (Turner & Avison, 2003) and back pain (Edwards, 2008) in the African American population. Chronic exposure to racism has been tied to problem drinking and to poor sleep quality (Oshri, Kogan, Liu, Sweet, & Mackillop, 2017), and to atypical cortisol reactivity and recovery (Tackett, Herzhoff, Smack, Reardon, & Adam, 2017).

Racism is not the only form of prejudice that contributes to poor health. Sexism predicts poor physical and mental health for women (Ryff, Keyes, & Hughes, 2003). Women have the best health in states in which their earnings, employment, and political participation are highest and the worst health in those states in which they score lowest on these indices (Jun, Subramanian, Gortmaker, & Kawachi, 2004). Discrimination against mothers is particularly rampant and difficult to combat (Biernat, Crosby, & Williams, 2004). Many people have multiple sources of potential discrimination, for example, an African American lesbian mother, and examining both the individual and total discrimination experienced may provide a clearer picture of health effects (Lewis & Van Dyke, 2018).

Negative stereotypes about aging may compromise health among older adults. In one study, simply exposing older adults to negative aging stereotypes increased cardiovascular responses to stress (Levy, Hausdorff, Hencke, & Wei, 2000). Perceived discrimination has been tied to poorer physical and cognitive functioning among the elderly (Shankar & Hinds, 2017). Suicide rates among ethnic immigrant groups have been tied to the amount of hate speech directed toward those groups (Mullen & Smyth, 2004) and the strain of trying to adjust to a new culture can produce adverse changes in stress-related biomarkers (Fang, Ross, Pathak, Godwin, & Tseng, 2014). Perceived discrimination is linked to substance abuse among Native American children (Whitbeck, Hoyt, McMorris, Chen, & Stubben, 2001) and to depression among Native American adults (Whitbeck, McMorris, Hoyt, Stubben, & LaFromboise, 2002). Exposure to stress and prejudice can adversely affect LGBT young adults' physical functioning (Niles, Valenstein-Mah, & Bedard-Gilligan, 2017), and exposure to weight stigma can affect biomarkers of stress in obese people (Schvey, Pulh, & Brownell, 2014). Converging evidence like this indicates clearly that the stressors associated with discrimination, racism, and prejudice can adversely affect health.

Work and Sedentary Lifestyle    The most common work that people undertook before the Industrial Revolution was agricultural production, which involves physical labor. As people have moved into sedentary office jobs, the amount of exercise they get in their work lives has declined substantially. Even jobs that require high levels of physical exertion, such as construction work and firefighting, may include so much stress that the benefits of exercise are eliminated. Because activity level is related to health, this change in the nature of work increases vulnerability to illness.

Overload    Work overload is a chief factor producing high levels of occupational stress. Workers required to work too long and too hard at too many tasks feel more stressed, have poorer health habits, and have more health risks than do workers not suffering from overload (Lumley et al., 2014). The chronic neuroendocrine activation and cardiovascular activation associated with overcommitment can contribute to cardiovascular disease (Steptoe, Siegrist, Kirschbaum, & Marmot, 2004; Von Känel, Bellingrath, & Kudielka, 2009).

An old rock song states, "Monday, Monday, can't trust that day." Monday may indeed be one of the most stressful days of the week. Weekdays more generally are associated with more worry and chronic work overload than weekends, resulting in altered cortisol levels (Schlotz, Hellhammer, Schulz, & Stone, 2004). Unfortunately, many people, particularly in the United States, don't use their weekends to recover and instead work through the weekend. Then they dump the work they did over the weekend onto their coworkers on Monday. Incomplete recovery from work contributes to death from cardiovascular disease (Kivimäki et al., 2006).

So well established is the relation between work overload and poor health that Japan, a country notorious for its long working hours, long work weeks, little sleep, and lack of vacations, has a term, *karoshi*, that refers to death from overwork. One study found that men who worked more than 61 hours a week experienced twice the risk of a heart attack as those working 40 hours or less; sleeping 5 hours or less at least 2 days a week increased this risk by two to three times (Liu & Tanaka, 2002). Under Japanese law, families are entitled to compensation if they can prove that the breadwinner died of *karoshi* (Martin, 2016). As a result, work hours have declined in Japan over the past 20 years.

Ambiguity and Role Conflict    Role conflict and role ambiguity are associated with stress. Role ambiguity occurs when a person has no clear idea of what to do and no idea of the standards used for evaluating work. **Role conflict** occurs when a person receives conflicting information about work tasks or standards

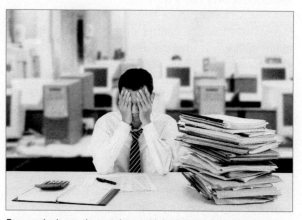

*Research shows that workers with high levels of job strain and low levels of control over their work are under great stress and may be at risk for coronary heart disease.*
Creativa Images/Shutterstock

from different individuals. For example, if a college professor is told by one colleague to publish more articles, is advised by another colleague to publish fewer papers but of higher quality, and is told by a third to improve teaching ratings, the professor may experience role ambiguity and conflict. Chronically high blood pressure and elevated heart rate have been tied to role conflict and role ambiguity (French & Caplan, 1973). When people receive clear feedback about the nature of their performance, they report lower levels of stress (Cohen & Williamson, 1988).

Social Relationships  The inability to develop satisfying social relationships at work has been tied to job stress (House, 1981), to psychological distress at work (Buunk, Doosje, Jans, & Hopstaken, 1993), and to poor physical and mental health (Shirom, Toker, Alkaly, Jacobson, & Balicer, 2011). Having a poor relationship with one's supervisor predicts job distress and may increase a worker's risk for coronary heart disease (Davis, Matthews, Meilahn, & Kiss, 1995).

To a degree, having an amicable social environment at work depends on being an amicable coworker. A study of air traffic controllers found that people who were not particularly well liked by their coworkers and who consequently did not have much social contact were more likely to become ill and to experience an accidental injury than were people who enjoyed and contributed to a more satisfying social climate (Niemcryk, Jenkins, Rose, & Hurst, 1987).

Social relationships not only combat stress in their own right, they also buffer other job stressors, such as low control over one's work.

Control  Lack of control over one's work life is a major stressor. It predicts dissatisfaction at work and absenteeism as well as physiological arousal that predicts disease. Lack of control at work has been tied to greater risk of coronary artery disease (Bosma et al., 1997) and to all-cause mortality. Job control, by contrast, can improve health (Smith, Frank, Bondy, & Mustard, 2008).

Karasek et al. (1981) developed a model of job strain that helps to explain its adverse effects on health. They maintain that high psychological demands on the job with little decision latitude (such as low job control) causes job strain, which, in turn, can lead to the development of coronary artery disease. Research generally supports this idea (Emeny et al., 2013). The chronic anger that can result from high strain jobs may

further contribute to coronary artery disease risk (Fitzgerald, Haythornthwaite, Suchday, & Ewart, 2003). When high demands and low control are combined with little social support at work, in what has been termed the **demand-control-support model,** risk for coronary artery disease is greater (Hintsanen et al., 2007; Muhonen & Torkelson, 2003). Other health-related outcomes, including heightened HPA axis reactivity (Eddy, Wertheim, Hale, & Wright, 2018) and even suicide, have been tied to high demands and low control at work (Milner et al., 2017). The perception that one's effort at work is insufficiently rewarded (effort–reward imbalance) is also associated with health risks, especially coronary heart disease (Aboa-Éboulé et al., 2011). Adverse health effects of job strain are stronger among blue-collar than white-collar workers (Joseph et al., 2016) and particularly strong among shift workers (Wirth, Shivappa, Burch, Hurley, & Hébert, 2017).

Unemployment  Unemployment is a major life stressor. It increases psychological distress (Burgard, Brand, & House, 2007), physical symptoms, physical illness (Hamilton, Broman, Hoffman, & Renner, 1990), alcohol abuse (Catalano et al., 1993), difficulty achieving sexual arousal, low birth weight of offspring (Catalano, Hansen, & Hartig, 1999), elevated inflammation (Janicki-Deverts, Cohen, Matthews, & Cullen, 2008), and compromised immune functioning (Cohen et al., 2007; Segerstrom & Miller, 2004).

For example, in a study of SES-related decline in the wake of Hurricane Katrina, those who suffered trauma or who lost their jobs and experienced other deprivations showed enduring health effects (Joseph, Matthews, & Myers, 2014).

Uncertainty over employment and unstable employment have also been tied to physical illness (Heaney, Israel, & House, 1994). For example, a study found that men who had held a series of unrelated jobs were at greater risk of dying than were men who remained in the same job or in the same type of job (Pavalko, Elder, & Clipp, 1993). Being stably employed is protective of health (Rushing, Ritter, & Burton, 1992).

Other Occupational Outcomes  Stress shows up in ways other than illness that may be extremely costly to an organization. Workers who cannot participate actively in decisions about their jobs show higher rates of absenteeism, job turnover, tardiness,

**TABLE 6.3 | Reducing Stress at Work**

Because work is such an important and time-consuming part of life, it can contribute to the joy but also to the stress that people experience each day. How can stress on the job be reduced?

1. Minimize physical work stressors, such as noise, harsh lighting, crowding, or temperature extremes.
2. Minimize unpredictability and ambiguity in expected tasks and standards of performance. When workers know what they are expected to do, they are less distressed.
3. Involve workers as much as possible in the decisions that affect their work.
4. Make jobs as interesting as possible.
5. Provide workers with opportunities to develop or promote meaningful social relationships.
6. Reward workers for good work, rather than focusing on punishment for poor work.
7. Look for signs of stress before stress has an opportunity to do significant damage. Supervisors can watch for negative affect, such as boredom, apathy, and hostility, because these affective reactions often precede more severe reactions to stress, such as poor health or absenteeism.
8. Add workplace perks that enhance quality of life. Some organizations, such as Google, go so far as to permit pets at work and provide high-quality food continuously throughout the day (Cosser, 2008).

*Source*: Cosser, Sandy. EzineArticles. "Google Sets The Standard For A Happy Work Environment." Last modified by February 11, 2008.

job dissatisfaction, sabotage, and poor performance on the job. Workers may take matters into their own hands and reduce stress by not working as long, as hard, or as well as their employers expect (Kivimäki, Vahtera, Ellovainio, Lillrank, & Kevin, 2002).

## Some Solutions to Workplace Stressors

A blueprint for change has been offered by several organizational stress researchers (i.e., Kahn, 1981) (Table 6.3).

## Combining Work and Family Roles

Much of the stress that people experience results not from one role in their lives but from the combination of several roles. As adults, most of us will be workers, partners, and parents. Each of these roles entails heavy obligations, and stress can result when one is attempting to combine multiple roles.

**Women and Multiple Roles**   These problems are particularly acute for women (Gilbert-Ouimet, Brisson, Milot, & Vezina, 2017). More than half of married women with young children are currently employed (U.S. Bureau of Labor Statistics, 2018). Managing multiple roles is most difficult when both work and family responsibilities are heavy (Emmons, Biernat, Teidje, Lang, & Wortman, 1990), and having many responsibilities at home has health risks of its own (Thurston, Sherwood, Matthews, & Blumenthal, 2011). Because concessions to working parents are rarely made at work and because mothers take on more household tasks and child care than fathers (Emmons et al., 1990), home and work responsibilities may conflict with each other, increasing stress.

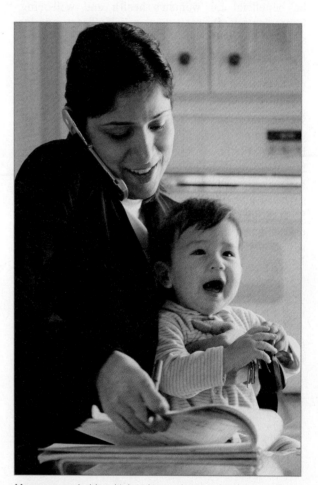

*Many women hold multiple roles, such as worker, homemaker, and parent. Although these multiple roles can provide much satisfaction, they also make women vulnerable to role conflict and role overload.*

Terry Vine/Blend Images LLC

Working women who have children at home have higher levels of cortisol, higher cardiovascular reactivity, and more home strain than those without children at home (Frankenhaeuser et al., 1989; Luecken et al., 1997). Single women raising children on their own are most at risk for health problems (Hughes & Waite, 2002), whereas women who are happily married are less likely to show these negative effects (Saxbe, Repetti, & Nishina, 2008).

Protective Effects of Multiple Roles    Despite the potential for working mothers to suffer role conflict and overload, there can be positive effects of combining home and work responsibilities (e.g., Janssen et al., 2012). Combining motherhood with employment can be beneficial for women's health and well-being, improving self-esteem, feelings of self-efficacy, and life satisfaction (Verbrugge, 1983; Weidner, Boughal, Connor, Pieper, & Mendell, 1997). Being a parent also confers resistance to colds (Sneed, Cohen, Turner, & Doyle, 2012).

Having control and flexibility over one's work environment (Lennon & Rosenfield, 1992), having a good income (Rosenfield, 1992), having someone to help with the housework (Krause & Markides, 1985), having adequate child care (Ross & Mirowsky, 1988), having a partner (Ali & Avison, 1997), and having a supportive, helpful partner (Klumb, Hoppmann, & Staats, 2006) all reduce the likelihood that multiple role demands will lead to stress and its psychological and physical costs (Ten Brummelhuis & Bakker, 2012).

Men and Multiple Roles    Men experience stress as they attempt to combine multiple roles as well. Studies show that men are more distressed by financial strain and work stress, whereas women are more distressed by adverse changes in the home (Barnett, Raudenbush, Brennan, Pleck, & Marshall, 1995).

Combining employment and marriage is protective for men's health and mental health (Burton, 1998), just as it is for women who have enough help. But multiple roles can take their toll on men, too. Repetti (1989) studied workload and interpersonal strain and how they affected fathers' interactions with the family at the end of the day. She found that after a demanding day at work (high workload strain) fathers were more withdrawn in their interactions with their children. After stressful interpersonal events at work (high interpersonal strain), conflict with children increased. Employed, unmarried fathers may be especially vulnerable to psychological distress (Simon, 1998).

For both men and women, the research on multiple roles is converging on the idea that stress is lower when one finds meaning in one's life. The protective effects of employment, marriage, and parenting on psychological distress and the beneficial effects of social support on health attest to the beneficial effects of social roles (Burton, 1998). When these sources of meaning and pleasure in life are challenged, as through role conflict and role overload, health may suffer (Stansfeld, Bosma, Hemingway, & Marmot, 1998).

Children    Children and adolescents also experience stress that can make home life stressful (Repetti, Wang, & Saxbe, 2011). One study found that social and academic failure experiences at school, such as being rejected by a peer or having difficulty with schoolwork, significantly increased a child's demanding and aversive behavior at home—specifically, acting out and making demands for attention (Repetti & Pollina, 1994). Children are also affected by their parents' work and family stressors, with consequences for the children's academic achievement and acting out in adolescence (Menaghan, Kowaleski-Jones, & Mott, 1997). Stress in children leads to adoption of an unhealthy lifestyle (Michels et al., 2015). •

# SUMMARY

1. Events are perceived as stressful when people believe that their resources (such as time, money, and energy) may not be sufficient to meet the harm, threat, or challenge posed by the stressor.

2. Whether an event is stressful depends on how it is appraised. Events that are negative, uncontrollable or unpredictable, ambiguous, overwhelming, and threatening to central life tasks are especially likely to be perceived as stressful.

3. Early research on stress examined how a person mobilizes resources to fight or flee from threatening stimuli (the fight-or-flight response). Selye proposed the General Adaptation Syndrome, maintaining that reactions to stress go through three phases: alarm, resistance, and exhaustion. Recent efforts have focused on social responses to stress, that is, the ways in which people tend-and-befriend others in times of stress.

4. The physiology of stress implicates the sympathetic adrenomedullary (SAM) system and the hypothalamic–pituitary–adrenocortical (HPA) axis. Over the long term, repeated activation of these and other physiological systems can lead to cumulative damage, termed allostatic load, which represents the premature physiological aging that chronic or recurrent stress can produce.

5. Usually, people can adapt to mild stressors, but severe stressors may cause chronic health problems. Stress can have disruptive aftereffects, including persistent physiological arousal, psychological distress, poor task performance, and, over time, declines in cognitive capabilities. Vulnerable populations—such as children, the elderly, and the poor—may be particularly adversely affected by stress.

6. Researchers study stress in the laboratory and through experimental research that manipulates exposure to pathogens. Research on stressful life events indicates that any event that forces a person to make a change increases stress and the likelihood of illness. Chronic stress, as well as the daily hassles of life, affects health adversely.

7. Studies of occupational stress suggest that work hazards, work overload, work pressure, role conflict and ambiguity, inability to develop satisfying job relationships, inability to exert control in one's job, and unemployment can lead to increased illness, job dissatisfaction, absenteeism, tardiness, and turnover. Some of these job stresses can be prevented or offset through intervention.

8. Combining multiple roles, such as those related to work and home life, can create role conflict and role overload, producing psychological distress and poor health. On the other hand, such role combinations may confer meaning and enhance well-being. Which of these effects occur depend, in large part, on available resources, such as time, money, and social support.

# KEY TERMS

acute stress paradigm
aftereffects of stress
allostatic load
chronic strain
daily hassles
demand-control-support model

fight-or-flight response
general adaptation syndrome
person–environment fit
primary appraisal
reactivity
role conflict

secondary appraisal
stress
stressful life events
stressors
tend-and-befriend

# Coping, Resilience, and Social Support

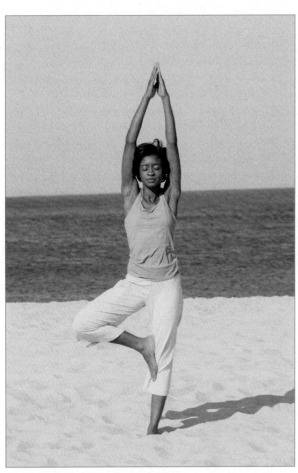

Jack Hollingsworth/Photodisc/Getty Images

In June 2012, wildfires swept through Colorado. Thousands of people were evacuated, and many lost their homes and personal property. Those whose homes survived intact often moved back into neighborhoods that were otherwise devastated. Even in cases where peoples' losses seemed similar, however, not everyone was affected the same way.

Consider four families, all of whom lost the better part of their homes and possessions to the fires. One family, newly arrived from Mexico, who had not yet found friends or employment, lost everything. They were devastated psychologically, uncertain whether to return to Mexico or remain. An older man with a heart condition succumbed to a heart attack, leaving his elderly wife behind. A third family, with financial resources and relatives in the area, were quickly taken in and began looking for another home. A young couple, wiped out by the experience, responded with resilience, determined to make a new start in Denver.

What these accounts illustrate is the degree to which stress is moderated by personal and circumstantial factors. People with many resources, such as money or social support, may find a stressful experience to be less so. Others, without resources or coping skills, may adjust poorly.

We term these factors **stress moderators** because they modify how stress is experienced and the effects it has. Moderators of the stress experience may have an impact on stress itself, on the relation between stress and psychological responses, on the relation between stress and illness, and on the degree to which a stressful experience intrudes into other aspects of life.

## ■  COPING WITH STRESS AND RESILIENCE

**Coping** is defined as the thoughts and behaviors used to manage the internal and external demands of situations that are appraised as stressful (Folkman & Moskowitz, 2004; Taylor & Stanton, 2007). Coping has several important characteristics. First, the relationship between coping and a stressful event is a dynamic process. Coping is a series of transactions between a person who has a set of resources, values, and commitments and a particular environment with its own resources, demands, and constraints (Folkman & Moskovitz, 2004). Thus, coping is not a one-time action that someone takes but rather a set of responses, occurring over time, by which the environment and the person influence each other.

A second important aspect of coping is its breadth. Emotional reactions, including anger or sadness, are part of the coping process, as are actions that are voluntarily undertaken to confront the event. Figure 7.1 presents a diagram of the coping process.

### Personality and Coping

The personality characteristics that each person brings to a stressful event influence how he or she will cope with that event.

**Negativity, Stress, and Illness**   Some people experience stressful events especially strongly, which increases their psychological distress, their physical symptoms, and their likelihood of illness. Research has especially focused on **negative affectivity** (Watson & Clark, 1984), a pervasive negative mood marked by anxiety, depression, and hostility. People high in negative affectivity (also called neuroticism) express distress, discomfort, and dissatisfaction in many situations.

Negative affectivity or neuroticism is related to poor health, including such chronic disorders as arthritis, diabetes, chronic pain, and coronary artery disease (Charles, Gatz, Kato, & Pedersen, 2008; Friedman & Booth-Kewley, 1987; Shipley, Weiss, Der, Taylor, & Deary, 2007; Strickhauser, Zell, & Krizan, 2017). Neuroticism coupled with social inhibition and isolation (sometimes referred to as the Type D or "distressed" personality) can be an especially toxic combination for health (Kupper & Denollet, 2018).

What links chronic negative affect to illness? One pathway is through stress generation; people with high negative affectivity can contribute to the occurrence of such stressful events as intimate relationship break-up and job loss, for example, which in turn prompt health problems (Iacovino, Bogdan, & Oltmanns, 2016). Negative affectivity also can prompt higher reactivity to stress, in its relation to elevated levels of stress indicators such as cortisol (Polk, Cohen, Doyle, Skoner, & Kirschbaum, 2005), heart rate (Daly, Delaney, Doran, Harmon, & MacLachlan, 2010), inflammation (Roy et al., 2010), and risk factors for coronary heart disease (Kupper & Denollet, 2018). Other links are unconstructive coping strategies and poor health habits. For example, people high in negative affectivity are more likely to cope with stress through avoidance (Carver & Connor-Smith, 2010), drink heavily and use drugs (Frances, Franklin, & Flavin, 1986), be sedentary (Allen, Walter, & McDermott, 2017), and experience

**FIGURE 7.1 | The Coping Process** *Sources:* Stone, George C., Frances Cohen, and Nancy E. Adler. *Health Psychology: A Handbook : Theories, Applications, and Challenges of a Psychological Approach to the Health Care System.* Canada: Jossey-Bass Publishers, 1979; Hamburg, David A. and John E. Adams. "A Perspective on Coping Behavior: Seeking and Utilizing Information in Major Transitions." *Archives of General Psychiatry* 17, no. 3 (1967): 277–84. Lazarus, Richard S., and Susan Folkman. *Stress, Appraisal, and Coping.* New York: Springer Publishing Company, 1984; Holahan, Charles J., & Rudolf H. Moos. "Personal and contextual determinants of coping strategies." *Journal of Personality and Social Psychology* 52, no. 5 (1987): 946–55. Taylor, Shelley E. "Adjustment to Threatening Events: A Theory of Cognitive Adaptation." *American Psychologist* 38, no. 11 (1983): 1161–1173."

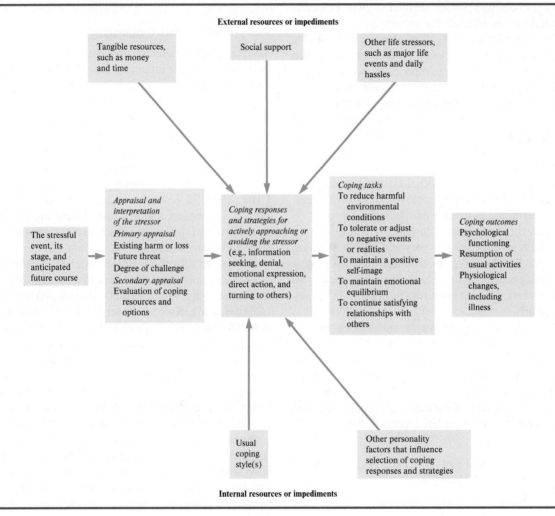

more disrupted sleep (Harvey, Gehrman, & Espie, 2014; Stephan, Sutin, Bayard, Križan, & Terracciano, 2018).

Although negative affectivity can compromise health, it can also create a false impression of poor health when none exists. People who are high in negative affectivity report more physical symptoms, such as headaches and other pains, especially under stress (Watson & Pennebaker, 1989). One reason may be that negative affect leads people to worry, be more aware of their symptoms, and attribute their symptoms to poor health (Mora, Halm, Leventhal, & Ceric, 2007). But in other cases, there is no evidence of an underlying physical disorder (Diefenbach, Leventhal, Leventhal, & Patrick-Miller, 1996). People high in negative affectivity may, nonetheless, use health services during stressful times more than people who are more positive (Cohen & Williamson, 1991). To summarize, people who are high in negative affect are more likely to get sick, but they also are distressed, experience physical symptoms, and seek medical attention even when they are not sick.

People vary in whether they are fundamentally optimistic or pessimistic about life. Scheier, Carver, and Bridges (1994) developed a scale of dispositional optimism to measure this pervasive individual difference. Items from the Life Orientation Test are as follows. (For each item, answer "true" or "false.")

1. In uncertain times, I usually expect the best.
2. It's easy for me to relax.
3. If something can go wrong for me, it will.
4. I'm always optimistic about my future.
5. I enjoy my friends a lot.
6. It's important for me to keep busy.
7. I hardly ever expect things to go my way.
8. I don't get upset too easily.
9. I rarely count on good things happening to me.
10. Overall, I expect more good things to happen to me than bad.

### Scoring

Sum how many "trues" you indicated for items 1, 4, and 10 and how many "falses" you indicated for items 3, 7, and 9 to obtain an overall score. Items 2, 5, 6, and 8 are filler items only.

———

**Positivity and Illness**   Positive emotional functioning promotes better mental and physical health (Cohen & Pressman, 2006; Wiest, Schüz, Webster, & Wurm, 2011) and a longer life (Okely, Weiss, & Gale, 2017; Xu & Roberts, 2010). Positive emotional states have been tied to lower levels of stress indicators such as cortisol and better immune responses to challenges such as exposure to a flu virus (Low, Matthews, & Hall, 2013; Steptoe, Demakakos, de Oliveira, & Wardle, 2012). When people are feeling positive, they also invest time and effort to overcome obstacles in pursuit of their goals (Haase, Poulin, & Heckhausen, 2012), which may accordingly affect their mood and lower their stress levels. In addition to promoting general well-being, positivity promotes several specific psychological resources that improve coping (Taylor & Broffman, 2011), to which we next turn.

## Psychosocial Resources

**Optimism**   An optimistic nature can help people cope more effectively with stress and reduce their risk for illness (Scheier, Carver, & Bridges, 1994). Scheier and colleagues developed a measure of dispositional optimism that identifies generalized positive expectations about the future. Box 7.1 lists the items on this measure, the Life Orientation Test (LOT-R).

How does optimism exert a positive impact on symptom expression, psychological adjustment, and health outcomes? Optimists have better physiological stress profiles on indicators such as cortisol, blood pressure, and systemic inflammation, which involves chronic activation of some components of the immune system (Scheier & Carver, 2018; Segerstrom & Sephton, 2010). Optimism also promotes active, **approach-oriented coping** efforts and healthy behaviors, which improve long-term prospects for psychological and physical health (Scheier & Carver, 2018; Segerstrom, Castañeda, & Spencer, 2003). Optimism fosters a sense of personal control, which has beneficial effects on physical functioning (Ruthig & Chipperfield, 2007). As noted in Chapter 1, meta-analysis is a particularly strong form of evidence because it includes many studies. A meta-analysis of 83 studies concerning the relation of optimism to physical health found effects not only on a broad array of health outcomes, but also on the physiological indicators that can predict them (Rasmussen, Scheier, & Greenhouse, 2009).

Optimism is usually beneficial for coping. But because optimists are persistent in pursuing their goals, they sometimes experience short-term physiological costs (Segerstrom, 2001). When optimists' expectations are not met, they may feel stressed, and compromised immune functioning may be a short-term consequence (Segerstrom, 2006a). Overall, though, optimism is a potent and valuable resource.

**Psychological Control**   **Psychological control** is the belief that one can determine one's own behavior, influence one's environment, and bring about desired outcomes. The belief that one can exert control over stressful events has long been known to help people cope with stress (Taylor, Helgeson, Reed, & Skokan, 1991; Thompson, 1981). Perceived control is closely related to self-efficacy, which is a more narrow belief that one's actions to obtain a specific outcome in a specific situation will be successful (Bandura, 1977). A related construct is collective control, which maintains that through collaboration with family and friends (Hou & Wan, 2012) or with medical practitioners, one may successfully cope with a stressful event. Thus control need not be personal to be adaptive: the perception that control is shared with significant other people in one's life can be beneficial (Hou & Wan, 2012).

Many studies show that the belief that one can exert control in stressful situations improves emotional well-being, coping with a stressful event, health behaviors (Gale, Batty, & Deary, 2008), and physiological stress indicators such as immune functioning and cardiovascular risk factors (Paquet, Dubé, Gauvin, Kestens, & Daniel, 2010). People who have a high sense of personal control may be protected from the elevated risk of death that typically is associated with high exposure to lifetime trauma (Elliot, Turiano, Infurna, Lachman, & Chapman, 2018). Perceived control fosters physical activity, which may be one reason why it contributes to good health (Infurna & Gerstorf, 2014).

So powerful are the effects of psychological control that they are the basis for interventions to promote good health habits (Chapters 4 and 5), to help people cope with stressful events, such as surgery and noxious medical procedures (Chapter 8), and to improve treatment effectiveness (Geers, Rose, Fowler, Rasinski, Brown, & Helfer, 2013). People going through unpleasant medical procedures, such as gastroendoscopic exams (Johnson & Leventhal, 1974), childbirth (Leventhal, Leventhal, Schacham, & Easterling, 1989), and chemotherapy (Burish & Lyles, 1979), have all benefitted from **control-enhancing interventions**. These interventions use information, relaxation, and cognitive–behavioral techniques, such as learning to think differently about the unpleasant sensations of a procedure, to reduce anxiety, improve coping, and promote recovery.

Like optimism, control is not a panacea for all aversive situations. People who desire control especially benefit from control-based interventions (Thompson, Cheek, & Graham, 1988). But control may actually be aversive if it gives people more responsibility than they want (Chipperfield & Perry, 2006). Nonetheless, the benefits of perceived control, especially in treatment settings, are clear.

Self-Esteem    High **self-esteem** is tied to effective coping. It seems to be most protective at low levels of stress; at higher levels of stress, the stressful events themselves can overwhelm the benefits of self-esteem (Whisman & Kwon, 1993). Nonetheless, typically self-esteem is associated with lower levels of stress indicators, such as HPA axis activity (Seeman et al., 1995), which may be the root by which self-esteem affects illness. In addition, people with stronger self-related resources have better health habits, being somewhat less likely to smoke or use alcohol to excess, for example (Friedman et al., 1995).

Additional Psychosocial Resources    Conscientiousness is a psychosocial resource that has health benefits. One study (Friedman et al., 1993) assessed young people in the early 1920s to see if differences in personality in childhood predicts who lived longer. Those people who were highly conscientious as children were more likely to live to an old age (Costa, Weiss, Duberstein, Friedman, & Siegler, 2014; Friedman et al., 1995; Hampson, Edmons, Goldberg, Dubanoski, & Hillier, 2013; Turiano, Chapman, Gruenwald, & Mroczek, 2015). Conscientious people may be more successful at avoiding harmful situations, they may think more about their health (Hill, Turiano, Hurd, Mroczek, & Roberts, 2011), they may be more adherent to treatment recommendations (Hill & Roberts, 2011), they practice good health habits (Hampson, Edmons, Goldberg, Dubanoski, & Hillier, 2015), and they use their cognitive abilities effectively (Hampson et al., 2015). They may consequently have lower stress-related biomarkers (Booth et al., 2014; Bogg & Slatcher, 2015; Mõttus, Luciano, Starr, Pollard, & Deary, 2013; Taylor et al., 2009).

Finding life deeply meaningful and purposeful, especially when accompanied by a sense of peace and harmony, can buffer against stress and promote health (Czekierda, Banik, Park, & Luszczynska, 2017; Hill, Sin, Turiano, Burrow, & Almeida, 2018; Visotsky, Hamburg, Goss, & Lebovits, 1961). The many routes to a sense of meaning and peace include engagement in cherished relationships, a chosen occupation, public service, religious affiliation (Box 7.2), and other pathways. Health benefits are documented across adulthood and in various groups, from healthy individuals

I just prayed and prayed and God stopped that thing just before it would have hit us.

—Tornado survivor

People going through stressful events have long turned to their faith and to God for solace, comfort, and insight. The majority of people in the United States believe in God (80 percent), attend church services at least once a month (55 percent), and say that religion is important in their personal lives (80 percent) (Gallup, 2009). Religion is especially important to women and to African Americans (Holt, Clark, Kreuter, & Rubio, 2003).

Religion (or spirituality, independent of organized religion) can promote well-being (Kashdan & Nezlek, 2012; McIntosh, Poulin, Silver, & Holman, 2011). People with strong spiritual beliefs have greater life satisfaction, greater personal happiness, fewer negative consequences of traumatic life events, and, for some disorders, a slower course of illness (George, Ellison, & Larson, 2002; Ironson et al., 2011; Romero et al., 2006). Surveys find that nearly half of people in the United States use prayer to deal with health problems (Zimmerman, 2005, March 15), and it seems to work. For example, surgery patients with stronger religious beliefs experienced fewer complications and had shorter hospital stays than people with less strong religious beliefs (Contrada et al., 2004).

Religion (or spirituality) may be helpful for coping with stress for several reasons. First, it provides a belief system and a way of thinking about stressful events that can lessen distress and enable people to find meaning in these events (Cheadle, Schetter, Lanzi, Vance, Sahadeo, Shalowitz, & the Community Child Health Network, 2015). Second, spiritual beliefs can lead to better health practices (Hill, Ellison, Burdette, & Musick, 2007). Third, organized religion can provide a sense of group identity for people because it provides a network of supportive individuals who share their beliefs (Gebauer, Sedikides, & Neberich, 2012; George et al., 2002). Fourth, religion has been tied to better health. For example, attending religious services has been tied to lower blood pressure (Gillum & Ingram, 2006), fewer complications from surgery (Ai, Wink, Tice, Bolling, & Shearer, 2009), and few adverse health symptoms (Berntson, Norman, Hawkley, & Cacioppo, 2008). Religion can lower cardiovascular, neuroendocrine, and immune responses to stressful events (Maselko, Kubzansky, Kawachi, Seeman, & Berkman, 2007; Seeman, Dubin, & Seeman, 2003).

Religious beliefs are not an unqualified blessing, however. Prayer itself does not appear to have health benefits (Masters & Spielmans, 2007; Nicholson, Rose, & Bobak, 2010). Moreover, if people see their health disorders as punishments from God, or if their health problems lead them to struggle with their faith, psychological and physical distress can be worsened (Park, Wortmann, & Edmondson, 2011; Reynolds, Mrug, Wolfe, Schwebel, & Wallander, 2016). Nonetheless, typically religion is not only a meaningful part of life but can offer emotional and physical health benefits as well (George et al., 2002; Powell, Shahabi, & Thoresen, 2003).

to those coping with such ailments as spinal cord injury, cancer, kidney transplant, and heart failure (Czekierda et al., 2017).

Being self-confident and having an easygoing disposition also facilitate coping (Holahan & Moos, 1990, 1991). Nonetheless, oddly, cheerful people die sooner than people who are not cheerful (Friedman et al., 1993). It may be that cheerful people grow up being more careless about their health and, as a result, experience health risks (Martin et al., 2002).

Being smart is good for you. More intelligent people have better physiological profiles across the life span (Calvin, Batty, Lowe, & Deary, 2011; Morozink, Friedman, Coe, & Ryff, 2010) and live longer (Wrulich, Brunner, Stadler, Schalke, Keller, & Martin, 2014).

Emotional stability also predicts longevity (Terracciano, Löckenhoff, Zonderman, Ferrucci, & Costa, 2008; Weiss, Gale, Batty, & Deary, 2009).

To summarize, coping resources are important because they help people manage the demands of daily stressful events with less emotional distress, fewer health risks, better health habits, and a higher quality of life. As such, coping resources are especially helpful to vulnerable populations, especially people low in socioeconomic status (Kiviruusu, Huurre, Haukkala, & Aro, 2013; Schöllgen, Huxhold, Schüz, & Tesch-Römer, 2011). These features are at the core of a health-prone personality, characterized by positivity, optimism, a sense of control, conscientiousness, and self-esteem.

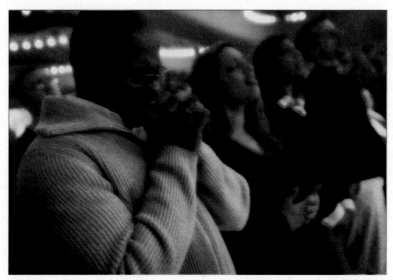

*Religion promotes psychological well-being, and people with religious faith may be better able to cope with aversive events.*

Kristy-Anne Glubish/Design Pics

## Resilience

Psychological resources such as these not only enable people to confront and cope with stressors but also help them bounce back from bad experiences and adapt flexibly to the changing demands of stressful situations (Fredrickson, Tugade, Waugh, & Larkin, 2003). This is called resilience (Dunkel Schetter & Dolbier, 2011).

A sense of coherence about one's life (Haukkala, Konttinen, Lehto, Uutela, Kawachi, & Laatikainen, 2013), a sense of humor (Cousins, 1979), trust in others (Barefoot et al., 1998), and a sense that life is worth living ("ikigai" in Japanese; Sone et al., 2008) are also resources that promote resilience, effective coping, and health.

In addition to these personality resources, taking opportunities for rest, relaxation, and renewal help people cope more effectively with stressors (Ong, Bergeman, Bisconti, & Wallace, 2006). Taking joy in positive events and celebrating them with other people improves mood not only immediately but also over the long term (Langston, 1994). Even taking a short vacation can be restorative (de Bloom, Geurts, & Kompier, 2012). Being able to feel positive emotions, even when going through intense stressors, is a coping resource that resilient people draw on (Tugade & Fredrickson, 2004).

## Coping Style and Coping Strategies

A seriously ill cancer patient was asked how she managed to cope with her disease so well. She responded, "I try to have cracked crab and raspberries every week." People have their favorite ways of coping, as this cancer patient described. There are also general styles of coping. **Coping style** is a propensity to deal with stressful events in a particular way. In contrast, **coping strategies** or processes are attempts to address the demands of a specific stressful experience. Most people engage in an assortment of coping strategies to manage stressful experiences. As another person coping with cancer said, "I do a bunch of things. I talk to my wife. I get as much information as I can about treatments and the latest research. I rely on my faith. I try to live each day as I want to" (Hoyt & Stanton, 2012; p. 232).

**Approach and Avoidance**    Some people cope with threatening events with an **avoidant (minimizing) coping style,** whereas others have an **approach-oriented (confrontive, vigilant) coping style,** by gathering information or taking direct action. **Avoidance-oriented coping** processes involve attempts to push away stressor-related thoughts and feelings, deny the existence or seriousness of the stressor, or distract oneself through other activities. Approach-oriented coping processes include efforts to

The Brief COPE assesses commonly used coping strategies for managing stressful events. People rate how they are coping with a stressful event by answering items on a scale from 0 ("I haven't been doing this at all") to 3 ("I've been doing this a lot"). Think of a stressful event that you are currently going through (a problem with your family, a roommate difficulty, problems in a course), and see which coping methods you use.

1. Active coping

   I've been concentrating my efforts on doing something about the situation I'm in.
   I've been taking action to try to make the situation better.

2. Planning

   I've been trying to come up with a strategy about what to do.
   I've been thinking hard about what steps to take.

3. Positive reframing

   I've been trying to see it in a different light, to make it seem more positive.
   I've been looking for something good in what is happening.

4. Acceptance

   I've been accepting the reality of the fact that it has happened.
   I've been learning to live with it.

5. Humor

   I've been making jokes about it.
   I've been making fun of the situation.

6. Religion

   I've been trying to find comfort in my religion or spiritual beliefs.
   I've been praying or meditating.

7. Using emotional support

   I've been getting emotional support from others.
   I've been getting comfort and understanding from someone.

8. Using instrumental support

   I've been trying to get advice or help from other people about what to do.
   I've been getting help and advice from other people.

9. Self-distraction

   I've been turning to work or other activities to take my mind off things.
   I've been doing something to think about it less, such as going to movies, watching TV, reading, daydreaming, sleeping, or shopping.

10. Denial

    I've been saying to myself "this isn't real."
    I've been refusing to believe that it has happened.

11. Venting

    I've been saying things to let my unpleasant feelings escape.
    I've been expressing my negative feelings.

12. Substance use

    I've been using alcohol or other drugs to make myself feel better.
    I've been using alcohol or other drugs to help me get through it.

13. Behavioral disengagement

    I've been giving up trying to deal with it.
    I've been giving up the attempt to cope.

14. Self-blame

    I've been criticizing myself.
    I've been blaming myself for things that happened.

---

*Source:* Carver (1997).

solve the problem at hand, seek support from others, and actively accept or find benefit in the stressful experience.

The Brief COPE is a measure that allows researchers to assess some of these more specific coping strategies (see Box 7.3). Another approach-oriented process is coping through emotional approach, which involves active attempts to acknowledge, understand, and express stressor-related emotions (Stanton et al., 2000).

Examples of the coping strategies used to combat the threat of AIDS appear in Box 7.4.

People who cope with threatening events through approach may pay a short-term price in anxiety and physiological reactivity as they confront stressful events, but be better off in the long term (Smith, Ruiz, & Uchino, 2000). Thus, the avoider or minimizer may cope well with a trip to the dentist but cope poorly

BOX 7.4    Coping with HIV

AIDS (acquired immune deficiency syndrome) has killed millions of people worldwide, and thousands more live, sometimes for years, with the knowledge that they have the disease. Here are some of the coping strategies that people with HIV infection have reported using.

### SOCIAL SUPPORT OR SEEKING INFORMATION

A key point in my program is that I have a really good support network of people who are willing to take the time, who will go the extra mile for me. I have spent years cultivating these friendships.

### DIRECT ACTION

My first concern was that, as promiscuous as I have been, I could not accept giving this to anyone. So I have been changing my lifestyle completely, putting everything else on the back burner.

### STRATEGIES OF DISTRACTION, ESCAPE, OR AVOIDANCE

I used to depend on drugs a lot to change my mood. Once in a while, I still find that if I can't feel better any other way, I will take a puff of grass or have a glass of wine, or I use music. There are certain recordings that can really change my mood drastically. I play it loud and I dance around and try to clear my head.

### EMOTIONAL REGULATION/VENTILATION

Sometimes I will allow myself to have darker feelings, and then I grab myself by the bootstraps and say, okay,

that is fine, you are allowed to have these feelings but they are not going to run your life.

### PERSONAL GROWTH

In the beginning, AIDS made me feel like a poisoned dart, like I was a diseased person and I had no self-esteem and no self-confidence. That's what I have been really working on, is to get the self-confidence and the self-esteem back. I don't know if I will ever be there, but I feel very close to being there, to feeling like my old self.

When something like this happens to you, you can either melt and disappear or you can come out stronger than you did before. It has made me a much stronger person. I literally feel like I can cope with anything. Nothing scares me, nothing. If I was on a 747 and they said we were going down, I would probably reach for a magazine.

### POSITIVE THINKING AND RESTRUCTURING

I have been spending a lot of time lately on having a more positive attitude. I force myself to become aware every time I say something negative during a day, and I go, "Oops," and I change it and I rephrase it. So I say, "Wonderful," about 42,000 times a day. Sometimes I don't mean it, but I am convincing myself that I do. The last chapter has not been written. The fat lady has not sung. I'm still here.

*Source:* Reed (1989).

---

with ongoing job stress. In contrast, the vigilant coper may fret over the visit to the dentist but take active efforts to reduce job stress.

Which coping processes people use and whether the processes are effective can depend on their general coping style and other attributes such as their level of optimism, aspects of the stressor such as its controllability, and the interpersonal and environmental context (Taylor & Stanton, 2007). For example, whether avoidant or approach-related coping is effective depends on how long the stressor lasts. People who cope with stress by minimizing or avoiding threatening events may deal effectively with short-term threats (Wong & Kaloupek, 1986). However, if stress persists over time,

avoidance is not as successful. For example, much of the American population reported high levels of post traumatic stress disorder symptoms following the 9/11 attacks. Those who used avoidant coping strategies fared worse psychologically over the long term, compared with those who used more active coping strategies (Silver, Holman, McIntosh, Poulin, & Gil-Rivas, 2002). People who cope using avoidance may not make enough cognitive and emotional efforts to anticipate and manage long-term problems (Suls & Fletcher, 1985; Taylor & Stanton, 2007).

Although both avoidant and approach-oriented coping can have advantages, on the whole, approach-oriented coping is more effective than avoidant coping, and it is tied to better mental and physical health outcomes (Taylor & Stanton, 2007). For example, avoidant coping with breast cancer in women recently diagnosed with the disease contributed to high levels of depression across 12 months (Stanton et al., 2018). On the other hand, increases in coping through active acceptance and emotional expression regarding cancer were linked to a low level of depression as well as recovery during the year from initially elevated depressive symptoms. In addition, trained clinicians' provision of early palliative care—aid in managing symptoms, as well as understanding and communicating prognosis and preferences of care—to adults newly diagnosed with incurable cancer improved psychological adjustment by increasing their use of approach-oriented coping (Greer et al., 2018). People who are able to alter their coping strategies to meet the demands of a stressful situation also adjust better than those who do not (Chen, Miller, Lachman, Gruenewald, & Seeman, 2012).

Just as stressful experiences often involve not only individuals but also their intimate others, coping processes also can be shared. A study of married couples, in which one partner had diabetes and both spouses completed daily diary assessments over 2 weeks, provides an example (Zajdel, Helgeson, Seltman, Korytkowski, & Hausmann, 2018). Couples who endorsed more communal coping—appraising one member's diabetes as the couple's rather than one partner's problem and coping collaboratively—reported better mood and the partner with diabetes had better self-care (e.g., medication adherence) over the 14 days than did partners who had lower communal coping.

The correspondence in partners' coping styles also can be important. For example, when partners' styles of coping with anger (e.g., suppression vs. expression) did not match, husbands and wives were at higher risk of an early death 32 years later (Bourassa, Sbarra, Ruiz, Karciroti, & Harburg, 2019).

### Problem-Focused and Emotion-Focused Coping

Another useful distinction is between problem-focused and emotion-focused coping (cf. Folkman, Schaefer, & Lazarus, 1979; Pearlin & Schooler, 1978). **Problem-focused coping** involves attempts to do something constructive about the stressful conditions that are harming, threatening, or challenging an individual. **Emotion-focused coping** involves efforts to regulate emotions experienced due to the stressful event.

Typically people use both problem-focused and emotion-focused coping to manage stressful events (Folkman & Lazarus, 1980).

The nature of the event contributes to which coping strategies will be used (Vitaliano et al., 1990). For example, work-related problems benefit from problem-focused coping, such as taking direct action or seeking help from others. Emotion-focused coping may be used more when a threat to one's health must be tolerated but may not be amenable to direct action. Overall, situations in which something constructive can be done will favor problem-focused coping, whereas those situations that are less controllable favor emotion-focused coping (Zakowski, Hall, Klein, & Baum, 2001).

**Proactive Coping**   Much coping is proactive; that is, people anticipate potential stressors and act in advance, either to prevent them or to reduce their impact (Aspinwall, 2011; Aspinwall & Taylor, 1997). Proactive coping requires first, the abilities to anticipate or detect potential stressors; second, coping skills for managing them; and third, self-regulatory skills, which are the ways that people control, direct, and correct their actions as they attempt to counter potential stressful events.

Proactive coping has been understudied because, by definition, if stressors are headed off in advance or reduced, they are less likely to occur or be experienced as intensely stressful. Clearly though, heading off a stressor is preferable to coping with it when it hits full force, and proactive coping merits additional attention (Aspinwall, 2011).

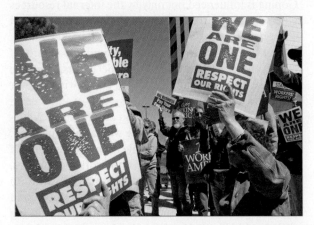

*Coping researchers have found that direct action often leads to better adjustment to a stressful event than do coping efforts aimed at avoidance of the issue or denial.*
Susan See Photography

**FIGURE 7.2 | Race- and Ethnicity-Adjusted Life Expectancy for 40-Year-Olds by Household Income Percentile, 2001 to 2014**    *Source:* Chetty, Raj, Michael Stepner, Sarah Abraham, Shelby Lin, Benjamin Scuderi, Nicholas Turner, Augustin Bergeron, and David Cutler. "The Association between Income and Life Expectancy in the United States, 2001–2014," *JAMA* 315, no. 16 (2016): 1750–66.

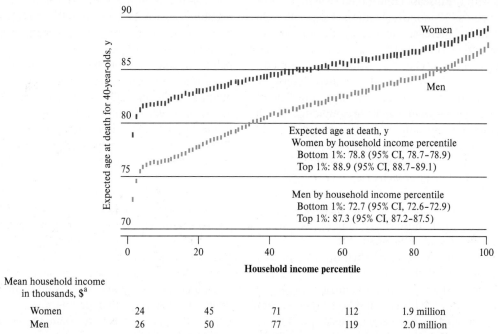

| Mean household income in thousands, $[a] | | | | | |
|---|---|---|---|---|---|
| Women | 24 | 45 | 71 | 112 | 1.9 million |
| Men | 26 | 50 | 77 | 119 | 2.0 million |

The difference between expected age at death in the top and bottom income percentiles is 10.1 years (95% CI, 9.9–10.3 years) for women and 14.6 years (95% CI, 14.4–14.8 years) for men. From Chetty et al. (2016).

## ■ COPING AND EXTERNAL RESOURCES

Coping is influenced not only by the internal resources a person brings to a stressor, such as coping style, but also by external resources. These include time, money, education, a decent job, friends, family, standard of living, the presence of positive life events, and the absence of other life stressors. People with greater resources typically cope with stressful events better, because time, money, friends, and other resources simply provide more ways of dealing with a stressful event. In Chapter 6, we saw an example of the moderation of stress by resources. Relative to nonworking mothers, working mothers who had adequate child care and whose husbands shared in household tasks benefited psychologically from their work, whereas working mothers without these resources showed higher levels of distress.

One of the most potent external resources with respect to health is socioeconomic status (SES). Peo-

ple who are high in SES have fewer medical and psychiatric disorders, and they show lower mortality from all causes of death. So strong is this relationship that, even in animals, higher-status animals are less vulnerable to infection than lower-status animals are (Cohen, Doyle, Skoner, Rabin, & Gwaltney, 1997). Figure 7.2 illustrates the relation between social class and mortality (see Adler, Boyce, Chesney, Folkman, & Syme, 1993).

## ■ COPING OUTCOMES

Throughout this discussion, we have referred to effective coping. What constitutes effective coping? Health psychologists typically assess whether the following outcomes have been achieved:

- Reducing or eliminating stressors
- Tolerating or adjusting to negative events or realities
- Maintaining a positive self-image

- Maintaining emotional equilibrium
- Continuing satisfying relationships with others
- Enhancing the prospects of recovery, if one is ill
- Keeping physiological, neuroendocrine, and immune reactivity relatively low or restoring these systems to pre stress levels (Karatsoreos & McEwen, 2011).

Another often-used criterion of effective coping is how quickly people can return to their prestress activities. Many stressors—especially severe ones, such as the death of a spouse, or chronic ones, such as excessive noise—interfere with daily life activities. If people's coping efforts help them resume usual activities, coping is judged to be effective. Following some stressors, though, life is actually improved; priorities may be reevaluated, and a person may seek to live a better and somewhat different life.

## ■ COPING INTERVENTIONS

People often can benefit from help to cope effectively. Fortunately, a number of interventions for coping with stress are supported by rigorous research.

### Mindfulness Meditation and Acceptance/Commitment Therapy

Mindfulness meditation teaches people how to adopt a state of mind marked by heightened awareness of the present moment, accepting and acknowledging it without becoming distracted or distressed by stress (Davidson & Kaszniak, 2015). Mindfulness can improve quality of life, reduce anxiety, and improve coping, and so it has been the basis of interventions (Schirda, Nicholas, & Prakash, 2015). Mindfulness-based stress reduction (MBSR) is a systematic training in mindfulness to help people manage their reactions to stress and the accompanying negative emotions (Dimidjian & Segal, 2015; Jacobs et al., 2013). Thus, the goal of mindfulness meditation is to help people approach stressful situations mindfully rather than reacting to them automatically (Hölzel et al., 2011).

How does mindfulness generate its positive effects? Mindfulness and MBSR can mute biological responses to stress (Hughes et al., 2013; Jacobs et al., 2013; Nyklíček, Mommersteeg, Van Beugen, Ramakers, & Van Boxtel, 2013). As studies in health neuroscience demonstrate, among other neural pathways, mindfulness

engages the prefrontal cortical regions of the brain, which regulate affect and downregulate activity in the limbic areas related to anxiety and other negative emotions (Creswell, Lindsay, Villalba, & Chin, 2019). Mindfulness meditation also promotes self-kindness, which in turn contributes to positive psychological adjustment in younger women with breast cancer, for example (Boyle, Stanton, Ganz, Crespi, & Bower, 2017). In addition, mindfulness training can reduce feelings of loneliness and increase social contact (Lindsay, Young, Brown, Smyth, & Creswell, 2019).

Acceptance and commitment therapy (ACT) is also an intervention that incorporates mindful awareness and acceptance, with the fundamental premise that pain, grief, and illness are inevitable elements of life (Hayes, 2016). ACT promotes psychological flexibility and committed pursuit of core values and life goals rather than constant striving to eliminate or escape life's troubles. Acceptance and mindfulness therapies can improve the quality of life while people are coming to grips with the stressors they experience. Promising evidence has accrued for the efficacy of mindfulness meditation and ACT for conditions such as chronic pain (Creswell, 2017; Hilton et al., 2017; Veehof, Trompetter, Bohlmeijer, & Schreurs, 2016).

### Expressive Writing

Disclosing emotions can have beneficial effects on health. For many years, researchers suspected that when people undergo traumatic events and cannot or do not communicate about them, those events may fester inside them, producing intrusive thoughts and feelings for years and even decades. This inhibition of traumatic events involves physiological work, and the more people are forced to inhibit their thoughts, emotions, and behaviors, the more their physiological activity may increase (Pennebaker, 1997). Consequently, the ability to confide in others or to consciously confront one's feelings may reduce the need to obsess about and inhibit the event, which may, in turn, reduce the physiological activity associated with the event. These insights have been explored through an approach called expressive writing (Pennebaker & Smyth, 2016).

In an early study, Pennebaker and Beall (1986) had 46 undergraduates write either about the most traumatic and stressful event ever in their lives or about trivial topics. Although the people writing about traumas were more upset immediately after they wrote their essays, there was no lasting psychological distress and, most important, they were less likely to visit the student health center during the following 6 months. Subsequent studies have found that when people have talked about or written about traumatic events, psychological and physiological indicators of stress can improve, as can direct indicators of health such as wound healing (Robinson, Jarrett, Vedhara, & Broadbent, 2017). The usefulness of expressive writing varies across studies and can depend on characteristics of the participants (e.g., culture, support in their environments), the focus of the writing, and other factors (Chu, Wong, & Lu, 2019; Jensen-Johansen et al., 2019; Korotana, Dobson, Pusch, & Josephson, 2016; Merz, Fox, & Malcarne, 2014; Travagin, Margola, & Revenson, 2015).

## Self-Affirmation

Earlier in this chapter we noted how self-related resources, such as self-esteem, can help people cope with stress. As noted in Chapter 3, a technique that makes use of this insight is called self-affirmation. When people positively affirm their values, they feel better about themselves and show lower physiological activity and distress (Cohen & Sherman, 2014). Writing about important social relationships appears to be the most impactful self-affirmation task (Shnabel, Purdie-Vaughns, Cook, Garcia, & Cohen, 2013). Self-affirmation can reduce defensiveness about personally relevant risk information and consequently make people more receptive to reducing their risk (Schüz, Schüz, & Eid, 2013). Consequently, researchers are now using self-affirmation as an intervention to help people cope with stress. In one study (Sherman, Bunyan, Creswell, & Jaremka, 2009), students wrote about an important personal value just before taking a stressful exam. Heart rate and blood pressure responses to the exam were attenuated by this self-affirmation. Self-affirmation can also undermine defensive reactions to threats (Harris, Mayle, Mabbott, & Napper, 2007; Van Koningsbruggen, Das, & Roskos-Ewoldsen, 2009).

## Relaxation Training

Whereas the techniques we have discussed so far give a person cognitive insights into the nature and control of stress, another set of techniques—relaxation training—affects the physiological experience of stress by reducing arousal.

Relaxation therapies include deep breathing, progressive muscle relaxation training, guided imagery, transcendental meditation, yoga, and self-hypnosis.

What are the benefits? These techniques can reduce heart rate, muscle tension, blood pressure, inflammatory activity, lipid levels, anxiety, and tension, among other physical and psychological benefits (Barnes, Davis, Murzynowski, & Treiber, 2004; Lutgendorf, Anderson, Sorosky, Buller, & Lubaroff, 2000; Scheufele, 2000; Speca, Carlson, Goodey, & Angen, 2000). Even 5 to 10 minutes of deep breathing and progressive muscle relaxation can be beneficial.

Yoga may have health benefits. One study found that people who regularly practiced yoga experienced more positive emotions and showed lower inflammatory responses to stress than those who were new to the practice. Yoga, then, may ameliorate the burden that stress places on an individual (Kiecolt-Glaser et al., 2010; Pascoe, Thompson, & Ski, 2017). Joyful music can also be a relaxing stress buster (Miller, Mangano, Beach, Kop, & Vogel, 2010).

## Coping Skills Training

Teaching people effective coping techniques is another beneficial intervention individually, in a group setting, or even by telephone (Blumenthal et al., 2014). Most of these interventions draw on principles from CBT (Antoni, Carrico, et al., 2006). Coping effectiveness training typically begins by teaching people how to appraise stressful events and disaggregate the stressors into specific tasks. The person learns to distinguish those aspects of a stressor that may be changeable from those that are not. Specific coping strategies are then practiced to deal with these specific stressors. Encouraging people to maintain their social support is also an important aspect of coping effectiveness training (Folkman et al., 1991). We will discuss several coping effectiveness interventions in the chapters on chronic diseases. Here, we highlight coping effectiveness training for managing the stress of college life.

Managing the Stress of College    Many people have difficulty managing stress themselves. Accordingly, health psychologists have developed techniques for **stress management.** Stress management programs typically involve three phases. In the first phase, participants learn what stress is and how to identify the stressors in their own lives. In the second phase, they acquire and practice skills for coping with stress. In the final phase, they practice these coping techniques in targeted stressful situations and monitor their effectiveness (Meichenbaum & Jaremko, 1983).

As an example, college can be an extremely stressful experience for many new students. For some, it is their first time away from home, and they must cope with living in a dormitory surrounded by strangers. They may have to share a room with another person from a very different background and with very different personal habits. High noise levels, communal bathrooms, institutional food, and rigorous academic schedules may all be trying experiences for new students. Recognizing that these pressures exist, college administrators have increasingly made stress management programs available to their students.

### A Stress Management Program

A program called Combat Stress Now (CSN) makes use of these various phases of education, skill acquisition, and practice (Taylor, 2003).

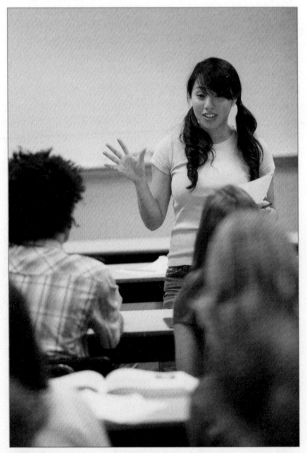

There are many stressful aspects of college life, such as speaking in front of large groups. Stress management programs can help students master these experiences.

Rob Melnychuk/Jupiterimages/Brand X/Alamy Stock Photo

### Identifying Stressors

In the first phase of the program, participants learn what stress is and how it creates physical wear and tear. In sharing their personal experiences of stress, many students find reassurance in the fact that other students have experiences similar to their own. They learn that stress is a process of psychological appraisal rather than a factor inherent in events themselves. Thus, college life is not inherently stressful but is a consequence of the individual's perceptions of it.

### Monitoring Stress

In the self-monitoring phase of the program, students are trained to observe their own behavior closely and to record the circumstances that they find most stressful. In addition, they record their physical, emotional, and behavioral reactions to those stresses as they experience them. Students also record any maladaptive efforts they undertook to cope with these stressful events, including excessive sleeping or eating, online activity, and alcohol consumption.

### Identifying Stress Antecedents

Once students learn to chart their stress responses, they are taught to examine the antecedents of these experiences. They learn to focus on what happens just before they experience feelings of stress. For example, one student may feel overwhelmed with academic life only when contemplating having to speak out in class, whereas another student may experience stress primarily before exams. By pinpointing exactly those circumstances that initiate feelings of stress, students can more precisely identify their own trouble spots.

### Avoiding Negative Self-Talk

Students are next trained to recognize and eliminate the negative self-talk they go through when they face stressful events. For example, the student who fears speaking out in class may recognize how self-statements contribute to this process: "I hate asking questions," "I always get tongue-tied," and "I'll probably forget what I want to say."

### Completing Take-Home Assignments

In addition to in-class exercises, students have take-home assignments. They keep a stress diary in which they record what events they find stressful and how they respond to them. As they become proficient in identifying stressful incidents, they are encouraged to record the negative self-statements or irrational thoughts that accompany the stressful experience.

Acquiring Skills    The next stage of stress management involves skill acquisition and practice. These skills include cognitive–behavioral management techniques, time management skills, and other stress-reducing interventions, such as exercise. Some of these techniques are designed to eliminate the stressful event; others are geared toward reducing the experience of stress without necessarily modifying the event itself.

Setting New Goals    Each student next sets several specific goals that he or she wants to meet to reduce the experience of college stress. For one student, the goal may be learning to speak in class without suffering overwhelming anxiety. For another, it may be going to see a particular professor about a problem.

Once the goals are set, specific behaviors to meet those goals are identified. In some cases, an appropriate response may be leaving the stressful event altogether. For example, the student who is having difficulty in a rigorous physics course may need to modify his goal of becoming a physicist. Alternatively, students may be encouraged to turn a stressor into a challenge. Thus, the student who fears speaking up in class may come to realize that she must not only master this fearful event but also actually come to enjoy it if she is to realize her long-term goal of becoming a professor.

Goal setting is important in effective stress management for two reasons. First, it prompts the person to distinguish among stressful events to be avoided, tolerated, or overcome. Second, it gets the person to be specific and concrete about exactly which stressors need to be tackled and what is to be done.

Engaging in Positive Self-Talk and Self-Instruction    Once students have set realistic goals and identified some target behaviors for reaching their goals, they learn how to engage in self-instruction and positive self-talk. Self-instruction involves reminding oneself of the specific steps that are required to achieve the goal. Positive self-talk involves providing the self with encouragement. For example, the student who is fearful of speaking out in class may learn to begin with simple questions or small points, or bring comments about the reading to class that can be used as a reminder of what point to raise. Once some proficiency in public speaking is achieved, students might encourage themselves by highlighting the positive aspects of the experience (e.g., holding the attention of the audience, making some points, and winning over a few converts to their positions).

Using Other Cognitive–Behavioral Techniques    In some stress management programs, contingency contracting and self-reinforcement (see Chapter 3) are encouraged. For example, the student who fears making oral presentations may define a specific goal, such as asking three questions in class in a week, which will be followed by a reward, such as tickets to a concert.

Several other techniques are frequently used in stress management interventions. **Time management** and planning help people set specific goals, establish priorities, avoid time-wasters, and learn what to ignore. Most stress management programs emphasize practicing good health habits and exercise at least 20 to 30 minutes at least 3 times a week. Assertiveness training is sometimes incorporated into stress management. The person is encouraged to identify the people in their environment who cause them special stress—called **stress carriers**—and develop techniques for confronting them. Because social support is so important to combating stress—a topic to which we next turn—ways of increasing warm social contact are encouraged as well.

Overall, stress management training imparts an array of valuable skills for living in a world with many sources of stress. Each person will find the particular techniques that work for him or her. Ultimately effectively dealing with stress improves mental and physical health.

# ◾ SOCIAL SUPPORT

The most vital of all protective psychosocial resources is social support. Social ties are emotionally satisfying, they mute the effects of stress, they reduce the likelihood that stress will lead to poor health, and they are linked to the longevity. Scientists in health psychology contend that close relationships are a sufficiently powerful contributor to health that promoting positive social connections should be a national public health priority (Holt-Lunstad, Robles, & Sbarra, 2017).

## What Is Social Support?

**Social support** is defined as information from others that one is loved and cared for, esteemed and valued, and part of a network of communication and mutual obligations. Social support can come from parents, a spouse or partner, other relatives, friends, social and community contacts (such as churches or clubs)

(Rietschlin, 1998), or even a devoted pet (McConnell, Brown, Shoda, Stayton, & Martin, 2011). Social support helps people thrive (Feeney & Collins, 2015). People with social support experience less stress when they confront a stressful experience, cope with it more successfully (Taylor, 2011), and even experience positive life events more positively (Gable, Gosnell, Maisel, & Strachman, 2012).

Not having social support in times of need is stressful, and social isolation and loneliness are powerful predictors of health and longevity (Cacioppo, Cacioppo, Capitanio, & Cole, 2015). For example, the elderly, the recently widowed, and victims of sudden, severe, uncontrollable life events may need support but have difficulty getting it (Sorkin, Rook, & Lu, 2002). People who have difficulty with social relationships, such as the chronically shy (Naliboff et al., 2004) or those who anticipate rejection by others (Cole, Kemeny, Fahey, Zack, & Naliboff, 2003), are at risk for isolating themselves socially. Just as social support has health benefits, loneliness and social isolation have risks for physical, cognitive, and emotional functioning (Shankar, Hamer, McMunn, & Steptoe, 2013). In a study of ex-prisoners of war (POWs), loneliness and a perceived lack of social support 18 years after returning to their own country was linked to greater cellular aging 24 years later (Stein et al., 2018). In addition, large studies conducted over many years demonstrate that the lonely and socially isolated die at younger ages (Beller & Wagner, 2018; Tabue Teguo et al., 2016).

Social support can take any of several forms. **Tangible assistance** involves the provision of material support, such as services, financial assistance, or goods. For example, the gifts of food that often arrive after a death in a family mean that the bereaved family members will not have to cook for themselves and visiting friends and family.

Family and friends can provide **informational support** about stressful events. For example, if an individual is facing an uncomfortable medical procedure, a friend who went through the same thing could provide information about the exact steps involved, the potential discomfort experienced, and how long it takes.

Supportive friends and family can provide **emotional support** by reassuring the person that he or she is a valuable individual who is cared for. The warmth and nurturance provided by other people can enable a person under stress to approach the stressful event with greater assurance (Box 7.5).

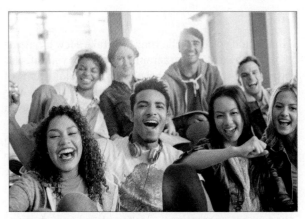

*Humor has long been thought to be an effective defense against stress.*
Caia Images/Glow Images

The types of social support just discussed have each been related to health indicators (e.g., Bowen et al., 2014). They all involve the actual provision of help and solace by one person to another. But in fact, many of the benefits of social support come from being socially integrated (Barger, 2013) and from the *perception* that social support is available. Simply believing that support is available (Smith, Ruiz, & Uchino, 2004) or contemplating the sources of support one typically has in life (Broadwell & Light, 1999) can yield beneficial effects.

Moreover, actually receiving social support from another person can have potential costs. First, one may use up another's time and attention, which can produce a sense of guilt and obligation. Needing to draw on others can also threaten self-esteem, because it suggests a dependence on others (Bolger, Zuckerman, & Kessler, 2000). These potential costs can undermine the distress-reducing benefits of social support. Indeed, research suggests that when one receives help from another but is unaware of it, that help is most likely to benefit the recipient (Bolger & Amarel, 2007). This kind of support is called **invisible support.**

## Effects of Social Support on Illness

Social support can lower the likelihood of illness, speed recovery from illness or treatment (Krohne & Slangen, 2005), and reduce the risk of mortality due to serious disease (House, Landis, & Umberson, 1988; Rutledge, Matthews, Lui, Stone, & Cauley, 2003). Hundreds of studies of people with both major and minor health disorders show that social support is beneficial for health.

How would you describe your life? Take a few moments to write down a few paragraphs about how your life has progressed so far. What have been the major events of your life? What has been important to you? Now go back to see how often you mention other people in those paragraphs.

Two psychologists, Sarah Pressman and Sheldon Cohen (2007), did precisely this. They looked at the autobiographies of 96 psychologists and 220 literary writers and counted how often the authors mentioned social relationships. Pressman and Cohen then related the number of mentions of relationships and emotions to how long the writer lived (Pressman & Cohen, 2011).

They found that the number of social words used in these autobiographies predicted a longer life. Why would this be the case? Pressman and Cohen reasoned that social words used in autobiographies provide an indirect measure of the social relationships with which these people were engaged. As we have seen, good social relationships are associated with longer life. The use of positive-emotion words in these autobiographical accounts also predicted longevity, although only positive emotions conveying activation, such as lively and vigorous, were associated with longevity and not positive statements that were peaceful or calm.

So, to the extent that you mentioned important social relationships in your autobiography, it reflects positively on your ability to experience social support and ultimately to enjoy good health and a long life.

Social support also typically benefits health behaviors as well (Cohen & Lemay, 2007). People with high levels of social support are more adherent to their medical regimens (DiMatteo, 2004), and they are more likely to use health services (Wallston, Alagna, DeVellis, & DeVellis, 1983). However, social support can lead to some bad health habits, as when one's peer group smokes, drinks heavily, or takes drugs (Wills & Vaughan, 1989) or when a lot of social contact is coupled with stress; under these circumstances, risk of minor illnesses such as colds or flus may actually increase because of contagion through the social network (Hamrick, Cohen, & Rodriguez, 2002).

Lonely and socially isolated people have poorer health and experience more adverse symptoms on a daily basis (Wolf & Davis, 2014). They also practice poorer health habits, which may contribute to risk for poor health (Crittenden, Murphy, & Cohen, 2018; Kobayashi & Steptoe, 2018).

### Biopsychosocial Pathways

The challenge for social support research is to identify the biopsychosocial pathways by which social contacts exert beneficial or health-compromising effects. Studies suggest that social support has beneficial effects on the cardiovascular, endocrine, and immune systems (Taylor, 2011). Social support can reduce physiological and neuroendocrine responses to stress. For example, in a study of the common cold, healthy volunteers reported their social ties, such as whether they had a spouse, living parents, friends, or workmates, and whether they were members of social groups, such as clubs. The volunteers were then given nasal drops containing a virus and were observed for the development of cold symptoms. People who had larger social networks were less likely to develop colds, and those who did have colds had less severe ones (Cohen et al., 1997).

Psychologists often study the effects of social support using the acute stress paradigm—that is, by taking people into the laboratory, putting them through

*In addition to being an enjoyable aspect of life, social support from family and friends helps keep people healthy and may help them recover faster when they are ill.*

Big Cheese Photo/Getty Images

stressful tasks, and then measuring their biological stress responses. In several studies, researchers have conducted these procedures, having some of the people bring a supportive companion and having others go through the procedures alone. When a supportive companion is present, physiological reactivity to the stressful tasks is usually more subdued (Christenfeld, 1997; Robinson et al., 2017; Smith, Loving, Crockett, & Campbell, 2009).

Social support is tied to reduced cortisol responses to stress, which can have beneficial effects on illness (Turner-Cobb, Sephton, Koopman, Blake-Mortimer, & Spiegel, 2000). Social support is also associated with better immune functioning (Herbert & Cohen, 1993) and lower inflammation (Uchino et al., 2018), with less accumulation of allostatic load (Brooks, Gruenewald, Karlmangla, Hu, Koretz, & Seeman, 2014), and with less cellular aging (Carroll, Diez Roux, Fitzpatrick, & Seeman, 2013). Integrated biopsychosocial pathways, then, provide the links between social support and reduced risk of illness (Uchino & Way, 2017).

Several studies have also shown that social support modifies the brain's responses to stress. For example, in one study (Coan, Schaefer, & Davidson, 2006), married women were exposed to the threat of electric shock while holding their husband's hand, the hand of an anonymous male experimenter, or no hand at all. Holding one's husband's hand led to reduced activation in neural systems related to threat responses: more limited attenuation occurred from just holding an anonymous person's hand. Of considerable interest, the higher the quality of the woman's marriage, the

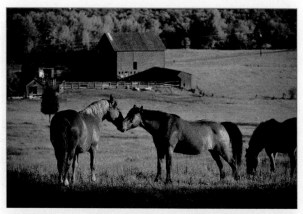

*Animals enjoy the benefits of social support just as humans do. For example, female horses who form relationships with unrelated females are more likely to give birth to foals that survive over the long term (Cameron, Setsaas, & Linklater, 2009).*

Comstock Images/Alamy Stock Photo

more reduction in neural activation there was (Coan, Schaefer, & Davidson, 2006). Even looking at a partner's picture can make a painful experience easier to endure (Master et al., 2009).

Over time, family members shape each other's biology including biological responses to stress (Laws, Sayer, Pietromonaco, & Powers, 2015; Saxbe et al., 2014). Dyadic coping, that is, the effects of each member of a couple on the other's coping, can be seen both in similar coping styles and in their underlying biology (e.g., Slatcher, Selcuk, & Ong, 2015).

## Moderation of Stress by Social Support

How does social support moderate the effects of stress? Two possibilities have been explored. The **direct effects hypothesis** maintains that social support is generally beneficial during nonstressful as well as stressful times. The **buffering hypothesis** maintains that the physical and mental health benefits of social support are chiefly evident during periods of high stress; when there is little stress, social support may offer few such benefits. According to this viewpoint, social support acts as a reserve and resource that blunts the effects of stress when it is at high levels.

Evidence suggests both direct and buffering effects of social support (Bowen et al., 2014; Cohen, & Hoberman, 1983; Cohen & McKay, 1984). Generally, when researchers have looked at social support in terms of the number of people one identifies as friends and the number of organizations one belongs to, direct effects social support on health are found. When social support is assessed qualitatively, such as by the number of people perceived to be available who will provide help if it is needed, buffering effects of social support have been found (House et al., 1988).

**Extracting Support**   The effectiveness of social support depends on how an individual uses a social support network. Some people are better than others at extracting the support they need. Research using twin study methodology has discovered genetic underpinnings in the ability either to construe social support as available or to establish supportive networks (Kessler, Kendler, Heath, Neale, & Eaves, 1992). During periods of high stress, genetic predispositions to draw on social support networks may be activated, leading to the perception that support will be available to mute stress.

Social skills influence the ability to develop social support as well. Cohen, Sherrod and Clark (1986) assessed incoming college freshmen as to their social competence, social anxiety, and self-disclosure skills to see if these skills influenced whether the students were able to develop and use social support effectively. The students with more social competence, lower social anxiety, and better self-disclosure skills developed more effective social support networks and were more likely to form friendships.

## What Kinds of Support Are Most Effective?

Not all aspects of social support are equally protective against stress. For example, having a confidant (such as a spouse or partner or close friend), particularly on a daily basis, may be the most effective social support (Stetler & Miller, 2008; Umberson, 1987). Marriage, especially a satisfying marriage, is one of the best protectors against stress (Robles, 2014). On average, men's health benefits substantially from marriage (e.g., Sbarra, 2009), whereas women's health benefits only slightly from marriage. Leaving a marriage, being unmarried, or being in an unsatisfying marriage all bring health risks, especially for women and especially when the relationship problems lead to depression (Kiecolt-Glaser, 2018; Liu & Umberson, 2008; Sbarra & Nietert, 2009). Marital strain, fighting, and separation and divorce have powerful negative effects on health (Nealey-Moore, Smith, Uchino, Hawkins, & Olson-Cerney, 2007).

Support from family is important as well. Receiving social support from one's parents in early life and living in a stable and supportive environment as a child have long-term effects on coping abilities and on health (Chen, Brody, & Miller, 2017; Puig, Englund, Simpson, & Collins, 2013; Repetti et al., 2002). Experiencing the divorce of one's parents in childhood predicts premature death in middle age (Friedman, Tucker, Schwartz, et al., 1995).

Support from one's community beneficially affects health. For example, an investigation in Indonesia found that mothers who were active in the community were more likely to get resources and information about health care for their children, resources that would otherwise not have been accessible (Nobles & Frankenberg, 2009). Thus, one mechanism linking community level support to health may be increased knowledge about resources.

Matching Support to the Stressor    Different kinds of stressful events create different needs, and social support is most effective when it meets those needs. This is called the **matching hypothesis** (Cohen &

McKay, 1984; Cohen & Wills, 1985). For example, if a person has someone he or she can talk to about problems but actually needs only to borrow a car, the presence of a confidant is useless. But if a person is upset about how a relationship is going and needs to talk it through with a friend, then the availability of a confidant is a very helpful resource. In short, support that is responsive to a person's needs is most beneficial (Maisel & Gable, 2009), and cultural factors can shape the source and nature of social support that are best-suited to the recipient's needs (Campos & Kim, 2017).

Support from Whom?    Providing effective social support is not always easy for the support network. It requires skill. When it is provided by the wrong person, support may be unhelpful or even rejected, as when a stranger tries to comfort a lost child.

Social support may also be ineffective if the type of support provided is not the kind that is needed. Emotional support is most beneficial when it comes from intimate others, whereas information and advice may be more valuable coming from experts. Thus, a person who desires solace from a family member but receives advice instead may find that, rather than being supportive, the family member actually makes the stressful situation worse (Dakof & Taylor, 1990). The benefits of social support are greater when the person from whom one is seeking support is perceived to be responsive to one's needs (Selcuk & Ong, 2013).

Threats to Social Support    Stressful events can interfere with obtaining social support. People who are

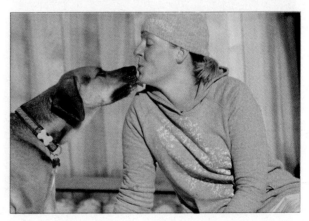

*Social support can come not only from family and friends but also from a loved pet. Research suggests that dogs are better at providing social support than cats or other animals.*
Ingram Publishing/SuperStock

Most people have at least one bad relationship. It might be a sibling with whom you are constantly feuding, a sloppy sullen roommate, a demanding partner, or even a parent. Even in usually good relationships, things can go wrong. But do these bad relationships affect health? The answer appears to be yes.

In a study by Jessica Chiang and colleagues (2012), college students completed daily diaries each evening for 8 days about their social experiences of that day. They recorded the number of positive social interactions, negative interactions, and competitive experiences they had had that day. For each interaction, the students briefly described the experience. A few days later, their levels of inflammation—an immunologic marker of stress and a pathway to several diseases—was assessed. Students who had experienced primarily positive interactions had normal levels of inflammation. But students who had experienced negative interactions, such as conflicts or arguments with others, had higher levels of inflammation.

Those who had gone through competitive social interactions had elevated inflammation levels as well, although only certain kinds of competition were tied to inflammation. Competitive leisure-time activities, such as tennis or an online game, did not increase levels of inflammation. However, academic and work-related competitive events and competing for the attention of another person, such as a romantic partner or friend, were both associated with heightened inflammation. The more of these negative and competitive events a person experienced, the higher their levels of inflammation.

Inflammation in response to a short-term stressor can be adaptive, as it can help heal wounds during competitive struggles. Chronic inflammation, however, is related to hypertension, heart disease, diabetes, depression, and some cancers. So people whose lives have

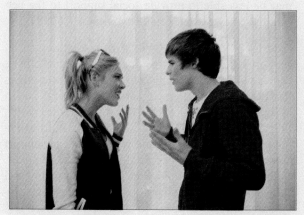

*A lot of relationships aren't all good or all bad, but instead, they make one feel ambivalent. Sometimes the person is there for you and sometimes not. Ambivalent relationships can compromise health (Uchino et al., 2012).*
funstock/iStockphoto/Getty Images

recurring conflict or competition may, over the long term, be at risk for these disorders.

Does it matter when in one's life the negative relationships occur? Research suggests that negative relationships early in life, during childhood, may be especially important for inflammation (Chen et al., 2017; Miller & Chen, 2010). When a person grows up in a harsh family, marked by conflict, neglect, or cold non nurturant parenting, that person shows a stronger inflammatory response to stress as early as adolescence, suggesting that by adulthood, the risk of chronic illness may already be established.

The evidence relating bad relationships to inflammation is strong enough to suggest a bit of advice: Decline bad relationships. They add stress to life and erode good health. Instead, populate your life with supportive and upbeat people. The beneficial effects of social support on mental and physical health are clear.

---

under stress may express distress to others and drive those others away, thus making a bad situation even worse (Alferi, Carver, Antoni, Weiss, & Duran, 2001).

Sometimes, would-be support providers do not provide the support that is needed and, instead, react in an unsupportive manner that aggravates the negative event (see Box 7.6).

Too much or overly intrusive social contact may actually make stress worse. When social support is

controlling or directive, it may have some benefits for health behaviors but produce psychological distress (Lewis & Rook, 1999). For example, people who belong to "dense" social networks (friendship or family groups that spend a lot of time together) can find themselves besieged by advice and interference in times of stress. As comedian George Burns once noted, "Happiness is having a large, loving, caring, close-knit family in another city." When family members or friends are also affected by the stressful event, they may be less able to provide social support to the person in greatest need (Melamed & Brenner, 1990).

**Giving Social Support** Most research on social support has focused on getting support from others, which has benefits. But giving social support to others has beneficial effects on mental and physical health as well (Inagaki & Orehek, 2017; Li & Ferraro, 2005; Piliavin & Siegl, 2007). For example, one study examined the effects of giving and receiving social support among older married people (Brown, Nesse, Vinokur, & Smith, 2003). People who provided instrumental support to friends, relatives, and neighbors or who provided emotional support to their spouses were less likely to die over the next 5 years. Volunteering, as by working at a soup kitchen or raising funds for others, has health benefits as well (Poulin et al., 2014). Thus, giving support can promote health, especially when the support is freely given and the support provider believes that it is useful (Inagaki & Orehek, 2017).

## Enhancing Social Support

Health psychologists view social support as an important resource in primary prevention. Increasingly, people are living alone for long periods during their lives, because they have never married, are divorced, or have lost a spouse to death (U.S. Census Bureau, 2012). Americans report that they have fewer close friends now than has been true in the past.

As of March 2019, Facebook has more than 2.4 billion active users per month, of which 1.5 billion log on at least once every day (Facebook, 2019).

Clearly, patterns of social support are shifting, but whether they are shifting in ways that continue to provide support remains to be seen. Networking may be an added source of social support for people, but those who use it to express distress may drive others away (Forest & Wood, 2012).

Finding ways to increase the effectiveness of existing or potential support from family, friends, and Internet buddies should be a high research priority. (Bookwala, Marshall, & Manning, 2014). A number of interventions have been undertaken to try to reduce loneliness. Some of these focus on improving social skills, whereas others attempt to enhance existing social support. Social support groups (Taylor, 2011) and Internet-based social support interventions (Haemmerli, Znoj, & Berger, 2010) show promise for enhancing access to socially supportive resources. Some focus on getting people to increase their opportunities for social contact, and others address the maladaptive internal monologues that people sometimes generate about themselves and their social adeptness that can drive other people away. Loneliness is often an emotional state, rather than purely a consequence of little social contact (Cacioppo, Grippo, London, Goossens, & Cacioppo, 2015). Poor quality of sleep and anxiety can lead to depression, negative social cognitions, and further loneliness (Zawadzki, Graham, & Gerin, 2013). Consequently, cognitive–behavioral interventions that target social cognitions and encourage people to attend to the positive aspects of the social environment have been most successful in reducing loneliness (Cacioppo et al., 2015). These interventions are covered more fully in Chapter 11. ●

## SUMMARY

1. Coping is the process of managing demands that tax or exceed a person's resources. Coping efforts are guided by internal resources such as optimism, personal control, and self-esteem and external resources such as time, money, the absence of simultaneous life stressors, and social support.

2. Coping styles are predispositions to cope with stress in particular ways. Coping strategies are attempts to address the demands of a specific stressful experience. An important distinction is between approach-oriented coping and avoidance-oriented coping. Although avoidance may be successful in the short run, on the whole, approach-related coping is more effective.

3. Coping efforts may be directed to solving problems or to regulating emotions. People most often use multiple types of coping strategies to manage stress.

4. Coping efforts are judged to be successful when they reduce physiological indicators of arousal, enable the person to resume desired activities, and free the individual from psychological distress.

5. Coping effectiveness training, which draws on the principles of cognitive–behavioral therapy, teaches effective coping skills. Emotional disclosure and expressive writing about stressful events also can be effective.

6. Stress management programs exist for those who need help in developing their coping skills. These programs teach people to identify sources of stress in their lives, to develop coping skills to deal with those stressors, and to practice these skills and monitor their effectiveness.

7. Social support involves tangible assistance, information, or emotional comfort that lets people know they are loved and cared for, esteemed and valued, and part of a social network.

8. Social support reduces psychological distress, can improve health habits, and has undeniable benefits on physical health. These benefits are chiefly gained because social support reduces psychological and physiological reactivity to stress.

9. Having a confidant such as a spouse or close friend is especially beneficial, as is support from family early in life. Social support is most effective when it matches one's needs and is from the person best able to provide it.

10. Increasing the quality and quantity of social support a person receives is an important goal of health psychology interventions.

## KEY TERMS

approach-oriented coping
avoidance-oriented coping
buffering hypothesis
control-enhancing interventions
coping strategies
coping style
direct effects hypothesis
emotion-focused coping

emotional support
informational support
invisible support
matching hypothesis
negative affectivity
problem-focused coping
psychological control
self-esteem

social support
stress carriers
stress management
stress moderators
tangible assistance
time management

# PART 4

# Seeking and Using Health Care Services

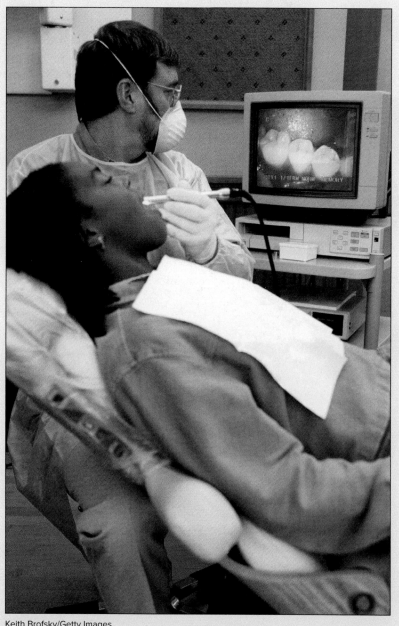

Keith Brofsky/Getty Images

8

# Using Health Services

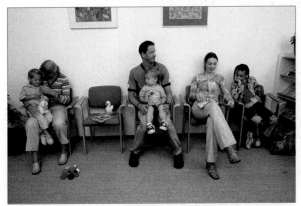

Picture Partners/Pixtal/age fotostock

On the surface, the questions of who uses health services and why would seem to be medical issues. The obvious answer is that people use services when they are sick. But this issue can also be psychological: When and how does a person decide that he or she is sick? When are symptoms dismissed as inconsequential? When does a person decide that a symptom requires treatment by a professional, and when do chicken soup, fluids, and bed rest seem to be all that is needed?

## ■ RECOGNITION AND INTERPRETATION OF SYMPTOMS

Although people have some awareness of what is going on in their bodies, that awareness may be limited. This limitation leaves a great deal of room for social and psychological factors to operate in the recognition and interpretation of illness.

### Recognition of Symptoms

> I have a tumor in my head the size of a basketball.
> I can feel it when I blink.
>
> —Woody Allen, *Hannah and Her Sisters*

Common observation reveals that some individuals maintain their normal activities in the face of debilitating symptoms, whereas others take to their beds the moment they detect any minor bodily disturbance.

**Individual Differences**   Hypochondriacs, like characters that Woody Allen has played, are convinced that normal bodily symptoms are indicators of illness. Although hypochondriacs are only 4 to 5 percent of the population, they make extensive use of medical services, and so understanding the symptom experience is important (Tomenson et al., 2012).

The most frequent symptoms experienced by people who convert their distress into physical symptoms are back pain, joint pain, pain in the extremities, headache, abdominal symptoms such as bloating, "allergies" to particular foods, and cardiovascular symptoms such as palpitations (Carmin, Weigartz, Hoff, & Kondos, 2003; Rief, Hessel, & Braehler, 2001). Contrary to stereotypes, women are not more likely than men to report these symptoms. But there are pronounced age effects, with older people reporting more symptoms than young people.

People who are high in neuroticism recognize their symptoms quickly and report their symptoms quickly (Feldman, Cohen, Doyle, Skoner, & Gwaltney, 1999), and they often erroneously believe that they have serious diseases. As we saw in Chapter 7, neuroticism is a pervasive negative way of viewing the world marked by negative emotions, self-consciousness, and a concern with bodily processes. Neurotic, anxious people may exaggerate their symptoms, or they may simply be more attentive to real symptoms (Howren, Suls, & Martin, 2009; Tomenson et al., 2012).

**Attentional Differences**   People who are focused on themselves (their bodies, their emotions, and their reactions in general) are quicker to notice symptoms than are people who are focused externally, on their environment and activities (Pennebaker, 1983). So, people who hold boring jobs, who are socially isolated, who keep house for a living, or who live alone report more physical symptoms than do people who have interesting jobs, have active social lives, work outside the home, or live with others. People who experience more distractions and attend less to themselves experience fewer symptoms than people who have little activity in their lives (Pennebaker, 1983).

**Situational Factors**   A boring situation makes people more attentive to symptoms than does an interesting situation. For example, people are more likely to notice itching or tickling in their throats and to cough in response during boring parts of movies than during interesting parts (Pennebaker, 1980). A symptom is more likely to be perceived on a day when a person is at home than on a day full of frenzied activity. Intense physical activity takes attention away from symptoms, whereas quiescence increases the likelihood of their recognition.

Any situational factor that makes illness or symptoms especially salient promotes their recognition. For example, a common phenomenon in medical school is **medical students' disease.** As they study each illness, many medical students imagine that they have it. Studying the symptoms leads the students to focus on their own fatigue and other internal states; as a consequence, symptoms consistent with the illness under study seem to emerge (Mechanic, 1972).

**Stress**   Stress can precipitate or aggravate the experience of symptoms. People who are under stress may believe that they are more vulnerable to illness and so attend more closely to their bodies. Financial strain, disruptions in personal relationships, and other stressors lead people to believe that they are ill (Ewart, Elder, Laird, Shelby, & Walker, 2014; val Gils, Janssens, & Rosmalen, 2014), perhaps because they experience stress-related physiological changes, such as accelerated heartbeat or fatigue, and interpret these changes as symptoms of illness (Cameron, Leventhal, & Leventhal, 1995).

**Mood and Emotions**     People who are in a good mood or who have positive expectations rate themselves as more healthy, report fewer illness-related memories, and report fewer symptoms. Even people who have diagnosed illnesses report fewer or less serious symptoms when they are in a good mood (Gil et al., 2004). People in a bad mood, or with negative expectations, report more symptoms, are more pessimistic that any actions they might take will relieve their symptoms, and perceive themselves as more vulnerable to future illness (Leventhal, Hansell, Diefenbach, Leventhal, & Glass, 1996). Positive and negative expectations can be modified, however, which may reduce the symptom experience and effects on mood (Crichton et al., 2014).

## Interpretation of Symptoms

The interpretation of symptoms is also a heavily psychological process. Consider the following incident. At a large metropolitan hospital, a man in his late 20s came to the emergency room with the sole symptom of a sore throat. He brought with him six of his relatives: his mother, father, sister, aunt, and two cousins. Because patients usually go to an emergency room with only one other person, and because a sore throat is virtually never seen in the emergency room, the staff were understandably curious about the reason for his visit. One particularly sensitive medical student reasoned that something more must have caused the man to come to the emergency room with his entire family in tow, so he probed cautiously but persistently during the intake interview with the patient. Gradually, it emerged that the young man's brother had died a year earlier of Hodgkin's disease, a form of cancer that involves the progressive infection and enlargement of the lymph nodes. The brother's first symptom had been a sore throat, which he and the family had allowed to go untreated.

This poignant incident illustrates how important social and psychological factors can be in understanding people's interpretations of their symptoms and their decisions to seek treatment.

**Prior Experience**     As the preceding incident attests, the interpretation of symptoms is heavily influenced by prior experience. Unless a symptom previously indicated a serious disease, people who have experience with a medical condition estimate the prevalence of their symptoms to be greater and often regard the condition as less serious than do people with no history of the condition (Jemmott, Croyle, & Ditto, 1988). Common disorders are generally regarded as less serious than are rare or distinctive risk factors and disorders (Croyle & Ditto, 1990).

**Expectations**     Expectations influence the interpretation of symptoms. People may ignore symptoms they are not expecting and amplify symptoms they do expect (Leventhal, Nerenz, & Strauss, 1982). When people feel vulnerable to disease, they are more likely to interpret bodily sensations as indicative of illness, and even regard other people in the environment as potential disease carriers (Miller & Maner, 2012). An example is described in Box 8.1.

**Seriousness of the Symptoms**     Symptoms that affect highly valued parts of the body are usually interpreted as more serious and as more likely to require attention than are symptoms that affect less valued organs. For example, people are especially anxious when their eyes or face are affected, but less so if the symptom involves part of the trunk. A symptom will prompt seeking treatment if it limits mobility or if it affects a highly valued organ, such as chest discomfort thought to be indicative of heart disease (Eifert, Hodson, Tracey, Seville, & Gunawardane, 1996). Above all, if a symptom causes pain, it will lead a person to seek treatment more promptly than if it does not cause pain.

## Cognitive Representations of Illness

People hold beliefs, or cognitive representations, about their illnesses that affect their treatment-seeking behavior. The **commonsense model of illness** argues that people hold implicit commonsense beliefs about their symptoms and illnesses that result in organized **illness representations** or schemas (Leventhal, Leventhal, & Breland, 2011; Leventhal, Weinman, Leventhal, & Phillips, 2008). These coherent conceptions of illness are acquired through the media, through personal experience, and from family and friends who have had experience with similar disorders.

## Can Expectations Influence Sensations? The Case of Premenstrual Symptoms

BOX **8.1**

Many women experience unpleasant physical and psychological symptoms just before the onset of menstruation, including swollen breasts, cramping, irritability, and depression. These symptoms clearly have a physiological basis, but psychological factors may contribute as well (Beal et al., 2014).

To test this idea, Ruble (1972) recruited a number of women to participate in a study. She told them she was using a new scientific technique that would predict their date of menstruation. She then randomly told participants that the technique indicated either that their period was due within the next day or two (premenstrual group) or that their period was not due for 7 to 10 days (intermenstrual group). In fact, all the women were approximately a week from their periods. The women were then asked to complete a questionnaire indicating the extent to which they were experiencing symptoms typically associated with the premenstrual state.

The women who had been led to believe that their period was due within the next day or two reported more psychological and physiological symptoms of premenstruation than did women who were told their periods were not due for 7 to 10 days.

Of course, the results of this study do not mean that premenstrual symptoms have no physical basis. Indeed, the prevalence and seriousness of premenstrual syndrome (PMS) bear testimony to the debilitating effect that premenstrual bodily changes can have on physiological functioning and behavior. Rather, the results suggest that women who believe themselves to be premenstrual may be more attentive to and reinterpret naturally fluctuating bodily states as consistent with the premenstrual state. These findings also illustrate the significance of psychological factors in the experience of symptoms more generally.

These commonsense models range from being quite sketchy and inaccurate to being extensive, technical, and complete. Their importance stems from the fact that they lend coherence to a person's comprehension of the illness experience. As such, they can influence people's preventive health behaviors, their reactions when they experience symptoms or are diagnosed with illness, their adherence to treatment recommendations, their expectations for their future health (Petrie & Weinman, 2012), and their health outcomes (Kaptein et al., 2010).

Commonsense models include basic information about an illness (Leventhal et al., 2008). The *identity,* or label, for an illness is its name; its *causes* are the factors that the person believes gave rise to the illness; its *consequences* are its symptoms, the treatments that result, and their implications for quality of life; *time line* refers to the length of time the illness is expected to last; and *control/cure* identifies whether the person believes that the illness can be managed or cured through appropriate actions and treatments; and *emotional representations* include how people feel about the illness and its possible course and treatment. *Coherence* refers to how well these beliefs hang together in a cogent representation of the disorder.

Most people have at least three models of illness (Leventhal et al., 2008):

- *Acute illness* is believed to be caused by specific viral or bacterial agents and is short in duration, with no long-term consequences. An example is the flu.

- *Chronic illness* is believed to be caused by multiple factors, including health habits, and is long in duration, often with severe consequences. An example is heart disease.

- *Cyclic illness* is marked by alternating periods during which there are either no symptoms or many symptoms. An example is herpes.

People's conceptions of illness vary and can greatly influence behavior related to a disease. For example, diabetes may be regarded by one person as an acute condition caused by a diet high in sugar, whereas another person with the same disease may see it as a lifelong condition with potentially catastrophic consequences. Not surprisingly, these people will treat their disorders differently, maintain different levels of vigilance toward symptoms, and show different patterns of seeking treatment (Petrie & Weinman, 2012). When an illness is relabeled either by a physician or by the person experiencing the symptoms, major changes in beliefs about the cause, nature of the disorder, and expectations regarding treatment can result (Petrie, MacKrill, Derksen, & Dalbeth, 2018). Ambiguity about one's illness has been tied to poor well-being (Hoth et al., 2013), and so conceptions of illness can be very useful. Those conceptions give people a basis for interpreting new information, influence their treatment-seeking decisions, lead them to alter or fail to adhere to their medication regimens (Coutu, Dupuis, D'Antono, & Rochon-Goyer, 2003), and influence expectations about future health (Leventhal et al., 2008). However, these effects can occur automatically and without awareness, leading to both inappropriate and unexamined interpretations of illness events as well (Lowe & Norman, 2017).

Sometimes patients' conceptions of their illnesses match those of their health care providers, but other times they do not. In these latter cases, misunderstandings or misinterpretation of information can result (Brooks, Rowley, Broadbent, & Petrie, 2012).

## Lay Referral Network

Sociologists have written at length about the **lay referral network,** an informal network of family and friends who offer their own interpretations of symptoms, often well before any medical treatment is sought (Freidson, 1961). The patient may mention the symptoms to a family member or coworker, who may then respond with personal views of what the symptom is likely to mean ("George had that, and it turned out to be nothing at all"). The friend or relative may offer advice about the advisability of seeking medical treatment ("All he got for going to see the doctor was a big bill") and recommendations for various home remedies ("Lemon and tequila will clear that right up").

In many communities, the lay referral network is the preferred mode of treatment. A powerful lay figure, such as an older woman who has had many children, may act as a lay practitioner; because of her years of experience, she is assumed to have personal wisdom in medical matters (Freidson, 1961; Hayes-Bautista, 1976). Within ethnic communities, the lay referral network will sometimes incorporate beliefs about the causes and cures of disease that would be regarded as supernatural or superstitious by traditional medicine. In addition, these lay referral networks often recommend home remedies regarded as more appropriate or more effective than traditional medicine.

## The Internet

The Internet constitutes a lay referral network of its own. The amount of health information on the Internet has risen exponentially in recent years. As a result, many people now investigate their own and others' symptoms and disorders online, often well before they seek medical attention, if they do. Estimates are that at least 80 percent of Internet users or 93 million people overall have searched a health-related topic on the Internet (Weaver, 2018), and more than half of them say it improved the way they took care of themselves (Dias et al., 2002).

Are these trends worrisome? According to a recent study of physicians, 96 percent believe that the Internet will affect health care positively, and many physicians turn to the Internet themselves for the most up-to-date information on illnesses, treatments, and the processing of insurance claims. Nonetheless, some of what is on the Internet is not accurate (Kalichman et al., 2006), and people who use the Web to get information about their illness sometimes get worse (Gupta, 2004, October 24). Telemedicine use, that is, virtual visits with a physician, has increased substantially, and a Kaiser Foundation study indicated that as of 2018, 74 percent of large employers provided coverage for telemedicine (Kiplinger, 2019).

## ■ WHO USES HEALTH SERVICES?

Just as illness is not evenly distributed across the population, neither is the use of health services.

## Age

The very young and the elderly use health services most frequently (Meara, White, & Cutler, 2004). Young children develop a number of infectious childhood diseases as they are acquiring their immunities; therefore, they frequently require the care of a pediatrician. Both illness frequency and the use of services decline in adolescence and throughout young adulthood. Use of health services increases again in late adulthood, when people begin to manifest chronic conditions and diseases of aging (Cherry, Lucas, & Decker, 2010).

## Gender

Women use medical services more than men do. Pregnancy and childbirth account for much of this gender difference in use, but not all. Various explanations have been offered, including the fact that women have better homeostatic mechanisms than men do: They report

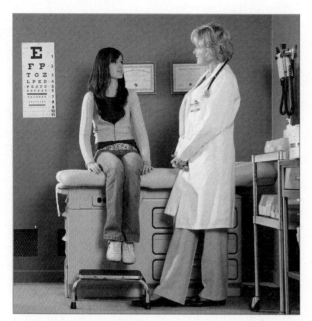

*Women use medical services more than men, they may be sick more than men, and their routine care requires more visits than men's.*

Radius Images/Getty Images

pain earlier, experience temperature changes more rapidly, and detect new smells faster. Thus, they may also be more sensitive to bodily disruptions, especially minor ones that may elude men (Leventhal, Diefenbach, & Leventhal, 1992).

Another possible explanation stems from social norms. Men are expected to project a tough, macho image, which involves being able to ignore pain and not give in to illness, whereas women are not subject to these same pressures (Klonoff & Landrine, 1992).

Women also use health care services more often because their medical care is more fragmented. Medical care for most men involves a trip to a general practitioner for a physical examination that includes preventive care. But women may visit a general practitioner or internist for a general physical, a gynecologist for Pap tests, and a breast cancer specialist or mammography service for breast examinations and mammograms. Thus, women may use services more than men in part because the medical care system is not particularly well structured to meet women's basic health needs.

## Social Class and Culture

The lower social classes use medical services less than do more affluent social classes (Adler & Stewart, 2010), in part because poorer people have less money to spend on health services or little or no insurance (Gindi & Jones, 2014; Gindi, Kirzinger, & Cohen, 2013). However, with Medicare for the elderly, Medicaid for the poor, and other inexpensive health services, the gap between medical service use by the rich and by the poor has narrowed somewhat, in part due to the Affordable Care Act.

In addition to cost, there are not as many high-quality medical services available to the poor, and what services there are, are often inadequate and understaffed (Kirby & Kaneda, 2005). Consequently, many poor people receive no regular medical care at all and see physicians only in the emergency room. The biggest gap between the rich and the poor is in the use of preventive health services, such as inoculations against disease and screening for treatable disorders, which lays the groundwork for poorer health across the life span.

## Social Psychological Factors

Social psychological factors—including an individual's attitudes toward life and his or her beliefs about symptoms and health services—influence who uses health services. As we saw in Chapter 3, the health belief model maintains that whether a person seeks treatment for a symptom can be predicted by whether the person perceives a threat to health and whether he or she believes that a particular health measure will be effective in reducing that threat. The health belief model explains people's use of services quite well. But the model does a better job of explaining the treatment-seeking behavior of people who have money and access to health care services than of people who do not.

The use of health care services is influenced by socialization—chiefly, by the actions of one's parents. Just as children and adolescents learn health behaviors from their parents, they also learn when and how to use health care services.

People who are socially isolated use health services more than people who are socially connected (Cruwys, Wakefield, Sani, Dingle, & Jetten, 2018). This is not because isolated people necessarily have poorer health (although they sometimes do). Rather, socially isolated people are motivated to seek care by a need for social contact. In one study, isolated people who joined a social group subsequently reduced their number of medical visits (Cruwys et al., 2018).

To summarize, health services are used by people who have the need, time, money, prior experience, beliefs that favor the use of services, and access to services.

# ■ MISUSING HEALTH SERVICES

Health services may be abused as well as used. One type of abuse occurs when people seek out health services for problems that are not medically significant, overloading the medical system. Another type of abuse involves delay, when people should seek health care for a problem but do not.

## Using Health Services for Emotional Disturbances

Physicians estimate that as much as half to two-thirds of their time is taken up by patients whose complaints are psychological or social rather than medical (Katon et al., 1990). This problem is more common for general practitioners than for specialists, although no branch of medicine is immune. College health services periodically experience this problem during exam time, when symptoms increase in response to stress.

These nonmedical complaints can be a result of trauma, relationship problems, and other stressors (Ziadni et al., 2018) and often stem from anxiety and depression, both of which, unfortunately, are widespread (Howren & Suls, 2011). Patients who come to the emergency room with chest pain or who visit their physicians with cardiac symptoms are especially likely to have complicating anxiety and depressive disorders, with 23 percent estimated to have a psychiatric disorder (Srinivasan & Joseph, 2004). Unfortunately, symptoms such as these can lead physicians to intervene with medical

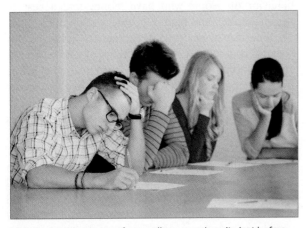

*Visit the health service of any college or university just before exams begin, and you will see a unit bracing itself for an onslaught. Admissions to health services can double or even triple as papers become due and exams begin.*

dolgachov/Getty Images

treatments that are inappropriate (Salmon, Humphris, Ring, Davies, & Dowrick, 2007).

Why do people seek a physician's care when their complaints should be addressed by a mental health specialist? Stress and emotional responses to it, such as anxiety, worry, and depression, are accompanied by a number of physical symptoms (Pieper, Brosschot, van der Leeden, & Thayer, 2007). Anxiety can produce diarrhea, upset stomach, sweaty hands, shortness of breath (sometimes mistaken for asthma symptoms), difficulty in sleeping, poor concentration, and general agitation. Depression can lead to fatigue, difficulty performing everyday activities, listlessness, loss of appetite, and sleep disturbances. People may mistake the symptoms of their mood disorder for a physical health problem and thus seek a physician's care (Vamos, Mucsi, Keszei, Kopp, & Novak, 2009). Psychologically-based complaints may not only influence seeking contact initially but also lead to multiple visits, slow recovery, and prolonged hospital stays as well (De Jonge, Latour, & Huyse, 2003; Rubin, Cleare, & Hotopf, 2004).

So problematic is the issue of seeking health care treatment for anxiety and depression that a study in the *Annals of Internal Medicine* suggested that physicians begin all their patient interviews with the direct questions, "Are you currently sad or depressed? Are the things that previously brought you pleasure no longer bringing you pleasure?" Positive answers to questions such as these would suggest that the patient may need treatment for depression as well as, or even instead of, other medical treatments (Means-Christensen, Arnau, Tonidandel, Bramson, & Meagher, 2005; Pignone et al., 2002; Rhee, Holditch-Davis, & Miles, 2005). Indeed, research has found that when medical services integrate mental health and physical health care, the number of medical visits can be reduced (Turner et al., 2018).

Another reason that people use health services for psychological complaints is that medical disorders are perceived as more legitimate than psychological ones. For example, a man who is depressed by his job and who stays home to avoid it will find that his behavior is more acceptable to both his employer and his spouse if he says he is ill than if he admits he is depressed. Many people still believe that it is shameful to see a mental health specialist or to have mental problems.

Illness brings benefits, termed **secondary gains,** including the ability to rest, to be freed from unpleasant tasks, to be cared for by others, and to take time off from work. These reinforcements can interfere with the process of returning to good health. (Some of these

One summer, a mysterious epidemic broke out in the dressmaking department of a southern textile plant, affecting 62 workers. The symptoms varied but usually included nausea, numbness, dizziness, and occasionally vomiting. Some of the ill required hospitalization, but most were simply excused from work for several days.

Almost all the affected workers reported having been bitten by a gnat or mite immediately before they experienced the symptoms. Several employees who were not afflicted said they had seen their fellow workers bitten before they came down with the disease. However, local, state, and federal health officials who were called in to investigate could obtain no reliable description of the suspected insect. Furthermore, careful inspection of the textile plant by entomologists and exterminators turned up only a small variety of insects—beetles, gnats, flies, an ant, and a mite—none of which could have caused the reported symptoms.

Company physicians and experts from the U.S. Public Health Service Communicable Disease Center began to suspect that the epidemic might be a case of hysterical contagion. They hypothesized that, although some of the afflicted individuals may have been bitten by an insect, anxiety or nervousness was more likely responsible for the onset of the symptoms. On hearing this conclusion, employees insisted that the "disease" was caused by a bite from an insect that was in a shipment of material recently received from England.

In shifting from a medical to a social explanation, health experts highlighted several points. First, the entire incident, from the first to the last reported case, lasted a period of 11 days, and 50 of the 62 cases (80 percent) occurred on 2 consecutive days after the news media had sensationalized earlier incidents. Second, most of the afflicted individuals worked at the same time and place in the plant. Third, the 58 working at the same time and place were all women; one other woman worked on a different shift, two male victims worked on a different shift, and one man worked in a different department. Moreover, most of these women were married and had children; they were accordingly trying to combine employment and motherhood, often an exhausting arrangement.

The epidemic occurred at a busy time in the plant—June being a crucial month in the production of fall fashions—and there were strong incentives for employees to put in overtime and to work at a high pace. The plant was relatively new, and personnel and production management were not well organized. Thus, the climate was ripe for high anxiety among the employees.

Who, then, got "bitten" by the "June bug," and why? Workers with the most stress in their lives (married women with children) who were trying to cope with the further demands of increased productivity and overtime were most vulnerable. Job anxieties, coupled with the physical manifestations of fatigue (such as dizziness), created a set of symptoms that, given appropriate circumstances, could be labeled as illness. The rumor of a suspicious bug and the presence of ill coworkers apparently provided the appropriate circumstances, legitimizing the illness and leading to the epidemic that resulted.

*Source:* Kerckhoff and Back (1968).

---

factors may have played a role in one famous case of hysterical contagion; see Box 8.2.)

Finally, the inappropriate use of health services can represent true malingering. A person who does not want to go to work may know all too well that the only acceptable excuse that will prevent dismissal for absenteeism is illness. Moreover, workers may be required to document their absences in order to collect wages or disability payments and may thus have to keep looking until they find a physician who is willing to "treat" the "disorder."

But errors can be made in the opposite direction as well: People with legitimate medical problems may be falsely assumed to be psychologically disturbed. Physicians are more likely to reach this conclusion about their female patients than their male patients (Redman, Webb, Hennrikus, Gordon, & Sanson-Fisher, 1991), even though objective measures suggest equivalent rates of psychological disturbance.

## Delay Behavior

A very different misuse of health services occurs when an individual should seek treatment for a symptom but puts off doing so. A lump, chronic shortness of breath, blackouts, skin discoloration, radiating chest pain, seizures, and severe stomach pains are serious

**FIGURE 8.1 | Stages of Delay in Seeking Treatment for Symptoms**    *Source:* Based on Andersen, B.L., J. T. Cacioppo, and D. C. Roberts. "Delay in Seeking a Cancer Diagnosis: Delay Stages and Psychophysiological Comparison Processes." *British Journal of Social Psychology* 34 (January 1995): 33–52. Fig. 1, p. 35.

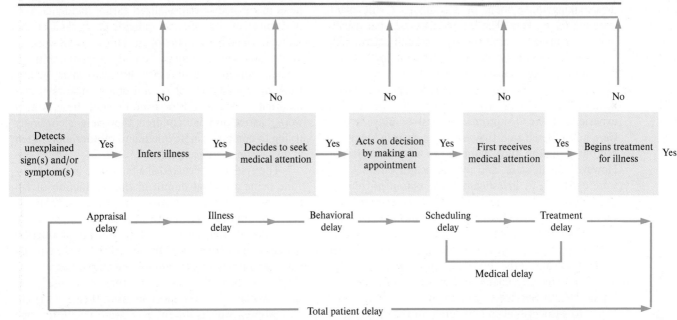

symptoms for which people should seek treatment promptly. Unfortunately, a person may live with one or more of these potentially serious symptoms for months without seeking care. This is called **delay behavior.** For example, a factor contributing to the high rate of death and disability from heart attacks is that patients often delay seeking treatment for its symptoms, instead normalizing them as gastric distress, muscle pain, and other, less severe disorders.

Delay is defined as the time between when a person recognizes a symptom and when the person obtains treatment. Delay is composed of several periods, diagrammed in Figure 8.1: **appraisal delay,** which is the time it takes an individual to decide that a symptom is serious; **illness delay,** which is the time between the recognition that a symptom implies an illness and the decision to seek treatment; **behavioral delay,** which is the time between deciding to seek treatment and actually doing so (Safer, Tharps, Jackson, & Leventhal, 1979); and **medical delay** (scheduling and treatment), which is the time that elapses between the person's calling for an appointment and his or her receiving appropriate medical care. Delay in seeking treatment for some symptoms is appropriate. For example, a runny nose or a mild sore throat usually will clear up on its own. However, in other

cases, symptoms may be debilitating for weeks or months, and to delay seeking treatment is inappropriate (Petrova et al., 2017).

**What Causes Delay?**    People who delay are very similar to people who do not use services more generally. For example, when money is not available, people may persuade themselves that the symptoms are not serious enough to seek treatment. Delay is more common among people with no regular contact with a physician and among people who are phobic about medical services. The elderly delay less than middle-aged people, especially if they believe that the symptoms may be serious (Leventhal, Easterling, Leventhal, & Cameron, 1995).

Symptoms predict delay as well. If a symptom is similar to one that previously turned out to be minor, the person will seek treatment less quickly than if the symptom is new. Symptoms that do not hurt or change quickly and that are not incapacitating are less likely to prompt a person to seek medical treatment (Safer et al., 1979). Symptoms that can be easily accommodated and do not provoke alarm may be delayed. For example, people have difficulty distinguishing between ordinary moles and melanomas (a potentially fatal skin cancer), and so may delay seeking treatment. Symptoms that are typical of a disorder, on the other hand, are more commonly treated (e.g., a lump for breast cancer) than atypical symptoms of the same disorder (Meechan, Collins, & Petrie, 2003).

Even after a consultation, up to 25 percent of patients delay taking recommended treatments, put off getting tests, or postpone acting on referrals. In some cases, patients have had their curiosity satisfied by the first visit and no longer feel any urgency about their condition. In other cases, patients become truly alarmed by the symptoms and, to avoid thinking about them, take no further action.

Delay on the part of the health care practitioner is also a significant factor, accounting for at least 15 percent of all delay behavior (Cassileth et al., 1988). In most cases, health care providers delay as a result of honest mistakes. For example, blackouts can indicate any of many disorders ranging from heat prostration or over-zealous dieting to diabetes or a brain tumor. A provider may choose to rule out the more common causes of a symptom before proceeding to the more invasive or expensive tests needed to rule out a less probable cause. Thus, when the more serious diagnosis is found to apply, the appearance of unwarranted delay exists.

Medical delay is more likely when a patient deviates from the profile of the average person with a given disease. •

## S U M M A R Y

1. The detection of symptoms, their interpretation, and the use of health services are heavily influenced by psychological processes.

2. Personality and culture, focus of attention, the presence of distracting or involving activities, mood, the salience of illness or symptoms, and individual differences in the tendency to monitor threats influence whether a symptom is noticed. The interpretation of symptoms is influenced by prior experience and expectations about their likelihood and meaning.

3. Commonsense models of illness (which identify the type of disease and its causes, consequences, timeline, controllability/cure, and coherence) influence how people interpret their symptoms

and whether they act on them by seeking medical attention.

4. Social factors, such as the lay referral network, can act as a go-between for the patient and the medical care system.

5. Health services are used disproportionately by the very young and very old, by women, and by middle- and upper-class people. The health belief model also influences the use of health services.

6. Health services can be abused. A large percentage of patients who seek medical attention are depressed or anxious and not physically ill. Also, people commonly ignore symptoms that are serious, resulting in dangerous delay behavior.

## K E Y   T E R M S

appraisal delay
behavioral delay
commonsense model of illness
delay behavior

illness delay
illness representations
lay referral network
medical delay

medical students' disease
secondary gains

# CHAPTER 9

# Patients, Providers, and Treatments

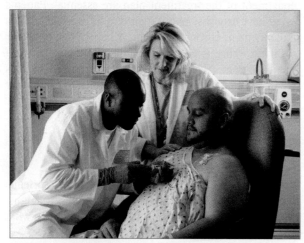

Rhoda Bear/National Cancer Institute

## CHAPTER OUTLINE

# ■ HEALTH CARE SERVICES

"I've had this cold for 2 weeks, so finally I went to the student health services to get something for it. I waited more than an hour! And when I finally saw a doctor, he spent a whole 5 minutes with me, told me what I had was viral, not bacterial, and that he couldn't do anything for it. He sent me home and told me to get a lot of rest, drink fluids, and take over-the-counter medications for the stuffiness and the pain. Why did I even bother?!" (Student account of a trip to the health services)

Much of the communication between patients and providers goes very well. Information is exchanged, treatment recommendations are made, and both patient and provider are satisfied. Sometimes, however, things do not go well. Nearly everyone has a horror story about a visit to a physician. Long waits, insensitivity, apparently faulty diagnoses, and treatments that have no effect are the themes of these stories. But in the same breath, the storyteller may expound on the virtues of his or her latest physician with an enthusiasm bordering on worship. To what do we attribute this seemingly contradictory attitude toward health care practitioners?

Health ranks among the values we hold dearest. Good health is a prerequisite to nearly every other activity, and poor health can interfere with nearly all aspects of life. Moreover, illness is usually uncomfortable, so people want to be treated quickly and successfully. Perhaps, then, it is no wonder that physicians and other health care professionals are alternately praised and vilified: Their craft is fundamental to the enjoyment of life. Some of the health care practitioners increasingly involved in patient care are described in Table 9.1.

## Patient Consumerism

At one time the physician's authority was accepted without question or complaint. Increasingly, though, patients have adopted consumerist attitudes toward their health care. This change is due to several factors.

First, patients are often presented with choices, and to make choices, one must be informed. The mere act of choice is empowering. Second, many illnesses, especially chronic ones, require a patient to be actively engaged in the treatment regimen. Consequently, the patient's full cooperation and participation in the development and enactment of the treatment plan are essential. Patients often have expertise about their illness, especially if it is a recurring or chronic problem. A patient will do better if this expertise is tapped and integrated into the treatment program. All of these factors contribute to patients regarding themselves as consumers of health care rather than passive recipients.

## Structure of the Health Care Delivery System

Until a few decades ago, the majority of Americans received their health care from private physicians, whom they paid directly on a visit-by-visit basis, in what was termed **private, fee-for-service care.**

That picture has changed. More than 92 million Americans now receive their health care through a prepaid financing and delivery system, termed a **health maintenance organization (HMO)** (Kaiser Family Foundation, February 2017, see Box 9.1). In this arrangement, an employer or employee pays an agreed-on

**TABLE 9.1 | Types of Health Care Providers**

| | | |
|---|---|---|
| Nearly half of all physicians are in practices that employ nurse practitioners, advanced practice nurses, or physician's assistants (Park, Cherry, & Decker, 2011). | | |
| | **Description** | **Responsibilities** |
| Nurse practitioners | Affiliated with physicians in private practice; see their own patients | Provide routine medical care; prescribe treatment; monitor progress of chronically ill patients; explain disorders and their origins, diagnoses, prognoses, and treatments |
| Advanced-practice nurses | Include certified nurse midwives, clinical nurse specialists, and certified nurse anesthetists | Some obstetrical care and births; cardiac or cancer care; administering anesthesia |
| Physician's assistants | Educated in 2-year programs in medical schools and teaching hospitals | Perform many routine health care tasks, such as taking down medical information or explaining treatment regimens to patients |

*Source:* Hing, Esther, and Sayeedha Uddin. "Physician Assistant and Advance Practice Nurse Care in Hospital Outpatient Departments: United States, 2008–2009." *National Center for Health Statistics* 77 (November 2011): 1–8.

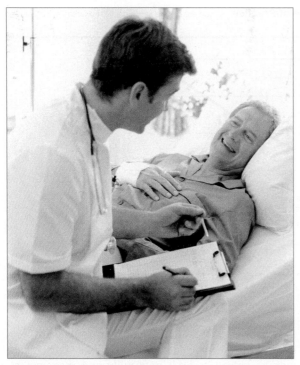

*When physicians treat patients in a warm, friendly, and confident manner, they are judged to be competent as well as nice.*
Digital Vision/SuperStock

monthly rate, and the employee can then use services at no additional (or a greatly reduced) cost. This arrangement is called **managed care.** In some cases, HMOs have their own staff, from which enrollees must seek treatment.

In **preferred-provider organizations (PPOs),** a network of affiliated practitioners have agreed to charge preestablished rates for services, and enrollees in the PPO must choose from these practitioners when seeking treatment. Table 9.2 describes the differences among types of health care plans.

## Patient Experiences with Managed Care

Although much patient contact with the health care system is positive, there are predictable ways in which communication goes awry, and we focus on those issues here. The changing structure of the health care delivery system can undermine patient–provider communication. Prepaid plans operate on a referral basis, so that the provider who first sees the patient determines what is wrong and then recommends specialists to follow up with treatment. Because providers are often paid according to the number of cases they see, referrals are desirable. Therefore, a **colleague orientation,** rather than a client or patient orientation, can develop (Mechanic, 1975). Because the patient no longer pays directly for service, and because the provider's income is not directly affected by whether the patient is pleased with the service, the provider may not be overly concerned with patient satisfaction. The provider is, however, concerned with what his or her colleagues think, because it is on their recommendations that he or she receives additional cases. In theory, such a system can produce high technical quality of care because providers who make errors receive fewer referrals; however, there is less incentive to offer emotionally satisfying care.

HMOs and other prepaid plans may inadvertently undermine care in other ways. When providers are pressured to see as many patients as possible, the consequences can be long waits and short visits. These

**TABLE 9.2 | Types of Health Care Plans**

| Name | How It Works |
| --- | --- |
| Health maintenance organization (HMO) | Members select a primary-care physician from the HMO's pool of doctors and pay a small fixed amount for each visit. Typically, any trips to specialists and nonemergency visits to HMO network hospitals must be preapproved. |
| Preferred-provider organization (PPO) | A network of doctors offers plan members a discounted rate. Patients usually don't need prior authorization to visit an in-network specialist. |
| Point-of-service plan (POS) | These are plans administered by insurance companies or HMOs that let members go to doctors and hospitals out of the network—for a price. Members usually need a referral to see a network specialist. |
| Traditional indemnity plan | Patients select their own doctors and hospitals and pay on a fee-for-service basis. They don't need a referral to see a specialist. |

*Sources:* National Committee for Quality Assurance. "Health Plans." Accessed June 28, 2019. https://reportcards.ncqa.org/#/health-plans/list.

**FIGURE 9.1 | Percentage of Physicians in Various Forms of Practice**    *Sources:* Bianco & Schine, 1997, March 24; Bureau of Labor Statistics, 2019.

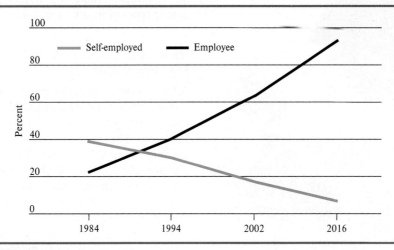

*Physicians and surgeons projected.

problems are compounded if a patient is referred to several specialists. Patients may feel that they are being shunted from provider to provider with no continuity in their care and no opportunity to build a personal relationship with any one individual.

Precisely because of some patient dissatisfaction, some HMOs have taken steps to reduce long waits, to allow for personal choice, and to make sure a patient sees the same provider at each visit. Changes such as these have resulted in **patient-centered care,** which involves providing patients with information, involving them in decisions regarding care, and consideration of psychosocial issues such as social support needs (Bergeson & Dean, 2006).

### ■ THE NATURE OF PATIENT–PROVIDER COMMUNICATION

As noted, patient–practitioner communication does not always go smoothly. Criticisms of providers usually center on jargon, lack of feedback, and depersonalized care. The quality of communication with a provider is important to patients, but it also affects care. Poor patient–provider communication has been tied to nonadherence to treatment recommendations and the initiation of malpractice litigation, for example.

Most of us are insufficiently knowledgeable about medicine and standards of practice to know whether we have been treated well medically. Consequently, we often judge technical quality on how care is delivered.

A warm, confident, friendly provider is judged to be both nice and competent, whereas a cool, aloof provider may be judged as both unfriendly and incompetent (Bogart, 2001). In reality, the technical quality of care and the manner in which care is delivered are unrelated. What factors affect quality of communication?

### Setting

In many ways, the medical office is an unlikely setting for effective communication. The average visit lasts only 12 to 15 minutes, and when you are trying to explain your symptoms, the physician will, on average, interrupt you before you get 23 seconds into your comments (Simon, 2003). Moreover, it is difficult to present your complaints effectively when you are in pain or have a fever, or if you are anxious or embarrassed about your condition.

The provider's role is a difficult one as well. He or she must extract significant information as quickly as possible from the patient. The provider is often on a tight schedule, with other patients backing up in the waiting room. The disorder may have been made more complicated by the patient's self-treatment, which can mask and distort the symptoms. Further, the patient's ideas of which symptoms are important may not correspond to the provider's knowledge, and so important signs may be overlooked. With the patient seeking solace and the provider trying to maximize the efficient use of time, there are clearly potential sources of strain.

## Provider Behaviors That Contribute to Faulty Communication

**Inattentiveness**    Communication between patient and physician can be eroded by certain provider behaviors. One problematic provider behavior is inattentiveness—that is, not listening. Typically, patients do not have the opportunity to finish their explanation of concerns before the provider begins the process of diagnosis.

**Use of Jargon**    Patients understand relatively few of the complex terms that providers often use. Providers learn a complex vocabulary for understanding illnesses and communicating about them to other professionals; they often find it hard to remember that patients do not share this expertise. In some cases, jargon-filled explanations may be used to keep the patient from asking too many questions or from discovering that the provider actually is not certain what the patient's problem is. The use of jargon may also stem from an inability to gauge what the patient will understand.

**Baby Talk**    Because practitioners may underestimate what their patients will understand about an illness and its treatment, they may resort to baby talk and simplistic explanations. One woman who is both a cancer researcher and a cancer patient reports that when she goes to see her cancer specialist, he talks to her in a very complex, technical manner until the examination starts. Once she is on the examining table, he shifts to very simple sentences and explanations. She is now a patient and no longer a colleague. The truth about what most patients can understand lies somewhere between the extremes of technical jargon and baby talk.

**Nonperson Treatment**    Depersonalization of the patient is another problem that impairs the quality of the patient–provider relationship (Kaufman, 1970). One patient—a psychologist—reports:

> When I was being given emergency treatment for an eye laceration, the resident surgeon abruptly terminated his conversation with me as soon as I lay down on the operating table. Although I had had no sedative, or anesthesia, he acted as if I were no longer conscious, directing all his questions to a friend of mine—questions such as, "What's his name? What occupation is he in? Is he a real doctor?" etc. As I lay there, these two men were speaking about me as if I were not there at all. The moment I got off the table

and was no longer a cut to be stitched, the surgeon resumed his conversation with me, and existence was conferred upon me again. (Zimbardo, 1969, p. 298)

Nonperson treatment may be employed at particularly stressful moments to keep the patient quiet and to enable the practitioner to concentrate. In that way, it may serve a valuable medical function. But patient depersonalization can also have adverse medical effects. For example, medical staff making hospital rounds often use either highly technical or euphemistic terms when discussing cases with their colleagues; these terms may confuse or alarm the nonparticipating but physically present patient, an effect to which the provider may be oblivious.

Patient depersonalization also provides emotional protection for the provider. It is difficult for a provider to work in a continual state of awareness that his or her every action influences someone's state of health and happiness (Cohen et al., 2003). Moreover, every provider has tragedies—as when a patient dies or is left incapacitated by a treatment—but the provider must find a way to continue to practice. Depersonalization helps provide such a way.

**Stereotypes of Patients**    Negative stereotypes of patients may contribute to poor communication and subsequent treatment. Physicians give less information, are less supportive, and demonstrate less proficient clinical performance with black and Hispanic patients and patients of lower socioeconomic class than is true for more advantaged patients, even in the same health care settings (van Ryn & Fu, 2003) (see Box 9.1) and often without realizing it (Schaa, Roter, Biesecker, Cooper, & Erby, 2015). When a person is seen by a physician of the same race or ethnicity, satisfaction with treatment tends to be higher (Laveist & Nuru-Jeter, 2002). Physicians, like many professionals, have personal biases and blind spots, but are likely to harbor an illusion of objectivity (Redelmeier & Ross, 2018), and so these blind spots and biases may go ignored.

Many physicians have negative perceptions of the elderly (Haug & Ory, 1987), and these beliefs can compromise care. Older patients are less likely than younger patients to be resuscitated in emergency rooms or given active treatment protocols for life-threatening diseases (Haug & Ory, 1987; Morgan, 1985). The negative attitudes of physicians seem to be reciprocated in the elderly, in that among people

More than 25.2 million people in the United States have limited English proficiency (Pandya, McHugh, & Batalova, 2011). Consequently, language barriers are a formidable problem in patient–provider communication. Increasingly, language barriers contribute to communication problems (Halim, Yoshikawa, & Amodio, 2013). Consider the experiences of a 12-year-old Latino boy and his mother attempting to communicate what was wrong:

> *"La semana pasada a él le dio mucho mareo y no tenía fiebre ni nada, y la familia por parte de papá todos padecen de diabetes."* (Last week, he had a lot of dizziness, and he didn't have fever or anything, and

his dad's family all suffer from diabetes.) "Uh hum," replied the physician. The mother went on. *"A mi me da miedo porque él lo que estaba mareado, mareado, mareado y no tenía fiebre ni nada."* (I'm scared because he's dizzy, dizzy, dizzy, and he didn't have fever or anything.) Turning to Raul, the physician asked, "OK, so she's saying you look kind of yellow, is that what she's saying?" Raul interpreted for his mother: *"Es que se me vi amarillo?"* (Is it that I looked yellow?) *"Estaba como mareado, como pálido"* (You were dizzy, like pale), his mother replied. Raul turned back to the doctor. "Like I was like paralyzed, something like that," he said (Flores, 2006, p. 229).

aged 65 or more years, only 54 percent express high confidence in physicians.

Sexism is a problem in medical practice as well. For example, in experimental studies that attributed reported chest pain and stress to either a male or female patient, medical intervention was perceived to be less important for the female patient (Martin & Lemos, 2002).

In comparison with male physicians, female physicians generally conduct longer visits, ask more questions, make more positive comments, and show more nonverbal support, such as smiling and nodding (Hall, Irish, Roter, Ehrlich, & Miller, 1994). The matching of gender between patient and practitioner fosters rapport and disclosure (Levinson, McCollum, & Kutner, 1984; Weisman & Teitelbaum, 1985). However, physicians of both genders prefer male patients (Hall, Epstein, DeCiantis, & McNeil, 1993).

Patients who are regarded as seeking treatment largely for depression, anxiety, or other forms of psychological disorder also evoke negative reactions from physicians. With these patients, physician attention may be cursory (Epstein et al., 2006). Physicians prefer healthier patients to sicker ones (Hall et al., 1993), and they prefer acutely ill to chronically ill patients; chronic illness poses uncertainties and raises questions about prognosis, which acute diseases do not. Chronic illness can also increase a physician's distress over having to give bad news (Cohen et al., 2003). Patients who are the objects of stereotypes are more likely to become distrustful and dissatisfied with their care.

## Patients' Contributions to Faulty Communication

Within a few minutes of having discussed their illness with a provider, as many as one-third of patients cannot repeat their diagnosis, and up to one-half do not understand important details about the illness or treatment (Golden & Johnston, 1970). Whereas dissatisfied patients complain about the incomplete or overly technical explanations they receive from providers, dissatisfied providers complain that even when they give clear, careful explanations to patients, the explanation goes in one ear and out the other.

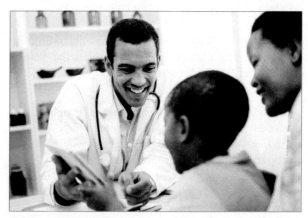

*Patients are often most comfortable interacting with a physician who is similar to themselves.*
Henk Badenhorst/Getty Images

With patients assuming more responsibility for their own care, the issue of health illiteracy has come to the fore. Although millions of young people graduate from high school each year, many of them lack the basic literacy skills needed to adhere to medical prescriptions, comprehend the meaning of their risk factors, or interpret the results of tests from physicians. Poorly educated people, the elderly, and non-English speakers have particular problems adopting the consumer role toward their care (Center for the Advancement of Health, May 2004). As people age, their number of medical problems usually increases, but their abilities to present their complaints effectively and follow treatment guidelines declines. About 40 percent of patients over age 50 have difficulty understanding their prescription instructions. Extra time and care may be needed to communicate this vital information to older patients.

### How Patients Compromise Communication

Several patient characteristics contribute to poor communication with providers. Neurotic patients often present an exaggerated picture of their symptoms (Ellington & Wiebe, 1999), compromising a physician's ability to gauge the seriousness of a patient's condition. When patients are anxious, their learning can be impaired (Graugaard & Finset, 2000). Anxiety makes it difficult to focus attention and process incoming information and retain it (Graugaard & Finset, 2000). Negative affectivity more generally compromises adherence (Molloy et al., 2012). To the extent that a practitioner can reduce anxiety, anger, and other negative emotions, communication may improve (Falkenstein, Tran, Ludi, Molkara, & Nguyen, 2016; Gerhart, Sanchez, Burns, Hobfoll, & Fung, 2015).

Some patients are unable to understand even simple information about their case (Galesic, Garcia-Retamero, & Gigerenzer, 2009; Link, Phelan, Miech, & Westin, 2008). Lack of intelligence or poor cognitive functioning impedes the ability to play a consumer role (Stilley, Bender, Dunbar-Jacob, Sereika, & Ryan, 2010). Patients for whom the illness is new and who have little prior information or experience with the disorder or the medication also have difficulty comprehending their disorders and treatments (DiMatteo & DiNicola, 1982; Rottman, Marcum, Thorpe, & Gellad, 2017).

**Patient Attitudes Toward Symptoms**   Patients respond to different symptoms of their illness than do practitioners (Greer & Halgin, 2006), especially ones that interfere with their activities. But providers are more concerned with the underlying illness, its severity, and treatment. Patients may consequently misunderstand the provider's emphasis on factors that they consider to be incidental, they may pay little attention, or they may believe that the provider has made an incorrect diagnosis. Patients typically want to be treated (Bar-Tal, Stasiuk, & Maksymiuk, 2012). If the physician prescribes bed rest and over-the-counter medications, patients may feel that their concerns have been ignored.

Patients sometimes give providers misleading information about their medical history or their current concerns. Patients may be embarrassed about their health history (such as having had an abortion) or their health practices (such as being a smoker), and so may not report this information.

### Interactive Aspects of the Communication Problem

Qualities of the interaction between practitioner and patient can perpetuate faulty communication. A major problem is that the patient–provider interaction does not provide the opportunity for feedback to the provider. The provider sees the patient, the patient is diagnosed, treatment is recommended, and the patient leaves. When the patient does not return, any number of things may have happened: The treatment may have cured the disorder; the patient may have gotten worse and decided to seek treatment elsewhere; the treatment may have failed, but the disorder may have cleared up anyway; or the patient may have died. Not knowing which of these alternatives has actually occurred, the provider does not know the impact and success rate of the advice given. Obviously, it is to the provider's psychological advantage to believe that the diagnosis was correct, that the patient followed the advice, and that the patient's disorder was cured by the recommended treatment. However, the provider may never find out for certain.

The provider may also find it hard to know when a satisfactory personal relationship has been established with a patient. Many patients are relatively cautious with providers. If they are dissatisfied, rather than complain about it directly, they may simply change providers. If a patient has stopped coming, the practitioner does not know if the patient has moved out of the area or switched to another practice. When providers do get feedback, it is more likely to be negative than positive: Patients whose treatments have failed are more likely to return than are patients whose treatments are successful (Rachman & Phillips, 1978).

Two points are important here. First, learning is fostered more by positive than by negative feedback; positive feedback tells one what one is doing right, whereas negative feedback may tell one what to stop doing but not necessarily what to do instead. Because providers get little feedback and more negative than positive feedback, this situation is not conducive to learning.

## Use of Artificial Intelligence

When you drill down to the root causes of poor communication between a patient and a practitioner, many problems may result from lack of time on the physician's part. Accordingly, any smart technological system that can relieve the burden on physicians is worth evaluating. Here are a few things that have been tried so far. In an article cleverly titled, "The Algorithm Will See You Now," physician Siddhartha Mukherjee points out how deep learning (machine learning that comes from many examples) can outperform experts, particularly in the task of inferring a diagnosis from a cluster of symptoms. It is possible for a machine to infer what can become a terminal disease: Can tiny hesitations and tremors be picked up early before full-blown Parkinson's disease symptoms set in? Can the early stages of Alzheimer's disease be inferred from particular changes in a person's speech patterns? Catching a disease in its early stages can improve treatment plans.

Repeat visits to evaluate already treated conditions are another time sink for both physicians and patients. Some such visits, however, may be forestalled by a picture from a cell phone. Is a rash clearing up? Is a surgical wound healing properly? Emailing or texting a photo can allow the physician to quickly determine if a patient needs to come in or if healing is progressing normally.

Given the communication problems already described, it is hard to know how well patients will respond to feedback from an algorithm or a "looks fine" text response to a picture from a physician. Will such treatment be perceived as depersonalized and remote? Evaluation of the psychosocial responses to these types of treatment will merit attention going forward. To the extent that the technology is integrated into personal contact with practitioners, such personal concerns may be avoided.

## ■ RESULTS OF POOR PATIENT–PROVIDER COMMUNICATION

The patient–provider communication problems would be little more than an unfortunate casualty of medical treatment were it not for the toll they take on health. Dissatisfied patients are less likely to comply with treatment recommendations or to use medical services in the future; they are more likely to turn to alternative services that satisfy emotional rather than medical needs; they are less likely to obtain medical checkups; and they are more likely to change doctors and to file formal complaints (Hayes-Bautista, 1976; Ware, Davies-Avery, & Stewart, 1978).

### Nonadherence to Treatment Regimens

Chapters 3 to 5 examined **adherence** to treatment regimens in the context of health behaviors and noted how difficult it can be to modify or eliminate poor health habits, such as smoking, or to achieve a healthy lifestyle. In this section, we examine adherence to treatment, the role of health institutions, and particularly the role of the provider, in promoting adherence.

Rates of Nonadherence    When patients do not adopt the behaviors and treatments their providers recommend, the result is **nonadherence** or noncompliance (DiMatteo, 2004). Estimates of nonadherence vary from a low of 15 percent to a staggering high of 93 percent. Even as many as 50 percent of people with chronic illnesses are not adherent to their treatments (Bruce et al., 2016). Averaging across all treatment regimens, nonadherence to treatment recommendations is about 26 percent (DiMatteo, Giordani, Lepper, & Croghan, 2002).

But adherence rates vary, depending on the treatment recommendations. For short-term antibiotic regimens, one of the most common prescriptions, about one-third of patients fail to comply adequately (see Rapoff & Christophersen, 1982). Between 50 and 60 percent of patients do not keep appointments for modifying preventive health behaviors (DiMatteo & DiNicola, 1982). More than 80 percent of patients who receive behavior-change recommendations from their doctors, such as stopping smoking or following a restrictive diet, fail to follow through. Even heart patients, such as patients in cardiac rehabilitation, who should be motivated to adhere, have an adherence rate of only 66 to 75 percent (Facts of Life, March 2003).

1. Make adult literacy a national priority.
2. Require that all prescriptions be typed on a keyboard.
3. Have secure electronic medical records for each person that document his or her complete medication history and that are accessible to both patients and their physicians.

4. Enforce requirements that pharmacists provide clear instructions and counseling along with prescription medication.
5. Develop checklists for both patients and doctors, so they can ask and answer the right questions before a prescription is written.

*Source:* The Center for the Advancement of Health (2009).

Overall, about 85 percent of patients fail to adhere completely to prescribed medications (O'Connor, 2006). Adherence is typically so poor that the benefits of many medications cannot be experienced (Haynes, McKibbon, & Kanani, 1996). Adherence is highest for treatments for HIV, arthritis, gastrointestinal disorders, and cancer, and poorest among patients with pulmonary disease, diabetes, and sleep disorders (DiMatteo et al., 2002).

Measuring Adherence    Asking patients about their adherence yields artificially high estimates (Kaplan & Simon, 1990; Turk & Meichenbaum, 1991). As a consequence, researchers draw on indirect measures of adherence, such as the number of follow-up or referral appointments kept, but even these measures can be biased. Overall, the research statistics probably underestimate the amount of nonadherence that is actually going on.

Factors in Communication    Adherence is highest when the patient receives a clear, jargon-free explanation of the etiology, diagnosis, and treatment recommendations. Especially among older patients, adherence is higher if the medication is perceived to be necessary and concerns about the medication itself are low (Dillon, Phillips, Gallagher, Smith, & Stewart, 2018). Adherence is higher among children when their parents are knowledgeable and conscientious (Lee et al., 2017), underscoring the need for clear explanations and treatment instructions. Adherence is higher if the patient has been asked to repeat the instructions, if the instructions are written down, if unclear recommendations are singled out and clarified, and if the instructions are repeated more than once (DiMatteo & DiNicola, 1982). Box 9.2 addresses some ways in which nonadherence may be reduced.

Treatment Regimen    Qualities of the treatment regimen also influence adherence. Treatment regimens that must be followed over a long time, that are complex, that require frequent dosage, and that interfere with other desirable activities in a person's life all show low levels of adherence (Ingersoll & Cohen, 2008; Turk & Meichenbaum, 1991). Keeping first appointments and obtaining medical tests show high adherence rates (Alpert, 1964; DiMatteo & DiNicola, 1982). Adherence is high (about 90 percent) when the advice is perceived as "medical" (e.g., taking medication) but lower (76 percent) if the advice is vocational (e.g., taking time off from work) and lower still (66 percent) if the advice is social or psychological (e.g., avoiding stressful social situations) (Turk & Meichenbaum, 1991).

People who enjoy the activities in their lives are more motivated to adhere to treatment. Adherence is substantially higher among patients who live in cohesive families but lower with patients whose families are in conflict (DiMatteo, 2004). Likewise, people who are depressed show poor adherence to treatment (DiMatteo, Lepper, & Croghan, 2000). Disorganized families with no regular routines have poorer adherence (Hall, Dubin, Crossley, Holmqvist, & D'Arcy, 2009; Jokela, Elovainio, Singh-Manoux, & Kivimäki, 2009; Schreier & Chen, 2010). Low IQ is tied to poor adherence. Nonadherent patients cite lack of time, no money, or distracting problems at home, such as instability and conflict, as impediments to adherence.

Often people cut back on their prescriptions to save money (Heisler, Wagner, & Piette, 2005). This can lead to **creative nonadherence,** namely modifying and supplementing a prescribed treatment regimen (Cohen, Kirzinger, & Gindi, 2013). For example, a poor patient may change the dosage level of a required medication to make the medicine last as long as possi-

**TABLE 9.3 | Why Do People Sue?**

Faulty communication can lead to malpractice litigation. Many suits are due to medical incompetence, but discretionary malpractice suits can be due to faulty communication. Typically,

1. Patients want to find out what happened
2. Patients want an apology from the doctor or hospital
3. Patients want to know that the mistake will not happen again

*Source:* Reitman, Valerie. "Healing Sound of a Word: 'Sorry'." Los Angeles Times, March 24, 2003.

ble or may keep some medication in reserve in case another family member develops the same disorder. One study of nonadherence among the elderly estimated that 73 percent of nonadherence was intentional rather than accidental (Cooper, Love, & Raffoul, 1982).

Creative nonadherence can also result from personal theories about a disorder and its treatment (Wroe, 2001). Patients supplement the treatment regimen with over-the-counter preparations to treat symptoms they think were ignored by the physician. Unfortunately, remedies can sometimes interact with prescribed drugs in unpredictable, even dangerous ways. Alternatively, the patient may alter the dosage requirement, reasoning, for example, that if four pills a day for 10 days will clear up the problem, eight pills a day for 5 days will do it twice as quickly. Creative nonadherence, then, is a widespread and potentially dangerous behavior.

Another costly consequence of poor patient-practitioner communication is malpractice suits. Table 9.3 shows some of the reasons why people sue in discretionary malpractice cases. The fallout from the costs of malpractice suits is that some physicians leave medicine altogether. For example, malpractice premiums are so high for obstetricians that some have decided to move to other specialties where malpractice insurance is lower (Eisenberg & Sieger, 2003, June 9).

## ■ IMPROVING PATIENT–PROVIDER COMMUNICATION AND INCREASING ADHERENCE TO TREATMENT

How can we improve communication so as to increase adherence to treatment? There are simple things that both practitioners and patients can do to improve communication.

## Teaching Providers How to Communicate

Given the motivation, any practitioner can be an effective communicator.

**Training Providers**    Many physicians are motivated to improve the communication process and to share in decision making, although they may not know how (Garcia-Retamero, Wicki, Cokely, & Hanson, 2014). Effective communication programs should teach skills that can be learned easily and incorporated in medical routines easily. Many communication failures in medical settings stem from violations of simple rules of courtesy. The practitioners should greet patients, address them by name, tell them where they can hang up their clothes, explain the purpose of a procedure while it is going on, say good-bye, and, again, use the patient's name. Such simple behaviors add a few seconds at most to a visit, yet they are seen as warm and supportive (DiMatteo & DiNicola, 1982). Nonverbal communication can create an atmosphere of warmth or coldness. A forward lean and direct eye contact, for example, can reinforce an atmosphere of supportiveness, whereas a backward lean, little eye contact, and a postural orientation leaning away from the patient can undercut verbal efforts at warmth by suggesting distance or discomfort (DiMatteo, Friedman, & Taranta, 1979; DiMatteo, Hays, & Prince, 1986). Effective nonverbal communication can improve adherence to treatment (Guéguen, Meineri, & Charles-Sire, 2010) (see Box 9.3).

Communication training needs to be practiced in the situations in which the skills will be used. Training

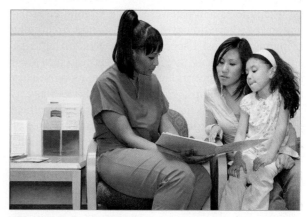

*When physicians present concrete advice about lifestyle change, patients are more likely to adhere.*
Image Source/Jupiterimages

1. Listen to the patient.
2. Ask the patient to repeat what has to be done.
3. Keep the prescription as simple as possible.
4. Give clear instructions on the exact treatment regimen, preferably in writing.
5. Make use of special reminder pill containers and calendars.
6. Call the patient if an appointment is missed.
7. Prescribe a self-care regimen in concert with the patient's daily schedule.
8. Emphasize at each visit the importance of adherence.
9. Gear the frequency of visits to adherence needs.
10. Acknowledge at each visit the patient's efforts to adhere.
11. Involve the patient's spouse or other partner.
12. Whenever possible, provide the patient with instructions and advice at the start of the information to be presented.
13. When providing the patient with instructions and advice, stress how important they are.
14. Use short words and short sentences.
15. Use explicit categorization where possible. (For example, divide information clearly into categories of etiology, treatment, or prognosis.)
16. Repeat things, where feasible.
17. When giving advice, make it as specific, detailed, and concrete as possible.
18. Find out what the patient's worries are. Do not confine yourself merely to gathering objective medical information.
19. Find out what the patient's expectations are. If they cannot be met, explain why.
20. Provide information about the diagnosis and the cause of the illness.
21. Adopt a friendly rather than a businesslike attitude.
22. Avoid medical jargon.
23. Spend some time in conversation about nonmedical topics.

_____
*Source:* Based on DiMatteo (2004).

that uses direct, supervised contact with patients and gives practitioners immediate feedback after a patient interview works well for training both medical and nursing students (Leigh & Reiser, 1986). Continuing education for physicians is an opportunity to address many of the communication issues that occur during patient–practitioner interactions (DeAngelis, 2019).

Training Patients    Interventions to improve patient communication include teaching patients skills for eliciting information from physicians. For example, a study by S. C. Thompson and colleagues (Thompson, Nanni, & Schwankovsky, 1990) instructed women to list three questions they wanted to ask their physician during their visit. Compared with a control group, women who listed questions in advance asked more questions during the visit and were less anxious. In a second study, Thompson and her colleagues added a third condition: Some women received a message from their physician encouraging question asking. These women, too, asked more of the questions they wanted to, had greater feelings of personal control, and were more satisfied with the office visit. Thus, listing one's own questions ahead of time can improve communication during office visits, leading to greater patient satisfaction.

Probing for Barriers to Adherence    Patients are remarkably good at predicting how compliant they will be with treatment regimens (Kaplan & Simon, 1990). By making use of this knowledge, the provider may discover what the barriers to adherence will be. For example, if the patient has been told to avoid stressful situations but anticipates several high-pressure meetings the following week at work, the patient and the provider together might consider how to resolve this dilemma. One option may be to have a coworker take the patient's place at some of the meetings.

Breaking advice down into manageable subgoals that can be monitored by the provider is another way to increase adherence. For example, if patients have been told to alter their diet and lose weight, modest weight-loss goals that can be checked at successive appointments might be established ("Try to exercise 3 times

**FIGURE 9.2 | The Information-Motivation-Behavioral Skills Model of Health Behavior**  The information-motivation-behavioral (IMB) skills model makes it evident that, to practice good health behaviors and adhere to treatment, a person needs the right information, the motivation to adhere, and the skills to perform the behavior.    *Sources:* Fisher, J. D., and W.A. Fisher. "Changing AIDS-Risk Behavior." *Psychological Bulletin* 111 (Spring 1992): 455–74; Fisher, J. D., W. A. Fisher, K. R. Amico, and J. J. Harman. "An Information-Motivation-Behavioral Skills Model of Adherence to Antiretroviral Therapy." *Journal of Health Psychology* 25 (July 2006): 462–73; Fisher, W. A., J. D. Fisher, and J. J. Harman. "Social Psychological Foundations of Health and Illness." In *The Blackwell Series in Health Psychology and Behavioral Medicine,* edited by J. Suls and K. Wallston, 82–105. Canada: John Wiley & Sons, 2008.

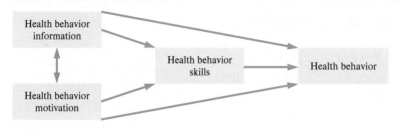

this week for 30 minutes"). In addition, making the medical importance of lifestyle changes clear can improve adherence.

When lifestyle change programs are "prescribed" for patients by physicians, patients show higher rates of adherence than if they are simply urged to make use of them (Kabat-Zinn & Chapman-Waldrop, 1988). Reasons why the health provider can change a patient's health behaviors are listed in Table 9.4.

**TABLE 9.4 | Why the Health Practitioner Can Be an Effective Agent of Behavior Change**

- The health practitioner is a highly credible source with knowledge of medical issues.
- The health practitioner can make health messages simple and tailor them to the individual needs and vulnerabilities of each patient.
- The practitioner can help the patient decide to adhere by highlighting the advantages of treatment and the disadvantages of nonadherence.
- The private, face-to-face nature of the interaction provides an effective setting for holding attention, repeating and clarifying instructions, extracting commitments from a patient, and assessing sources of resistance to adherence.
- The personal nature of the interaction enables a practitioner to establish referent power by communicating warmth and caring.
- The health practitioner can enlist the cooperation of other family members in promoting adherence.
- The health practitioner has the patient under at least partial surveillance and can monitor progress during subsequent visits.

Overall, the best way to improve adherence is to first provide patients with information about their treatment, listen to their concerns, encourage their partnership, build trust, and enhance recall. Second, practitioners can help patients believe in their treatment and become motivated to adhere to it. And finally, patients may need assistance in overcoming any practical barriers to the management of their diseases, which can include such factors as cost or little time (DiMatteo, Haskard-Zolnierek, & Martin, 2012). Figure 9.2 illustrates these processes, as they apply to health behavior.

Innovations in technology can make communication more efficient and effective. Smartphone apps, e-mail, and texting can be efficient ways to send messages from patient to physician and vice versa (*The Economist,* May 2015). Patients can even send pictures of rashes or wounds to help with treatment and follow-up.

## ■ THE PATIENT IN THE HOSPITAL SETTING

More than 36 million people are admitted yearly to the nearly 6,000 hospitals in this country (American Hospital Association, 2019). As recently as 60 or 70 years ago, hospitals were thought of primarily as places where people went to die (Noyes et al., 2000). Now, however, the hospital serves many treatment functions. The average length of a hospital stay has decreased, as Figure 9.3 illustrates, largely because outpatient visits have increased (American Hospital Association, 2009a); the number of deaths in the hospital have declined as well (Hall, Levant, & DeFrances, 2013).

**FIGURE 9.3** | **Average Length of Stay in Community Hospitals, 1995 to 2016**   *Source:* American Hospital Association. "Trendwatch Chart Book 2018 Trends Affecting Hospitals and Health Systems." Accessed April 11, 2019. https://www.aha.org/system/files/2018-07/2018-aha-chartbook.pdf.

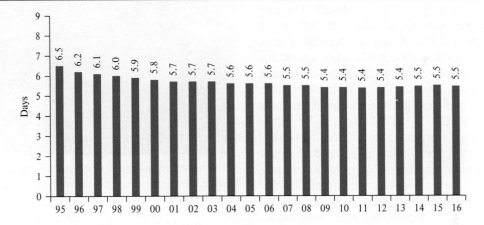

**Inpatient Admissions in Community Hospitals, 1995 to 2016**   *Source:* American Hospital Association. "Trendwatch Chart Book 2018 Trends Affecting Hospitals and Health Systems." Accessed April 11, 2019. https://www.aha.org/system/files/2018-07/2018-aha-chartbook.pdf.

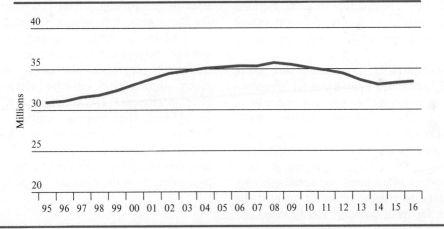

## Structure of the Hospital

The structure of hospitals depends on the health program under which care is delivered. For example, some HMOs and other prepaid health care systems have their own hospitals and employ their own physicians. In the case of the private hospital, there are two lines of authority—a medical line, which is based on technical skill and expertise, and an administrative line, which runs the business of the hospital.

**Cure, Care, and Core**   The functioning of the hospital typically revolves around three goals—cure, care, and core—which may sometimes conflict with each other. *Cure* is typically the physician's responsibility, through performing any treatment action that has the potential to restore patients to good health—that is, to cure them. Patient *care,* in contrast, is more the orientation of the nursing staff, and it involves the humanitarian side of medicine, that is, to do as much as possible to keep the patient's emotional and physical state in balance. The administration of the hospital is concerned with maintaining the *core* of the hospital: ensuring the smooth functioning of the system and the flow of resources, services, and personnel (Mauksch, 1973).

These goals are not always compatible. For example, a clash between the cure and care orientations might occur when deciding whether to administer chemotherapy to an advanced-cancer patient. The cure orientation might maintain that chemotherapy should be initiated even if the chance for survival is slim, whereas the care orientation might argue against the chemotherapy on the grounds that it causes patients great physical and emotional distress. In short, then, the different professional goals in a hospital treatment setting can conflict.

Occupational segregation in the hospital is high: Nurses talk to other nurses, physicians to other physicians, and administrators to other administrators. Physicians have access to some information that nurses may not see, whereas nurses interact with patients daily and know a great deal about their day-to-day progress, yet often their notes on charts may go unread by physicians. The U.S. health care system has been likened to a construction team trying to put up a building in which the construction workers, the electricians, and the plumbers all have different sets of plans, and no one knows what anyone else's plans look like.

An example of the problems associated with lack of communication is provided by nosocomial infection—that is, infection that results from exposure to disease in the hospital setting (Raven, Freeman, & Haley, 1982). Each day approximately 1 in every 31 U.S. patients contracts at least 1 infection during his or her hospital care (Centers for Disease Control and Prevention, 2017).

Hospital workers often break the seemingly endless rules designed to control infection, such as the strict guidelines for hand washing, sterilization, and waste disposal. Of all hospital workers, physicians are the most likely to commit such infractions. However, they are rarely corrected by those under them.

The preceding discussion has emphasized potential sources of conflict and ambiguity in hospital functioning. Burnout, another problem that can result in part from these issues, is described in Box 9.4. However, it is important to remember that hospital functioning is remarkably effective, given the changing realities to which it must accommodate. Thus, structural ambiguities, goal conflicts, and communication problems occur within a system that generally functions quite well.

The Role of Health Psychologists    The number of health psychologists who work in hospital settings has more than doubled over the past 10 years,

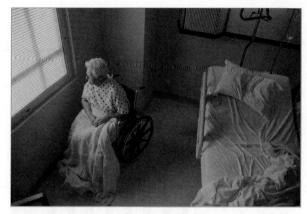

*The hospital can be a lonely and frightening place for many patients, leading to feelings of helplessness, anxiety, or depression.*
Ingram Publishing

and their roles have expanded. Psychologists participate in the diagnosis of patients and assess patients' level of functioning, which can help form the basis for therapeutic intervention. Psychologists are also involved in pre- and postsurgery preparation, pain control, interventions to increase medication and treatment adherence, and behavioral programs to teach appropriate self-care following discharge (Enright, Resnick, DeLeon, Sciara, & Tanney, 1990). In addition, they diagnose and treat psychological problems that can complicate patient care, including anxiety and depression. As our country's medical care system evolves over the next decades, the role of psychologists in the hospital will continue to evolve.

## The Impact of Hospitalization on the Patient

The patient comes unbidden to a large organization that awes and irritates him, even as it also nurtures and cares. As he strips off his clothing so he strips off, too, his favored costume of social roles, his favored style, and his customary identity in the world.

> He becomes subject to a time schedule and a pattern of activity not of his own making. (Wilson, 1963, p. 70)

Patients arrive at the hospital anxious about their disorder, anxious and confused over the prospect of hospitalization, and concerned with all the role obligations they must leave behind unfulfilled. The admission is often conducted by a clerk, who asks about scheduling, insurance, and money. The patient is then ushered into

Burnout is an occupational risk for anyone who works with needy people (Maslach, 2003), including physicians, nurses, and other medical personnel who work with sick and dying people (Rutledge et al., 2009). Burnout is marked by three components: emotional exhaustion, cynicism, and a low sense of efficacy in one's job. Staff members suffering from burnout show a cynical and seemingly callous attitude toward those whom they serve. Their view of clients is negative, and they often treat clients in detached ways (Maslach, 2003).

Burnout has been linked to absenteeism, high job turnover, lengthy breaks during working hours, and even suicide (Schernhammer, 2005). When burned-out workers go home, they are often irritable with their families. They are more likely to suffer from insomnia as well as drug and alcohol abuse, and they have a higher rate of psychosomatic disorders. Thus, burnout has substantial costs for both the institution and the person. Burnout has also been tied to elevated stress hormones (Pruessner, Hellhammer, & Kirschbaum, 1999), changes in immune functioning (Lerman et al., 1999), and poor health including coronary heart disease (Toker, Melamed, Berliner, Zeltser, & Shapira, 2012).

Why does burnout develop? Burnout develops when a person is required to provide services for highly needy people who may not be helped by those services: The problems may be just too severe. Moreover, such jobs often require the staff member to be consistently empathic, an unrealistic expectation. Caregivers may perceive that they give much more than they get back from their patients, and this imbalance aggravates burnout as well (Van Yperen, Buunk, & Schaufelli, 1992). Too much time spent with clients, little feedback, little sense of control or autonomy, little perception of success, role conflict, and role ambiguity are job factors that all aggravate burnout (Maslach, 1979).

High rates of burnout are found among nurses who work in stressful environments, such as intensive care, emergency rooms, or terminal care (Mallett, Price, Jurs, & Slenker, 1991; Moos & Schaefer, 1987). Many nurses find it difficult to protect themselves from

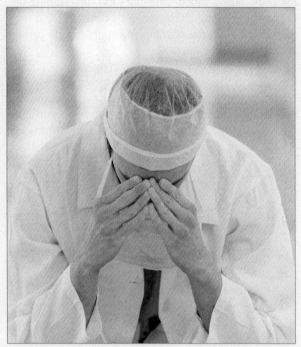

Erproductions Ltd/Blend Images LLC

the pain they feel from watching their patients suffer or die. The stress of the work environment, including the hectic pace of the hospital and the hurried, anxious behavior of coworkers also contributes to burnout (Parker & Kulik, 1995).

How can burnout be avoided? Group interventions can provide workers with an opportunity to meet informally with others to deal with burnout, to obtain emotional support, reduce their feelings of being alone, share feelings of emotional pain about death and dying, and vent emotions in a supportive atmosphere. In so doing, they may improve client care (Duxbury, Armstrong, Dren, & Henley, 1984) and control current feelings of burnout, as well as head off future episodes (Rowe, 1999). For example, seeing what other people do to avoid burnout can provide a useful model for one's own situation.

a strange room, given strange clothes, provided with an unfamiliar roommate, and subjected to tests. The patient must entrust him- or herself completely to strangers in an uncertain environment in which all procedures are new.

Hospital patients can have problematic psychological symptoms, especially anxiety and depression. Nervousness over tests or surgery can produce insomnia, nightmares, and an inability to concentrate. Hospital care can be fragmented, with as many as 30 different staff passing through a patient's room each day, conducting tests, taking blood, bringing food, or cleaning up. Often, the staff members have little time to spend with the patient beyond exchanging greetings, which can be alienating for the patient.

Improving sensitivity to these types of issues in the emergency room (ER) has been a target in recent years. Unrecognized and consequently untreated panic-like anxiety, panic attacks, and asthma attacks occur in as many as 44 percent of ER patients awaiting care (Foldes-Busque et al., 2018). Crowded, slow facilities that, on average, result in a wait of over 2 hours, have led to efforts to streamline the ER process (The Wall Street Journal, September 13, 2017, p. R1). Efforts can include increasing use of digital diagnosis, that is, use of artificial intelligence to infer a tentative diagnosis from symptoms and consequent prioritization for care.

At one time, patients complained bitterly about the lack of communication they had about their disorders and their treatments. Because of these concerns, hospitals have now tried to ameliorate this problem. Patients are now typically given a road map of what procedures they can expect and what they may experience as a result.

## ■ INTERVENTIONS TO INCREASE INFORMATION IN HOSPITAL SETTINGS

Many hospitals now provide interventions that help prepare patients generally for hospitalization and for the procedures they will undergo.

In 1958, psychologist Irving Janis conducted a landmark study that would forever change how patients are prepared for surgery. Janis was asked by a hospital to study its surgery patients to see if something could be done to reduce the stress that many of them experienced both before and after operations. Janis first grouped the patients according to the level of fear they experienced before their operations (high, medium, and low). Then he studied how well they understood and used the information the hospital staff gave them to help them cope with the aftereffects of surgery. Highly fearful patients generally remained fearful and anxious after surgery and showed many negative side effects, such as vomiting, pain, urinary retention, and difficulty with eating (see also Montgomery & Bovbjerg, 2004). Patients who initially had little fear also showed unfavorable reactions after surgery, becoming angry or upset or complaining. Of the three groups, the moderately fearful patients coped with postoperative stress most effectively.

In interpreting these results, Janis reasoned that highly fearful patients had been too absorbed with their own fears preoperatively to process the preparatory information adequately, and patients with little fear were insufficiently vigilant to understand and process the information effectively. Patients with moderate levels of fear, in contrast, were vigilant enough but not overwhelmed by their fears, so they were able to develop realistic expectations of what their postsurgery reactions would be; when they later encountered these sensations and reactions, they expected them and were ready to deal with them.

Subsequent studies have built on Janis's observations to create interventions. For example, in one study (Mahler & Kulik, 1998), patients awaiting coronary artery bypass graft (CABG) were exposed to one of three preparatory videotapes or to no preparation. One videotape conveyed information from a health care expert; the second not only featured the health care expert but also included clips of interviews with patients who reported on their progress; and the third presented information from a health care expert plus interviews with patients who reported that their recovery consisted of "ups and downs." Compared with patients who did not receive videotaped preparation, patients who saw one of the videotapes felt significantly better prepared for the recovery period, reported higher self-efficacy during the recovery period, were more adherent to recommended dietary and exercise changes during their recovery, and were released sooner from the hospital.

Research on the role of preparatory information in adjustment to surgery overwhelmingly shows that such preparation has beneficial effects on hospital patients (Salzmann et al., 2018). Patients who have been prepared are typically less emotionally distressed, regain their functioning more quickly, and are often able to leave the hospital sooner. One study (Kulik & Mahler, 1989) even found that the person who becomes your postoperative roommate can influence how you cope with the aftermath of surgery (Box 9.5). Preparation for patients is so beneficial that many hospitals show videotapes to patients to prepare them for upcoming procedures.

## ■ THE HOSPITALIZED CHILD

Were you ever hospitalized as a child? If so, think back over the experience. Was it frightening and disorienting? Did you feel alone and uncared for? Or was it a more positive experience? Perhaps your parents were

Patients who are hospitalized for serious illnesses or surgery often experience anxiety. From the earlier discussion of social support (see Chapter 7), we know that emotional support from others can reduce distress when people are undergoing stressful events. Accordingly, Kulik and Mahler (1987) developed a social support intervention for patients about to undergo cardiac surgery. Some of the patients were assigned a roommate who was also waiting for surgery (preoperative condition), whereas others were assigned a roommate who had already had surgery (postoperative condition). In addition, patients were placed with a roommate undergoing a surgery that was either similar or dissimilar to their own.

The researchers found that patients who had a postoperative roommate profited from this contact (see also Kulik, Moore, & Mahler, 1993). Patients with a postoperative roommate were less anxious before surgery, were able to move around after surgery, and were released more quickly from the hospital than were patients who had been paired with a roommate who was also awaiting surgery. Whether the type of surgery was similar or dissimilar made no difference, only whether the roommate's surgery had already taken place.

Why was having a postoperative roommate helpful for patients awaiting surgery? Possibly roommates were able to provide relevant information about the postoperative period. They may have acted as role models for how to cope postoperatively. Whatever the reason, social contact with a postoperative roommate clearly had a positive impact on the pre- and postoperative adjustment of these surgery patients (Kulik & Mahler, 1993; Kulik et al., 1993).

---

able to room in with you, or other children were around to talk to. You may have had either of these experiences because procedures for managing children in the hospital have changed dramatically over the past few decades.

Hospitalization can be hard on children. It is difficult for a child to be separated from family and home. Some children may not understand why they have been taken away from their families and mistakenly infer that they are being punished for some misdeed. The hospital environment can be lonely and isolating. Physical confinement in bed or confinement due to casts or traction keeps children from discharging energy through physical activity. Some children may become socially withdrawn, wet their beds, or have extreme emotional reactions ranging from fear to temper tantrums. The dependency that is fostered by bed rest and reliance on staff can also lead to regression. Children, especially those just entering puberty, can be embarrassed or ashamed by having to expose themselves to strangers. The child may also be subject to confusing or painful tests and procedures.

### Preparing Children for Medical Interventions

Just as adults are benefited by preparation, so children are as well (Jay, Elliott, Woody, & Siegel, 1991; Manne et al., 1990). In one study (Melamed & Siegel, 1975),

children about to undergo surgery were shown either a film of another child being hospitalized and receiving surgery or an unrelated film. Those children exposed to the relevant film showed less pre- and postoperative distress than did children exposed to the irrelevant film. Moreover, parents of the children exposed to the modeling film reported fewer problem behaviors after hospitalization than did parents of children who saw the control film.

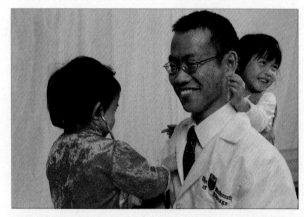

*Recent changes in hospitalization procedures for children have made hospitals less frightening places to be. Increasingly, medical personnel have recognized children's needs for play and have provided opportunities for play in hospital settings.*
2007 Keith Eng

Coping skills preparation can be helpful to children. For example, Zastowny and colleagues gave children and their parents information describing typical hospitalization and surgery experiences, relaxation training to reduce anxiety, or a coping skills intervention to teach children constructive self-talk (Zastowny, Kirschenbaum, & Meng, 1986). Both the anxiety reduction and the coping skills interventions reduced children's fearfulness and parents' distress. Overall, the children exposed to the coping skills intervention exhibited the fewest maladaptive behaviors during hospitalization, less problem behavior in the week before admission, and fewer problems after discharge. A meta-analysis of 723 studies showed that children and their parents who saw audiovisual preparation videos for surgery were less anxious before surgery, and the children were able to leave the hospital earlier after surgery (Chow et al., 2018).

Some preparation can be undertaken by parents. If a parent prepares a child for admission several days before hospitalization—explaining why it is necessary, what it will be like, who will be there, how often the parent will visit, and so on—this preparation may ease the transition. During admission procedures, a parent or another familiar adult can remain with the child until the child is settled into the new room and engaged in some activity.

The presence of parents during stressful medical procedures is not an unmitigated benefit. Parents do not always help reduce children's fears, pain, and discomfort (Manne et al., 1992). When present during invasive medical procedures, some parents can become distressed and exacerbate the child's own anxiety (Wolff et al., 2009). Nonetheless, parental support is important, and most hospitals now provide opportunities for extended parental visits, including 24-hour parental visitation rights. Despite some qualifications, the benefits of preparing children for hospitalization are now so widely acknowledged that it is more the rule than the exception.

# ■ COMPLEMENTARY AND ALTERNATIVE MEDICINE

Thus far, our discussion of treatment has focused on traditional treatment venues, including the physician's office and the hospital. However, nearly two-thirds of adults in the United States use **complementary and alternative medicine (CAM)** in addition to or instead of traditional medicine (Barnes, Powell-Griner, McFann,

**TABLE 9.5 | Ten Most Common CAM Therapies Among U.S. Adults**

1. Prayer—43%
2. Natural products (herbs, vitamins, and minerals)—17.7%
3. Deep breathing—12.7%
4. Meditation—9.4%
5. Chiropractic and Osteopathic—8.6%
6. Massage—8.3%
7. Yoga—6.1%
8. Diet-based therapies—3.6%
9. Progressive relaxation—2.9%
10. Guided imagery—2.2%

*Source:* U.S. Department of Health & Human Services, National Institute of Health, 2016. "Nationwide Survey Reveals Widespread Use of Mind and Body Practices." *News Release.* Last modified February 10, 2015. https://www.nih.gov/news-events/news-releases/nationwide-survey-reveals-widespread-use-mind-body-practices."

& Nahin, 2004; Neiberg et al., 2011). Complementary and alternative medicine is a diverse group of therapies, products, and medical treatments that include prayer, potions, natural herb products, meditation, yoga, massage, homeopathic medicines, and acupuncture, among other treatments. Table 9.5 lists the most common CAM practices. Until the 1990s, CAM was not a thriving business. Now, however, about two-thirds of people in the United States use CAM each year. More than $50 billion a year is spent on CAM therapies, much of which comes out of pocket; that is, it is not reimbursed by insurance companies.

The drugs and treatments of traditional medicine must be evaluated according to federal standards. Medications, for example, are typically evaluated through clinical trials and licensed by the Food and Drug Administration. However, the same is not true of CAM treatments, and so CAM represents a vast and often unevaluated aspect of care. This does not mean that CAM treatments do not work, but only that many have not been formally tested or have been evaluated only in very narrow contexts. For this reason, the National Center for Complementary and Alternative Medicine (NCCAM), now called the National Center for Complementary and Integrative Health, was created within the National Institutes of Health in 1998. Its mission is to evaluate the usefulness and safety of CAM therapies through rigorous scientific investigation and to discern what roles such therapies might have in improving health and health care (NCCAM, 2012). We begin this section with an overview of the philosophical origins of complementary and alternative medicine. We then turn to the most common CAM therapies and evaluate them where evidence is available.

## Philosophical Origins of CAM

CAM is rooted in **holistic medicine,** an approach to treatment that deals with the physical, psychological, and spiritual needs of the person. In many respects, this is a logical extension of the biopsychosocial model introduced in Chapter 1, which also seeks to treat the whole person. Perhaps the earliest approach to healing was prayer. As we saw in Chapter 1, medicine evolved from religion, in which the healing of the body was believed to result from expelling evil spirits from the body. CAM's origins lie in ancient African, European, and Middle Eastern religions and Asian cultures.

Traditional Chinese Medicine   **Traditional Chinese Medicine (TCM)** began more than 2,000 years ago and enjoys wide use throughout Asia. Recently, it has gained adherents in the United States. This approach to healing is based on the idea that a vital force, called qi (pronounced "chee"), flows throughout the body through channels called meridians that connect the parts of the body to each other and to the universe. Qi is considered the vital life force, and so if it is blocked or stagnant, disease can result. Keeping qi in balance is important both for maintaining good health and for improving health when it has been compromised.

TCM also strives to balance two forces, yin and yang. Yin is cold, passive, and slow-energy, whereas yang is hot, active, and rapid. Balancing the two is believed to be important for good health and attaining mental and physical harmony. Stress, infectious disorders, and environmental stressors can lead to imbalances between these forces, and thus the goal of intervention is to restore the balance.

To do so, TCM draws on such techniques as acupuncture, massage, diet, exercise, and meditation. It also draws on a variety of herbal preparations, including ginseng, wolfberry, gingerroot, dong quai, cinnamon, astragalus, and peony. Dietary intervention, which includes foods that shift the yin–yang balance, is a staple of TCM. Once on the wane, TCM is growing rapidly in popularity in China (*The Economist,* September, 2017).

There has been relatively little formal evaluation of TCM and its treatments, in large part because multiple treatments are often combined for individualized care based on a person's particular problem. Without standardized treatments received by a large number of people, formal evaluation is difficult. However, there is some formal support for certain aspects of TCM.

One theory that is gaining traction, if not yet substantial evidence, is the idea that the activities of TCM, especially its herbal preparations, have anti-inflammatory properties, and thus affect the immune system in a generally beneficial way that may have implications for a broad array of illnesses (Pan, Chiou, Tsai, & Ho, 2011). Whether traditional Chinese medicinal herbs and practices do indeed have anti-inflammatory actions is as yet unknown, but this is a promising evaluative pathway to pursue.

Ayurvedic Medicine   A related tradition that developed in India around 2,000 years ago is **ayurvedic medicine.** Like TCM, the goal is balance among the body, mind, and spirit (National Center for Complementary and Alternative Medicine, 2009a). Although people are born into a state of balance, events in their lives can disrupt it, compromising health, and so bringing these forces back into balance alleviates illness and maintains good health. As in TCM and holistic medicine more generally, information about lifestyle and behavior is elicited from the patient and family members to identify treatment goals to achieve harmony and balance. Diet, exercise, and massage are important elements of ayurvedic medicine, as are the use of herbs, oils, spices, and various minerals, to keep the person in balance. Ayurvedic medicine has been used to treat a variety of disorders, but little formal evaluation has been conducted.

Homeopathy and Naturopathy   **Homeopathy** is a philosophy developed in Europe in the 1700s, which likewise interprets disease and illness as caused by disturbances in a vital life force. Practitioners of homeopathy typically treat patients using diluted preparations that cause symptoms similar to those from which the patient suffers. When highly diluted, homeopathic remedies are typically safe, although when not sufficiently diluted, they can put patients at risk for illness. For some disorders, such as influenza-like syndromes, homeopathy may alleviate symptoms, but in other cases, the evidence is weak or mixed (Altunç, Pittler, & Ernst, 2007; Linde et al., 1999). At present, with respect to the standards of evidence-based medicine, the success of homeopathic treatments is still in question (Bellavite, Marzotto, Chirumbolo, & Conforti, 2011).

Other early origins of CAM include naturopathy, a medical system developed in the 1800s, whose central tenet is that the body can heal itself through diet, exercise, sunlight, and fresh air.

In summary, the origins of complementary and alternative medicine are at least 2,000 years old and arose from ancient religions and traditional healing practices in China and India, as well as from more recent health movements in Europe and the United States. All have as a fundamental principle the idea that the mind, body, spirit, and environment operate together to influence health. Intervention through prayer or meditation, diet, exercise, massage, herbal potions, and specific treatments, such as acupuncture, provide the impetus for the body to return itself to full health.

## ■ CAM TREATMENTS

In this section we review some of the most commonly used CAM therapies, and when possible, evaluate their effects. We begin with the most common CAM therapies, dietary supplements and prayer. We then discuss a central therapy of TCM, namely acupuncture, following which we consider several therapies that have their basis in meditation. These are sometimes called mind–body interventions, and they include yoga, hypnosis, mindfulness meditation, and guided imagery. Finally, we turn to massage therapy, chiropractic medicine, and osteopathy, which involve the manipulation of soft tissue or spine and joints.

### Dietary Supplements and Diets

**Dietary supplements** contain nutrients in amounts that are as high or higher than levels recommended by the U.S. National Academy of Medicine's daily recommendations. Over one-half of the U.S. population regularly uses dietary supplements, the most common being multivitamins (Gahche et al., 2011). Calcium is taken by nearly 61 percent of women over age 60, and consumption of folic acid and vitamin D supplements has also substantially increased in recent years (Gahche et al., 2011). People who do not get enough vitamins and minerals from food alone, or have certain medical conditions, might benefit from multivitamins, but there is little evidence that multivitamins prevent illness or improve health for most people (National Institutes of Health, 2018). Moreover, supplements that contain iron are associated with increased risk of death among older women (Mursu, Robien, Harnack, Park, & Jacobs, 2011). Accordingly, some practitioners maintain that

dietary supplements should be reserved for people who have symptomatic nutrient deficiency disorders; in these cases, dietary supplements have clear health benefits.

Overall, the use of dietary supplements is not related to improved health (Rabin, 2012). Many people who take supplements believe that they can stave off chronic disease, but until recently this has been more claim than substance. However, a recent study found that among older men who took a multivitamin daily, cancer rates were reduced by 8 percent (Gaziano et al., 2012). This well-designed study provides some evidence that dietary supplements may have health benefits for at least some groups of healthy people.

Vitamin D supplements may reduce symptoms of depression (Shaffer et al., 2014). However, because supplements are perceived to improve health, at least some people use them as insurance against their unhealthy behaviors. For example, in two studies, people who took placebo dietary supplements were less likely to exercise and more likely to eat unhealthy foods, compared with people who knew that the drug they had received was a placebo (Chiou, Yang, & Wan, 2011). Thus, at least in some people, dietary supplements may confer an illusory sense of invulnerability that may have hidden costs.

Increasingly, people are eating specific foods (and avoiding others) to achieve good health. Foods that affect the microbiome in the gut are among them (Sonnenburg & Sonnenburg, 2015). Beginning in infancy with mother's milk and continuing into old age, how we feed ourselves can influence the microbiotica in the gut, and probiotic supplements are often used to augment these effects. Whether health risks are affected is hard to evaluate, in part because each person's microbiome is individual, influenced by genetics, food consumption, and other aspects of the environment (Sonnenburg & Sonnenburg, 2015).

Specific diets have also been used in an effort to improve health. These include macrobiotic and vegetarian diets. Vegetarian diets involve reducing or eliminating meat and fish and increasing consumption of vegetables, fruits, grains, and plant-based oils. As we saw in Chapter 4, reduced consumption of meat is widely recommended for health. However, vegetarians run a risk of consuming insufficient protein and nutrients, and so careful attention to the components of vegetarian diets is vital. Macrobiotic diets, which restrict vegetarian consumption primarily to grains, cereals, and vegetables, require even greater attention to nutritional content (American Cancer Society, 2008).

## Prayer

When prayer is included as a CAM therapy, the number of adults in the United States who report using CAM yearly totals two-thirds. Surveys (Gallup Poll, 2009) indicate that the majority of people in the United States believe in God (80 percent), report attending church services at least once a month (55 percent), and say that religion is important in their personal lives (80 percent). Nearly half the population in the United States uses prayer to deal with health problems (Zimmerman, 2005, March 15).

Prayer may have some benefits for coping with illness. For example, in one study, surgery patients with strong religious beliefs experienced fewer complications and had shorter hospital stays than those with less strong religious beliefs (Contrada et al., 2004). Spiritual beliefs have been tied to better health practices (Hill, Ellison, Burdette, & Musick, 2007), better health (Krause, Ingersoll-Dayton, Liang, & Sugisawa, 1999), and longer life (Koenig & Vaillant, 2009; McCullough, Friedman, Enders, & Martin, 2009; Schnall et al., 2010). Religious attendance can protect against high blood pressure (Gillum & Ingram, 2006), complications from surgery (Ai, Wink, Tice, Bolling, & Shearer, 2009), and headache (Wachholtz & Pargament, 2008), among other disorders and symptoms (Berntson, Norman, Hawkley, & Cacioppo, 2008), perhaps because of its promotion of a healthy lifestyle (Musick, House, & Williams, 2004). However, religious beliefs do not appear to retard the progression of cancer or speed recovery from acute illness (Powell, Shahabi, & Thoresen, 2003).

Prayer is unusual in that health psychologists have actually evaluated its efficacy with respect to evidence-based medicine standards. On the whole, despite some benefits, many of which may come from the sense of calm or relaxation that religion can provide, prayer itself does not appear to reliably improve health (Masters & Spielmans, 2007; Nicholson, Rose, & Bobak, 2010). The social support that comes from religious attendance, as noted in Chapter 7, can lead to health benefits, but reliable effects of prayer on health have not been found.

## Acupuncture

**Acupuncture** has been in existence in China for more than 2,000 years. In acupuncture treatment, long, thin needles are inserted into designated areas of the body that theoretically influence the areas in which a patient is experiencing a disorder. Although the main goal of acupuncture is to cure illness, it may also have an analgesic effect. In China, some patients are able to undergo surgery with only the analgesia of acupuncture. During surgery, these patients are typically conscious, fully alert, and able to converse while the procedures are going on.

Acupuncture is often used to control pain (Cherkin et al., 2009), although how it does so is not fully known. Acupuncture may function partly as a counterirritation pain management technique. It is typically accompanied by relaxation, a belief that acupuncture will work, and preparation regarding what sensations the needles will cause and how to tolerate them. All of these factors by themselves can reduce pain. Acupuncture may also be distracting, and it is often accompanied by analgesic drugs that also reduce pain. Some benefits may also be due to placebo effects. Finally, acupuncture may trigger the release of endorphins, which reduces the experience of pain.

An evaluation of the effectiveness of acupuncture is difficult because of its limited use in the United States. Of 32 reviews of the acupuncture literature, 25 of them failed to demonstrate its effectiveness with respect to many disorders (Ernst, 2009). There may be some benefits for certain kinds of pain (Birch, Hesselink, Jonkman, Hekker, & Bos, 2004), especially short-term pain, but it is not as effective for chronic pain.

The broad claims for acupuncture have not yet been upheld scientifically (Ernst, 2009; Ernst, Lee, & Choi, 2011). Moreover, there are some risks of adverse effects, such as bleeding or infection (Ernst, Lee, & Choi, 2011). As is true for many other evaluations of CAM therapies, studies of acupuncture's effectiveness are typically limited by small samples, poor controls, and poor design (Ahn et al., 2008). Consequently, using the standards of evidence-based medicine, conclusions regarding the effectiveness of acupuncture for disorders other than management of acute pain are not definitive.

## Yoga

**Yoga** has been practiced for more than 5,000 years, although it has only recently become popular in the United States. Yoga is a general term that includes breathing techniques, posture, strengthening exercises, and meditation. Originating in spiritual traditions in India, yoga is now practiced by nearly 15 percent of people in the United States in 2017 (National Center for Complementary and Integrative Health, 2018). The yoga market is a multi billion dollar industry in the United States, and yoga is now used to treat chronic pain, bronchitis, symptoms associated with menopause, and a variety of mental and physical ailments related to stress, including anxiety and depression. Because stress and anxiety contribute to many chronic disorders and lower quality of life, a non pharmacologic therapy that can reduce stress and anxiety has much promise, and yoga is one popular option (Li & Goldsmith, 2012).

In studies that have evaluated its effectiveness, most people report lower stress and anxiety, although many studies have small numbers of participants and are not well controlled (Li & Goldsmith, 2012; Lin, Hu, Chang, Lin, & Tsauo, 2011; Smith & Pukall, 2009). Yoga has also been used to treat cancer-related fatigue. In one study of breast cancer survivors, a yoga intervention significantly reduced fatigue and improved vigor (Bower et al., 2011). There is, as yet, however, no strong evidence that yoga improves physical health.

## Hypnosis

**Hypnosis** is one of the oldest CAM techniques. Old medical textbooks and anthropological accounts of healing rituals provide anecdotal evidence of such extreme interventions as surgery conducted with no apparent pain while the patient was under a hypnotic trance.

Hypnosis involves a state of relaxation; relaxation alone can help reduce stress and discomfort. Typically, the client is explicitly told that the hypnosis will be successful: Expectations can reduce discomfort via the placebo effect. Hypnosis is itself a distraction, and distraction can reduce discomfort. The patient is usually instructed to think about the discomfort differently, and the meaning attached to discomfort influences the experience. And finally, in the case of pain management, the patient undergoing hypnosis is often given painkillers or other drug treatments.

The effects of hypnosis are mixed. The beneficial effects of hypnosis in reducing pain may be due at least in part to the composite effects of relaxation, reinterpretation, distraction, and drugs. The effects of self-hypnosis on chronic pain are roughly comparable with those of progressive muscle relaxation and similar relaxation therapies (Jensen & Patterson, 2006). The use of hypnosis for other health-related issues has not been formally evaluated.

## Meditation

Meditation refers to a variety of therapies that aim to focus and control attention (National Center for Complementary and Integrative Health, 2016). For example, in transcendental meditation, the person focuses his or her awareness on a single object (such as a flower) or on a word or short phrase called a mantra. Meditators often achieve an advanced state of relaxation and control of bodily processes.

Mindfulness meditation, which was discussed in Chapter 7, teaches people to strive for a state of mind marked by awareness and to focus on the present moment, accepting and acknowledging it without becoming distracted or distressed by stress. Thus, the goal of mindfulness meditation is to help people approach stressful situations mindfully, rather than reacting to them automatically (Bishop, 2002; Hölzel et al., 2011).

More empirical investigations have been conducted on mindfulness meditation than on most other CAM therapies. Certain aspects of meditation may be helpful for managing pain (Perlman, Salomons, Davidson, & Lutz, 2010). On the whole, it appears to be successful in controlling stress and anxiety (Chiesa & Serretti, 2009; Grossman, Niemann, Schmidt, & Walach, 2004) and managing HPA reactivity and blood pressure responses to stress (Jacobs et al., 2013; Nykliček, Mommersteeg, Van Beugen, Ramakers, & Van Boxtel, 2013). Mindfulness meditation may also be an effective treatment for certain functional disorders such as fibromyalgia (Grossman, Tiefenthaler-Gilmer, Raysz, & Kesper, 2007). Most studies of mindfulness meditation, however, compare those who have been trained in the practice with waitlist controls, that is, people who are motivated to learn mindfulness but have not yet had the opportunity. True control groups are rare. In one of the few studies to date that has randomly assigned people to mindfulness meditation or to a control group, mindfulness training had some impact on alleviating pain but not on distress (MacCoon et al., 2012). In non experimental studies, mindfulness-based interventions have been effective in treating depression, anxiety, and other psychiatric disorders (Ivanovski & Malhi, 2007; Keng, Smoski, & Robins, 2011). Still, as is true of most CAM therapies, the quality of the evidence remains inconsistent (Chiesa & Serretti, 2009).

## Guided Imagery

**Guided imagery** is a meditative procedure that has been used to control discomfort related to illness and treatment, especially cancer. In guided imagery, a patient is instructed to conjure up a picture that he or she holds in mind during a procedure or during the experience of discomfort. Some practitioners of guided imagery use it primarily to induce relaxation. The patient is encouraged to visualize a peaceful, relatively unchanging scene, to hold it in mind, and to focus on it fully.

This process brings on a relaxed state, concentrates attention, and distracts the patient—all techniques that have been shown to reduce discomfort.

An example of using guided imagery to control the discomfort of a medical procedure is provided by a patient undergoing radiation therapy:

> When I was taking the radiation treatment, I imagined I was looking out my window and watching the trees and seeing the leaves go back and forth in the wind. Or, I would think of the ocean and watch the waves come in over and over again, and I would hope, "Maybe this will take it all away."

A different visualization technique may be used by patients trying to take a more aggressive stance toward illness and discomfort. Instead of using imagery to calm and soothe themselves, these patients use it to rouse themselves into a confrontive stance by imagining a combative, action-filled scene. The following example is from a patient who used aggressive imagery in conjunction with chemotherapy treatment:

> I imagined that the cancer was this large dragon and the chemotherapy was a cannon, and when I was taking the chemotherapy, I would imagine it blasting the dragon, piece by piece.

One chemotherapy patient profited from the use of both types of imagery:

> It was kind of a game with me, depending on my mood. If I was peaceful and wanted to be peaceful, I would image a beautiful scene, or if I wanted to do battle with the enemy, I would mock up a battle and have my defenses ready.

How effective is guided imagery? Early claims that guided imagery can cure diseases such as cancer have no foundation. However, the practice of guided imagery can alleviate stress and induce relaxation. There is some evidence that guided imagery can reduce pain (Abdoli, Rahzani, Safaie, & Sattari, 2012; Posadzki, Lewandowski, Terry, Ernst, & Stearns, 2012), but on the whole, like other CAM therapies, there are too few rigorous randomized clinical trials that test its effectiveness (Posadzki & Ernst, 2011).

## Chiropractic Medicine

**Chiropractic medicine** was founded by Daniel Palmer in 1895 and involves performing adjustments on the spine and joints to correct misalignments that are believed to both prevent and cure illness. Chiropracty is a popular intervention in the United States, and several schools of chiropractic education train practitioners. About 20 percent of people in the United States will make use of chiropractic services at some point in their lives, primarily for the treatment of pain (Barnes, Powell-Griner, McFann, & Nahin, 2004). Most of the evidence for beneficial effects of chiropractic management is limited to a few small-scale studies (Pribicevic, Pollard, Bonello, & de Luca, 2010; Stuber & Smith, 2008). Accordingly, more formal evaluation of these techniques for specific disorders is needed.

## Osteopathy

Osteopathy is an alternative medical practice that draws on the body's ability to heal itself. Using manual and manipulative therapy, the osteopath seeks to facilitate healing. There is little scientific evidence for the principles of osteopathy, and little empirical evidence that it is effective except for managing lower back pain (New York University Langone Medical Center, 2012).

## Massage

In contrast to chiropracty, massage involves manipulation of soft tissue. In TCM, massage (tui na) is used to manipulate the flow of qi. Massage reduces stress and is believed to boost immune functioning and flush waste out of the system. Certain forms of exercise such as tai chi, which are methodical and stylized, may induce a meditative state and balance the life force.

Massage is also used to control stress and pain, and about 5 percent of people in the United States use massage as CAM (Barnes, Powell-Griner, McFann, & Nahin, 2004). Some studies have found massage to be effective for persistent back pain, but the studies are limited by small samples, poor controls, and weak designs (Cherkin, Sherman, Deyo, & Shekelle, 2003).

## Who Uses CAM?

Many people who use CAM do not disclose that fact, perhaps because they are embarrassed about it or think they will be thought foolish by others. But those who have tried it and achieved beneficial physical or psychological effects readily share their reactions (Sirois, Riess, & Upchurch, 2017). Most people who use CAM use only one form. That is, people who take dietary supplements do not necessarily also practice yoga or seek treatment from chiropractors. About 20 percent of adults use two different CAM therapies, but only

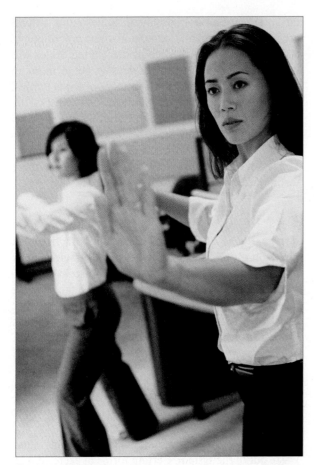

Tai chi is a Chinese martial art and form of stylized, meditative exercise, characterized by methodically slow circular and stretching movements and positions of bodily balance.
Image Source/Blend Images

treated through traditional medicine (Frass et al., 2012). Experiencing delays in receiving medical care and high costs of medical care can also lead to the use of CAM therapies. Use of CAM therapies, particularly chiropractic care, massage, and acupuncture, increases significantly when access to conventional care has been restricted (Su & Li, 2011).

CAM therapies are used more by white people than by minorities, and are especially used by non-Hispanic white, middle-aged, and older women (Frass et al., 2012; Gahche et al., 2011). The typical CAM therapy for this group is a dietary supplement containing calcium. Overall, the use of CAM therapies has grown in the past two decades, especially among non-Hispanic whites (Gahche et al., 2011).

## Complementary and Alternative Medicine: An Overall Evaluation

There is currently insufficient evidence to evaluate the effectiveness of most CAM therapies. In many cases, formal studies have not been undertaken, and when they have, the samples are often small, the controls poor, and the designs weak. The verdict, accordingly, is out on many of these treatments (*The Economist,* April 2012), except in particular cases (e.g., specific dietary supplements provide benefits for nutrient deficiencies).

It is difficult to evaluate CAM therapies because they are often highly individualized. Thus, formal standards of evidence-based medicine run against the philosophy that guides CAM treatment recommendations, namely that each patient's therapeutic regimen addresses that person's specific problems. One patient's pain may be treated through one set of CAM therapies, whereas another patient's pain may be treated through a different set of individualized therapies.

Because many CAM therapies have not been formally evaluated, the conflict posed by these therapies is this: They are now so widely used that they have become a standard part of health care, yet when and why they work is often in question. Moreover, many of these therapies, like traditional interventions, have a placebo component, which means that the mere taking of an action can ameliorate a disorder largely by improving mental and physical adjustment to it. Of course, many therapies that are now established as active treatments were once considered alternative treatments. For example, dietary change (Chapter 4) and even surgery were once considered alternative medicine, but now are often well integrated into health care. This is because

5 percent use three or more. Most commonly, those who use more than one CAM therapy combine herbal or dietary supplements with prayer or meditation (Neiberg et al., 2011).

Why do people use complementary and alternative medicines? People often turn to CAM if they have disorders that are not successfully treated by traditional medicine. These include functional disorders that are not well managed by traditional medicine, such as chronic fatigue syndrome; chronic conditions whose existence or treatment create side effects, such as cancer; and intractable pain problems, such as back problems or neck pain (Barnes, Powell-Griner, McFann, & Nahin, 2004). Depression, anxiety, stress, insomnia, severe headaches, and stomach and intestinal disorders also prompt the use of CAM therapies, particularly when these conditions have not been successfully these treatments have been subject to the standards of evidence-based medicine, which is now the standard for making the transition from CAM to medical intervention (Committee on the Use of Complementary and Alternative Medicine, 2005).

Some CAM therapies such as massage and some forms of yoga are intrinsically enjoyable, and so asking if they "work" is akin to asking whether reading a book, gardening, or raising tropical fish "works." They don't need to work medically to have a beneficial impact on well-being. Moreover, if people feel less "stressed out" after having practiced some CAM therapies, such as meditation or guided imagery, that may be benefit enough. Overall, though, as patients insist on having more of these alternative therapies included in their treatment, as they pester their physicians and insurance companies to have CAM therapies covered, and as they expend billions of dollars on CAM therapies, the pressure to formally evaluate these treatments through more rigorous research mounts.

Thus, at present, the importance of CAM derives from the fact that millions of people worldwide use these therapies and spend billions of dollars doing so (*The Economist,* April 2012). Moreover, more people use self-care and CAM therapies to treat themselves when they are ill than use traditional medicine (Suzuki, 2004), and millions of these people practice **integrative medicine,** that is, the combination of alternative medicine with conventional medicine. Given widespread use, the effectiveness and safety of these therapies are essential, and so continued evaluation of their effectiveness is critical (Selby & Smith-Osborne, 2013). Moreover, because some use of CAM therapies results from unmet treatment and emotional needs, these need greater consideration in the treatment process as well.

## ▣ THE PLACEBO EFFECT

Consider the following:

- Inhaling a useless drug improved lung function in children with asthma by 33 percent.
- People exposed to fake poison ivy develop rashes.
- Forty-two percent of balding men who took a placebo maintained or increased their hair growth.
- Sham knee surgery reduces pain as much as real surgery (Blakeslee, 1998, October 13).

All of these surprising facts are due to one effect— the placebo.

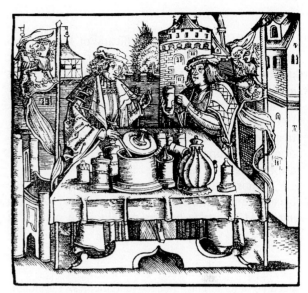

*This 16th-century woodcut shows the preparation of theriac, a supposed antidote to poison. If theriac was a successful treatment, it was entirely due to the placebo effect.*
INTERFOTO/Alamy Stock Photo

## History of the Placebo

In the early days of medicine, few drugs or treatments gave any real physical benefit. As a consequence, patients were treated with a variety of bizarre, largely ineffective therapies. Egyptian patients were medicated with "lizard's blood, crocodile dung, the teeth of a swine, the hoof of an ass, putrid meat, and fly specks" (Findley, 1953), concoctions that were not only ineffective but also dangerous. If the patient did not succumb to the disease, he or she had a good chance of dying from the treatment. Medical treatments of the Middle Ages were somewhat less lethal, but not much more effective. These European patients were treated with ground-up "unicorn's horn" (actually, ground ivory), bezoar stones (supposedly a "crystallized tear from the eye of a deer bitten by a snake" but actually an animal gallstone or other intestinal piece), theriac (made from ground-up snake and between 37 and 63 other ingredients), and, for healing wounds, powdered Egyptian mummy (Shapiro, 1960). As late as the 17th and 18th centuries, patients were subjected to bloodletting, freezing, and repeatedly induced vomiting to bring about a cure (Shapiro, 1960).

Such accounts make it seem miraculous that anyone survived these early medical treatments. But people did; moreover, they often seemed to get relief from these

A dramatic example of the efficacy of the placebo effect is provided by the case history of a cancer patient, Mr. Wright. The patient thought he was being given injections of a controversial drug, Krebiozen, about which his physician was highly enthusiastic. In fact, knowing that Krebiozen was not an effective treatment, the physician gave Mr. Wright daily injections of nothing but fresh water. The effects were astonishing:

Tumor masses melted. Chest fluid vanished. He became ambulatory and even went back to flying again. At this time he was certainly the picture of health. The water injections were continued since they worked such wonders. He then remained symptom-free for over 2 months. At this time the final AMA announcement appeared in the press—"Nationwide Tests Show Krebiozen to Be a Worthless Drug in Treatment of Cancer."

Within a few days of this report, Mr. Wright was readmitted to the hospital in extremis; his faith was now gone, his last hope vanished, and he succumbed in less than 2 days.

_____

*Source:* Klopfer (1959, p. 339).

peculiar and largely ineffective remedies. Physicians have for centuries been objects of great veneration and respect, and this was no less true when few remedies were actually effective. To what can one attribute the success that these treatments provided? The most likely answer is that these treatments are examples of the **placebo effect.**

## What Is a Placebo?

A **placebo** is "any medical procedure that produces an effect in a patient because of its therapeutic intent and not its specific nature, whether chemical or physical" (Liberman, 1962, p. 761). The word comes originally from Latin, meaning "I will please." Any medical procedure, ranging from drugs to surgery to psychotherapy, can have a placebo effect.

Placebo effects extend well beyond the beneficial results of ineffective substances (Stewart-Williams, 2004; Webb, Simmons, & Brandon, 2005). Much of the effectiveness of active treatments that produce real cures on their own includes a placebo component. For example, in one study (Beecher, 1959), patients complaining of pain were injected with either morphine or a placebo. Although morphine was substantially more effective in reducing pain than was the placebo, the placebo was a successful painkiller in 35 percent of the cases. In summarizing placebo effects, A. K. Shapiro (1964) stated:

Placebos can be more powerful than, and reverse the action of, potent active drugs. . . . The incidence of placebo reactions approaches 100% in some studies. Placebos can have profound effects on organic illnesses, including incurable malignancies. . . .

Placebos can mimic the effects usually thought to be the exclusive property of active drugs. (p. 74)

How does a placebo work? People do not get better only because they think they are going to get better, although expectations play an important role (Geers, Wellman, Fowler, Rasinski, & Helfer, 2011). Nor does a placebo work simply because the patient is distracted from the condition (Buhle, Stevens, Friedman, & Wager, 2012). The placebo response is a complex, psychologically-mediated chain of events that often has physiological effects. For example, if the placebo reduces a negative mood, then activation of stress systems may be reduced (Aslaksen & Flaten, 2008). Placebos may also work in part by stimulating the release of opioids, the body's natural painkillers (Levine, Gordon, & Fields, 1978).

Research that examines brain activity using fMRI (functional magnetic resonance imaging) technology reveals that when patients report reduced pain after taking a placebo, they also show decreased activity in pain-sensitive regions of the brain (Wager et al., 2004). Evidence like this suggests that placebos may work via some of the same biological pathways as "real" treatments (Lieberman et al., 2004; Petrovic, Kalso, Peterson, & Ingvar, 2002). Box 9.6 describes a case of a successful placebo effect with a cancer patient. What factors determine when placebos are most effective?

## Provider Behavior and Placebo Effects

The effectiveness of a placebo varies depending on how a provider treats the patient and how much the provider seems to believe in the treatment (Kelley et al., 2009).

Providers who exude warmth, confidence, and empathy get stronger placebo effects than do more remote and formal providers (Howe, Goyer, & Crum, 2017). Placebo effects are strengthened when the provider radiates competence and provides reassurance to the patient that the condition will improve. Taking time with patients and not rushing them also strengthens placebo effects (Liberman, 1962; Shapiro, 1964). Signs of doubt or skepticism may be communicated subtly, even nonverbally, to a patient, and these signs will reduce the effect.

## Patient Characteristics and Placebo Effects

Some patients show stronger placebo effects than others. People who have a high need for approval or low self-esteem and who are persuadable in other contexts show stronger placebo effects. Anxious people experience stronger placebo effects. This effect seems to result less from personality than from the fact that anxiety produces physical symptoms, including distractibility, racing heart, sweaty palms, nervousness, and difficulty sleeping. When a placebo is administered, anxiety may be reduced, and this overlay of anxiety-related symptoms may disappear (Sharpe, Smith, & Barbre, 1985). When patients are informed that the placebo they will take has no active medicine, the placebo may not work as well or at all (Mathur, Jarrett, Broadbent, & Petrie, 2018).

## Patient–Provider Communication and Placebo Effects

As previously noted, good communication between provider and patient is essential if patients are to follow through on their prescribed treatment regimens. This point is no less true for placebo responses. For patients to show a placebo response, they must understand what the treatment is supposed to do and what they need to do.

One benefit of the placebo is the symbolic value it has for the patient. When patients seek medical treatment, they want an expert to tell them what is wrong and what to do about it. When a disorder is diagnosed and a treatment regimen is prescribed, however ineffective, the patient has tangible evidence that the provider knows what is wrong and has done something about it (Shapiro, 1964).

## Situational Determinants of Placebo Effects

A setting that has the trappings of medical formality (medications, machines, uniformed personnel) will induce stronger placebo effects than will a less formal setting. If all the staff radiate as much faith in the treatment as the physician, placebo effects will be heightened.

The shape, size, color, taste, and quantity of the placebo also influence its effectiveness: The more a drug seems like medicine, the more effective it will be (Shapiro, 1964). Treatment regimens that seem medical and include precise instructions produce stronger placebo effects than regimens that do not seem very medical. Thus, for example, foul-tasting, peculiar-looking little pills that are taken in precise dosages ("take two" as opposed to "take two or three") and at prescribed intervals will show stronger placebo effects than will good-tasting, candy-like pills with dosage levels and intervals that are only roughly indicated ("take one or two anytime you feel discomfort"). People taking placebos can experience side effects, especially if other people apparently do (Faasse, Parkes, Kearney, & Petrie, 2018). Interestingly, changing from a branded to a generic drug appears to reduce the drug's effectiveness and increase side effects, despite no change in the active ingredients (Faasse, Cundy, Gamble, & Petrie, 2013). Not being given a choice of placebos when two alternatives are available also reduces the placebo response (Bartley, Faasse, Horne, & Petrie, 2016).

The nocebo effect refers to the fact that information about potential adverse effects of a condition or treatment may help produce those adverse effects (Webster, Weinman, & Rubin, 2018). The nocebo effect relies on many of the same mechanisms as placebo effects do. That is, negative expectations and lack of choice can influence mood and symptoms just as positive expectations and choice do (Crichton, Dodd, Schmid, Gamble, Cundy, & Petrie, 2014). For example, one study found that exposing people to information suggesting that wind farm noise can have adverse health effects found an increase in symptoms and negative mood (Crichton et al., 2014).

## Social Norms and Placebo Effects

The placebo effect is facilitated by norms that surround treatment regimens—that is, the expected way in which treatment will be enacted. Drug taking is a normative behavior. In 2017, people in the United States spent approximately $333.4 billion on prescription drugs and an additional $64.1 billion on non durable medical products such as over-the-counter drugs (Centers for Medicare and Medicaid Services, 2018). About 40 percent of Americans use at least one prescription medication regularly, and 12 percent use

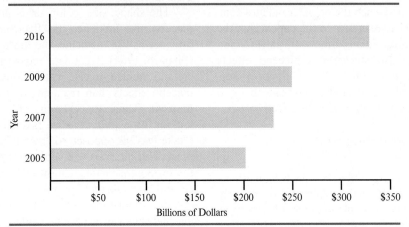

**FIGURE 9.4 | Prescription Drug Spending 2005 to 2016**

*Source:* Centers for Medicare and Medicaid Services, 2011; Hartman, Martin, Espinosa, Catlin, and The National Health Care Spending Team, 2017.

three or more (National Center for Health Statistics, 2009) (Figure 9.4). When people see a physician for an ailment, they may expect and even demand a prescription, which can lead to overprescription (Sirota, Round, Samaranayaka, & Kostopoulou, 2017).

A large number of people are killed or seriously injured each year by overzealous drug taking. Forty-eight percent of people in the United States take at least one prescription drug each month and 11 percent take five or more (Gu, Dillon, & Burt, 2010). There are more than 2.5 million ER visits due to adverse side effects or disabilities in the United States each year (Centers for Disease Control and Prevention, October 2015), which cost hospitals at least $3 billion in longer hospital stays and other complications (Hansen, Oster, Edelsberg, Woody, & Sullivan, 2011). The more general cost to society of adverse drug reactions is estimated to be $55.7 billion a year (Centers for Disease Control and Prevention, October 2015). However, the drug-taking epidemic continues unabated. Clearly, there is enormous faith in medications, and the psychological if not the physical benefits can be quite substantial. Thus, placebos are effective in part because people believe that drugs work and because they have a great deal of experience with drug taking.

Equally important is the fact that most people have no experience that disconfirms their drug taking. If one is ill, takes a drug, and subsequently gets better, as most of us do most of the time, one does not in reality know exactly what caused this result. A drug may be responsible; the disease may have run its course; or

one's mood may have picked up, altering the body's physiological balance and making it no longer receptive to an invader. Probably a combination of factors is at work. Regardless of the actual cause of success, the patient acting as his or her own naïve physician will probably attribute success to whatever drug he or she took, however erroneous that conclusion may be.

## The Placebo as a Methodological Tool

The placebo response is so powerful that no drug can be marketed in the United States unless it has been evaluated against a placebo. The standard method for so doing is termed a **double-blind experiment.** In such a test, a researcher gives one group of patients a drug that is supposed to cure a disease or alleviate symptoms; another group receives a placebo. The procedure is called double-blind because neither the researcher nor the patient knows whether the patient received the drug or the placebo; both are "blind" to the procedure. Once the effectiveness of the treatment has been measured, the researcher looks in the coded records to see which treatment each patient received. The difference between the effectiveness of the drug and the effectiveness of the placebo is considered to be a measure of the drug's effectiveness (America & Milling, 2008). Comparison of a drug against a placebo is essential for accurate measurement of a drug's effect. Drugs may look four or five times more successful than they really are if there is no effort to evaluate them against a placebo (Miller, 1989). •

| S U M M A R Y |
| --- |

1. Patients evaluate their health care based more on the quality of the interaction they have with the provider than on the technical quality of care.

2. Many factors can impede effective patient–provider communication. The office setting and the structure of the health care delivery system are often designed for efficient rather than supportive health care.

3. Providers contribute to poor communication by not listening, using jargon-filled explanations, alternating between overly technical explanations and infantilizing baby talk, communicating negative expectations, and depersonalizing the patient.

4. Patients contribute to poor communication by failing to learn details of their disorder and treatment, failing to give providers correct information, and failing to follow through on treatment recommendations. Patient anxiety, lack of education, and lack of experience with the disorder interfere with effective communication as well.

5. Because the provider usually receives little feedback about whether the patient followed instructions or the treatments were successful, it is difficult to identify and correct problems in communication.

6. Poor communication leads to nonadherence to treatment and, potentially, the initiation of malpractice litigation.

7. Adherence to treatment is lower when recommendations do not seem medical, when lifestyle modification is needed, when complex self-care regimens are required, and when patients hold theories about the nature of their illness or treatment that conflict with medical theories.

8. Adherence is increased when patients have decided to adhere, when they feel the provider cares about them, when they understand what to do, and when they have received clear written instructions.

9. Efforts to improve communication include training in communication skills. Patient-centered communication improves adherence. Face-to-face communication with a physician can enhance adherence to treatment because of the personalized relationship that exists.

10. The hospital is a complex organizational system buffeted by changing medical, organizational, and financial climates. Different groups in the hospital have different goals, such as cure, care, or core, which may occasionally conflict. Such problems are exacerbated by communication barriers.

11. Hospitalization can be a frightening and depersonalizing experience for patients. The adverse reactions of children in hospitals have received particular attention.

12. Information and control-enhancing interventions improve adjustment to hospitalization and to stressful medical procedures such as surgery in both adults and children.

13. Nearly two-thirds of adults in the United States use complementary and alternative medicine (CAM) instead of or in conjunction with traditional medicine. The most common of these are prayer and herbal or vitamin supplements. Other common CAM therapies include meditation, yoga, massage, acupuncture, chiropracty, osteopathy, hypnosis, and guided imagery.

14. People are more likely to turn to CAM therapies if their disorders have not been successfully treated by traditional medicine. Evaluation of CAM therapies has been difficult because they are often individualized, and thus, treatment does not conform to standards required for formal evaluation using standards of evidence-based medicine.

15. Overall, the evidence for CAM therapies suggests success of certain therapies for the management of pain. For other disorders, there is not yet sufficient evidence.

16. A placebo is any medical procedure that produces an effect in a patient because of its therapeutic intent and not its actual nature. Virtually every medical treatment shows some degree of placebo effect.

17. Placebo effects are enhanced when the physician shows faith in a treatment, the patient is

predisposed to believe that it will work, these expectations are successfully communicated, and the trappings of medical treatment are in place.

18. Placebos are also a vital methodological tool in evaluating drugs and other treatments.

## KEY TERMS

acupuncture
adherence
ayurvedic medicine
chiropractic medicine
colleague orientation
complementary and alternative medicine (CAM)
creative nonadherence
dietary supplements

double-blind experiment
guided imagery
health maintenance organization (HMO)
holistic medicine
homeopathy
hypnosis
integrative medicine
managed care

nonadherence
patient-centered care
placebo
placebo effect
preferred-provider organization (PPO)
private, fee-for-service care
Traditional Chinese Medicine
yoga

# CHAPTER 10

# The Management of Pain and Discomfort

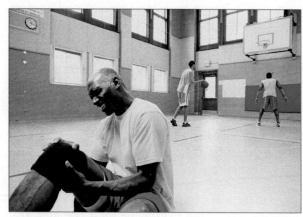

Andersen Ross/Blend Images LLC

Pain hurts, and it can be so insistent that it overwhelms other basic needs. But the significance of pain goes beyond the disruption it produces. Although we think of pain as an unusual occurrence, we actually live with minor pains all the time. These pains are critical for survival because they provide low-level feedback about the functioning of our bodily systems. We use this feedback, often unconsciously, as a basis for making minor adjustments, such as shifting our posture, rolling over while asleep, or crossing and uncrossing our legs.

Pain also has medical significance. It is the symptom most likely to lead a person to seek treatment (see Chapter 8). It can complicate illnesses and hamper recovery from medical procedures (McGuire et al., 2006). Complaints of pain often accompany mental and other physical disorders, and this comorbidity

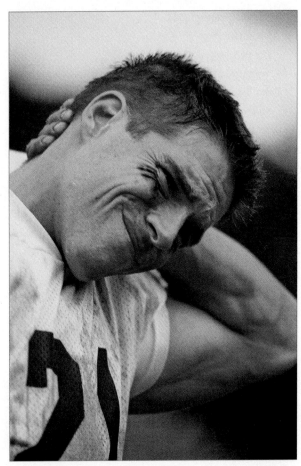

*Pain is a valuable cue that tissue damage has occurred and activities must be curtailed.*

Eyewire/Getty Images

further complicates diagnosis and treatment (Berna et al., 2010; Kalaydjian & Merikangas, 2008). Unfortunately, the relationship between pain and the severity of an underlying problem can be weak. For example, a cancerous lump rarely produces pain, at least in its early stages, yet it is of great medical importance.

Pain is also medically significant because it can be a source of misunderstanding between a patient and the medical provider. From the patient's standpoint, pain is the problem. To the provider, pain is a by-product of a disorder. In fact, pain is often considered by practitioners to be so unimportant that until recently many medical schools had little systematic coverage of pain in their curricula. This lack of attention to pain is misguided. Although the practitioner focuses attention on symptoms, which, from a medical standpoint, may be more meaningful, the patient may feel that pain is the important problem and it is not getting sufficient attention. As we saw in Chapter 9, patients may choose not to comply with their physician's recommendations if they think they have been misdiagnosed or if their chief symptoms have been ignored.

Pain has psychological as well as medical significance. When patients are asked what they fear most about illness and its treatment, the common response is pain. The dread of not being able to reduce one's suffering arouses more anxiety than the prospect of surgery, the loss of a limb, or even death. In fact, inadequate relief from pain is the most common reason for a patient's request for euthanasia or assisted suicide (Cherny, 1996). Moreover, depression, anxiety, guilt, and anger worsen the experience of pain (Burns et al., 2016; Serbic, Pincus, Fife-Schaw, & Dawson, 2016).

Pain has social causes and consequences (Burns et al., 2016). Although social support is usually helpful to people undergoing chronic problems, social support for pain can inadvertently act as reinforcement of pain behaviors, which then become part of the pain problem. Moreover, physical pain overlaps with social pain (Eisenberger, 2012a, 2012b). That is, social pain, namely the feeling of social rejection or loss, relies on the same pain-related neurocircuitry that physical pain relies on, suggesting that there are meaningful similarities in the way that social and physical pain are experienced. These insights may also help explain why psychological distress is such a key component of physical pain.

No introduction to pain would be complete without a consideration of its prevalence and cost. Chronic

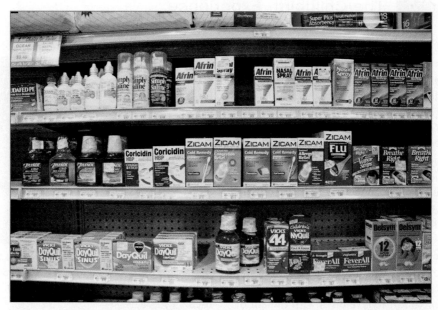

At least $2.6 billion is spent annually in the United States on over-the-counter remedies to reduce the temporary pain of minor disorders.
Erica Simone Leeds

pain lasting at least 6 months or longer affects nearly 116 million people in the United States (Jensen & Turk, 2014), and costs in disability and lost productivity add up to more than $560 billion annually (The Wall Street Journal, February 7, 2019). Fifty-four percent of people in the United States suffer from chronic back pain for 5 years or longer, 54 million people suffer from daily arthritis pain, around 2 to 4 percent of the world's adult population suffers from chronic headaches, and one in three people treated for cancer suffer moderate to severe pain (American Cancer Society, May 2017; Centers for Disease Control and Prevention, January 2019; World Health Organization, April 2016). Over 40 percent of people who live in nursing homes have chronic pain (Hunnicutt, Ulbricht, Tjia, & Lapane, 2017). Even children can experience chronic pain (Palermo, Valrie, & Karlson, 2014). In 2017, there were about 58 opioid prescriptions for pain modulation written for every 100 Americans (Centers for Disease Control and Prevention, 2018). In the United States, the use of addictive pain killers contributes to declining life expectancy among poorly educated whites (Case & Deaton, 2015). The pain business is big business, reflecting the suffering, both chronic and temporary, that millions of people experience.

## ■ THE ELUSIVE NATURE OF PAIN

Pain is one of the more elusive aspects of illness and its treatment. It is fundamentally a psychological experience, and the degree to which it is felt and how incapacitating it is depend in large part on how it is interpreted. Howard Beecher (1959), a physician, was one of the first to recognize this. During World War II, Beecher served in the medical corps, where he observed many wartime injuries. In treating soldiers, he noticed a curious fact: Only 25 percent of them requested morphine (a widely used painkiller) for what were often severe and very likely painful wounds. When Beecher returned to his Boston civilian practice, he often treated patients who sustained comparable injuries from surgery. However, in contrast to the soldiers, 80 percent of the civilians appeared to be in great pain and demanded painkillers. To make sense of this apparent discrepancy, Beecher concluded that the meaning attached to pain substantially determines how it is experienced. For the soldier, an injury meant that he was alive and was likely to be sent home. For the civilian, the injury represented an unwelcome interruption of valued activities.

Pain is also heavily influenced by the context in which it is experienced. Sports lore is full of accounts

BOX 10.1

# A Cross-Cultural Perspective on Pain: The Childbirth Experience

Although babies are born in every society, the childbirth experience varies dramatically from culture to culture, and so does the experience of pain associated with it. Among Mexican women, for example, the word for labor (dolor) means sorrow or pain, and the expectation of giving birth can produce a great deal of fear. This fear and the anticipation of pain can lead to a more painful experience with more complications than is true for women who do not bring these fears and expectations to the birthing experience (Scrimshaw, Engle, & Zambrana, 1983).

In contrast is the culture of Yap in the South Pacific, where childbirth is treated as an everyday occurrence. Women in Yap perform their normal activities until they begin labor, at which time they retire to a childbirth hut to give birth with the aid of perhaps one or two other women. Following the birth, there is a brief period of rest, after which the woman resumes her activities. Problematic labors

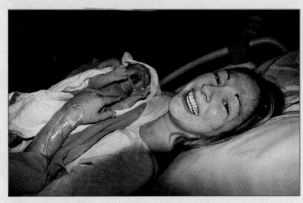

*The meaning attached to an experience substantially determines whether it is perceived as painful. For many women, the joy of childbirth can mute the pain associated with the experience.*
Digital Vision/Getty Images

and complications during pregnancy are reported to be low (Kroeber, 1948).

---

of athletes who injured themselves on the playing field but stayed in the game, apparently oblivious to their pain. One reason is that sympathetic arousal, as occurs in response to vigorous sports, diminishes pain sensitivity (Fillingham & Maixner, 1996; Zillman, de Wied, King-Jablonski, & Jenzowsky, 1996). In contrast, stress and psychological distress aggravate the experience of pain (Strigo, Simmons, Matthews, Craig, & Paulus, 2008).

Pain has a substantial cultural component. People from some cultures report pain sooner and react more intensely to it than individuals from other cultures (Lu, Zeltzer, & Tsao, 2013; Palit et al., 2013). An example of these kinds of cultural differences appears in Box 10.1. There are gender differences in the experience of pain as well, with women typically showing greater sensitivity to pain (Burns, Elfant, & Quartana, 2010).

## Measuring Pain

One barrier to the treatment of pain is the difficulty people have in describing it objectively. If you have a lump, you can point to it; if a bone is broken, it can be seen in an X-ray. But pain does not have these objective referents.

**Verbal Reports**    One solution to measuring pain is to draw on the large, informal vocabulary that people use for describing pain. Medical practitioners usually use this information to understand patients' complaints. A throbbing pain, for example, has different implications than does a shooting pain or a constant, dull ache.

Researchers have developed pain questionnaires to assess pain (Osman, Breitenstein, Barrios, Gutierrez, & Kopper, 2002) (Figure 10.1). Such measures typically ask about the nature of pain, such as whether it is throbbing or shooting, as well as its intensity (Dar, Leventhal, & Leventhal, 1993; Fernandez & Turk, 1992). Measures also address the psychosocial components of pain, such as how much fear it causes and how much it has taken over a person's life (Osman et al., 2000). Measures like these can help practitioners get a full picture of the patient's pain. A novel effort to assess pain appears in Box 10.2.

Methodological tools from neuroscience have yielded insights about pain. Patients with chronic pain disorders show significant loss of gray matter in the brain regions involved in the processing of pain, specifically the prefrontal, cingular, and insular cortex (Valet et al., 2009). These structural markers not only provide objective neural information about changes in the brain due to pain, but may also be useful for

**FIGURE 10.1 | The McGill Pain Questionnaire**   *Source:* Melzack, Ronald. *Pain Measurement and Assessment*. New York: Raven Press, 1983.

Patient's name _____   Date _____   Time _____ A.M./P.M.

| | | | | |
|---|---|---|---|---|
| **1** Flickering —<br>Quivering —<br>Pulsing —<br>Throbbing —<br>Beating —<br>Pounding —<br>**2** Jumping —<br>Flashing —<br>Shooting —<br>**3** Pricking —<br>Boring —<br>Drilling —<br>Stabbing —<br>Lancinating —<br>**4** Sharp —<br>Cutting —<br>Lacerating —<br>**5** Pinching —<br>Pressing —<br>Gnawing —<br>Cramping —<br>Crushing —<br>**6** Tugging —<br>Pulling —<br>Wrenching —<br>**7** Hot —<br>Burning —<br>Scalding —<br>Searing —<br>**8** Tingling —<br>Itchy —<br>Smarting —<br>Stinging —<br>**9** Dull —<br>Sore —<br>Hurting —<br>Aching —<br>Heavy —<br>**10** Tender —<br>Taut —<br>Rasping —<br>Splitting — | **11** Tiring —<br>Exhausting —<br>**12** Sickening —<br>Suffocating —<br>**13** Fearful —<br>Frightful —<br>Terrifying —<br>**14** Punishing —<br>Grueling —<br>Cruel —<br>Vicious —<br>Killing —<br>**15** Wretched —<br>Blinding —<br>**16** Annoying —<br>Troublesome —<br>Miserable —<br>Intense —<br>Unbearable —<br>**17** Spreading —<br>Radiating —<br>Penetrating —<br>Piercing —<br>**18** Tight —<br>Numb —<br>Drawing —<br>Squeezing —<br>Tearing —<br>**19** Cool —<br>Cold —<br>Freezing —<br>**20** Nagging —<br>Nauseating —<br>Agonizing —<br>Dreadful —<br>Torturing —<br>PPI<br>**0** No pain —<br>**1** Mild —<br>**2** Discomforting —<br>**3** Distressing —<br>**4** Horrible —<br>**5** Excruciating — | Brief —<br>Momentary —<br>Transient — | Rhythmic —<br>Periodic —<br>Intermittent — | Continuous —<br>Steady —<br>Constant — |

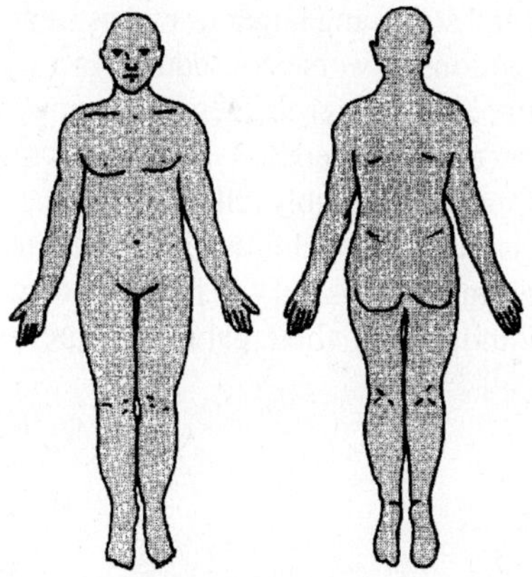

E = External
I = Internal

Comments:

charting functional pain disorders, such as fibromyalgia, in which no clear tissue damage is present.

Pain Behavior   Other assessments of pain have focused on **pain behaviors**—behaviors that arise from chronic pain, such as distortions in posture or gait, facial and audible expressions of distress, and avoidance of activities (Turk, Wack, & Kerns, 1995). Pain behaviors provide a basis for assessing how pain has disrupted a person's life. Because pain behavior is observable and

BOX **10.2** Headache Drawings Reflect Distress and Disability

A recent way that psychologists have come to understand people's experiences with pain is through their drawings. In one study, students who experienced persistent headaches were asked to draw a picture of how their headaches affected them. The psychologists (Broadbent, Niederhoffer, Hague, Corter, & Reynolds, 2009) analyzed these drawings for their size, darkness, and content.

They found that darker drawings were associated with greater emotional distress and larger drawings were associated with perceptions of worse consequences and symptoms, more pain, and greater sadness. Drawings, then, offer a novel way to assess people's experiences of their headaches and appear to reliably reflect illness perceptions and distress (Kirkham, Smith, & Havsteen-Franklin, 2015). These may be a useful way for practicing clinicians to better understand their patients' experiences of pain.

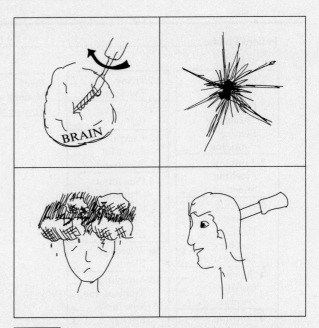

*Source:* Broadbent, E., Kate Niederhoffer, Tiffany Hague, Arden L. Corter, and L. Reynolds. "Headache Sufferers' Drawings Reflect Distress, Disability and Illness Perceptions." *Journal of Psychosomatic Research* 66, no. 5 (2009): 465–470. doi:10.1016/j.jpsychores.2008.09.006.

measurable, the focus on pain behaviors has helped define the characteristics of different kinds of pain syndromes.

## The Physiology of Pain

Pain has psychological, behavioral, and sensory components, and this perspective is useful for making sense of the manifold pathways and receptors involved in the pain experience.

**Overview** The experience of pain is a protective mechanism to bring tissue damage into conscious awareness. At the time of the pain experience, however, it is unlikely to feel very protective. Unlike other bodily sensations, the experience of pain is accompanied by motivational and behavioral responses, such as withdrawal, and intense emotional reactions, such as crying or fear, and both verbal and nonverbal communications to others who can ameliorate or enhance the pain experience (Hadjistavropoulos et al., 2011). All of these factors are an integral part of the pain experience and are important to diagnosis and treatment.

Emotional factors are greatly intertwined with the experience of pain. Negative emotions exacerbate pain, and pain exacerbates negative emotions (Gilliam et al., 2010). As will be seen, these emotions often need to be targeted alongside the management of pain itself.

Scientists have distinguished among three kinds of pain perception. The first is mechanical **nociception**— pain perception—that results from mechanical damage to the tissues of the body. The second is thermal damage, or the experience of pain due to temperature exposure. The third is referred to as polymodal nociception, a general category referring to pain that triggers chemical reactions from tissue damage.

**Gate-Control Theory of Pain** Originally, the scientific understanding of pain was developed in the **gate-control theory of pain** (Melzack & Wall, 1982). Although our knowledge of the physiology of pain has now progressed beyond that early model, it was central to the progress that has been made in recent decades. Many of its insights are reflected in our current knowledge of the physiology of pain.

**FIGURE 10.2** | **The Experience of Pain**   The signal from an injured area goes to the spinal cord, where it passes immediately to a motor nerve (1) connected to a muscle, in this case, in the arm. This causes a reflex action that does not involve the brain. But the signal also goes up the spinal cord to the thalamus (2), where the pain is perceived.

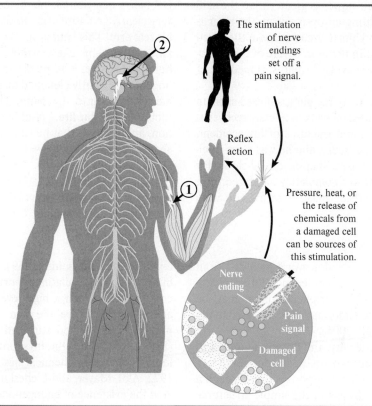

Nociceptors in the peripheral nerves first sense injury and, in response, release chemical messengers, which are conducted to the spinal cord, where they are passed directly to the reticular formation and thalamus and into the cerebral cortex. These regions of the brain, in turn, identify the site of the injury and send messages back down the spinal cord, which lead to muscle contractions, which can help block the pain, and changes in other bodily functions, such as breathing.

Two major types of peripheral nerve fibers are involved in nociception. A-delta fibers are small, myelinated fibers that transmit sharp pain. They respond especially to mechanical or thermal pain, transmitting sharp, brief pains rapidly. C-fibers are unmyelinated nerve fibers, involved in polymodal pain, that transmit dull, aching pain. (Myelination increases the speed of transmission, so sudden, intense pain is more rapidly conducted to the cerebral cortex than is the slower, dull, aching pain of the C-fibers.)

Peripheral nerve fibers enter the spinal column at the dorsal horn. Sensory aspects of pain are heavily determined by activity in the A-delta fibers, which project onto areas in the thalamus and the sensory areas of the cerebral cortex (see Figure 10.2). The motivational and affective elements of pain appear to be influenced more strongly by the C-fibers, which project onto different thalamic, hypothalamic, and cortical areas. The experience of pain, then, is determined by the balance of activity in these nerve fibers, which reflects the pattern and intensity of stimulation.

Several other regions of the brain are involved in the modulation of pain (Derbyshire, 2014). The periaqueductal gray, a structure in the midbrain, has been tied to pain relief when it is stimulated. Neurons in the periaqueductal gray connect to the reticular formation in the medulla, which makes connections with the neurons in the substantia gelatinosa of the dorsal horn of the spinal cord. Sensations are modulated by the dorsal horn

Nerve injury of the shoulder is becoming increasingly common because motorcycles are widely accessible and, all too often, their power is greater than the skill of their riders. On hitting an obstruction, the rider is catapulted forward and hits the road at about the speed the bike was traveling. In the most severe of these injuries, the spinal roots are avulsed—that is, ripped out of the spinal cord—and no repair is possible.

C. A., age 25, an Air Force pilot, suffered such an accident. After 8 months, he had completely recovered from the cuts, bruises, and fractures of his accident. There had been no head injury, and he was alert, intelligent, and busy as a student shaping a new career for himself. His right arm was completely paralyzed from the shoulder down, and the muscles of his arm were

thin. In addition, the limp arm was totally anesthetic so that he had no sensation of any stimuli applied to it. On being questioned, he stated that he could sense very clearly an entire arm, but it had no relationship to his real arm. This "phantom" arm seemed to him to be placed across his chest, while the real, paralyzed arm hung at his side. The phantom never moved and the fingers were tightly clenched in a cramped fist, with the nails digging into the palm. The entire arm felt "as though it was on fire." Nothing has helped his condition, and he finds that he can control the pain only by absorbing himself in his work.

*Source:* Melzack & Wall (1982, pp. 21–22).

in the spinal column and by downward pathways from the brain that interpret the pain experience. Inflammation that originally occurs in peripheral tissue may be amplified, as pain-related information is conveyed to the dorsal horn (Ikeda et al., 2006).

Pain sensation, intensity, and duration interact to influence the experience of pain, its perceived unpleasantness, and emotional responses to it through a central network of pathways in the limbic structures and the thalamus, which direct their inputs to the cortex. In the cortical regions of the brain, nociceptive input is integrated with contextual information about the painful experience. Processes in the cerebral cortex are involved in cognitive judgments about pain, including the evaluation of its meaning, which contributes to the strong emotions often experienced during pain and which can themselves exacerbate pain. The overall experience of pain, then, is a complex outcome of the interaction of these elements of the pain experience (Figure 10.2). An example of just how complex pain and its management can be is provided in Box 10.3.

## Neurochemical Bases of Pain and Its Inhibition

The brain controls the amount of pain an individual experiences by transmitting messages down the spinal cord to block the transmission of pain signals. One landmark study that confirmed this hypothesis was

conducted by Reynolds (1969). He demonstrated that by electrically stimulating a portion of a rat brain, one could produce such a high level of analgesia that the animal would not feel the pain of abdominal surgery, a phenomenon termed stimulation-produced analgesia (SPA). Reynolds's findings prompted researchers to look for the neurochemical basis of this effect, and in 1972, Akil, Mayer, and Liebeskind (1972, 1976) uncovered the existence of endogenous opioid peptides.

What are **endogenous opioid peptides**? Opiates, including heroin and morphine, are pain control drugs manufactured from plants. Opioids are opiate-like substances, produced within the body, that constitute a neurochemically based, internal pain regulation system. Opioids are produced in many parts of the brain and glands of the body, and they project onto specific receptor sites in various parts of the body.

Endogenous opioid peptides are important because they are the natural pain suppression system of the body. Clearly, however, this pain suppression system is not always in operation. Particular factors must trigger its arousal. Stress is one such factor. Acute stress reduces sensitivity to pain, a phenomenon termed stress-induced analgesia (SIA), and SIA can be accompanied by an increase in brain endogenous opioid peptides (Lewis, Terman, Shavit, Nelson, & Liebeskind, 1984). The release of endogenous opioid peptides may also be one of the mechanisms underlying various techniques of pain control (Bolles & Fanselow, 1982).

## ■ CLINICAL ISSUES IN PAIN MANAGEMENT

Historically, pain has been managed by physicians and other health care workers. Traditional pain management methods include pharmacological, surgical, and sensory techniques. Increasingly, psychologists have become involved in pain management, adding techniques that include a heavily psychological component. These techniques include relaxation, hypnosis, acupuncture, biofeedback, distraction, and guided imagery. As these methods have gained prominence, the importance of patients' self-management, involving responsibility for and commitment to the course of pain treatment, has assumed centrality in pain management.

### Acute and Chronic Pain

There are two main kinds of clinical pain: acute and chronic. **Acute pain** typically results from a specific injury that produces tissue damage, such as a wound or broken limb. As such, it typically disappears when the tissue damage is repaired. Acute pain is usually short in duration and is defined as pain that goes on for 6 months or less. Although it can produce substantial anxiety, anxiety dissipates once painkillers are administered or the injury begins to heal. **Chronic pain** typically begins with an acute episode, but unlike acute pain, it does not decrease with treatment and the passage of time.

There are several different kinds of chronic pain. **Chronic benign pain** typically persists for 6 months or longer and is relatively unresponsive to treatment. The pain varies in severity and may involve any of several muscle groups. Chronic low back pain, which affects about one-third of people in the United States, is an example (Pegram, Lumley, Jasinski, & Burns, 2016).

**Recurrent acute pain** involves intermittent episodes of pain that are acute in character but chronic inasmuch as the condition recurs for more than 6 months. Migraine headaches, temporomandibular disorder (involving the jaw), and trigeminal neuralgia (involving spasms of the facial muscles) are examples.

**Chronic progressive pain** persists longer than 6 months and increases in severity over time. Typically, it is associated with malignancies or degenerative disorders, such as cancer or rheumatoid arthritis. About 116 million Americans suffer from chronic pain at any given time (Jensen & Turk, 2014), with back pain being the most common (Table 10.1). Chronic pain is not necessarily present every moment, but the fact that it

**TABLE 10.1 | Common Sources of Chronic Pain**

- Back pain—70–85 percent of Americans have back trouble at some point in their lives.
- Headaches—approximately 45 million Americans have chronic recurrent headaches.
- Cancer pain—the majority of advanced cancer patients suffer moderate to severe pain.
- Arthritis pain—arthritis affects 40 million Americans.
- Neurogenic pain—pain resulting from damage to peripheral nerves or the central nervous system.
- Psychogenic pain—pain not due to an identifiable physical cause.

*Source:* U.S. Department of Health & Human Services. National Institute of Neurological Disorders and Stroke. "Pain: Hope Through Research." Last Modified August 08, 2018.

is chronic virtually forces sufferers to organize their lives around it.

**Acute Versus Chronic Pain**    The distinction between acute and chronic pain is important in clinical management for several reasons. First, acute pain and chronic pain present different psychological profiles. Chronic pain often carries an overlay of psychological distress, which complicates diagnosis and treatment. Depression, anxiety, and anger are common and may exacerbate pain and pain-related behaviors (Bair, Wu, Damush, Sutherland, & Kroenke, 2008; Burns et al., 2008). One study found that pain is present in two-thirds of patients who seek care from physicians with primary symptoms of depression (Bair et al., 2004). Thus, pain and depression appear to be especially heavily intertwined.

Some chronic pain patients develop maladaptive coping strategies, such as catastrophizing their illness, engaging in wishful thinking, or withdrawing socially, which can complicate treatment and lead to more care seeking (Özkan, Zale, Ring, & Vranceanu, 2017). When patients have endured their pain for long periods of time without any apparent relief, it is easy to imagine that the pain will only get worse and be a constant part of the rest of their life—beliefs that magnify the distress of chronic pain and feed back into the pain itself (Tennen, Affleck, & Zautra, 2006; Vowles, McCracken, & Eccleston, 2008). When these psychological issues are effectively treated, this fact may in itself reduce chronic pain (Fishbain, Cutler, Rosomoff, & Rosomoff, 1998).

A second reason to distinguish between acute pain and chronic pain is that most pain control techniques

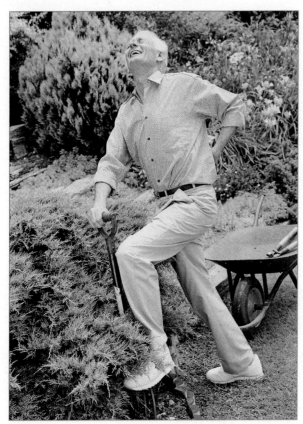

*More than 116 million Americans, many of them elderly, suffer from chronic pain.*

BananaStock/Alamy Stock Photo

work well to control acute pain but are less successful with chronic pain, which requires individualized techniques for its management.

Third, chronic pain involves the complex interaction of physiological, psychological, social, and behavioral components, more than is the case with acute pain. For example, chronic pain patients often experience social rewards from the attention they receive from family members, friends, or even employers; these social rewards, or secondary gains, can help maintain pain behaviors (McClelland & McCubbin, 2008).

The psychological and social components of pain are important because they are an integral aspect of the pain experience and influence the likelihood of successful pain control (Burns, 2000). As such, chronic pain management is complicated and must be thought of not as merely addressing a pain that simply goes on for a long time but as an unfolding complex physiological, psychological, and behavioral experience that evolves over time into a syndrome (Jensen & Turk, 2014).

**Who Becomes a Chronic Pain Patient?**    All chronic pain patients were once acute pain patients. What determines who makes the transition to chronic pain? Chronic pain may result from a predisposition to react to a bodily insult with a specific bodily response, such as tensing one's jaw or altering one's posture (Glombiewski, Tersek, & Rief, 2008). This response can be exacerbated by stress or even by efforts to suppress pain (Quartana, Burns, & Lofland, 2007). Chronic pain patients may experience pain especially strongly because of high sensitivity to noxious stimulation, impairment in pain regulatory systems, and an overlay of psychological distress (Sherman et al., 2004).

Unlike acute pain, chronic pain usually has been treated through a variety of methods, used both by patients themselves and by physicians. Chronic pain may be exacerbated by inappropriate prior treatments, by misdiagnosis, and/or by inappropriate prescriptions of medications (Kouyanou, Pither, & Wessely, 1997).

**The Lifestyle of Chronic Pain**    By the time a pain patient is adequately treated, this complex, dynamic interaction of physiological, psychological, social, and behavioral components is often tightly integrated, making it difficult to modify (Flor et al., 1990). The following case history suggests the disruption and agony that can be experienced by the chronic pain sufferer:

> A little over a year ago, George Zessi, 54, a New York furrier, suddenly began to have excruciating migraine headaches. The attacks occurred every day and quickly turned Zessi into a pain cripple. "I felt like I was suffering a hangover each morning without even having touched a drop. I was seasick without going near a boat," he says. Because of the nausea that often accompanies migraines, Zessi lost fifty pounds. At his workshop, Zessi found himself so sensitive that he could not bear the ringing of a telephone. "I was incapacitated. It was difficult to talk to anyone. On weekends, I couldn't get out of bed," he says. A neurologist conducted a thorough examination and told Zessi he was suffering from tension. He took several kinds of drugs, but they did not dull his daily headaches. (Clark, 1977, p. 58)

As this case history suggests, chronic pain can entirely disrupt a person's life (Karoly, Okun, Enders, & Tennen, 2014). Many chronic pain patients have left their jobs, abandoned their leisure activities, withdrawn from their families and friends, and developed an entire lifestyle around pain. Because their income is often reduced, their standard of living may decline, and they may need public assistance. Economic hardship increases the experience of pain as well (Rios & Zautra, 2011). The pain lifestyle becomes oriented around the experience of pain and its treatment. A good night's sleep is often elusive for months or years at a time; lack of sleep makes pain worse, and pain leads to sleep loss in a vicious cycle (Gasperi, Herbert, Schur, Buchwald, & Afari, 2017). Work-related aspirations and personal goals may be set aside because life has become dominated by chronic pain (Karoly & Ruehlman, 1996). The loss of self-esteem that is experienced by these patients can be substantial.

Some patients receive compensation for their pain because it resulted from an injury, such as an automobile accident. Compensation can actually increase the perceived severity of pain, the amount of disability experienced, the degree to which pain interferes with life activities, and the amount of distress that is reported (Ciccone, Just, & Bandilla, 1999; Groth-Marnat & Fletcher, 2000), because it provides an incentive for being in pain.

**The Toll of Pain on Relationships**   Chronic pain takes a toll on marriage and other family relationships. Chronic pain patients may not communicate well with their families, and sexual relationships almost always deteriorate. A meta-analysis of 103 pain experiences revealed that, although family and health care professionals have a rough idea of what the patient is going through, they typically underestimate the patient's pain (Ruben, Blanch-Hartigan, & Shipherd, 2018). Among those chronic pain patients whose spouses are supportive, such positive attention may inadvertently maintain the pain and disability (Ciccone, Just, & Bandilla, 1999; Turk, Kerns, & Rosenberg, 1992). Adolescent chronic pain patients may be rejected or even bullied by their peers (Fales, Rice, Aaron, & Palermo, 2018). Nonetheless, as it does for so many other negative experiences, social support can buffer the adverse effects of chronic pain (Matos, Bernardes, Goubert, & Beyers, 2017).

**Chronic Pain Behaviors**   Chronic pain leads to a variety of pain-related behaviors that can also maintain the pain experience. For example, sufferers may avoid loud noises and bright lights, reduce physical activity, and shun social contacts. These alterations in lifestyle then become part of the pain problem and may persist and interfere with successful treatment

(Philips, 1983). Understanding what pain behaviors an individual engages in and knowing whether they persist after the treatment of pain are important factors in treating the total pain experience.

## Pain and Personality

Because psychological factors are so clearly implicated in the experience of pain, and because pain serves psychological functions for some chronic pain sufferers, researchers have examined whether there is a **pain-prone personality**—a constellation of personality traits that predispose a person to experience chronic pain.

This hypothesis is too simplistic. First, pain itself can produce alterations in personality and behavior that are consequences, not causes, of the pain experience. For example, memories of previous painful experiences can affect subsequent ones (Noel, Rabbitts, Fales, Chorney, & Palermo, 2017). Second, individual experiences of pain are too varied and complex to be explained by a single profile. Nonetheless, certain personality attributes are reliably associated with chronic pain, including neuroticism, introversion, and the use of passive coping strategies (Ramirez-Maestre, Lopez-Martinez, & Zarazaga, 2004). Pre existing psychological distress, including anxiety, PTSD, loneliness, depression, and fatigue, can also aggravate the pain process (Jaremka et al., 2014; Ruiz-Párraga & López-Martínez, 2014; Vassend, Røysamb, Nielsen, & Czajkowski, 2017).

**Pain Profiles**   Developing psychological profiles of different groups of pain patients has proven to be helpful for treatment. To develop profiles, researchers have drawn on personality instruments, such as the Minnesota Multiphasic Personality Inventory (MMPI) (Johansson & Lindberg, 2000). Chronic pain patients typically show elevated scores on three MMPI subscales: hypochondriasis, hysteria, and depression. This constellation of traits is commonly referred to as the "neurotic triad."

Depression reflects the feelings of despair or hopelessness that can accompany long-term experience with unsuccessfully treated pain. Depression increases perceptions of pain (Dickens, McGowan, & Dale, 2003), and so it can feed back into the total pain experience, increasing the likelihood of pain behaviors such as leaving work (Linton & Buer, 1995). Interventions with depressed pain patients must address both depression and pain (Ingram, Atkinson, Slater, Saccuzzo, & Garfin, 1990).

Chronic pain can lead to a sense of injustice. The frustration of having goals and interests thwarted and the fact that other people cannot help much can lead to anger and ultimately social isolation (Sturgeon, Carriere, Kao, Rico, & Darnall, 2016).

People who suppress their anger may experience pain more strongly than people who manage anger more effectively or people who do not experience as much anger (Burns, Quartana, & Bruehl, 2008; Quartana, Bounds, Yoon, Goodin, & Burns, 2010). The relation of anger suppression and pain may be due to a dysfunction in the opioid system that controls pain or to psychological processes involving hypervigilance (Bruehl, Burns, Chung, & Quartana, 2008).

Chronic pain can also be associated with other complicating disorders, including anxiety disorders, substance use disorders, and PTSD (Nash, Williams, Nicholson, & Trask, 2006; Turk & Gatchel, 2018; Vowles, Zvolensky, Gross, & Sperry, 2004). The reason chronic pain and psychiatric disorders are so frequently associated is not fully known. One possibility is that chronic pain activates latent psychological vulnerabilities (Dersh, Polatin, & Gatchel, 2002).

## ■ PAIN CONTROL TECHNIQUES

What is **pain control**? Pain control can mean that a patient no longer feels anything in an area that once hurt. It can mean that the person feels sensation but not pain. It can mean that he or she feels pain but is no longer concerned about it. Or it can mean that the person is still hurting but is now able to tolerate it.

Some pain control techniques work because they eliminate feeling altogether (e.g., spinal blocking agents), whereas others succeed because they reduce pain to sensation (such as sensory control techniques), and still others succeed because they enable patients to tolerate pain more successfully (such as psychological approaches). It will be useful to bear these distinctions in mind as we evaluate the success of specific pain control techniques.

### Pharmacological Control of Pain

The traditional and most common method of controlling pain is through the administration of drugs. Morphine (named after Morpheus, the Greek god of sleep) has been the most popular painkiller for decades (Melzack & Wall, 1982). A highly effective painkiller, morphine has the disadvantage of addiction, and patients may build up a tolerance to it. Currently, opioid medications are widely prescribed for chronic pain, but their side effects, risks, possibility of addiction, and

even effectiveness raise cautions about their widespread use (Gatchel et al., 2014).

Any drug that influences neural transmission is a candidate for pain relief. Some drugs, such as local anesthetics, can affect the transmission of pain impulses from the peripheral receptors to the spinal cord. The application of an analgesic to a wound is an example of this approach. The injection of drugs, such as spinal blocking agents, is another method.

Pharmacological relief from pain may also be provided by drugs that act directly on higher brain regions. Antidepressants, for example, combat pain not only by reducing anxiety and improving mood but also by affecting the downward pathways from the brain that modulate pain.

Sometimes pharmacological treatments make the pain worse rather than better. Patients may consume large quantities of painkillers that are only partially effective and that have undesirable side effects, including inability to concentrate and addiction. Drug-poisoning deaths involving opioid analgesic drugs have been rising steadily over the past 15 years (Chen, Hedegaard, & Warner, 2014). Nerve-blocking agents may be administered to reduce pain, but these can also produce side effects, including anesthesia, limb paralysis, and loss of bladder control; moreover, even when they are successful, the pain will usually return within a short time.

The main concern practitioners have about the pharmacological control of pain is addiction, and a subset of pain patients are very vulnerable to addiction. Additional information on the **opioid crisis** brought on by opioid addiction is found in Box 10.4. On the other hand, even long-term use of prescription pain drugs for such conditions as arthritis appears to produce very low rates of addiction.

The concern over addiction can lead to undermedication. One estimate is that about 15 percent of patients with cancer-related pain and as many as 80 percent with noncancer chronic pain do not receive sufficient pain medication, leading to a cycle of stress, distress, and disability (Chapman & Gavrin, 1999).

### Surgical Control of Pain

The surgical control of pain also has a long history. Surgical treatment involves cutting or creating lesions in the so-called pain fibers at various points in the body so that pain sensations can no longer be conducted. Some surgical techniques attempt to disrupt the transmission of pain from the periphery to the spinal cord;

At one time, practitioners believed that pain was under treated as a clinical problem. A new class of drugs, called opioids, arose to manage acute and chronic pain. Opioids include some prescription painkillers and illicit drugs such as heroin, and synthetic drugs that have pain-reducing properties, such as fentanyl and the very powerful carfentanil. The most recently released data suggest that nearly 400,000 people in the United States have overdosed on these drugs since 2000, and about 50,000 to 60,000 people die each year as a result of their use. Moreover, opioids do not seem to be particularly good for treating chronic pain, but because they are highly addictive, people continue to take them.

Opioids began to be prescribed for pain on a widespread basis in the 1990s. It is estimated that a third of people in the United States have been given a prescription for opioids and that 20 percent of people who start a 10-day course will become long-term users (The Hartford.com, *The Opioid Crisis*, downloaded March 7, 2019). Drug overdoses are now the leading cause of death among people under 50 in the United States (The New York Times, June 6, 2017).

How can we get ahead of this expanding problem? Federal guidelines to reduce over prescription is one point of attack. The treatment of pain through non-drug means such as acupuncture may help (The Wall Street Journal, February 14, 2017). Making changes to the drugs can help, such as reformulating OxyContin (an opioid) so it cannot be crushed and snorted (The Economist, June, 2, 2018). Medication-based treatment, such as methadone, may be the most promising avenue. But as new synthetic drugs emerge, the difficulty of getting ahead of this epidemic is clear.

others are designed to interrupt the flow of pain sensations from the spinal cord upward to the brain.

Although these surgical techniques are sometimes successful in reducing pain temporarily, the effects are often short-lived. Therefore, many pain patients who have submitted to operations to reduce pain may gain only short-term benefits, at substantial cost: the risks, possible side effects, and tremendous expense of surgery. It is now believed that the nervous system has substantial regenerative powers and that blocked pain impulses find their way to the brain via different neural pathways.

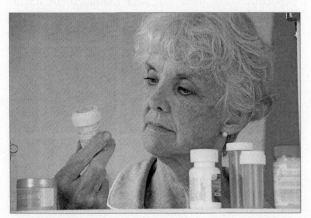

*About 116 million people in the United States experience chronic pain that requires treatment.*

Ariel Skelley/Blend Images

Moreover, surgery can worsen the problem because it damages the nervous system, and this damage can itself be a chief cause of chronic pain. Hence, whereas surgical treatment for pain was once relatively common, researchers and practitioners are increasingly doubtful of its value, even as a treatment of last resort.

## Sensory Control of Pain

One of the oldest known techniques of pain control is **counterirritation.** Counterirritation involves inhibiting pain in one part of the body by stimulating or mildly irritating another area. The next time you hurt yourself, you can demonstrate this technique on your own (and may have done so already) by pinching or scratching an area of your body near the part that hurts. Typically, the counterirritation produced when you do this will suppress the pain to some extent.

This common observation has been incorporated into the pain treatment process. An example of a pain control technique that uses this principle is spinal cord stimulation (North et al., 2005). A set of small electrodes is placed or implanted near the point at which the nerve fibers from the painful area enter the spinal cord. When the patient experiences pain, he or she activates a radio signal, which delivers a mild electrical stimulus to that area of the spine, thus inhibiting pain. Sensory control techniques have had some success in reducing the experience of pain. However, their effects are often only short-lived, and they may therefore be appropriate primarily for temporary relief from acute pain or as part of a general regimen for chronic pain.

In recent years, pain management experts have turned increasingly to exercise and other ways of increasing mobility to help the chronic pain patient. At one time, it was felt that the less activity, the better, so that healing could take place. In recent years, however, exactly the opposite philosophy has held sway, with patients urged to stay active to maintain their functioning.

We now turn to psychological techniques for the management of pain. Unlike the pharmacological, surgical, and sensory pain management techniques considered so far, these more psychological techniques require active participation and learning on the part of the patient (Jensen & Turk, 2014). Therefore, they are more effective for managing slow-rising pains, which can be anticipated and prepared for than, for sudden, intense, or unexpected pains.

## Biofeedback

**Biofeedback,** a method of achieving control over a bodily process, has been used to treat a variety of health problems, including pain (see Chapter 6) and hypertension (see Chapter 13).

What Is Biofeedback?    Biofeedback involves providing biophysiological feedback to a patient about some bodily process of which the patient is usually unaware. Biofeedback training can be thought of as an operant learning process. First, the target function to be brought under control, such as an aching pain or high heart rate, is identified. This function is then tracked by a machine, which provides information to the patient. For example, heart rate might be converted into a tone, so the patient can hear how quickly or slowly his or her heart is beating. The patient then attempts to change the bodily process. Through trial and error and continuous feedback from the machine, the patient learns what thoughts or behaviors will modify the bodily function.

Biofeedback has been used to treat a number of chronic pain syndromes, including headaches (Duschek, Schuepbach, Doll, Werner, & Reyes del Paso, 2011), Raynaud's disease (a disorder in which

the small arteries in the extremities constrict, limiting blood flow and producing a cold, numb aching), temporomandibular joint pain (Glaros & Burton, 2004), and pelvic pain (Clemens et al., 2000).

How successful is biofeedback in treating pain patients? Despite widely touted claims for its efficacy, there is only modest evidence that it is effective in reducing pain (White & Tursky, 1982). Even when biofeedback is effective, it may be no more so than less expensive, more easily used techniques, such as relaxation (Blanchard, Andrasik, & Silver, 1980; Bush, Ditto, & Feuerstein, 1985).

## Relaxation Techniques

Relaxation training has been employed with pain patients extensively, either alone or in concert with other pain control techniques. One reason for teaching pain patient relaxation techniques is that it enables them to cope more successfully with stress and anxiety, which may ameliorate pain. Relaxation may also affect pain directly. For example, the reduction of muscle tension or the diversion of blood flow induced by relaxation may reduce pains that are tied to these physiological processes.

What Is Relaxation?    In relaxation, an individual shifts his or her body into a state of low arousal by progressively relaxing different parts of the body. Controlled breathing is added, in which breathing shifts from relatively short, shallow breaths to deeper, longer breaths. Anyone who has been trained in prepared childbirth techniques will recognize that these procedures are used for pain management during early labor.

Meditation, slow breathing, and mindfulness also reduce pain sensitivity and can produce analgesic effects, possibly through a combination of relaxation and self-regulatory skills (Grant & Rainville, 2009; Zautra, Fasman, Davis, & Craig, 2010). Spiritual meditation tied to religious beliefs can aid in the control of some pains such as migraine headaches (Wachholtz & Pargament, 2008).

Does Relaxation Work?    Relaxation is modestly successful for controlling some acute pains and may be useful in treating chronic pain when used with other methods of pain control. Some of the beneficial physiological effects of relaxation training may be due to the release of endogenous opioids (McGrady

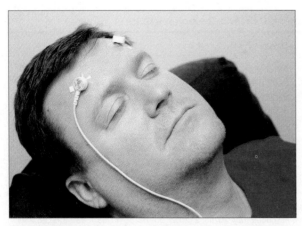

*Biofeedback has been used successfully to treat muscle-tension headaches, migraine headaches, and Raynaud's disease. However, evidence to date suggests that other, less expensive relaxation techniques may be equally successful.*
ftwitty/Getty Images

et al., 1992; Van Rood, Bogaards, Goulmy, & von Houwelingen, 1993).

## Distraction

People who are involved in intense activities, such as sports or military maneuvers, can be oblivious to painful injuries. These are extreme examples of a commonly employed pain technique: **distraction.** By focusing attention on an irrelevant and attention-getting stimulus or by distracting oneself with a high level of activity, one can turn attention away from pain (Dahlquist et al., 2007). But being in pain often orients a person to pain-relevant information, potentially making distraction difficult (Todd, van Ryckeghem, Sharpe, & Crombez, 2018).

### How Does Distraction Work?
There are two quite different mental strategies for controlling discomfort. One is to distract oneself by focusing on another activity. For instance, an 11-year-old boy described how he reduced pain by distracting himself while in the dentist's chair:

> When the dentist says, "Open," I have to say the Pledge of Allegiance to the flag backwards three times before I am even allowed to think about the drill. Once he got all finished before I did. (Bandura, 1991)

The other kind of mental strategy for controlling stressful events is to focus directly on the events but to reinterpret the experience. The following is a description from an 8-year-old boy who confronted a painful event directly:

> As soon as I get in the dentist's chair, I pretend he's the enemy and I'm a secret agent, and he's torturing me to get secrets, and if I make one sound, I'm telling him secret information, so I never do. I'm going to be a secret agent when I grow up, so this is good practice. (Bandura, 1991)

### Is Distraction Effective?
Distraction is a useful technique of pain control, especially with acute pain (Dahlquist et al., 2007). For example, in one study, 38 dental patients were exposed to one of three conditions. One-third of the group heard music during the dental procedure; one-third heard the music coupled with a suggestion that the music might help them reduce stress; and the third group heard no music. Patients in both music groups reported experiencing less discomfort than did patients in the no-treatment group (Anderson, Baron, & Logan, 1991).

Distraction is most effective for coping with low-level pain. Its practical significance for chronic pain management is limited by the fact that such patients cannot distract themselves indefinitely. Moreover, distraction by itself lacks analgesic properties (McCaul, Monson, & Maki, 1992). Thus, while effective, distraction may be most useful when used in conjunction with other pain control techniques.

## Coping Skills Training

Coping skills training helps chronic pain patients manage pain. For example, one study with burn patients found that brief training in cognitive coping skills, including distraction and focusing on the sensory aspects of pain instead of its painful qualities, led to reduced reported pain, increased satisfaction with pain control, and better pain coping skills (Haythornthwaite, Lawrence, & Fauerbach, 2001). Active coping skills can reduce pain in patients with a variety of chronic pains (Bishop & Warr, 2003; Mercado, Carroll, Cassidy, & Cote, 2000), and passive coping has been tied to poor pain control (Walker, Smith, Garber, & Claar, 2005).

### Do Coping Techniques Work?
Is any particular coping technique effective for managing pain? The answers depend on how long patients have had their pain. In a study of 30 chronic pain patients

**TABLE 10.2 | Cognitive–Behavioral Methods for Controlling Pain and Responses to It**

| Cognitive Techniques | Behavior |
|---|---|
| Cognitive restructuring, such as reframing negative thoughts about the pain.<br>Problem solving, such as defining pain-related problems and generating possible solutions. | Relaxation<br>Pacing, such as breaking up activities into smaller chunks.<br>Behavioral activation, such as gradually increasing one's activity level. |
| **Education** | **Other** |
| Providing information about pain, its causes, and its treatment.<br>Psychotherapy, such as motivational interviewing. | Hypnosis<br>Biofeedback<br>Relapse Prevention |

*Source:* Based on Skinner, Michelle, Hilary D. Wilson, and Dennis C. Turk. "Cognitive–Behavioral Perspective and Cognitive–Behavioral Therapy for People with Chronic Pain: Distinctions, Outcomes, and Innovations." *Journal of Cognitive Psychotherapy* 26, no. 2 (2012): 93–113. doi:10.1891/0889-8391.26.2.93.

and 30 recent-onset pain patients, researchers found that those with recent-onset pain experienced less anxiety and depression and less pain when employing avoidant coping strategies rather than attentional strategies. Because the pain was short term, putting it out of mind worked (Mullen & Suls, 1982).

In contrast, for chronic pain patients, attending directly to the pain, rather than avoiding it, was more adaptive (Holmes & Stevenson, 1990). Such studies suggest that pain patients might be trained in different coping strategies, avoidant versus attentive, depending on the expected duration of their pain (Holmes & Stevenson, 1990).

## Cognitive–Behavioral Therapy

Practitioners now typically use cognitive–behavioral therapy to control chronic pain (Ehde, Dillworth, & Turner, 2014). Cognitive–behavioral methods for pain management and responses to it can be found in Table 10.2. These interventions build on several objectives. First, they encourage patients to reconceptualize the problem from overwhelming to manageable. The pain problem must be perceived to be modifiable for cognitive and behavioral methods to have any impact. Acceptance and mindfulness-based treatments have been successful in helping people move outside their pain, fostering objectivity, detachment, and better functioning (McCracken & Vowles, 2014).

Second, clients must be convinced that the skills necessary to control the pain can and will be taught to them, thereby enhancing their expectations that the outcome of this training will be successful (Gil et al., 1996). For example, slow breathing, which is a part of relaxation therapy, works to manage pain much of the time, but

chronic pain patients may require special guidance to get benefits from these techniques (Zautra et al., 2010).

Third, clients are encouraged to reconceptualize their own role in the pain management process, from being passive recipients of pain to being active, resourceful, and competent individuals who can aid in the control of pain. These cognitions promote feelings of self-efficacy.

Fourth, clients learn how to monitor their thoughts, feelings, and behaviors to break up maladaptive behavioral syndromes that accompany chronic pain. As we noted in Chapter 3, patients often inadvertently undermine behavior change by engaging in discouraging self-talk. Helping pain patients develop more positive monologues increases the likelihood that cognitive–behavioral techniques will be successful.

Fifth, patients are taught how and when to employ overt and covert behaviors to make adaptive responses to the pain problem. This skills-training component of the intervention may include relaxation.

Sixth, clients are encouraged to attribute their success to their own efforts. By making internal attributions for success, patients come to see themselves as efficacious agents of change who are in a better position to monitor subsequent changes in the pain and bring about successful pain modification.

Seventh, just as relapse prevention is an important part of health habit change, it is important in pain control as well. Patients may be taught to identify situations likely to give rise to their pain and to develop alternative ways of coping with the pain, rather than engaging in the pain behaviors they have used in the past, such as withdrawing from social contact.

Finally, patients are often trained in therapies that can help them control their emotional responses to pain (Turk & Gatchel, 2018). Acceptance and commitment therapy, which involves a mindful distancing from the pain experience, as well as therapies for depression or anger implicated in the pain experience, can be helpful (McCracken & Vowles, 2014). Self-determination theory also provides guidelines for intervening with chronic pain patients by increasing autonomy, feelings of competence, and the experience of support (Uysal & Lu, 2011). Mindfulness interventions have also shown success for some chronic pain patient groups. A meta-analysis of 38 mindfulness meditation interventions with pain patients found a modest reduction in pain and improvement in quality of life, including a reduction in depression (Hilton, Hempel, Ewing, Apaydin, & Xenakis, 2017). The ability to take a nonjudgmental stance toward the pain situation may be one benefit of mindfulness (Ciere et al., 2018)

### Do Cognitive–Behavioral Interventions Work?

Evaluation of cognitive–behavioral interventions suggests that these techniques can be successful for managing chronic pain (Turk & Gatchel, 2018).

Hypnosis (Jensen & Patterson, 2014), acupuncture, and guided imagery are also used by some practitioners and patients to manage pain. These techniques are used more generally to combat the effects and side effects of illness and treatment, and so they were covered in Chapter 9. Their role in pain management requires additional evaluations, but as noted in Chapter 9, acupuncture appears to be successful for treating some kinds of pain.

### ■ PAIN MANAGEMENT PROGRAMS

Only a half century ago, the patient who suffered from chronic pain had few treatment avenues available, except for the possibilities of addiction to morphine or other painkillers and rounds of only temporarily successful surgeries. Now, however, a coordinated form of treatment has developed to treat chronic pain (Gatchel, McGeary, McGeary, & Lippe, 2014).

These interventions are termed **pain management programs,** and they make available to patients all that is known about pain control. The first pain management program was founded in Seattle at the University of Washington by physician John Bonica in 1960. The earliest pain treatment programs were inpatient, multiweek endeavors designed to decrease use of pain medication and restore daily living skills. Presently, however, most chronic pain management efforts are outpatient programs, because they can be successful and are less costly.

Typically, these programs are interdisciplinary efforts, bringing together neurological, cognitive, behavioral, and psychological expertise concerning pain (Gatchel et al., 2014). As such, they involve the expertise of physicians, psychologists, or psychiatrists, and physical therapists, with consultation from specialists in neurology, rheumatology, orthopedic surgery, internal medicine, and physical medicine.

### Initial Evaluation

Initially, patients are evaluated with respect to their pain and pain behaviors. This includes a qualitative and quantitative assessment of the pain, including its location, sensory qualities, severity, and duration, as well as its onset and history. Functional status is then assessed, with patients describing how work and family life have been impaired. Exploring how the patient has coped with the pain in the past helps establish treatment goals for the future. For example, patients who withdraw from social activities in response to their pain may need to increase their involvement in social activities and their family life. Chronic pain patients are often deficient in self-regulatory skills, such as self-control and the ability to cognitively reappraise situations, and so coping skills training may be useful. The willingness to accept pain improves self-regulation and can diminish side effects of pain (Eisenlohr-Moul, Burris, & Evans, 2013).

Evaluation of psychological distress, illness behavior, and psychosocial impairment is often a part of this phase of pain management, as failure to attend to emotional distress can undermine patients' self-management (Damush, Wu, Bair, Sutherland, & Kroenke, 2008). Treatment for depression can both improve mental health and ameliorate the chronic pain experience (Teh, Zasylavsky, Reynolds, & Cleary, 2010).

### Individualized Treatment

Individualized programs of pain management are next developed. Such programs are typically structured and time limited. They provide concrete aims, rules, and endpoints so that the patient has specific goals to achieve.

Typically, these goals include reducing the intensity of the pain, increasing physical activity, decreasing reliance on medications, improving psychosocial functioning, reducing perception of disability, returning to full work status, and reducing the use of health care services (Vendrig, 1999).

## Components of Programs

Pain management programs include several common features. The first is patient education. Often conducted in a group setting, the educational component of the intervention may include discussions of medications; assertiveness or social skills training; ways of dealing with sleep disturbance; depression as a consequence of pain; nonpharmacological measures for pain control, such as relaxation skills and distraction; posture, weight management, and nutrition; and other topics related to the day-to-day management of pain.

Most patients are then trained in a variety of measures to reduce pain, such as relaxation training, exercise, and coping skills. The program may include components tailored to specific pains, such as stretching exercises for back pain patients.

Because many pain patients are emotionally distressed, group therapy is often conducted to help them gain control of their emotional responses, especially catastrophic thinking. Catastrophic thinking enhances the pain experience, possibly by its effects on muscle tension and blood pressure reactivity (Shelby et al., 2009; Wolff et al., 2008). Interventions are aimed at the distorted negative perceptions patients hold about their pain. For example, writing interventions have been undertaken with pain patients to get them to express their anger and make meaning from the experience; reductions in both distress and pain have been found (Graham, Lobel, Glass, & Lokshina, 2008). Publicly committing to coping well with pain in a group setting can improve psychological adjustment and beneficially affect treatment outcomes (Gilliam et al., 2013).

## Involvement of Family

Many pain management programs involve families. On the one hand, chronic pain patients often withdraw from their families, and efforts by the family to be supportive can sometimes inadvertently reinforce pain behaviors. Working with the family to reduce such counterproductive behaviors may be necessary. Helping family members develop more positive perceptions of each other is also a goal of family therapy, as families can often be frustrated and annoyed by the pain patient's complaints and inactivity (Williamson, Walters, & Shaffer, 2002).

## Relapse Prevention

Finally, relapse prevention is included so that patients will not backslide once they are discharged from the program. The incidence of relapse following initially successful treatment of persistent pain ranges from about 30 to 60 percent (Turk & Rudy, 1991). Consequently, relapse prevention techniques that help patients continue their pain management skills can maintain posttreatment pain reduction (Turk & Rudy, 1991).

## Evaluation of Programs

Pain management programs appear to be successful in helping control chronic pain. Studies that have evaluated behavioral interventions in comparison with nontreatment have found reductions in pain, disability, and psychological distress (Center for the Advancement of Health, 2000c; Haythornthwaite et al., 2001; Keefe et al., 1992). These interventions can improve social functioning as well (Stevens, Peterson, & Maruta, 1988). However, barriers, including cost and the difficulty of coordinating multiple professionals' services, are obstacles to implementing these programs (Gatchel et al., 2014). •

## SUMMARY

1. Pain is the symptom of primary concern to patients and leads them to seek medical attention. However, pain is often considered of secondary importance to practitioners.

2. Pain is subjective and, consequently, has been difficult to study. It is heavily influenced by the context in which it is experienced. To objectify the experience of pain, pain researchers have developed questionnaires to assess its dimensions and the pain behaviors that often accompany it.

3. According to the gate-control theory of pain, A-delta fibers conduct fast, sharp, localized pain; C-fibers conduct slow, aching, burning, and long-lasting pain; higher-order brain processes influence the experience of pain through the central control mechanism.

4. Neurochemical advances in the understanding of pain center around endogenous opioid peptides, which regulate the pain experience.

5. Acute pain is short term and specific to a particular injury or disease, whereas chronic pain does not decrease with treatment and time. Nearly 116 million Americans suffer from chronic pain, which may lead them to disrupt their entire lives in an effort to manage it.

6. Chronic pain is difficult to treat because it has a functional and psychological overlay. Chronic pain patients have elevated scores on the neurotic triad (hyperchondriasis, hysteria, and depression). Anger management is also implicated in pain control.

7. Pharmacological (e.g., morphine), surgical, and sensory stimulation techniques were once the mainstays of pain control, but increasingly, treatments with psychological components, including biofeedback, relaxation, hypnosis, acupuncture, distraction, and guided imagery, have been added to the pain control arsenal.

8. Cognitive–behavioral techniques that help instill a sense of self-efficacy have been used successfully in the treatment of pain.

9. Chronic pain can be treated through coordinated pain management programs oriented toward managing the pain, extinguishing pain behavior, and re establishing a viable lifestyle. These programs employ a mix of techniques in an effort to develop an individualized treatment program for each patient—a truly biopsychosocial approach to pain.

## KEY TERMS

acute pain
biofeedback
chronic benign pain
chronic pain
chronic progressive pain
counterirritation

distraction
endogenous opioid peptides
gate-control theory of pain
nociception
opioid crisis
pain behaviors

pain control
pain management programs
pain-prone personality
recurrent acute pain

# PART 5

# Management of Chronic and Terminal Health Disorders

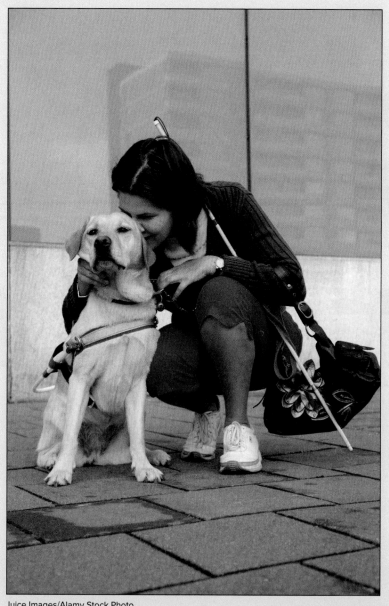

Juice Images/Alamy Stock Photo

# CHAPTER 11

# Management of Chronic Health Disorders

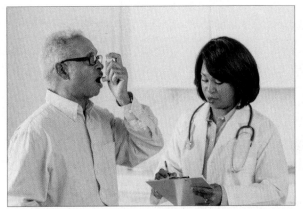

Terry Vine/Blend Images LLC

During a race at a high school track meet, a young runner stumbled and fell to the ground, caught in the grip of an asthma attack. As her mother frantically clawed through her backpack looking for the inhaler, three other girls on the track team offered theirs.

As this account implies, asthma rates have skyrocketed in recent years, particularly among children and adolescents. Nearly 6.3 million children have asthma, and nearly a third of those children require treatment in a hospital emergency room for an asthma attack each year (Centers for Disease Control and Prevention, 2016). Scientists are not entirely sure why asthma is on the increase, but the complications that it creates for young adults are evident. Caution, medication, and inhalers become a part of daily life. Psychosocial factors are clearly an important part of this adjustment, helping us answer such questions as "What factors precipitate an asthma attack?" and "What does it mean to have a chronic disease so early in life?"

At any given time, 60 percent of the adult population has a chronic condition, and the medical management of these chronic disorders, including psychological disorders, accounts for 90 percent of the nation's health spending (Centers for Disease Control and Prevention, 2019). People with chronic health disorders account for 90 percent of home care visits, 83 percent of prescription

drug use, 80 percent of the days spent in hospitals, 66 percent of doctor visits, and 55 percent of visits to hospital emergency rooms. And as the opening example implies, these conditions are not confined to older adults (see Figure 11.1). More than one-third of young adults age 18 to 44 have at least one chronic condition (Strong, Mathers, Leeder, & Beaglehole, 2005).

Chronic conditions range from moderate ones, such as partial hearing loss, to life-threatening disorders, such as cancer, coronary artery disease, and diabetes. For example, in the United States, arthritis in its various forms afflicts 53 million people (Centers for Disease Control and Prevention, 2016, April); 20 million people have had cancer (Centers for Disease Control and Prevention, 2016); diabetes afflicts 29 million people (American Diabetes Association, April 2016); 33 million people worldwide have sustained a stroke; 0.8 million people suffer from heart attacks each year (American Heart Association, 2015, December); and 80 million people have diagnosed hypertension (American Heart Association, December 2015).

Moreover, nearly half of adults aged 45 to 65 have two or more chronic conditions that require medical care or limit daily activities (Buttorff, Ruder, & Bauman, 2017; Gerteis et al., 2014; Suls, Green, & Davidson, 2016). Adults who live with **multimorbidity** have more

**FIGURE 11.1 | The Prevalence of Physical Limitations Increases with Age**   *Source:* J., Holmes, Powell-Griner, E., Lethbridge-Cejku, M., & Heyman, K. "Aging differently: Physical limitations among adults aged 50 years and over: United States, 2001–2007." NCHS Data Brief 20., U.S. Department of Health & Human Services, 2009. https://www.cdc.gov/nchs/data/databriefs/db20.pdf.

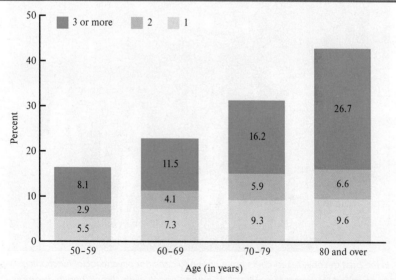

NOTE: The sum of the stacked sections in the bar for each age group represents the total percentage of adults in that age group with one or more physical limitations.

complicated treatment regimens, substantially higher health care costs, lower quality of life, and shorter lives than do individuals with no or one chronic condition (Gerteis et al., 2014; Suls et al., 2016). The fields of medicine and health psychology, even when a biopsychosocial model of health is adopted, have devoted far greater attention to single disease than multimorbidity. Research on the causes, experience, and treatment of multimorbidity is vital.

# ■ QUALITY OF LIFE

"The simple idea that is transforming health care: a focus on quality of life helps medical providers see the big picture and make for healthier, happier patients" (Landro, 2012, p. R1). Until recently, **quality of life** was not considered an issue of medical importance, except in terms of length of survival and signs of disease. There was virtually no consideration of the psychosocial consequences of health disorders and treatments. However, that picture is changing.

Medical measures are only weakly related to patients' or relatives' assessments of quality of life. In fact, one classic study of a hypertension medication (Jachuck, Brierley, Jachuck, & Willcox, 1982) found that although 100 percent of the physicians reported that their patients' quality of life had improved with the medication, only half the patients agreed and virtually none of the relatives did. Moreover, some health disorders and treatments are perceived by patients to be "fates worse than death" because they threaten valued life activities so completely (Ditto, Druley, Moore, Danks, & Smucker, 1996).

## What Is Quality of Life?

Because of findings like these, quality of life is now given attention in the management of chronic health disorders. Quality of life has several components—physical functioning, psychological status, social functioning, and disease- or treatment-related symptoms (Kahn & Juster, 2002; Power, Bullinger, Harper, & the World Health Organization Quality of Life Group, 1999). Researchers focus on how much the disease and its treatment interfere with the activities of daily living, such as sleeping, eating, going to work, and engaging in recreational activities. For patients with more advanced diseases, such assessments include whether the patient is able to bathe, dress, use the toilet, be mobile, be continent, and eat without assistance. Essentially, then, quality-of-life assessments gauge the extent to which a patient's normal life activities have been compromised by disease and treatment. A broad array of measures is available for evaluating quality of life in both adults (see, e.g., Cella & Stone, 2015; Molina et al., 2019) and children (Varni et al., 2018).

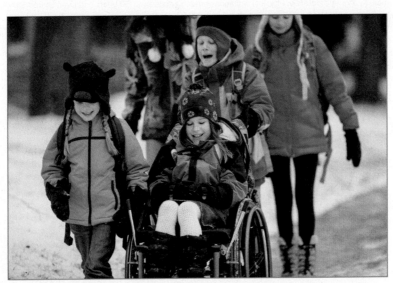

*In the past decade, researchers have begun to consider psychosocial functioning as an important aspect of quality of life among people with chronic health disorders and the disabled.*

Christopher Futcher/Stockphoto/Getty Images

## Why Study Quality of Life?

Why should we study quality of life among people with chronic health disorders? There are several reasons.

- Documentation of how health disorders affect domains of quality of life can guide interventions designed to improve those domains.

- Quality-of-life measures can help pinpoint which problems are likely to emerge for patients with which diseases.

- Quality-of-life measures assess the impact of treatments. For example, if a cancer treatment has slim survival benefit and produces severe side effects, the treatment may be more harmful than the disease.

- Quality-of-life measures can be less expensive and more convenient than other measures of functioning, with equivalent accuracy (Baumhauer, 2017).

- Quality-of-life data can be used to compare therapies. For example, if two therapies produce approximately equivalent survival rates but one lowers quality of life substantially, the treatment that keeps quality of life high is preferable.

- Quality-of-life data can help patients and the health care team know what to expect after a medical procedure and the likely course of recovery (Baumhauer, 2017).

- Quality-of-life information can inform practitioners about care that will maximize long-term health with the highest quality of life possible (Kaplan, 2003) (see Table 11.1).

- High quality of life can reduce the rate of illness progression (Rauma et al., 2014), symptoms experienced, and need for treatment (Detford, Taylor, Campbell, & Geaves, 2014).

## ■ EMOTIONAL RESPONSES TO CHRONIC HEALTH DISORDERS

Immediately after a chronic health disorder is diagnosed, a patient can be in a state of crisis marked by physical, social, and psychological disequilibrium. If the patient's usual coping efforts fail to resolve these problems, the result can be an exaggeration of symptoms and their meaning, indiscriminate efforts to cope, an increasingly negative attitude, and worsening health (Drossman et al., 2000; Epker & Gatchel, 2000). The uncertainty and ambiguity inherent in many chronic disorders (e.g., Will it get worse? If so, how quickly?) affects quality of life adversely (Hoth et al., 2013). People with chronic health disorders are more likely to suffer from depression, anxiety, and generalized distress (De Graaf & Bijl, 2002; Mittermaier et al., 2004). These psychological changes are important because they compromise quality of life, predict lower adherence to treatment, and increase the risk of dying early (Bruce, Hancock, Arnett, & Lynch, 2010; Christensen, Moran, Wiebe, Ehlers, & Lawton, 2002).

### Denial

**Denial** is a defense mechanism by which people avoid the implications of a disorder, especially one that may be

**TABLE 11.1 | Quality-of-Life Scores for U.S. Population and Several Groups of People with Chronic Health Disorders**

A look at the typical score for the U.S. population indicates how each of several chronic conditions affects functioning in each area. For example, pain and vitality are most problematic for migraine sufferers, osteoarthritis compromises physical activities related to roles, and diabetes undermines general health.

| | Physical Functioning | Role-Physical | Bodily Pain | General Health | Vitality | Social Functioning | Role-Emotional | Mental Health |
|---|---|---|---|---|---|---|---|---|
| **U.S. Population*** | **92.1** | **92.2** | **84.7** | **81.4** | **66.5** | **90.5** | **92.1** | **81.0** |
| Clinical depression | 81.8 | 62.8 | 73.6 | 63.6 | 49.0 | 68.5 | 47.8 | 53.8 |
| Migraine | 83.2 | 54.0 | 51.3 | 70.1 | 50.9 | 71.1 | 66.5 | 66.4 |
| Hypertension | 89.5 | 79.0 | 83.8 | 72.6 | 67.2 | 92.1 | 79.6 | 77.3 |
| Osteoarthritis | 81.9 | 66.5 | 69.7 | 70.4 | 57.0 | 90.1 | 85.5 | 76.5 |
| Type 2 diabetes | 86.6 | 76.8 | 82.8 | 66.9 | 61.4 | 89.4 | 80.7 | 76.6 |

*U.S. population estimates are for those reporting no chronic conditions. Scores take into account other chronic conditions, age, gender.

*Source:* Based on Ware, J. E., Jr. Norm-based interpretation. Medical Outcomes Trust Bulletin, 2, 3, 1994.

life-threatening. It is a common early reaction to chronic health disorders (Krantz & Deckel, 1983; Meyerowitz, 1983). Patients may act as if the health disorder is not severe, it will shortly go away, or it will have few long-term implications. Immediately after the diagnosis of the health disorder, denial can serve a protective function by keeping the patient from having to come to terms with problems posed by the health disorder when he or she is least able to do so (Hackett & Cassem, 1973; Lazarus, 1983).

Over time, however, any benefit of denial gives way to its costs. It can interfere with taking in necessary treatment information and compromise health (Mund & Mitte, 2012).

## Anxiety

Following the diagnosis of a chronic health disorder, anxiety is also common. Many patients are overwhelmed by the potential changes in their lives and, in some cases, by the prospect of dying. Anxiety is especially high when people are waiting for test results, receiving diagnoses, awaiting invasive medical procedures, and anticipating or experiencing adverse side effects of treatment (Rabin, Ward, Leventhal, & Schmitz, 2001).

Anxiety is a problem not only because it is intrinsically distressing but also because it interferes with treatment. For example, anxious patients cope more poorly with surgery (Mertens, Roukema, Scholtes, & De Vries, 2010); anxious diabetic patients have poor glucose control (Lustman, 1988); anxiety complicates managing a host of chronic conditions (Favreau, Bacon, Labrecque, & Lovoie, 2014), and is especially prevalent among people with asthma and pulmonary disorders (Katon, Richardson, Lozano, & McCauley, 2004).

Symptoms of anxiety may also be mistaken for symptoms of the underlying disease and thus interfere with assessments of the disease and its treatment (Chen, Hermann, Rodgers, Oliver-Welker, & Strunk, 2006). Intervening to treat anxiety is increasingly recommended (Rollman & Huffman, 2013).

## Depression

**Depression** is a common reaction to chronic health disorders. Up to one-third of all medical inpatients with chronic disease report symptoms of depression, and up to one-quarter suffer from severe depression (Moody, McCormick, & Williams, 1990). Depression is especially common among stroke patients, cancer patients, and heart disease patients, as well as among

people with multimorbidity (Egede, 2005; see Taylor & Aspinwall, 1990, for a review).

At one time, depression was regarded only as an emotional disorder, but its medical significance is increasingly recognized. People who experience depression are more likely to develop anxiety and vice versa (Jacobson & Newman, 2017), and both predict onset of chronic health disorders (Niles & O'Donovan, 2019). Depression predicts death from all causes (Cuijpers et al., 2014; Houle, 2013; Morin, Galatzer-Levy, Maccallum, & Bonanno, 2017). People who have intermittent bouts of depression are more likely to get heart disease, atherosclerosis, hypertension, stroke, dementia, osteoporosis, and type 2 diabetes, and at younger ages. Depression exacerbates the course of several chronic disorders, most notably coronary heart disease. Depression complicates treatment adherence and medical decision making (Hilliard, Eakin, Borelli, Green, & Riekert, 2015). It interferes with patients adopting a comanagerial role, and it can increase the use of health services for treatment (Ahmedani, Peterson, Wells, & Williams, 2013).

Depression is sometimes a delayed reaction to chronic health disorders, because it takes time for patients to understand the full implications of their condition. For example, a stroke patient comments on his discharge from the hospital:

> That was a glorious day. I started planning all the things I could do with the incredible amount of free time I was going to have, chores I had put off, museums and galleries to visit, friends I had wanted to meet for lunch. It was not until several days later that I realized I simply couldn't do them. I didn't have the mental or physical strength, and I sank into a depression. (Dahlberg, 1977, p. 121)

**Assessing Depression** Depression is so prevalent among chronically ill patients that experts recommend routine screening for depressive symptoms during medical visits (Jha, Qamar, Vaduganathan, Charney, & Murrough, 2019; Löwe et al., 2003). Yet assessing depression in the chronically ill can be complicated. Many symptoms of depression, such as fatigue, sleeplessness, and weight loss, can also be symptoms of disease or side effects of a treatment. If depressive symptoms are attributed to illness or treatment, their significance may be less apparent, and, consequently, depression may go untreated (Ziegelstein et al., 2005).

Mollie Kaplan can remember half a century ago when she was 12 and met her husband, Samuel, at a Halloween party in the Bronx. What she can't remember is whether she had breakfast, so sometimes she eats it twice. She doesn't cook much anymore because if the recipe calls for salt, she can't remember whether she added it. "It's so frustrating," she said. "I can't read a book anymore, because if I stop and put a bookmark where I leave off, when I pick the book up again, I don't know what I have read." (Larsen, 1990, pp. E1, E8)

Mollie Kaplan has Alzheimer's disease. Alzheimer's is the sixth leading cause of death among U.S. adults, accounting for 121,404 deaths in 2017 (Alzheimer's Association, 2019). Currently, about 5.8 million Americans have the disease, with numbers projected to double by 2050 (Alzheimer's Association, 2019). Typical symptoms of Alzheimer's (named after Dr. Alois Alzheimer, who described it in 1906) include gradual progression of memory loss or other cognitive losses (language problems, motor skills), personality

change, and eventually loss of function (Mattson, 2004). Increasing frailty may foreshadow the onset of the disorder (Buchman, Boyle, Wilson, Tang, & Bennett, 2007). Personality changes include hostility, withdrawal, inappropriate laughing, agitation, and paranoia.

The strain of Alzheimer's disease on both the patient and the caregiver can be great. Approximately two-thirds of dementia caregivers are women (Alzheimer's Association, 2019). For the patient, being unable to do simple, routine tasks or remember an activity just completed is frustrating and depressing. For caregivers, the emotional toll is substantial. The family may be left with little alternative but to place the loved one in a nursing home, and the effect on family finances can be huge. Despite this grim picture, many treatments for Alzheimer's are in development, and many are currently being tested. As neuroscientists learn more about the cellular and molecular changes in the brain that lead to neurodegeneration, progress in prevention and treatment will be made.

**Who Gets Depressed?** Depression increases with the severity of the health disorder (Cassileth et al., 1985; Moody et al., 1990) and with pain and disability (Turner & Noh, 1988; Wulsin, Vaillant, & Wells, 1999). These problems are aggravated in people who are experiencing other negative life events and lack of social support (Bukberg, Penman, & Holland, 1984; Thompson et al., 1989). Other factors can protect people with chronic health conditions from depressive symptoms. For example, a sense of gratitude, which involves thankfulness to others and appreciation for what one has in life, predicted lower depressive symptoms in adults with arthritis or inflammatory bowel disease (Sirois & Wood, 2017).

Cognitive–behavioral and other evidence-based interventions are effective for the depression that so frequently accompanies chronic health disorders (van Straten, Geraedts, Verdonck-de Leeuw, Andersson, & Cuijpers, 2010). Even telephone-administered cognitive-behavioral therapy (CBT) can improve depression (Beckner, Howard, Vella, & Mohr, 2010). Treatment for depression may not only alleviate psychological distress but also reduce symptoms associated with the health disorder (Mohr, Hart, & Goldberg, 2003).

## ■ PERSONAL ISSUES IN CHRONIC HEALTH DISORDERS

To fully understand reactions to chronic health disorders requires a consideration of the self, its sources of resilience, and its vulnerabilities. The self is one of the central concepts in psychology. Psychologists refer to the **self-concept** as a stable set of beliefs about one's personal qualities and attributes. Self-esteem refers to the evaluation of the self-concept—namely, whether one feels good or bad about one's personal qualities and attributes.

A chronic health disorder can produce severe changes in self-concept and self-esteem (Ferro & Boyle, 2013). Many of these changes will be temporary, but some may be permanent, such as the mental deterioration that is associated with certain diseases (Box 11.1). The self-concept is a composite of self-evaluations regarding many aspects of life, which include body image, achievement, social functioning, and the private self.

### The Physical Self

**Body image** is the perception and evaluation of one's physical functioning and appearance. Body image can plummet during illness. Not only is the affected part

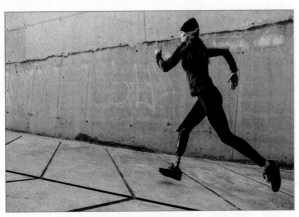

*Chronic health disorders or disability can interfere with some life activities, but a sense of self that is based on broader interests and abilities will sustain self-esteem.*

Dean Drobot/Shutterstock

of the body evaluated negatively, the whole body image may deteriorate. For patients with acute health disorders, changes in body image are short-lived; however, for people with chronic health disorders, negative evaluations may last. These changes in body image are important. First, a poor body image increases risk for depression and anxiety. Second, body image may influence how adherent a person is to the course of treatment and how willing he or she is to adopt a comanagement role. Finally, body image is important because it can be improved through interventions such as exercise (Wenninger, Weiss, Wahn, & Staab, 2003).

Perceived health is also an important dimension of physical health. Self-rated health predicts death over and above objective health indicators. It may also promote effective self-care, which requires active engagement (Denford, Taylor, Campbell, & Greaves, 2014). The first line of defense for most people with chronic disorders is self-care, and so promoting the coping resources to make it possible is essential (Hwang, Moser, & Dracup, 2014).

### The Achieving Self

Achievement through vocational and avocational activities is also an important source of self-esteem and the self-concept. Many people derive their primary life satisfaction from their job or career; others take great pleasure in their hobbies and leisure activities. If chronic health disorders threaten these valued aspects of the self, the self-concept may be damaged. The converse is also true: When work and hobbies are not threatened or curtailed by health disorders, the patient has these sources of satisfaction from which to derive self-esteem, and they can come to take on new meaning.

### The Social Self

Social resources, such as family and friends, can provide people with chronic health disorders with badly needed information, help, and emotional support. A breakdown in the support system has implications for all aspects of life (Barlow, Liu, & Wrosch, 2015). Perhaps for these reasons, fears about being abandoned by others are among the most common worries of people with chronic health disorders. Consequently, family participation in the health disorder management process and social activities is generally more widely encouraged.

### The Private Self

The residual core of a patient's identity—ambitions, goals, and desires for the future—are also affected by chronic health disorders (e.g., Smith, 2013). Adjustment can be impeded because the patient has an unrealized dream, which is now out of reach, or at least appears to be. For example, the dream of retiring to a cabin on a lake in the mountains may not be viable if the management of a chronic condition requires living near a major medical center. Encouraging the patient to discuss this difficulty may reveal alternative paths to fulfillment and awaken new ambitions, goals, and plans for the future.

## ■ COPING WITH CHRONIC HEALTH DISORDERS

Although most patients with chronic health disorders experience some distress, most do not seek formal or informal treatment for their symptoms. Instead, they draw on their internal and social resources for solving problems and alleviating psychological distress. How do they cope so well?

### Coping Strategies and Chronic Health Disorders

Numerous researchers systematically investigate the cognitive appraisals and coping strategies of people with chronic health disorders. In an early study (Dunkel-Schetter, Feinstein, Taylor, & Falke, 1992), cancer patients were asked to identify the aspect of cancer they found to be most stressful. Fear and uncertainty about the future were most common (41 percent), followed by limitations in physical abilities, appearance, and lifestyle (24 percent), and pain management (12 percent). Patients were then asked to indicate the coping strategies they had used to deal with these problems. The five most commonly used strategies were social support/direct problem solving ("I talked to someone to find out more about the situation"), distancing ("I didn't let it get to me"), positive focus ("I came out of the experience better than I went in"), cognitive escape/avoidance ("I wished that the situation would go away"), and behavioral escape/avoidance (efforts to avoid the situation by eating, drinking, or sleeping). These strategies are similar to those employed to manage other stressful events (see Chapter 7).

### Which Coping Strategies Work?

Do any particular coping strategies facilitate psychological adjustment among people with chronic health disorders? As is true for coping with other stressful events, avoidant coping is tied to greater psychological distress and is a risk factor for adverse responses to health disorders (Heim, Valach, & Schaffner, 1997). It may also exacerbate the disease process itself (Frenzel, McCaul, Glasgow, & Schafer, 1988).

In contrast, coping that involves actively approaching one's chronic illness experience often predicts good adjustment. People who cope using positive, confrontative responses to stress; who solicit health-related information about their condition (Christensen, Ehlers, Raichle, Bertolatus, & Lawton, 2000); who have a strong sense of control (Burgess, Morris, & Pettingale, 1988); and who believe that they can personally direct control over a health disorder (Taylor, Helgeson, Reed, & Skokan, 1991) all show better psychological adjustment. Because of the diversity of problems that chronic disorders pose, people who are flexible copers may cope better than do people who engage in a predominant coping style (Cheng, Hui, & Lam, 2004).

Virtually all chronic health disorders require some degree of self-management. For example, diabetic patients must control their diet and perhaps take daily injections of insulin. Both stroke and heart patients must make alterations in their daily activities if they have impairments. Patients who do not incorporate chronic health disorders into their self-concept may fail to be effective co-managers. They may not follow their treatment regimen. They may not be attuned to signs of recurrent or worsening disease. They may engage in foolhardy behaviors that pose a risk to their health, such as smoking. Thus, developing a realistic sense of one's health disorder, the restrictions it imposes, and the regimen that is required is an important process of coping with chronic health disorders.

## Patients' Beliefs About Chronic Health Disorders

### Beliefs About the Nature of the Health Disorder

In Chapter 8, we described the common-sense model of health disorders and the fact that patients develop coherent theories about their health disorder, including its identity, causes, consequences, timeline, and controllability. One of the problems that often arises in adjustment to chronic health disorders is that patients adopt an unhelpful model for their disorder—most notably, an acute model (see Chapter 8). For example, hypertensive patients may believe incorrectly that, if they feel all right, they no longer need to take medication (Hekler et al., 2008). Thus, it is important for health care providers to probe patients' beliefs about their health disorder to check for significant gaps and misunderstandings in their knowledge that may interfere with self-management (Stafford, Jackson, & Berk, 2008).

### Beliefs About the Cause of the Health Disorder

People with chronic health disorders often develop theories about how it arose (Costanzo, Lutgendorf, Bradley, Rose, & Anderson, 2005). These theories about origins of the health disorder include stress, physical injury, disease-causing bacteria, and God's will. Of perhaps greater significance is where patients ultimately place the blame for their health disorder. Do they blame themselves, another person, the environment, or a quirk of fate?

Self-blame for chronic health disorders is widespread. Patients frequently perceive themselves as having brought on their health disorder through their own actions. For example, they may blame their poor health habits, such as smoking or diet. What are the consequences of self-blame? Some researchers have found that self-blame can lead to guilt, self-recrimination, or depression (Bennett, Compas, Beckjord, & Glinder, 2005; Friedman et al., 2007). But perceiving the cause of one's health disorder as self-generated may alternatively represent an effort to assume control over the disorder. Self-blame may be adaptive under certain conditions, but not others (Schulz & Decker, 1985; Taylor et al., 1984a).

Blaming another person for one's health disorder is maladaptive (Affleck et al., 1987; Taylor et al., 1984a). For example, some patients believe that their health disorder was brought about by stress caused by family members, ex-spouses, or colleagues at work. Blame of this other person or persons may be tied to unresolved hostility, which can interfere with adjustment to the disease. Forgiveness, by contrast, is a healthier response (Worthington, Witvliet, Pietrini, & Miller, 2007).

Beliefs About the Controllability of the Health Disorder    Patients develop a number of control-related beliefs. They may believe, as do many cancer patients, that they can prevent a recurrence of the disease through good health habits or even sheer force of will. They may believe that by complying with treatments and physicians' recommendations, they achieve vicarious control over their health disorder.

People who have a sense of control or self-efficacy with respect to their health disorders are better adjusted to their circumstances. This relationship has been found for a broad array of health disorders, ranging from asthma in children (Lavoie et al., 2008) to functional disability in old age (Wrosch, Miller, & Schulz, 2009). The experience of control or self-efficacy may even prolong life (Kaplan, Ries, Prewitt, & Eakin, 1994).

## ■ COMANAGEMENT OF CHRONIC HEALTH DISORDERS

### Physical and Behavioral Rehabilitation

**Physical rehabilitation** involves several goals: to learn how to use one's body as much as safely possible, to learn how to sense changes in the environment to make the appropriate physical accommodations, to learn new physical management skills, to learn a necessary treatment regimen, and to learn how to control energy expenditure. Not all chronic health disorders require physical rehabilitation, but some do. Exercise goes a long way in reducing the symptoms of many chronic disorders (van der Ploeg et al., 2008). Physical activity can, in turn, pave the way for more general changes in self-efficacy (Motl & Snook, 2008).

Many patients who require physical rehabilitation have problems resulting from prior injuries or participation in athletic activities earlier in life, including knee problems, shoulder injuries, and the like. Most such problems worsen with age. Disabilities are more common among African Americans and Hispanics than among whites (Ward & Schiller, 2011). Functional decline in the frail elderly who live alone is a particular problem (Gill, Baker, Gottschalk, Peduzzi, Allore, & Byers, 2002). Physical therapy can ameliorate these age-related declines and can also help patients recover from treatments designed to alleviate them, such as surgery (Stephens, Druley, & Zautra, 2002). Robots are increasingly being used to help disabled people maximize their functioning (Broadbent, 2017). Some chronic functional disorders have origins that still baffle scientists; they are described in Box 11.2.

Patients may need a pain management program for the alleviation of discomfort. They may require prosthetic devices, such as an artificial limb after amputation related to diabetes. They may need training in the use of adaptive devices; for example, a patient with multiple sclerosis or a spinal cord injury may need to learn how to use a wheelchair. Certain cancer patients may elect cosmetic surgery, such as breast reconstruction after a mastectomy or the insertion of a synthetic jaw after head and neck surgery. Disorders such as stroke, diabetes, and high blood pressure may compromise cognitive functioning, requiring active intervention (Zelinski, Crimmins, Reynolds, & Seeman, 1998). Because stress exacerbates so many chronic disorders, stress management programs are increasingly incorporated into the physical treatment regimens as well.

The Impact on Sexuality    Many chronic health disorders—including heart disease, stroke, and cancer—compromise sexual activity. In many cases, the decline can be traced to psychological factors (such as loss of desire, fears about aggravating the chronic condition, or erectile dysfunction). The ability to continue physically intimate relations can improve relationship satisfaction among people with chronic health disorders and improve emotional functioning (Perez, Skinner, & Meyerowitz, 2002).

Adherence    As with all lifestyle intervention, adherence to treatment is problematic with people who have chronic health disorders. A first step in increasing adherence is education. Some patients may not realize that lifestyle aspects of their treatment regimen, such as exercise, are important to their recovery and functioning. As discussed in Chapter 9, education alone often is not sufficient to guarantee adherence, however. High expectations for controlling one's health and self-efficacy, coupled with knowledge of the treatment regimen, predict adherence to chronic disease regimens (Schneider, Friend, Whitaker, & Wadhwa, 1991).

In recent years, health psychologists have explored the causes and consequences of functional somatic syndromes. These syndromes are marked by symptoms, suffering, and disability, but not by any demonstrable tissue abnormality. In short, we don't know why people have these disorders. Functional somatic syndromes include chronic fatigue syndrome (CFS), irritable bowel syndrome, and fibromyalgia, as well as chemical sensitivity, sick building syndrome, repetitive stress injury, complications from silicone breast implants, Gulf War syndrome, and chronic whiplash.

CFS, one of the most common, involves debilitating fatigue present for at least 6 months. People with CFS show slowed thinking, reduced attention, and impairments in memory (Majer et al., 2008). For many years, no biological cause for CFS could be found. However, a viral agent and immune system changes have now been implicated as potential causes (Centers for Disease Control and Prevention, 2019).

Fibromyalgia is an arthritic syndrome involving widespread pain with tenderness in multiple sites. About 4 million individuals suffer from this disorder. The origins of fibromyalgia are unclear and the symptoms are varied, but the disorder is associated with sleep disturbance, disability, and high levels of psychological distress (Finan, Zautra, & Davis, 2009; Zautra et al., 2005).

Functional disorders are extremely difficult to treat inasmuch as their etiology is not well understood. Because of their insidious way of eroding quality of life, the functional syndromes typically cause psychological distress, including depression, and the symptoms of the health disorders are sometimes misdiagnosed as depression (Mittermaier et al., 2004; Skapinakis, Lewis, & Mavreas, 2004).

Who develops functional somatic disorders? Functional somatic syndromes are more common in women than in men, and people who have a prior history of emotional disorders, especially anxiety and depression (Bornschein, Hausteiner, Konrad, Förstl, & Zilker, 2006; Nater et al., 2009). A history of infections is also implicated (Lacourt, Houtveen, Smeets, Lipovsky, & van Doornen, 2013). People who are low in socioeconomic status, who are unemployed, and who are members of minority groups have a somewhat elevated likelihood of developing chronic fatigue (Taylor, Jason, & Jahn, 2003). Twin studies of CFS suggest that there may be genetic underpinnings of these disorders (Buchwald et al., 2001). A history of family disruption, childhood maltreatment and abuse, or childhood trauma may also be implicated (Afari et al., 2014; van Gils, Janssens, & Rosmalen, 2014).

The functional syndromes overlap heavily in symptoms (Kanaan, Lepine, & Wessely, 2007). Many of the disorders are marked by abdominal distention, headache, fatigue, and disturbances in the sympathetic and HPA axis stress systems (Reyes del Paso, Garrido, Pulgar, Martín-Vázquez, & Duschek, 2010). Among the common factors implicated in their development are a pre existing viral or bacterial infection and a high number of stressful life events (Fink, Toft, Hansen, Ornbol, & Olesen, 2007).

These similarities should not be interpreted to mean that these disorders are psychiatric in origin or that the care of these patients should be shifted exclusively to psychology and psychiatry. Instead, this overlap suggests that breakthroughs in understanding the etiology and developing treatments for these disorders may be made by pooling knowledge from all these syndromes, rather than by treating them as separate disorders (Fink et al., 2007). Although each disorder has distinctive features (Moss-Morris & Spence, 2006), the core symptoms of fatigue, pain, sick-role behavior, and negative affect are all associated with chronic, low-level inflammation, and possibly this sustained immune response is what ties these disorders together.

How are these disorders treated? Generally, practitioners combine pharmacological interventions for such symptoms as sleep deprivation and pain with behavioral interventions, including exercise and cognitive–behavioral therapy, efforts that appear to achieve some success (Rossy et al., 1999). Coping interventions such as written emotional expression can produce health benefits as well (Broderick, Junghaenel, & Schwartz, 2005). Simultaneous attention to the medical symptoms and the psychosocial distress generated by these disorders is essential for successful treatment. Social support in the family improves functioning as well (Band, Barrowclough, & Wearden, 2014).

BOX 11.3    Epilepsy and the Need for a Job Redesign

In infancy, Colin S. developed spinal meningitis, and although he survived, the physician expressed some concern that permanent brain damage might have occurred. Colin was a normal student in school until approximately age 11, when he began to have spells of blanking out. At first, his parents interpreted these as a form of acting out, the beginnings of adolescence. However, it became clear that Colin had no recollection of these periods and became angry when questioned about them. His parents took him to a physician for evaluation, and after a lengthy workup, the doctor concluded that Colin was suffering from epilepsy.

Shortly thereafter, Colin's blanking out (known as petit mal seizures) became more severe and frequent; soon after that, he began to have grand mal seizures, involving severe and frightening convulsions. The doctors tried several medications before finding one that controlled the seizures. Indeed, so successful was the medication that Colin eventually was able to obtain a driver's license, having gone 5 years without a seizure. After he completed high school and college, Colin chose social work as his career and became a caseworker. His livelihood depended on his ability to drive because his schedule involved visiting many clients for in-home evaluations. Moreover, Colin was married, and he and his wife were supporting two young children.

In his early 30s, Colin began to experience seizures again. At first, he and his wife tried to pretend that nothing was wrong, but they quickly realized that the epilepsy was no longer under control. Colin's epilepsy represented a major threat to the family's income because Colin could no longer do his job as a caseworker. Moreover, his ability to find reemployment was compromised by the revocation of his driver's license. With considerable anxiety, Colin went to see his employer, the director of the social services unit.

After consultation, Colin's supervisor determined that he had been a valuable worker and they did not want to lose him. They therefore redesigned his position so that he could have a desk job that did not require the use of a car. By having his responsibilities shifted away from the monitoring to the evaluation of cases, and by being given an office instead of a set of addresses to visit, Colin was able to use the skills he had worked so hard to develop. In this case, then, Colin's employer responded sympathetically and effectively to the compromises that needed to be made in Colin's job responsibilities.

## Vocational Issues in Chronic Health Disorders

Many chronic health disorders create problems for patients' vocational activities and work status (Grunfeld, Drudge-Coates, Rixon, Eaton, & Cooper, 2013). Some patients need to restrict or change their work activities. Patients with spinal cord injuries who previously held positions that required physical activity will need to acquire skills that will let them work from a seated position. This kind of creative job change is illustrated in Box 11.3.

### Discrimination Against People with Chronic Health Disorders    Some people with chronic health disorders, such as heart patients, cancer patients, and AIDS patients, face job discrimination (Heckman, 2003). Because of these potential problems, job difficulties that the patient may encounter should be assessed early in the recovery process. Job counseling, retraining programs, and advice on how to avoid or combat discrimination can then be initiated promptly. Box 11.4 focuses on some health care professionals who deal with such problems.

### The Financial Impact of Chronic Health Disorders    Chronic health disorders can have a substantial financial impact on the patient and the family. Many people are not covered by insurance sufficient to meet their needs. Patients who must cut back on their work or stop working altogether may lose their insurance coverage. Thus, many people with chronic health disorders are hit by a double whammy: Income may be reduced, and simultaneously, the benefits that would have helped shoulder the costs of care may be cut back. The United States is the only developed country in which this problem still exists. The Affordable Care Act (ACA) has helped to reduce this problem.

## Social Interaction Problems in Chronic Health Disorders

After diagnosis, some people with chronic health disorders have trouble re-establishing satisfying social relations.

### Negative Responses from Others    Acquaintances, friends, and relatives may have problems adjusting to the patient's altered condition. Many

In addition to clinical health psychologists, a variety of professionals work with people with chronic health disorders.

## PHYSICAL THERAPISTS

**Physical therapists** typically receive their training as undergraduates or in a master's program, which is preparation for required licensure. About 239,800 people work as licensed physical therapists in hospitals, nursing homes, rehabilitation centers, and schools for disabled children (U.S. Bureau of Labor Statistics, 2019). Physical therapists help people with muscle, nerve, joint, or bone diseases or injuries overcome their disabilities. They work primarily with accident victims, disabled children, and older people. Physical therapists administer and interpret tests of muscle strength, motor development, functional capacity, and respiratory and circulatory efficiency. Using these tests, they develop individualized treatment programs, the goals of which are to increase strength, endurance, coordination, and range of motion. Physical therapists also conduct ongoing evaluations and modification of these programs in light of treatment goals. In addition, they help patients learn to use adaptive devices and become accustomed to new ways of performing old tasks.

## OCCUPATIONAL THERAPISTS

**Occupational therapists** work with people who are emotionally and physically disabled to determine skills, abilities, and limitations. In 2016, there were 130,400 occupational therapists (U.S. Bureau of Labor Statistics, 2019). They evaluate the existing capacities of patients, help them set goals, and plan a therapy program with other members of a rehabilitation team to build on and expand these skills. They help patients regain physical, mental, or emotional stability; relearn daily routines, such as eating, dressing, writing, or using a telephone; and prepare for employment. They plan and direct educational, vocational, and recreational activities to help patients become more self-sufficient.

Patients who are seen by occupational therapists range from children involved in crafts programs to adults who must learn new skills, such as working on a computer or using power tools. In addition, occupational therapists teach creative tasks, such as painting or crafts, which help relax patients, provide a creative outlet, and offer some variety to those who are institutionalized.

Occupational therapists obtain training through occupational therapy training programs located in universities and colleges around the country, and they must be formally licensed.

## DIETITIANS

Many of the country's 68,000 **dietitians** and nutritionists work with people with chronic health disorders (U.S. Bureau of Labor Statistics, 2019). Dietitians are formally licensed and must complete a 4-year degree program and clinically supervised training to be registered with the American Dietetic Association. Many dietitians are administrators who apply the principles of nutrition and food management to meal planning for hospitals, universities, schools, and other institutions. Dietitians also work directly with people with chronic health disorders to help plan and manage special diets. These clinical dietitians assess the dietetic needs of patients, supervise the service of meals, instruct patients in the requirements and importance of their diets, and suggest ways of maintaining adherence to diets after discharge. Many dietitians help people with diabetes control their calorie intake and food choices.

## SOCIAL WORKERS

**Social workers** help patients and their families with social problems that can develop while they are dealing with their health disorder and recovery by providing therapy, making referrals to other services, and engaging in general social planning. They may work in hospitals, clinics, community mental health centers, rehabilitation centers, and nursing homes.

A medical social worker might help a patient understand the health disorder more fully and deal with emotional responses such as depression or anxiety, through therapy. A social worker can also help the patient and family find the resources they need to solve their problems, such as household cleaning services or transportation.

In 2016, approximately 682,100 individuals were employed as social workers; one-third worked for the local or state government (U.S. Bureau of Labor Statistics, 2019). The minimum qualification for social work is a bachelor's degree, but for many positions a master's degree (MSW) is required. More than 500 colleges nationwide offer accredited undergraduate programs in social work, and more than 200 colleges and universities offer graduate programs (U.S. Bureau of Labor Statistics, 2019).

people hold negative stereotypes about certain groups of people with chronic health disorders, including those with cancer or AIDS (Fife & Wright, 2000).

People with disabilities may elicit ambivalence. Friends and acquaintances may give verbal signs of warmth and affection while nonverbally conveying rejection through their gestures, contacts, and postures. Distant relationships with friends and acquaintances appear to be more adversely affected than close relationships (Dakof & Taylor, 1990).

The Impact on the Family    Most often, individuals alone do not experience chronic diseases; their families and other loved ones also do. The family is a social system, and disruption in the life of one family member invariably affects the lives of others. One of the chief changes brought about by chronic health disorders is an increased dependency of the person with the chronic illness on other family members. If the patient is married, the health disorder inevitably places increased responsibilities on the spouse. While trying to provide support for the patient, the family's own social support needs may go unmet.

New responsibilities may fall on children and other family members living at home. Consequently, the patient's family may feel that their lives have gone out of control (Compas, Worsham, Ey, & Howell, 1996). Role strains can emerge as family members find themselves assuming new tasks and simultaneously realize that their time to pursue recreational and other leisure-time activities has declined (Pakenham & Cox, 2012). Although they often are eager to understand and help,

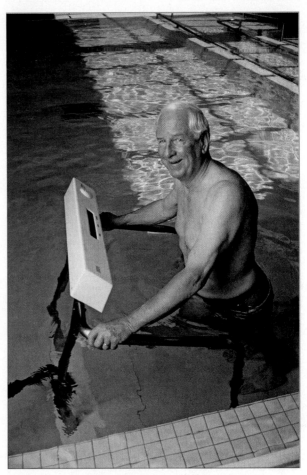

*Physical rehabilitation concentrates on enabling people to use their bodies as much as possible, to learn new physical management skills if necessary, and to pursue an integrated treatment regimen.*

Don Tremain/Getty Images

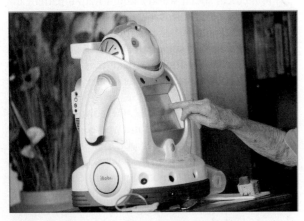

*Robots, like the one seen here, are increasingly being used to help disabled people maximize their functioning.*

Elizabeth Broadbent, The University of Auckland, New Zealand

children and adolescents who assume more responsibilities than normal for their age group can react by rebelling or acting out. Problem behaviors may include regression (such as bed-wetting), difficulties at school, truancy, sexual activity, drug use, and antagonism toward other family members.

If family members' resources are already stretched to the limit, accommodating new tasks is difficult. The wife of one stroke patient suggested some of the burdens such patients can create for their families:

> In the first few weeks, Clay not only needed meals brought to him, but countless items he wanted to use, to look at, and so forth. He was not aware of how much Jim [the patient's son] and I developed our leg muscles

in fetching and carrying. When he was on the third floor I would say "I am going downstairs. Is there anything you want?" No, he couldn't think of a thing. When I returned he remembered something, but only one thing at a time. There are advantages to a home with stairs, but not with a stroke victim in the family. (Dahlberg, 1977, p. 124)

For people with chronic health disorders, their quality of life depends quite heavily on the quality of life that their partner experiences (Segrin, Badger, & Harrington, 2012). Consequently, dyadic or communal coping whereby intimate partners take a "we" approach to maintain their relationship while jointly managing the stress of a chronic disorder helps manage the strain of chronic and life-threatening health disorders (Badr, Carmack, Kashy, Cristofanilli, & Revenson, 2010). Couple-oriented interventions for people with chronic health disorders have generally positive effects on couple functioning and patients' abilities to manage their symptoms (Martire & Helgeson, 2018).

Despite the strains that develop when a family member has a chronic health disorder, there is no evidence that such strains are catastrophic (Rini et al., 2008). Moreover, some families actually become closer as a consequence of chronic health disorders.

The Caregiving Role   Care for people with chronic health disorders is notoriously irregular. Few facilities provide the custodial care that may be needed, and so the burden of care often falls on a family member. Women more commonly become caregivers than men. The typical caregiver is a woman in her 60s caring for an elderly spouse, but caregivers also provide help for their own parents and for disabled children.

Some caregiving is short term or intermittent, but caregiving for patients with Alzheimer's disease, Parkinson's disease, advancing multiple sclerosis, and stroke can be long term and grueling. Family members who provide intense caregiving are at risk for distress, depression, and declining health (Mausbach, Patterson, Rabinowitz, Grant, & Schulz, 2007). Caregivers are often elderly, and, consequently, their own health may be threatened when they become caregivers (Gallagher, Phillips, Drayson, & Carroll, 2009). Many studies attest to the risks that caregiving poses for immune functioning (Li et al., 2007), endocrine functioning (Mausbach et al., 2005), depression (Mintzer et al., 1992), poor quality of sleep (Brummett et al., 2006), cardiovascular diseases (Mausbach et al., 2007;

Roepke et al., 2011), risk of infectious disease, and even death (Schulz & Beach, 1999). Caregivers who are experiencing other stressors in their lives or whose caregiving burden is especially great are at particular risk for mental and physical health declines (Brummett et al., 2005; Kim, Knight, & Longmire, 2007). It has been estimated that women lose, on average, more than $324,000 in wages, pensions, and social security benefits due to caring for family members; the comparable figure for men is approximately $284,000 (Greene, 2011).

Caregiving can also strain the relationship between patient and caregiver (Martire, Stephens, Druley, & Wojno, 2002). Patients are not always appreciative of the help they receive and resent the fact that they need help. Their resentment can contribute to the depression often seen in caregivers (Newsom & Schulz, 1998). Caregivers fare better when they have a strong sense of personal mastery and active coping skills (Aschbacher et al., 2005), as well as good family functioning (Deatrick et al., 2014).

Caregivers themselves may be in need of interventions (Mausbach et al., 2012). The demands of caregiving may tie them to the home and give them little free time; depression and compromised physical health are common problems (Mausbach et al., 2012). Engaging in pleasant experiences and little activity restriction both promote quality of life and may reduce physical health threats related to caregiving (Chattillion et al., 2013; Mausbach et al., 2017). The Internet can provide support to caregivers. One study (Czaja & Rubert, 2002) reported that caregivers who were able to communicate online with other family members, a therapist, and an online discussion group found the services to be very valuable, suggesting that Internet interventions have promise (DuBenske et al., 2014). Physical activity interventions improve caregivers' quality of life and other outcomes (Lambert et al., 2016). Brief daily yoga meditation practice by caregivers may also improve mental health and cognitive functioning and lower symptoms of depression (Lavretsky et al., 2013).

But caregiving can also be a positive time when relationships deepen and the caregiver and recipient become closer, deriving meaning in their relationship (Horrell, Stephens, & Breheny, 2015).

## Gender and the Impact of Chronic Health Disorders

Women with chronic health disorders experience more deficits in social support than do men with chronic health disorders. One study found that disabled women receive less social support because they are less likely to be married or get married than disabled men (Kutner, 1987). Because women with chronic health disorders and/or elderly women may experience reduced quality of life for other reasons as well, such as low income and high levels of disability (Haug & Folmar, 1986), problems in social support may exacerbate these existing differences.

Even when women with chronic health disorders are married, they are more likely to be institutionalized for their health disorder than are husbands. Married men spend fewer days in nursing homes than do married women (Freedman, 1993). It may be that husbands feel less capable of providing care than wives, or, because husbands are older than wives, they may be more disabled than are wives of husbands with chronic health disorders.

## Positive Changes in Response to Chronic Health Disorders

Throughout the chapter, we have focused on problems that chronic health disorders can create. This focus obscures an important point—namely, that human beings are fundamentally resilient (Taylor, 1983; Zautra, 2009). As people strive to overcome the challenges posed by chronic health disorders, they often find that health disorders confer positive as well as negative outcomes (Arpawong, Richeimer, Weinstein, Elghamrawy, & Milam, 2013; Taylor, 1983, 1989). People may experience positive emotions such as joy (Levy, Lee, Bagley, & Lippman, 1988) and optimism (Cordova, Cunningham, Carlson, & Andrykowski, 2001; Scheier, Weintraub, & Carver, 1986). They may perceive that having narrowly escaped death, they should reorder their priorities in a more satisfying way. They may also find more meaning in the daily activities of life (Low, Stanton, & Danoff-Burg, 2006).

In one study (Collins, Taylor, & Skokan, 1990), more than 90 percent of cancer patients reported at least some beneficial changes in their lives as a result of the cancer, including an increased ability to appreciate each day and the inspiration to do things now rather than postponing them. These patients said that they were putting more effort into their relationships and believed they had acquired more awareness of others' feelings and more empathy and compassion for others. They reported feeling stronger and more self-assured as well.

How do people with chronic health disorders so often manage to achieve such a high quality of life?

Many people with chronic health disorders perceive that they have some control over what happens to them, hold positive expectations about the future, and have a positive view of themselves. These beliefs are adaptive for mental and physical health much of the time (Taylor, 1983), but they become especially important when a person faces a chronic health disorder. Helgeson (2003) examined these beliefs in men and women treated for coronary artery disease with an angioplasty and then followed them over 4 years. These positive beliefs not only predicted positive adjustment to disease but also were associated with a lower likelihood of a repeat cardiac event (see Figure 11.2).

## When a Child Has a Chronic Health Disorder

Chronic health disorders are especially problematic when the person with the chronic illness is a child. First, children may not fully understand their diagnosis and treatment and thus experience confusion as they try to cope (Strube, Smith, Rothbaum, & Sotelo, 1991). Second, because children with chronic health disorders cannot follow their treatment regimen by themselves, the family must participate actively in the treatment process. Such interdependence can lead to tension between parent and child (Manne, Jacobsen, Gorfinkle, Gerstein, & Redd, 1993). Sometimes, children must be exposed to isolating and terrifying procedures to treat their condition (Kellerman, Rigler, & Siegel, 1979). All these factors can create distress for children, siblings, and parents (Silver, Bauman, & Ireys, 1995).

Children suffering from chronic health disorders can exhibit a variety of behavioral problems, including rebellion and withdrawal (Alati et al., 2005). They may suffer low self-esteem because they believe that the chronic health disorder is a punishment for bad behavior. They may feel cheated because their peers are healthy. Nonadherence to treatment, underachievement in school, and regressive behavior, such as bedwetting or temper tantrums, are fairly common. Children with chronic health disorders may develop maladaptive coping styles involving repression, which interfere with their understanding of and ability to comanage their disorders (Phipps & Steele, 2002). Like other chronic diseases, childhood chronic diseases can be exacerbated by stress. These problems can be further aggravated if families do not have adequate styles

**FIGURE 11.2 | Positive Life Changes Experienced by MI Patients and Breast Cancer Patients in Response to Their Health Disorders**   Most of the benefits reported by heart attack patients involve lifestyle changes, reflecting the fact that heart disease yields to changes in health habits. Cancer patients, in contrast, report changes in their social relationships and meaning attached to life; cancer may not be as directly influenced by health habits as heart disease, but may be amenable to finding purpose or meaning in other life activities.   *Source:* K. J., Petrie, Buick, D. L., Weinman, J., & Booth, R. J. "Positive effects of illness reported by myocardial infarction and breast cancer patients." Journal of Psychosomatic Research 47, no. 6, 537–543.

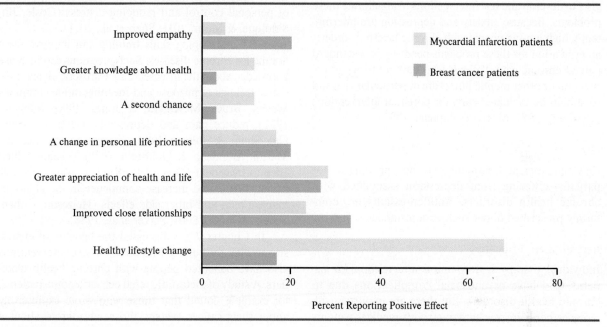

*Percent Reporting Positive Effect*

of communicating with each other and of resolving conflict (Chen, Bloomberg, Fisher, & Strunk, 2003; Manne et al., 1993).

**Improving Coping**   Several factors can improve a child's ability to cope with a chronic health disorder. Parents with realistic attitudes toward the disorder and its treatment can soothe the child emotionally and provide an informed basis for care. If the parents are not depressed, have a sense of mastery over the child's health disorder, and can remain calm, especially during treatments (DuHamel et al., 2004), the child's adjustment will be better (Timko, Stovel, Moos, & Miller, 1992). If children are encouraged to engage in self-care as much as possible, and only realistic restrictions are placed on their lives, adjustment will also be better. Encouraging regular school attendance and reasonable physical activities is particularly beneficial.

When families are unable to provide help for their child diagnosed with a chronic health disorder or are overcome by their own distress, interventions may be

needed. Providing family therapy and training the family in the treatment regimen can improve family functioning (Bakker, Van der Heijden, Van Son, & Van Loey, 2013).

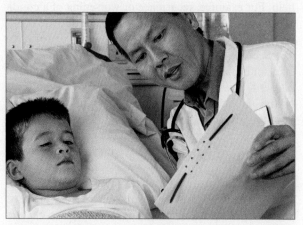

*Children's needs to be informed about their illness and to exert control over illness-related activities and over their lives have prompted interventions to involve children in their own care.*
Cathy Yeulet/123RF

## ■ PSYCHOLOGICAL INTERVENTIONS AND CHRONIC HEALTH DISORDERS

Most people with chronic health disorders achieve a fairly high quality of life. However, adverse effects of chronic disease and treatments have led health psychologists to develop and test interventions to ameliorate these problems. Because anxiety and depression are intermittently high among people with chronic health disorders, an evaluation for these problems needs to be a standard part of chronic care. Patients who have a history of depression or other mental illness are at particular risk and so should be evaluated early for potential interventions (Goldberg, 1981; Morris & Raphael, 1987).

### Pharmacological Interventions

Pharmacological treatment may be appropriate for patients suffering from depression associated with chronic health disorders. Antidepressants are commonly prescribed under such circumstances.

### Individual Therapy

Individual therapy is a common intervention for patients who have psychosocial complications due to chronic health disorders. But there are important differences between psychotherapy with medical patients and psychotherapy with patients who have primarily psychological disorders.

First, therapy with medical patients is more likely to be episodic than continuous. Chronic health disorders raise crises and issues intermittently that may require help. For example, recurrence or worsening of a condition may present a crisis that needs to be addressed with a therapist.

Second, collaboration with the ill person, physician, and family members is advisable with the patient's consent. The physician can inform the psychologist of the patient's current physical condition, and the psychologist can promote helpful communication between the physician and the patient.

Third, the therapist working with a medical patient must have a comprehensive understanding of the patient's health disorder and its modes of treatment. Health disorders and treatments themselves produce psychological problems (e.g. depression due to chemotherapy), and a therapist who is ignorant of this fact may make incorrect interpretations.

Individual therapy is often guided by CBT, targeting specific problems, such as fatigue, mood disorders,

functional impairments, or stress. For example, an 8-week CBT intervention directed to reducing fatigue was effective with patients under treatment for multiple sclerosis (Van Kessel et al., 2008). Relaxation therapy was also effective, although CBT was somewhat more so. Even briefer therapies, such as CBT conducted over the telephone, can benefit patients, enhancing a sense of personal control and reducing distress (Cosio, Jin, Siddique, & Mohr, 2011; Shen et al., 2011).

CBT and coping skills training can improve functioning for chronic diseases. Such programs can increase knowledge about the disease, reduce anxiety, increase patients' feelings of purpose and meaning in life (Brantley, Mosley, Bruce, McKnight, & Jones, 1990; Johnson, 1982), reduce pain and depression (Lorig, Chastain, Ung, Shoor, & Holman, 1989), improve coping (Lacroix, Martin, Avendano, & Goldstein, 1991), promote adherence to treatment (Greenfield, Kaplan, Ware, Yano, & Frank, 1988), and increase confidence in the ability to manage pain and other side effects (Helgeson, Cohen, Schulz, & Yasko, 2001; Parker et al., 1988).

In Chapter 7, we discussed the benefits of expressive writing for coping with stress. These interventions also have benefited people with chronic health disorders. A study of metastatic renal cell carcinoma patients, for example, found that those who wrote expressively about their cancer (versus those who wrote about a neutral topic) had less sleep disturbance and better sleep quality and duration and fewer problems with activities of daily life (de Moor et al., 2002).

With the move toward efficient and targeted therapies has come a focus on brief self-management interventions directed to debilitating symptoms such as fatigue (Friedberg et al., 2013) or needs, such as exercise (Pilutti, Greenlee, Motl, Nickrent, & Petruzzello, 2013).

The Internet poses exciting possibilities for providing interventions in a cost-effective manner. Information about health disorders can be presented in a clear and simple way, and recommendations for coping with common health disorder-related problems can be posted on websites for use by patients and their families (Budman, 2000). In one study, breast cancer patients who used the Internet for medical information experienced greater social support than those who did not. Moreover, patients spent less than an hour a week online at the site, suggesting that psychological benefits may result from a minimal time commitment (Fogel, Albert, Schnabel, Ditkoff, & Neugut, 2002). Other online interventions have been targeted to more general issues facing people with chronic disorders, such as

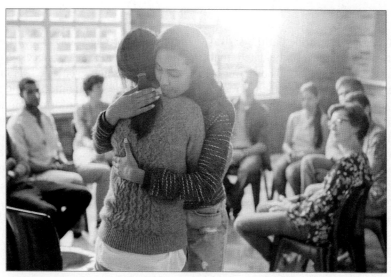

*Social support groups can satisfy unmet needs for social support from family and friends and can enable people to share their personal experiences with others like themselves.*

Caia Image/Image Source

altering diet in a healthy direction and increasing physical activity (McKay, Seeley, King, Glasgow, & Eakin, 2001).

Health behavior interventions delivered via the telephone directed to improving diet and increasing physical activity also can be successful (Gorst, Coates, & Armitage, 2016). In one study, several patient groups with chronic conditions significantly improved several health behaviors via telephone intervention (Lawler et al., 2010).

## Relaxation, Stress Management, and Exercise

Relaxation training is a widely used intervention with people with chronic health disorders, including asthma, cancer, and multiple sclerosis, among others. Combining relaxation training with stress management and blood pressure monitoring has proven useful in the treatment of hypertension (Agras, Taylor, Kraemer, Southam, & Schneider, 1987).

Mindfulness-based stress reduction (MBSR) can improve adjustment to chronic health disorders (Brown & Ryan, 2003). Mindfulness meditation teaches people to be highly focused on the present moment, acknowledging and accepting thoughts and feelings without becoming distracted or distressed by them. Acceptance and commitment therapy (ACT) is also used with people

with chronic health disorders and helps patients to accept their health disorder experiences without avoidance or fruitless striving (Lundgren, Dahl, & Hayes, 2008).

Exercise also improves quality of life among people who have chronic health disorders (Sweet, Martin Ginis, Tomasone, & SHAPE-SCI Research Group, 2013). Combined CBT and physical activity interventions for adults with chronic diseases do not appear more effective than either intervention alone, however (Bernard et al., 2018).

## Social Support Interventions

Social support is an important resource for people who have chronic health disorders. The benefits of social support are well documented for virtually every chronic health disorder in which this resource has been examined, including cancer, spinal cord injury, end-stage renal disease, and cardiovascular disease. Adult day service facilities can provide such support when help with activities of daily living is needed. Older adults, including those with Alzheimer's disease, are especially likely to make use of such services when they are available and affordable (Dwyer, Harris-Kojetin, & Valverde, 2014).

**Family Support**  Family support is especially important: It enhances the patient's physical and

Janet and Peter Birnheimer were thrilled at the arrival of their newborn but learned almost immediately that he had cystic fibrosis (CF). Shocked at this discovery—they had no idea that they both were carrying the recessive gene for CF—they tried to learn as much as they could about the disease. Their hometown physician was able to provide them with some information, but they realized from newspaper articles that there was breaking news as well. Moreover, they wanted help dealing with the coughing, wheezing, and other symptoms so they could provide their youngster with the best possible care.

The couple turned to the Internet, where they found a website for parents of children with CF. Online, they learned much more about the disease, found out where they could get articles providing additional information, chatted with other parents about the best ways to manage the symptoms, and shared the complex and painful feelings they had to manage every day (Baig, 1997, February 17).

As this account implies, the Internet is increasingly becoming a source of information and social support to people who have chronic health disorders. Websites provide instant access to other people going through the same events. CF is not a common disorder, and so the Birnheimers found that the website was their best source of information about breakthroughs in the causes and treatments of the disease, as well as the best source for advice from other parents about the psychosocial issues that arose. Websites have created opportunities for bringing together people who were once isolated, so that they can solve their problems through shared knowledge.

Websites are only as good as the information they contain, of course, and there is always the risk of misinformation. However, some of the better known websites are scrupulously careful about the information they post. Among services currently available is WebMD, a commercial website devoted to providing consumer and health information on the Internet. The National Institutes of Health (https://www.nih.gov/health-information) provides accurate and current information on hundreds of diseases.

---

emotional functioning, it promotes adherence to treatment (Martire, Lustig, Schulz, Miller, & Helgeson, 2004), and it can improve the course of health disorders (Walker & Chen, 2010). Family members can remind the patient about activities that need to be undertaken and even participate in them, so that adherence is more likely. For example, one of our students whose father was newly diagnosed with diabetes made it a point to take brisk walks with him just before breakfast 5 days a week.

Sometimes family members need guidance in the well-intentioned actions they should avoid because such actions actually make things worse (Dakof & Taylor, 1990; Martin, Davis, Baron, Suls, & Blanchard, 1994). For example, some family members think they themselves and their loved one who has a chronic health disorder should be relentlessly cheerful, which can have the unintended effect of leaving the patient unable to share distress or concerns with others. At different times during the course of a health disorder, patients may be best served by different kinds of support. Tangible aid, such as being driven to and from medical appointments, may be important at some points in time. At other times, however, emotional support may be more important (Dakof & Taylor, 1990; Martin et al., 1994).

Teaching families about the nature of the chronic health disorder experienced by one family member can be helpful not only to family functioning but also to the patient's course of the health disorder (Walker & Chen, 2010).

### Support Groups

Social **support groups** represent a resource for people who have chronic health disorders. Some of these groups are facilitated by a therapist, and in some cases, they are patient-led. Support groups discuss issues of mutual concern that arise as a consequence of health disorders. They provide specific information about how others have dealt with the problems and give people an opportunity to share their emotional responses and useful coping strategies with others facing the same problems. Social support groups can satisfy unmet needs for social support from family and caregivers, or they may act as an additional source of support provided by those going through the same event. The Internet now provides manifold opportunities for giving and receiving social support and information online (Box 11.5). •

## SUMMARY

1. At any given time, 50 percent of the population has at least one chronic condition that requires medical management. Quality-of-life measures pinpoint problems associated with diseases and treatments and help in policy decision making regarding the effectiveness and cost-effectiveness of interventions.

2. People with chronic health disorders can experience denial, intermittent anxiety, and depression. But these reactions, especially anxiety and depression, can be underdiagnosed, confused with symptoms of disease or treatment, or presumed to be normal and so not appropriate for intervention.

3. Anxiety is reliably tied to health disorder events, such as awaiting test results or obtaining regular checkups. Depression increases with the severity of disease, pain, and disability.

4. Active coping and flexible coping efforts are more effective than avoidance, passive coping, or use of one predominant coping strategy.

5. Patients develop concepts of their health disorder, its cause, and its controllability that relate to their coping and adjustment. Perceived personal control over health disorders and/or treatment is associated with good adjustment.

6. The management of chronic health disorders centers around physical problems, especially recovery of functioning and adherence to treatment; vocational retraining, job discrimination, financial hardship, and loss of insurance; gaps and problems in social support; and psychological reactions and personal losses, such as the threat that disease poses for long-term goals.

7. Most patients experience some benefits as well as negative effects from chronic health disorders. These positive outcomes may occur in part because patients compensate for losses in some areas of their lives with value placed on other aspects of life.

8. Interventions with people with chronic health disorders include pharmacological interventions; CBT; brief psychotherapeutic interventions; relaxation, stress management, exercise; social support interventions; family therapy; and support groups. Support groups, including online groups, can provide a helpful resource for people with chronic health disorders.

## KEY TERMS

body image
denial
depression
dietitians

multimorbidity
occupational therapists
physical rehabilitation
physical therapists

quality of life
self-concept
social workers
support groups

# CHAPTER 12

# Psychological Issues in Advancing and Terminal Illness

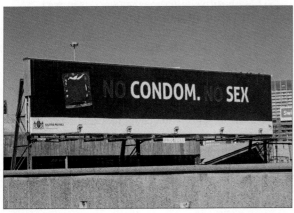

Rob Crandall/Alamy Stock Photo

At the first assembly of freshman year in a suburban high school, the principal opened his remarks by telling the assembled students, "Look around you. Look to your left, look to your right, look in front of you, and look in back of you. Four years from now, one of you will be dead." Most of the students were stunned by this remark, but one boy in the back feigned a death rattle and slumped to the floor in a mock display of the principal's prophecy. He was the one. Two weeks after he got his driver's license, his car spun out of control at high speed and crashed into a stone wall.

The principal, of course, had not peered into the future but had simply drawn on the statistics showing that even adolescents die, especially from accidents. By the time most of us reach age 18, we will have known at least one person who has died, whether it be a high school classmate, a grandparent, or a family friend. Many of these causes of death are preventable. Many children die from accidents in the home. Adolescents, as well as children, die in car crashes often related to risky driving, drugs, alcohol, or a combination of factors. Even death in middle and old age is most commonly due to the cumulative effects of bad health habits, such as smoking, poor diet, lack of exercise, and obesity. Overall, the risk of dying at any given time has decreased dramatically since 1900 for all age groups. A mere 100 years ago, people died primarily from infectious diseases, such as tuberculosis, influenza, or pneumonia. Now those diseases are much less widespread owing to major advances in public health measures, such as improved sanitation and education, as well as preventive medical technologies, such as vaccination, which were developed in the twentieth century. Today, when death does come, it will most likely stem from a chronic disease, such as cancer or heart disease, rather than from an acute disorder, especially in higher-income countries, as Tables 12.1 and 12.2 indicate. This fact means that, instead of facing a rapid, unanticipated death, the average adult may know what he or she will probably die of for 5, 10, or even more years.

Global life expectancy at birth in 2016 was 72 years (World Health Organization, May 2019), and in the United States it was 78.6 years (Xu, Murphy, Kochanek, Bastian, & Arias, 2018). Although favorable compared with some of the rest of the world, life expectancy in the United States lags behind that of many industrialized countries. The complex contributors include the relatively high rates of maternal and infant mortality, homicide, and unmet health care needs due to financial and structural barriers in the United States (Kontis,

**TABLE 12.1  |  Deaths: Leading Causes in the United States, 2016**

| Rank and Cause | Number of Deaths |
|---|---|
| 1. Heart disease | 635,260 |
| 2. Cancer | 598,038 |
| 3. Accidents (unintentional injuries) | 161,374 |
| 4. Chronic respiratory diseases | 154,596 |
| 5. Stroke (cerebrovascular diseases) | 142,142 |
| 6. Alzheimer's disease | 116,103 |
| 7. Diabetes | 80,058 |
| 8. Influenza/pneumonia | 51,537 |
| 9. Nephritis* | 50,046 |
| 10. Intentional self-harm (suicide) | 44,965 |

*Includes nephrotic syndrome and nephrosis.

Source: Xu, J., S. L. Murphy, K. D. Kochanek, B. Bastian, and Elizabeth Arias. "Deaths: Final Data for 2016." *National Vital Statistics Report* 67, no. 5 (2018): 1–76. www.cdc.gov/nchs/products/databriefs/db293.htm.

Bennett, Mathers, Li, Foreman, & Ezzati, 2017). In turn, these problems are related to social disparities, in that health burdens fall inequitably as a function of people's race and socioeconomic status (National Research Council and Institute of Medicine, 2013).

Moreover, overall gains in longevity have stalled or reversed during 2015 through 2017 in the United States, driven in part by rising deaths from opioid overdose (see Chapter 10, Box 10.4) and suicide (Bernstein, November 2018). Although suicide remains a rare behavior (14 of 100,000 people in 2017), it is the second leading cause of death in 10- to 34-year-olds (National Institute of Mental Health, May 2019). American Indian/Alaska Native and non-Hispanic white men have the highest suicide rates. Males have nearly four times the suicide rate of females, explained in part by access to guns, which accounts for 56 percent of suicide deaths in males and 31 percent in females. The toll-free National Suicide Prevention Lifeline at 1-800-273-TALK (8255) is available to anyone 24 hours a day, 7 days a week (for additional resources, see http://www.suicidepreventionlifeline.org).

## ■ DEATH ACROSS THE LIFE SPAN

Comedian Woody Allen remarked, "I'm not afraid of death. I just don't want to be there when it happens." Understanding the psychological issues associated with death and dying first requires an overview of

**TABLE 12.2** | Leading Causes of Mortality Among Adults, Worldwide, 2016

| Mortality, Low-income Countries | | | Mortality, High-income Countries | | |
|---|---|---|---|---|---|
| Rank | Cause | Deaths | Rank | Cause | Deaths |
| 1 | Lower respiratory infections | 76 | 1 | Ischaemic heart disease | 147 |
| 2 | Diarrheal diseases | 58 | 2 | Stroke | 63 |
| 3 | Ischaemic heart disease | 53 | 3 | Alzheimer's and other dementias | 61 |
| 4 | HIV/AIDS | 44 | 4 | Trachea, bronchus, lung cancers | 49 |
| 5 | Stroke | 42 | 5 | Chronic obstructive pulmonary disease | 47 |
| 6 | Malaria | 38 | 6 | Lower respiratory infections | 37 |
| 7 | Tuberculosis | 34 | 7 | Colon and rectum cancers | 28 |
| 8 | Preterm birth complications | 32 | 8 | Diabetes mellitus | 23 |
| 9 | Birth asphyxia and birth trauma | 30 | 9 | Kidney diseases | 19 |
| 10 | Road injury | 29 | 10 | Breast cancer | 16 |

*Source:* World Health Organization. "The Top 10 Causes of Death." Last Modified May 24, 2018. https://www.who.int/news-room/fact-sheets/detail/the-top-10-causes-of-death.

death itself. What is the most likely cause of death for a person of any given age, and what kind of death will it be?

### Death in Infancy and Childhood

Although the United States is one of the most technologically developed countries in the world, our **infant mortality rate** is still fairly high (5.87 per 1,000) (Xu et al., 2018), higher than that in most Western European nations. Although these figures represent a substantial decline in infant mortality since 1980 (from 12.6 per 1,000) (Centers for Disease Control and Prevention, 2012, January) (Figure 12.1), Black infants are still more than twice as likely to die during the first year as non-Hispanic white infants are (Xu et al., 2018).

**FIGURE 12.1** | Life Expectancy and Infant Mortality in the United States, 1900–2013

(*Source:* Xu, Jiaquan, Sherry L. Murphy, Kenneth D. Kochanek, and Brigham A. Bastian. "Deaths: Final Data for 2013." *Centers for Disease Control and Prevention* 64, no. 2 (2016): 01–119.)

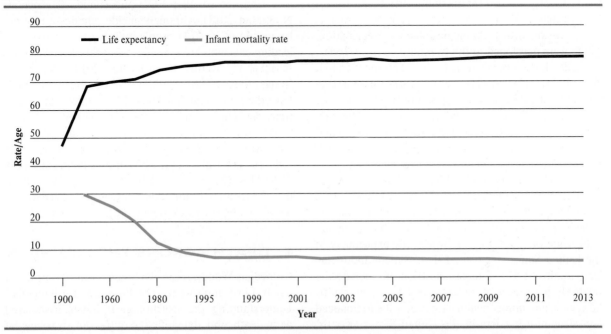

Causes of Death   The countries that have a lower infant mortality rate than the United States have national medical programs that provide free or low-cost maternal care during pregnancy. When infants are born prematurely or die at birth, the problems can frequently be traced to poor prenatal care for the mother. Fifteen percent of women in the United States receive inadequate prenatal care, which is related to being younger, having less education, and lacking financial access to care (Osterman & Martin, 2018).

During the first year of life, the main causes of death are congenital malformations, disorders related to preterm birth (before 37 weeks of pregnancy) and low birth weight, and **sudden infant death syndrome (SIDS)** (Xu et al., 2018). The causes of SIDS are not entirely known—the infant simply stops breathing—but brain and genetic problems appear to combine with environmental causes, such as the baby sleeping on its stomach or side, being exposed to maternal smoking in utero or early in infancy, and being fed only formula rather than being breastfed (Eunice Kennedy Shriver National Institute of Child Health and Development, January 2017). Mercifully, SIDS appears to be a gentle death for the child, although not for parents: The confusion, self-blame, and suspicion from others who do not understand this phenomenon can exact an enormous psychological toll on the parents. National resources are available on what parents and other caregivers can do to reduce the risk of SIDS (https://safetosleep. nichd.nih.gov/; https://www.nichd.nih.gov/health/topics/ sids/).

After the first year, the main cause of death among children under age 15 is accidents, which account for more than 30 percent of all deaths in this group. Congenital problems and cancer are the other leading causes of death in young children, and the most common cancer in children is leukemia.

Leukemia is a form of cancer that strikes the bone marrow, producing an excessive number of white blood cells and leading to severe anemia and other complications. Because of advances in treatment, including chemotherapy and bone marrow transplants, over 80 percent of children treated for cancer survive the disease for 5 years or more (National Cancer Institute, October 2018). Unfortunately, these procedures, especially bone marrow transplants, can be painful and produce unpleasant side effects. Overall, the mortality rates for most causes of death in infants and children have declined. However, suicide is now the second leading cause of death in children aged 10 to 14 years, and it is on the rise (Heron, 2018).

Children's Understanding of Death   The child's conception of death occurs gradually, with a

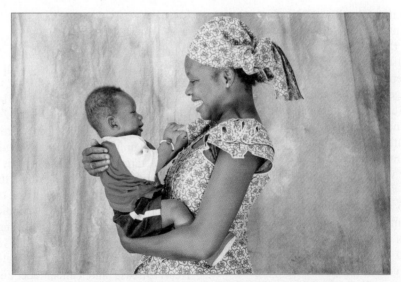

*A huge decline in child mortality is now occurring throughout Africa. Broad economic growth and public health policies such as the use of insecticide-treated bed nets to discourage mosquitoes and improvements in diet are among the reasons for this good news.*   (*Source: The Economist*, May 19, 2012)
commerceandculturestock/Moment/Getty Images

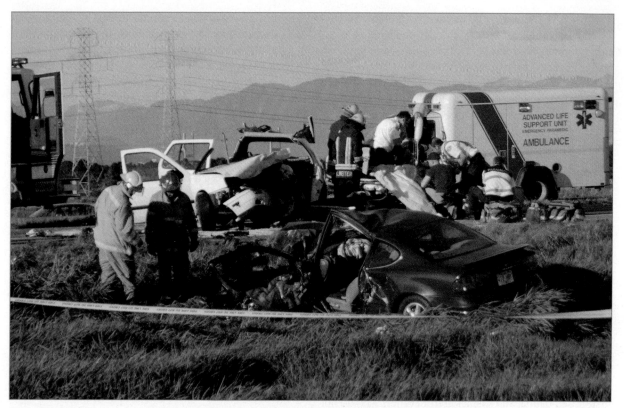

*One of the chief causes of death among adolescents and young adults is vehicle accidents.*
Sergei Bachlakov/Shutterstock

mature understanding of death—that it is final, occurs to all living things, and involves the permanent end of all capabilities of the physical body—developing at least through age 10 (Speece & Brent, 1996). Up to age 5, most children think of death as a great sleep. Children at this age are often curious about death rather than frightened or saddened by it, partly because they may not understand that death is final and irreversible. Rather, the dead person is thought to be still around, but in an altered state, like Snow White or Sleeping Beauty waiting for the prince (Bluebond-Langner, 1977).

Between ages 5 and 9, the idea that death is final develops, although most children do not have a biological understanding of death. For some of these children, death is personified into a shadowy figure, such as a ghost or devil who comes to take the person away. By ages 7 to 10, children typically develop an understanding of the processes involved in death (such as burial and cremation), know that the body decomposes, and realize that the person who has died will not return (Speece & Brent, 1996).

## Death in Adolescence and Young Adulthood

When asked their view of death, most young adults envision a trauma or fiery accident. This perception is realistic. Although the death rate in adolescence and young adulthood is low (about 0.51 and 0.97 per 1,000 for people ages 15 to 19 and 20 to 24, respectively), the major cause of death in this age group is unintentional injury, mainly involving automobiles (Heron, 2018). Suicide, largely through firearms, is the second leading cause of death in this age group. Homicide is the third leading cause of death overall and the leading cause of death for young Black men. The rates of accidents and suicide are disturbingly high in young American Indian/Alaska Native men aged 20 to 24 years (Heron, 2018) approximately 1.3 times more likely than the average. Heart disease and cancer account for most of the remaining deaths in this age group.

### Reactions to Young Adult Death   Next to the death of a child, the death of a young adult is considered the most tragic. Understandably, when young

adults do receive a diagnosis of a terminal illness, such as cancer, they can feel shock, outrage, and an acute sense of injustice. Their friends and family often have similar feelings. Because they are otherwise in good health, young adults may face a long and drawn-out period of dying. For them, unlike older people, there are fewer biological competitors for death, so they do not quickly succumb to complications, such as pneumonia or kidney failure.

## Death in Middle Age

As adults approach middle age, their leading causes of death in the United States shift toward chronic diseases. Cancer and heart disease replace accidents as the leading causes of death of adults aged 35 through 64 (Heron, 2018). In middle age, then, death begins to assume more realistic and, in some cases, fearful proportions, both because it is more common and because people develop chronic health problems that may ultimately kill them. The fear of death may be represented in a fear of loss of physical appearance, sexual prowess, or athletic ability. Or it may be focused on one's work: One might question its meaningfulness or acknowledge that youthful ambitions might not be realized (Gould, 1972).

Most adults evidence sound or increasing life satisfaction during midlife, even as some dimensions of health and cognitive performance decline (Lachman, Teshale, & Agrigoroaei, 2015). **Premature death**—that is, death that occurs before the average age for the population—increases during middle age. From 2011 to 2014 in the United States, American Indians and Alaska Natives had the highest premature mortality, followed by Black individuals. Protective factors in midlife for healthy physical functioning and lower premature mortality years later include having supportive social relationships, exercising regularly, and having a strong sense of personal control and purpose in life (Hill & Turiano, 2014; Lachman et al., 2015).

When asked, most people reply that they would prefer a sudden, painless, and nonmutilating death. Although sudden death has the disadvantage of not allowing people to prepare their exit, in some ways it facilitates a more graceful departure, because the dying person does not have to cope with physical deterioration, pain, and loss of mental faculties. Sudden death is, in some ways, kinder to family members as well. The family does not have to go through the emotional torment of witnessing the person's worsening condition, and

finances and other resources are not as severely taxed. A risk is that families may be poorly prepared to cope with the loss financially and otherwise, or family members may be estranged, with reconciliation now impossible.

## Death in Old Age

Dying is not easy at any time during the life cycle, but it may be easier in old age. People over age 65 are generally more prepared to face death than are the young. They have seen friends and relatives die and may have thought about their death and made some initial preparations.

Older people most often die of degenerative diseases, such as heart disease, cancer, stroke, Alzheimer's disease, and chronic lower respiratory disease (Heron, 2018), or simply from general physical decline that predisposes them to infectious disease or organ failure. The terminal phase of illness is generally shorter for older adults because there is often more than one biological competitor for death.

Why do some individuals live only into their 60s and others live into their 90s or longer? Health psychologists have investigated the factors that predict mortality in older people. Obviously, new illnesses and the worsening of pre-existing conditions account for many of these differences. But changes in psychosocial factors are also important. Poor mental health and reduced satisfaction with life predict decline among older adults (Myint et al., 2007; Rodin & McAvay, 1992; Zhang, Kahana, Kahana, Hu, & Pozuelo, 2009), whereas a sense of purpose is tied to a longer life (Boyle, Barnes, Buchman, & Bennett, 2009). Close family relationships also are protective of health.

In part because of such findings, health goals for older adults now focus less on reducing mortality and more on improving quality of life. In the United States, people age 65 and up are healthier due to lifestyle changes. However, the worldwide picture is quite different. People are living longer, about 61 years in some developing countries, but the prevalence of chronic diseases due to smoking, poor diet, sedentary lifestyle, and alcohol abuse means that many older people live poor-quality lives.

One curious fact is that women typically live longer than men—women, on average, live to 81 and men only to 76 (Xu et al., 2018). Box 12.1 explores some of the reasons for this difference in mortality rates between men and women. Table 12.3 provides a formula for roughly calculating personal longevity. Another website that offers projections about how likely you are to live is www.livingto100.com.

BOX 12.1    Why Do Women Live Longer Than Men?

On average, women live 5 years longer than men in the United States, and the difference in longevity applies worldwide (World Health Organization, 2019). Only in underdeveloped countries, in which childbirth technology is poorly developed, or in countries where women are denied access to health care, do men live longer. Why?

Women seem to be biologically more fit than men. Although more male than female fetuses are conceived, more males are stillborn or miscarried than are females, and male babies are more likely to die than females. In fact, the male death rate is higher at all ages, so that there are more females than males left alive by the time young people reach their 20s. Exactly what biological mechanisms make females more fit are still unknown. Some factors may be genetic; others may be hormonal. For example, when a gene on the X chromosome undergoes mutation, women have a second X to compensate. And women's greater estrogen may act to protect the heart.

Another reason why men die earlier than women is that men engage in more risky behaviors (Williams, 2003). Chief among these is smoking, which accounts for as much as 40 percent of the mortality difference between men and women through its causal role in heart disease, several cancers, and other life-limiting diseases (Beltrán-Sánchez, Finch, & Crimmins, 2015). Men are exposed to more occupational hazards and hold more hazardous jobs, such as construction work, police work, or firefighting. Men's alcohol consumption is greater than women's, exposing them to liver damage and alcohol-related accidents, and they consume more drugs than do women. Men are more likely to participate in hazardous sports and to use firearms recreationally. Men's greater access to firearms, in turn, makes them more likely to use guns to commit suicide—a method that is more effective than the methods typically favored by women (such as poison). Men also use automobiles and motorcycles more than women, contributing to their high death rate from accidents. Men's tendencies to cope with stress through fight (aggression) or flight (social withdrawal or withdrawal through drugs and alcohol) may thus also account for their shorter life span; women are more likely to tend and befriend instead (Taylor, Kemeny, Reed, Bower, & Gruenewald, 2000). Men engage in less preventive health care, and this is more true of men with strong masculinity beliefs (Springer & Mouzon, 2011). Macho men, then, live shorter lives.

Social support may be more protective for women than for men. On the one hand, being married benefits men more than women (Kiecolt-Glaser & Newton, 2001). However, women have more close friends and participate in more group activities, such as church or women's groups, that may offer support. Social support keeps stress systems at low levels and so may prevent some of the wear and tear that men, especially unattached men, sustain. All of these factors seem to play a role in women's advantage in longevity.

**TABLE 12.3 | How Long Will You Live?**

Longevity calculators are rough guides for calculating your personal longevity. Although many longevity calculators exist, one of the most popular is the True Vitality Test. This calculator asks questions such as:

Compared with a year ago, how has your overall health changed?
During the past month, how many days have you felt sad or depressed?
In the past week, during how many days did you exercise or engage in vigorous physical activity for at least 20 minutes?
On average, how many hours a night do you sleep?
On average, how many alcoholic drinks do you have in a typical day?
During the past week, how many servings of fresh vegetables did you eat?
During the past week, how many times did you consume sweets?
How satisfied are you with your work life?
How often do you attend religious activities?

After these questions are answered, you are provided with four scores: your biological age (your body's age given your habits), your life expectancy, your healthy life expectancy (years free of cancer, heart disease, and diabetes), and your accrued years (how many years you are gaining or losing as a result of your habits).

To get your score, go to http://apps.bluezones.com/vitality.

*Source:* Vitality Compass, http://apps.bluezones.com/vitality.

# ■ PSYCHOLOGICAL ISSUES IN ADVANCING ILLNESS

Although many people die suddenly, many people who are terminally ill know that they are going to die for some time before their death. As a consequence, a variety of medical and psychological issues arise for the person.

## Continued Treatment and Advancing Illness

Advancing and terminal illnesses frequently bring the need for continued treatments with debilitating and unpleasant side effects. For example, radiation therapy and chemotherapy for cancer may produce discomfort, nausea and vomiting, chronic diarrhea, hair loss, skin discoloration, fatigue, and loss of energy. The patient with advancing diabetes may require amputation of extremities, such as fingers or toes. The patient with advancing cancer may require removal of an organ to which the illness has now spread, such as a lung or part of the liver. The patient with degenerative kidney disease may be given a transplant, in the hope that it will forestall further deterioration.

There may, consequently, come a time when the question of whether to continue treatments becomes an issue. In some cases, refusal of treatment may indicate depression and feelings of hopelessness, but in many cases, the patient's decision may be supported by thoughtful choice.

### Is There a Right to Die?

In recent years, the right to die has assumed importance due to several legislative and social trends. In 1990, Congress passed the Patient Self-Determination Act, requiring that Medicare and Medicaid health care facilities have written policies and procedures concerning patients' wishes for life-prolonging therapy. These policies include the provision of a Do Not Resuscitate (DNR) order, which patients may choose to sign or not, in order to provide explicit guidance regarding their preferences for medical response to cardiopulmonary arrest.

An important social trend affecting terminal care is the right-to-die movement, which maintains that dying should become more a matter of personal choice and personal control. Derek Humphry's book *Final Exit* virtually leaped off bookstore shelves when it appeared in 1991. A manual of how to commit suicide or assist in suicide for the dying, it was perceived to give dying people the means for achieving a dignified death at a time of one's choosing.

Receptivity to such ideas as the right to die and assisted death for the terminally ill has increased in the American population. In a 1975 Gallup Poll, only 41 percent of respondents believed that someone in great pain with no hope of improvement had the moral right to commit suicide. In 2018, 72 percent agreed that doctors should be allowed by law to end a patient's life if the patient and family request it. Many European countries, as well as Australia and Canada, have much higher levels of support for assisted dying, with several approaching 90 percent (*The Economist*, October 20, 2012). Although some experts found that these preferences may change when people realize that they are facing death (Sharman, Garry, Jacobson, Loftus, & Ditto, 2008), declines in functioning appear to lead to reduced interest in life-prolonging treatments (Ditto et al., 2003). Only about one-quarter of adults in the United States say they have their preferences for end-of-life medical treatment in a written document (Kaiser Family Foundation, 2017) (see Box 12.2).

### Moral and Legal Issues

Increasingly, societies must grapple with the issue of **euthanasia** and **assisted death.** *Euthanasia* comes from the Greek word meaning "good death" (Pfeifer & Brigham, 1996). Euthanasia, which is legal in some countries, but not the United States, involves a physician administering a lethal dose of medication to a person. **Physician-assisted death,** which as of 2019 is legal in eight states of the United States (including the District of Columbia jurisdiction), involves a person voluntarily ending his or her life with a lethal dose of medication prescribed by a physician.

In 1997, Oregon became the first state to enact a law permitting physician-assisted dying, the Death with Dignity Act. To exercise this option, the adult must be mentally competent and have a terminal illness with less than 6 months to live. He or she must also be informed about alternatives, such as pain control and hospice care. He or she must make the request at least three times, and the case must be reviewed by a second physician for accuracy and to ensure that family members are not pressuring the patient to die (*The Economist,* October, 2012). Since the law was enacted, more than 2,000 Oregonians have received a prescription; most had cancer and 66 percent died from ingesting the drug. Patients who received the prescription most frequently reported concerns about losing autonomy, losing the ability to take part in activities that

(This is an example of the kind of letter that might be given by a patient to his or her physician.)

Dear Dr. _____.

I wish to maintain the last weeks of my life with dignity and to die an appropriate death.

To that end, I ask:

- That my health care choices (or those of the person designated to choose for me) be respected.

- That if palliative care is warranted, you will recommend a plan or facility.

- That I may be allowed to die with dignity and that extraordinary life saving measures will not be taken.

- That my "do not resuscitate" request will be honored.

I appreciate the opportunity to communicate my wishes with respect to the end of my life and your willingness to honor my requests so as to minimize the burden on me and my family.

Sincerely,

Signature                                    Date

---

make life enjoyable, and losing dignity (Oregon Health Authority, 2018). Although a 1997 Supreme Court ruling did not find physician-assisted dying to be a constitutional right, the Court nonetheless left legislation to individual states.

More passive measures to terminate life have also received attention. A number of states have now enacted laws enabling people with terminal diseases to write a **living will,** or provide advance directives, requesting that extraordinary life-sustaining procedures not be used if they are unable to make this decision on their own. Advance directives provide instructions and legal protection for the physician, so that life-prolonging interventions, such as the use of respirators, will not be indefinitely undertaken in a vain effort to keep the patient alive. This kind of document also helps to ensure that the patient's preferences, rather than a surrogate's (such as a relative), are respected (Ditto & Hawkins, 2005; Fagerlin, Ditto, Danks, Houts, & Smucker, 2001). Overall, 88 percent of hospice care patients, 65 percent of nursing home residents, but only 28 percent of home health care patients have filed at least one advanced directive with their physicians, usually a DNR order or a living will (Jones, Moss, & Harris-Kojetin, 2011).

Unfortunately, research suggests that many physicians do not follow the wishes of their dying patients, which can prolong pain and suffering. One study (Seneff, Wagner, Wagner, Zimmerman, & Knaus, 1995) found that although one-third of the patients had asked not to be revived with cardiopulmonary resuscitation, half the time this request was not indicated on their charts. Thus, at present, the living will and related tools are not completely successful in allowing patients to express their wishes and ensure that they are met. Box 12.3 presents a case on the question of assisted death.

The complex moral, legal, and ethical issues surrounding death are relatively new to our society. As researchers and clinicians, health psychologists can add to the discussion (Sears & Stanton, 2001). These issues are assuming increasing importance with the aging of the population.

## Psychological and Social Issues Related to Dying

Advancing and terminal illness raises a number of important psychological and social issues.

Changes in the Patient's Self-Concept    Advancing illness can threaten the self-concept. As the disease progresses, patients are increasingly less able to present themselves effectively. It may become difficult for them to maintain control of biological and social functioning. They may be incontinent (unable to control urination or bowel movements); they may drool, have distorted facial expressions, or shake uncontrollably. These changes can be difficult for the person and others.

People with advanced disease may also be in intermittent pain, may suffer from uncontrollable retching or vomiting, and may experience a shocking deterioration in appearance due to weight loss, the stress of treatments, or the sheer drain of illness. Even more threatening to some patients is mental regression and

May Harvey, age 60, was dying slowly and painfully of gastric cancer. She no longer had the energy to see friends and needed help for every daily activity, including basic hygiene. She decided to take her own life and asked her physician to help her. He refused, explaining that the law was very clear about not assisting a suicide. She turned to her husband who had been a medic overseas, but he also refused. He would lose his license to practice nursing and could go to prison.

So May decided she would have to do it herself. She began hoarding her sleeping pills and complained of insomnia, so her physician would increase the dosage. One day, May decided she had accumulated enough pills, and so she swallowed them all with water, expecting to slip into sleep and away from life. Instead, within the hour she threw them all up.

Frantic, she gathered them up, dried off what remained, and put them away for another try. Soon she had accumulated a few more pills. She picked a day when she was feeling better and swallowed them all again. The same thing happened. This time her husband realized what she was trying to do. He informed her physician who reduced her sleep medication. It did not matter because May was now too weak to try it a third time.

A few days later, May's daughter came in to help, and May told her what she had tried to do. "I don't see why they can't help me. When they put the dog to sleep, it was so easy and painless. Why can't they do the same for me?" May lived a few more weeks until finally she got the death she sought.

the inability to concentrate. Cognitive decline accelerates in the years prior to death (Wilson, Beck, Bienias, & Bennett, 2007). Losses in cognitive function may also be due either to the progressive nature of disease or to the tranquilizing and disorienting effects of painkillers and other medications.

Issues of Social Interaction    These issues spill over into social interactions. Although terminally ill people often want and need social contact, they may

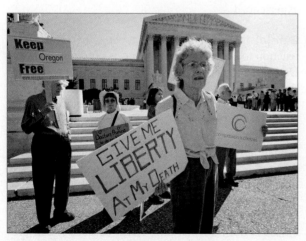

*In recent years, grassroots movements expressing the rights to die and to physician-assisted death have gained strength in the United States.*

CHARLES DHARAPAK/AP Images

be afraid that their obvious mental and physical deterioration will upset visitors. Thus, they may begin a process of social withdrawal, whereby they gradually restrict visits to only a few trusted others. Family and friends can help make this withdrawal less extreme: They can prepare visitors in advance for the person's state so that visitors do not upset the dying person with their reactions. They can control the place, time, and number of visitors to correspond to the terminally ill person's preferences.

Some disengagement from the social world is normal and may represent both end-of-life biological processes and the grieving process through which the final loss of family and friends is anticipated. This period of anticipatory grieving may compromise communication because it is hard for the patient to express affection for others while simultaneously preparing to leave them.

Communication Issues    As long as a patient's prognosis is favorable, communication is usually open; however, as the prognosis worsens and treatment becomes more drastic, communication may break down. Medical staff may become evasive when questioned about the patient's status. Family members may be cheerfully optimistic with the person, but confused and frightened when they try to elicit information from medical staff. Each person involved may believe that others do not want to talk about the death and try to protect each other, which can preclude

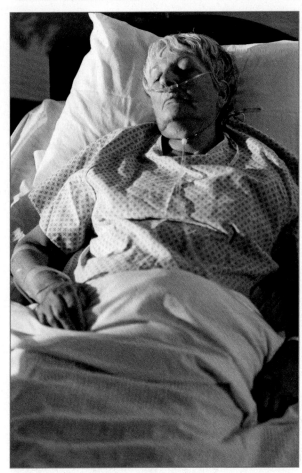

*Many terminally ill patients who find themselves repeated objects of intervention become worn out and eventually refuse additional treatment.*

Photodisc/Getty Images

communication. Death itself is still a taboo topic in our society. The issue is generally avoided in polite conversation; little research is conducted on death; and even when death strikes within a family, the survivors often try to bear their grief alone. The right thing to do, many people feel, is not to bring it up.

### The Issue of Nontraditional Treatment

As both health and communication deteriorate, some terminally ill patients turn away from traditional medical care. Many such patients fall victim to remedies with no basis in scientific evidence offered outside the formal health care system. Frantic family members, friends who are trying to be helpful, and patients themselves may scour fringe publications for seemingly

effective remedies or cures; they may invest thousands of dollars in their generally unsuccessful search.

What prompts people to take these often uncomfortable, inconvenient, costly, and worthless measures? Some patients are so frantic at the prospect of death that they will use up both their own savings and those of the family in the hope of a miracle cure. In other cases, turning to nontraditional medicine may be a symptom of a deteriorating relationship with the health care system and the desire for more humanistic care. This is not to suggest that a solid patient–practitioner relationship can prevent every patient from turning to quackery. However, when the patient is well informed and feels cared for by others, he or she is less likely to look for alternative remedies.

### ■ ARE THERE STAGES IN ADJUSTMENT TO DYING?

Do people pass through a predictable series of **stages of dying**?

### Kübler-Ross's Five-Stage Theory

Elisabeth Kübler-Ross, a pioneer in the study of death and dying, suggested that people pass through five stages as they adjust to the prospect of death: denial, anger, bargaining, depression, and acceptance. Although research shows that people who are dying do not necessarily pass through each of these stages in the exact order, all of these reactions are commonly experienced.

**Denial**    Denial is thought to be a person's initial reaction to learning of the diagnosis of terminal illness. Denial is a defense mechanism by which people avoid the implications of an illness. They may act as if the illness were not severe, it will shortly go away, and it will have few long-term implications. In extreme cases, the patient may even deny that he or she has the disease, despite having been given clear information about the diagnosis (Ditto, Munro, et al., 2003). Denial, then, is the subconscious blocking out of the full realization of the reality and implications of the disorder.

Denial early on in adjustment to life-threatening illness is both normal and useful because it can protect the patient from the full realization of impending death (Lazarus, 1983). Usually it lasts only a few days. When it lasts longer, it may require psychological intervention.

Anger   A second reaction to the prospect of dying is anger. The angry person is asking, "Why me? Considering all the other people who could have gotten the illness, all the people who had the same symptoms but got a favorable diagnosis, and all the people who are older, dumber, more bad-tempered, less useful, or just plain evil, why should I be the one who is dying?" Kübler-Ross quotes one of her dying patients:

> I suppose most anybody in my position would look at somebody else and say, "Well, why couldn't it have been him?" and this has crossed my mind several times. An old man whom I have known ever since I was a little kid came down the street. He was eighty-two years old, and he is of no earthly use as far as we mortals can tell. He's rheumatic, he's a cripple, he's dirty, just not the type of person you would like to be. And the thought hit me strongly, now why couldn't it have been old George instead of me? (quoted in Kübler-Ross, 1969, p. 50)

The angry patient may show resentment toward anyone who is healthy, such as hospital staff, family members, or friends. Angry patients who cannot express their anger directly by being irritable may do so indirectly by becoming embittered. Bitter patients show resentment through death jokes, cracks about their deteriorating appearance and capacities, or pointed remarks about all the exciting things that they will not be able to do because those events will happen after their death.

Anger is one of the harder responses for family and friends to deal with. They may feel they are being blamed by the patient for being well. The family may need to work together with a therapist to understand that the patient is not really angry with them but at fate; they need to see that this anger will be directed at anyone who is nearby, especially people with whom the patient feels no obligation to be polite and well behaved. Unfortunately, family members often fall into this category.

Bargaining   Bargaining is the third stage of Kübler-Ross's formulation. At this point, the person abandons anger in favor of a different strategy: trading good behavior for good health. Bargaining may take the form of a pact with God, in which the patient agrees to engage in good works or at least to abandon selfish ways in exchange for better health or more time. A sudden rush of charitable activity or uncharacteristically pleasant behavior may be a sign that the patient is trying to strike such a bargain.

Depression   Depression, the fourth stage in Kübler-Ross's model, may be viewed as coming to terms with lack of control. The terminally ill person acknowledges that little can now be done to stay the course of illness. This realization may be coincident with a worsening of symptoms, tangible evidence that the illness is not going to be cured. At this stage, people may feel nauseated, breathless, and tired. They may find it hard to eat, to control elimination, to focus attention, and to escape pain or discomfort.

Kübler-Ross refers to the stage of depression as a time for "anticipatory grief," when patients mourn the prospect of their own deaths. This grieving process may occur in two stages, as the person first comes to terms with the loss of past valued activities and friends and then begins to anticipate the future loss of activities and relationships. Depression, though far from pleasant, can be functional in that patients begin to prepare for the future. Depression can nonetheless require treatment, so that symptoms of depression can be distinguished from symptoms of physical deterioration.

Acceptance   The final stage in Kübler-Ross's theory is acceptance. At this point, the dying person may be too weak to be angry and too accustomed to the idea of dying to be depressed. Instead, a tired, peaceful, though not necessarily pleasant calm may descend. Some patients use this time to make preparations, deciding how to divide up their remaining possessions and saying goodbye to old friends and family members.

## Evaluation of Kübler-Ross's Theory

How good an account of the process of dying is Kübler-Ross's stage theory? As a description of the reactions of dying patients, her work was invaluable. She chronicled nearly the full array of reactions to death, as those who work with the dying are quick to acknowledge. Her work is also of inestimable value in pointing out the counseling needs of the dying. Finally, along with other researchers, she broke through the silence and taboos surrounding death, making it an object of both scientific study and sensitive concern. Nonetheless, it bears mention, again, that patients do not typically go through five stages in a predetermined order, but rather may experience the stages in a varying order or not at all.

Kübler-Ross's stage theory also does not fully acknowledge the importance of anxiety, which, next to depression, is one of the most common responses. What people fear most is not being able to control pain; they may welcome or even seek death to avoid it (Hinton, 1967). Other symptoms, such as difficulty breathing or uncontrollable vomiting, likewise produce anxiety, which may exacerbate the dying person's already deteriorating physical and mental condition.

## ■ PSYCHOLOGICAL ISSUES AND THE TERMINALLY ILL

Approximately 20 percent to one-third of Americans who die each year die in hospitals (Centers for Disease Control and Prevention, 2016; Teno et al., 2018).

### Medical Staff and the Terminally Ill Patient

Unfortunately, death in the institutional environment can be depersonalized and fragmented. Wards may be understaffed, with the staff unable to provide the kind of emotional support a patient needs. Hospital regulations may restrict the number of visitors or the length of time that they can stay, thereby reducing the availability of support from family and friends. Pain is one of the chief symptoms in terminal illness, and in the busy hospital setting, the ability of patients to get the amount of pain medication they need may be compromised.

The Significance of Hospital Staff to the Patient    Physical dependence on hospital staff is great because the patient may need help for even the smallest activity, such as turning over in bed. Patients are entirely dependent on medical staff for amelioration of their pain. And staff may be the only people to see a dying patient on a regular basis if he or she has no friends or family members who visit regularly.

Moreover, staff may be the only people who know the patient's actual physical state; hence, they are the patient's only source of realistic information. The patient may welcome communication with staff because he or she can be fully candid with them. Finally, staff are important because they are privy to one of the patient's most personal and private acts, the act of dying.

Risks of Terminal Care for Staff    **Terminal care** is hard on hospital staff. It is the least interesting physical care because it is often **palliative care**—that is, care designed to make the patient feel comfortable—rather than **curative care**—that is, care designed to cure the patient's disease. Terminal care involves a lot of unpleasant custodial work, such as feeding, changing, and bathing the patient, and sometimes symptoms go undertreated. The staff may burn out from watching patient after patient die, despite their best efforts.

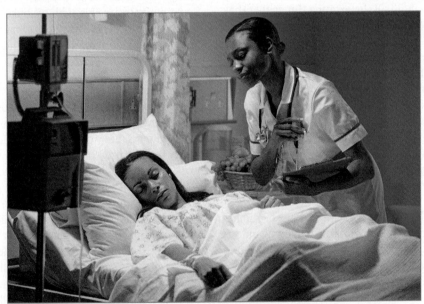

*Medical staff can be very significant to a dying patient because they see the patient on a regular basis, provide realistic information, and are privy to the patient's last personal thoughts and wishes.*
Flying Colours Ltd./Getty Images

Staff may be tempted to withdraw into a crisply efficient manner rather than a warm and supportive one so as to minimize their personal pain. Physicians, in particular, want to reserve their time for patients who can most profit from it and, consequently, may spend little time with a terminally ill patient. Unfortunately, terminally ill patients may interpret such behavior as abandonment and take it very hard. Accordingly, a continued role for the physician in the patient's terminal care in the form of brief but frequent visits is desirable.

Achieving an Appropriate Death   Psychiatrist Avery Weisman (1972, 1977), a distinguished clinician who worked with dying patients for many years, outlined a useful set of goals for medical staff in their work with the dying:

- *Informed consent*–Patients should be told the nature of their condition and treatment and, to some extent, be involved in their own treatment.

- *Safe conduct*–The physician and other staff should act as helpful guides for the patient through this new and frightening stage of life.

- *Significant survival*–The physician and other medical staff should help the patient use his or her remaining time as well as possible.

- *Anticipatory grief*–Both the patient and his or her family members should be aided in working through their anticipatory sense of loss and depression.

- *Timely and appropriate death*–The patient should be allowed to die when and how he or she wants to, as much as possible. The patient should be allowed to achieve death with dignity.

These guidelines, established many years ago, still provide the goals and means for terminal care. Unfortunately, a "good death" is still not available to all. A survey of the survivors of 1,500 people who had died revealed that dying patients often had not received enough medication to ease their pain and had not experienced enough emotional support. Lack of open communication and lack of respect from medical staff are two other common complaints (Teno, Fisher, Hamel, Coppola, & Dawson, 2002).

## The Promise of Palliative Care

The availability of palliative care in hospitals and medical clinics is surging in the United States. Palliative care teams typically include specialists in pain and symptom management, psychological health, social work, and spiritual care. In 2000, such teams provided care in only 25 percent of mid-size to large hospitals, but by 2015, the figure had tripled to 75 percent (Center to Advance Palliative Care, 2018).

From a meta-analysis of 43 randomized, controlled trials conducted in hospital and outpatient settings, palliative care produced improvements in patients' quality of life, advance care planning, and patient and caregiver satisfaction, and it lowered other medical care utilization (Kavalieratos et al., 2016). Many palliative care teams have too few resources to meet the demand, indicating that greater funding and more training of specialists are needed.

## Counseling with the Terminally Ill

Many dying patients need the chance to talk a counselor. Therapy is typically short term and the nature and timing of the visits typically depend on the desires and energy level of the patient. Moreover, patients typically set the agenda.

Therapy with the dying is different from typical psychotherapy in several respects. First, for obvious reasons, it is likely to be short term. The format of therapy with the dying also varies from that of traditional psychotherapy. The nature and timing of visits must depend on the inclination and energy level of the patient, rather than on a fixed schedule of appointments. The agenda should be set at least partly by the patient. And if an issue arises that the patient clearly does not wish to discuss, this wish should be respected.

Terminally ill patients may also need help in resolving unfinished business. Uncompleted activities may prey on the mind, and preparations may need to be made for survivors, especially dependent children. Through careful counseling, a therapist may help the patient come to terms with the need for these arrangements, as well as with the need to recognize that some things will remain undone.

Some **thanatologists**–that is, those who study death and dying–have suggested that behavioral and cognitive–behavioral therapies can be constructively employed with dying patients (Sobel, 1981). For example, progressive muscle relaxation can ameliorate discomfort and instill a renewed sense of control. Positive self-talk, such as focusing on one's life achievements, can undermine the depression that often accompanies dying. Family therapy can also be an appropriate way to deal with issues raised by terminal illness, to help the family and patient recognize and plan for the future. Therapies that center on helping the person with advanced disease focus on meaning and purpose in life, actions consistent with core values, and self-worth have evidence of efficacy (Martínez et al., 2017; Vos & Vitali, 2018).

## The Management of Terminal Illness in Children

Working with terminally ill children is perhaps the most stressful of all terminal care. As a result, family members, friends, and even medical staff may be reluctant to talk openly with a dying child about his or her situation.

Nonetheless, terminally ill children often know more about their situation than they are given credit for (Spinetta, 1982). Children use cues from their treatments and from the people around them to infer what their condition must be. As their own physical condition deteriorates, they develop a conception of their own death and the realization that it may not be far off, as this exchange shows:

> TOM: Jennifer died last night. I have the same thing. Don't I?
>
> NURSE: But they are going to give you different medicines.
>
> TOM: What happens when they run out?
> (Bluebond-Langner, 1977, p. 55)

It may be difficult to know what to tell a child. Unlike adults, children may not express their knowledge, concerns, or questions directly. They may communicate the knowledge that they will die only indirectly, as by wanting to have Christmas early so that they will be around for it. Or they may suddenly stop talking about their future plans.

One child, who when first diagnosed said he wanted to be a doctor, became quite angry with his doctor when she tried to get him to submit to a procedure by explaining the procedure and telling him, "I thought you would understand, Sandy. You told me once you wanted to be a doctor." He screamed back at her, "I'm not going to be anything," and then threw an empty syringe at her. She said, "OK, Sandy." The nurse standing nearby said, "What are you going to be?" "A ghost," said Sandy, and turned over (Bluebond-Langner, 1977, p. 59).

Counseling with a terminally ill child may be required and typically follows some of the same guidelines as is true with dying adults, but therapists can take cues about what to discuss from the child, talking only about those issues the child is ready to discuss. Parents, too, may need counseling to help them cope with the impending death. They may blame themselves for the child's illness or feel that there is more they could have done. The needs of other children may be passed over in the process of dealing with the dying child's situation. A counselor working with the family can help restore balance.

Parents of dying children experience an enormous stress burden to the degree that they sometimes have the symptoms of post traumatic stress disorder. The emotional distress of parents with dying children may require supportive mental health services and meetings with the physician to help the parents make sense of and derive meaning from the child's terminal illness, especially during the first few months after the child's diagnosis (Dunn et al., 2012) and death (Meert et al., 2015).

## ■ ALTERNATIVES TO HOSPITAL CARE FOR THE TERMINALLY ILL

Hospital care for the terminally ill is palliative, emotionally wrenching, and demanding of personalized attention in ways that often go beyond the resources of the hospital. Consequently, hospice care in one's own home or in a hospice facility is an increasingly elected option for dying people.

### Hospice Care

The idea behind **hospice care** is the acceptance of death, emphasizing the relief of suffering rather than the cure of illness. Hospice care is designed to provide palliative care and emotional support to dying patients and their family members. About 1.43 million people received services from hospices in 2015, making hospice care a significant contributor to the delivery of services to terminally ill patients (Harris-Kojetin, Sengupta, Lendon, Rome, Valverde, & Caffrey, 2019).

In medieval Europe, a **hospice** was a place that provided care and comfort for travelers. In keeping with this original goal, hospice care is both a philosophy concerning a way of dying and a system of care for the terminally ill. Typically, painful or invasive therapies are discontinued. Instead, care is aimed toward managing pain and symptoms such as nausea, weakness, and confusion.

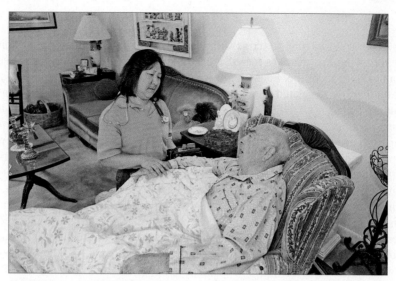

*Hospice care, an alternative to hospital and home care for the terminally ill, is designed to provide personalized palliative treatment without the strains that home care can produce.*

Rick Brady/McGraw-Hill Education

Most important, the patient's psychological comfort is emphasized. Patients are encouraged to personalize their living areas as much as possible by bringing in their own familiar things. Thus, in institutional hospice care, each room may look very different, reflecting the personality and interests of its occupant. Patients also typically wear their own clothes and determine their own activities.

Hospice care is oriented toward improving a patient's social support system. Restrictions on visits from family or friends are removed as much as possible. Staff are especially trained to interact with patients in a warm, emotionally caring way. Usually, counselors are available for individual, group, or family intervention.

### Home Care

Recent years have seen renewed interest in **home care** for dying patients. Home care appears to be the care of choice for most terminally ill people (National Hospice and Palliative Care Organization, 2015, September), and for many patients, it may be the only economically feasible care. The psychological advantages of home care are that the patient is surrounded by personal items and by family rather than medical staff. Some degree of control can be maintained over such activities as what to eat or what to wear.

Although home care is often easier on the patient psychologically, it can be very stressful for the family. Even if the family can afford around-the-clock nursing, often at least one family member's energies must be devoted to the patient on an almost full-time basis. The designated caregiver must often stop working and also face the additional stress of constant contact with the prospect of death. The caregiver may be torn between wanting to keep the patient alive and wanting the patient's and their own suffering to end.

### ■ PROBLEMS OF SURVIVORS

The death of a family member may be the most upsetting and dreaded event in a person's life. For many people, the death of a loved one is a more terrifying prospect than their own death or illness. Even when a death is anticipated and, on some level, wished for in order to end suffering, it may be very hard for survivors to cope.

The weeks just before the patient's death are often a period of frenzied activity. Visits to the hospital increase, preliminary legal or funeral preparations may be made, last-minute therapies may be initiated, or the patient may be moved to another facility. Family members are kept busy by the sheer amount of work that must be done. After the patient dies, there are activities related to the death and settling the estate

BOX **12.4** Cultural Attitudes Toward Death

Each culture has its own way of coming to terms with death. Although in some cultures death is feared, in others it is seen as a normal part of life. Each culture, accordingly, has developed death-related ceremonies that reflect these cultural beliefs.

In traditional Japanese culture, death is regarded as a process of traveling from one world to another. When someone dies, that person goes to a purer country, and the function of death rituals is to help the spirit make the journey. A series of rites and ceremonies takes place, aided by a minister, to achieve this end. The funeral events begin with a bedside service, in which the minister consoles the family. The next service is the Yukan, the bathing of the dead. An appreciation service follows the funeral, with food for all who have traveled long distances to attend. When the mourning period is over, a final party is given for friends and relatives as a way of bringing the mourners back into the community (Kübler-Ross, 1975).

In Hinduism, which is the main religion of India, death is not viewed as separate from life or as an ending. Rather, it is considered a continuous, integral part of life. Because Hindus believe in reincarnation, they believe that birth is followed by death and death by rebirth; every moment one is born and dies again. Thus, death is like any transition in life. The Hindus teach that one should meet death with tranquility and meditation. Death is regarded as the chief fact of life and a sign that all earthly desires are in vain. Only when an individual neither longs for nor fears death is that person capable of transcending both life and death and achieving nirvana—merging into

unity with the Absolute. In so doing, the individual is freed from the fear of death, and death comes to be seen as a companion to life (Kübler-Ross, 1975).

What would people from another culture think about attitudes toward death in the United States if they were to witness our death practices? First, they would see that many deaths take place in the hospital without the presence of close relatives. Once death has occurred, the corpse is promptly removed without the help of the bereaved, who see it, if at all, only after morticians have made it acceptable for viewing. In some cases, the corpse is cremated shortly after death and is never again seen by the family. A paid organizer, often a director of a funeral home, takes over much of the direction of the viewing and burial rituals, deciding matters of protocol and the timing of services. In most subcultures within the United States, a time is set aside when the bereaved family accepts condolences from visiting sympathizers. A brief memorial service is then held, after which the bereaved and their friends may travel to the cemetery, where the corpse or ashes are buried. Typically, there are strong social pressures on the friends and relatives of the deceased to show little sign of emotion. The family is expected to establish this pattern, and other visitors are expected to follow suit. A friend or relative who is out of control emotionally will usually withdraw from the death ceremony or will be urged to do so by others. Following the ceremony, there may be a brief get-together at the home of the bereaved, after which the mourners return home (Huntington & Metcalf, 1979).

(Box 12.4 describes some of the ways in which cultures vary in reactions to death and the formalities that follow). Then, very abruptly, the activities cease. Visitors return home, the patient has been cremated or buried, and the survivor is left alone.

## The Survivor

The aftermath of a death creates demands of its own. The typical survivor is a widow in her 60s or older, who may have physical problems of her own. If she has lived in a traditional marriage, she may find herself with tasks, such as preparing her income tax return and making household repairs, which she has never had to do before. Survivors may be left with few resources to turn to.

**Grief,** which is the psychological response to bereavement, is a feeling of hollowness, often marked by preoccupation with the image of the deceased person, expressions of hostility toward others, and guilt over the death. Especially during the first 6 months, bereaved people often experience restlessness and an inability to concentrate on activities, bothersome physical symptoms, more acute cardiac problems, more hospitalizations, and an increased risk of mortality (Rook & Charles, 2017).

A study of more than 200 bereaved adults from 1 to 24 months after losing a loved one to a health condition or disease provides insight into whether survivors' experience of grief corresponds to that described by Kübler-Ross (1975). In that sample (Maciejewski, Zhang, Block, & Prigerson, 2007), participants' disbelief peaked at 1 month after the loss, followed by peaks in yearning for the loved one, anger, and then depression, which peaked at 6 months. Acceptance increased over time through 24 months after the loved one's death. On average, yearning and acceptance were the most common reactions.

As with terminally ill individuals, however, people who lose a loved one neither invariably experience these reactions nor do they experience them in the same order. One of your textbook's authors (Stanton) once consulted with a bereaved woman who was troubled because her best friend, who had read a book by Kübler-Ross, told her that she was supposed to be experiencing anger and that she could not get through her grief without being angry. The woman expressed great relief when she learned that Kübler-Ross did not intend her ideas to be a prescription for "correct" grieving.

It may be difficult for outsiders to appreciate the degree of a survivor's grief. They may feel, especially if the death was a long time coming, that the survivor should be ready for it and thus show signs of recovery shortly after the death. Widows say that often, within a few weeks of their spouse's death, friends are urging them to pull out of their melancholy and get on with life. In some cases, the topic of remarriage is brought up within weeks after the death. However, normal grieving may go on for months (Maciejewski et al., 2007).

Whether it is adaptive to grieve or not to grieve has been debated. In contrast to psychologists' usual caution that the avoidance of negative emotions can be problematic, some evidence suggests that emotional avoidance (Bonanno, Keltner, Holen, & Horowitz, 1995) and positive appraisals (Stein, Folkman, Trabasso, & Richards, 1997) actually lead to better adjustment in the wake of a death. Bereaved adults who ruminate on the death are less likely to get good social support, they have higher levels of stress, and they are more likely to be depressed (Nolen-Hoeksema, McBride, & Larson, 1997). By contrast, extraverts seem to be good at martialing their social support and on the whole, extraverted and conscientious people seem to get through the bereavement period with less depression than people without these qualities (Pai & Carr, 2010).

The grief response may be more aggravated in men, in caregivers, and in those whose loss was sudden and unexpected (Aneshensel, Botticello, & Yamamoto-Mitani, 2004; Stroebe & Stroebe, 1987). Nonetheless,

the majority of widows and widowers are resilient in response to their loss (Vahtera et al., 2006), especially if the partner's death had been expected and they have had the opportunity to accept its inevitability (Bonanno et al., 2002; Wilcox et al., 2003). Among women who are depressed in widowhood, financial strain appears to be the biggest burden. For men, the strains associated with household management can lead to distress (Umberson, Wortman, & Kessler, 1992). Grief may be especially pronounced in mothers of children who have died (Li, Laursen, Precht, Olsen, & Mortensen, 2005), and it may be complicated by depression (Wijngaards-Meij et al., 2005).

As we will see in Chapter 14, the experience of bereavement can lead to adverse changes in immunologic functioning, increasing the risk of disease and even death. Increases in alcohol and drug abuse and inability to work can occur (Aiken & Marx, 1982). Programs designed to provide counseling to the bereaved can offset these adverse reactions (Aiken & Marx, 1982).

For child survivors, the death of a sibling raises particular complications, because many children have fervently wished, at one time or another, that a sibling was dead. When the sibling actually does die, the child may feel that he or she caused it. Possibly, the surviving child did not get much attention during the sibling's illness and may feel some temporary elation when the sibling is no longer around as a source of competition (Lindsay & McCarthy, 1974). As one child remarked on learning of his sibling's death, "Good. Now I can have all his toys" (Bluebond-Langner, 1977, p. 63).

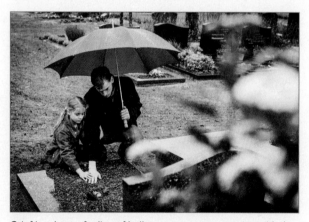

*Grief involves a feeling of hollowness, a preoccupation with the deceased person, and guilt over death. Often, outsiders fail to appreciate the depth of a survivor's grief or the length of time it takes to get over the bereavement.*
Marcel de Grijs/123RF

In helping a child to cope with the death of a parent or a sibling, it is best not to wait until the death has actually occurred. Rather, the child should be prepared for the death, perhaps by drawing on the death of a pet or a flower to aid understanding (Bluebond-Langner, 1977). The child's questions about death should be answered as honestly as possible, but without unwanted detail. Providing only what is asked for when the timing is right is the best course.

## Death Education

Because death has been a taboo topic, many people have misconceptions about it, including the idea that the dying wish to be left alone and not talk about their situation. Because of these concerns, some courses on dying, which may include volunteer work with dying patients, have been developed on some college campuses. A potential problem with such courses is that they may attract the occasional suicidal student and provide unintended encouragement for self-destructive leanings. Accordingly, some instructors have recommended confronting such problems head-on, in the hopes that they can be forestalled.

Whether college students are the best and the only population that should receive death education is another concern. Unfortunately, organized means of educating people outside the university system are few, so college courses remain one of the more viable vehicles for death education. Yet a book about death and dying, *Tuesdays with Morrie* (Albom, 1997), was a best seller for years, a fact that underscores how much people want to understand death. Moreover, causes of death, especially diseases with high mortality, dominate the news (Adelman & Verbrugge, 2000). At present, though, the news and a few books are nearly all there is to meet such needs. Through **death education,** it may be possible to develop realistic expectations, both about what modern medicine can achieve and about the kind of care the dying want and need.  •

# S U M M A R Y

1. Causes of death vary over the life cycle. In infancy, congenital abnormalities and sudden infant death syndrome (SIDS) account for most deaths. From ages 1 to 15, the causes shift to accidents and childhood leukemia. In adolescence and young adulthood, death is typically due to auto accidents, homicide, suicide, cancer, and heart disease. In adulthood, cancer and heart disease are the most common causes of death. Death in old age is usually due to heart disease, stroke, cancer, or physical degeneration.

2. Concepts of death change over the life cycle. In childhood, death is conceived of first as a great sleep and later as a ghostlike figure that takes a person away. Later, death is recognized to be an irreversible biological stage. Middle age is the time when many people first begin to come to terms with their own death.

3. Advancing disease raises psychological issues, including treatment-related discomfort and decisions of whether to continue treatment. Issues concerning the patient's directive to withhold extreme life-prolonging measures, assisted death, and euthanasia have been topics of concern in both medicine and law.

4. Patients' self-concepts must continually adapt in response to the progression of illness, change in appearance, energy level, control over physical processes, and degree of mental alertness. The patient may withdraw from family and friends as a result. Thus, issues of communication can be a focal point for intervention.

5. Kübler-Ross's theory of dying suggests that people go through stages, progressing through denial, anger, bargaining, depression, and finally acceptance. Research shows that patients do not necessarily go through these stages in sequence but that all these states describe reactions of dying people to a degree.

6. Much of the responsibility for psychological management of terminal illness falls on medical staff. Medical staff can provide information, reassurance, and emotional support when others cannot. Training in palliative care is important.

7. Psychological counseling needs to be made available to terminally ill patients, because many people need a chance to develop a perspective on their lives. Developing methods for training therapists in clinical thanatology, then, is an educational priority. Family therapy may be needed to soothe the problems of the family and to help the patient and family say goodbye to each other.

8. Counseling terminally ill children is especially important because both parents and children may be confused and frightened.

9. Hospice care and home care are alternatives to hospital care for the dying. Palliative and psychologically supportive care in the home or in a homelike environment can have beneficial psychological effects on dying patients and their survivors.

10. Grief is marked by a feeling of hollowness, preoccupation with an image of the deceased person, guilt over the death, expressions of hostility toward others, restlessness, and an inability to concentrate. Many people do not realize how long normal grieving takes.

# K E Y   T E R M S

curative care
death education
euthanasia
grief
home care
hospice

hospice care
infant mortality rate
living will
palliative care
physician-assisted death
premature death

stages of dying
sudden infant death syndrome (SIDS)
terminal care
thanatologists

# CHAPTER 13

# Heart Disease, Hypertension, Stroke, and Type 2 Diabetes

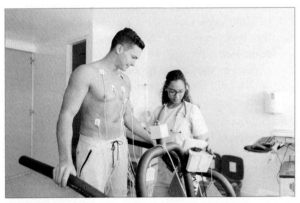

andresr/Getty Images

In this chapter, we consider four major chronic disorders: heart disease, hypertension, stroke, and diabetes. All four involve the circulatory and/or metabolic system and often represent co-occurring disorders, especially in older adults. Moreover, due to their frequency, they affect large numbers of people. For example, 29 percent of American adults have hypertension, 32 percent have elevated cholesterol, and 9 percent have diabetes (Centers for Disease Control and Prevention, 2017).

## ■ CORONARY HEART DISEASE

Coronary heart disease (CHD) is the number-one killer in the United States, accounting for one out of every three deaths (American Heart Association, 2018). It was not a major cause of death until the 20th century because, prior to that time, most people did not live long enough to develop heart disease; most people died of infectious diseases.

CHD is a disease of modernization, due at least in part to the changes in diet and reduced activity level that have accompanied modern life. Because of these factors, around the turn of the 20th century, the rate of CHD began to increase. Although it has recently begun to decline, it is estimated that 92.1 million adults in the United States are living with some form of cardiovascular disease (American Heart Association, 2018). Thirty-three percent of CHD-related deaths are considered premature; that is, they occur well before age 78.5, the expected age of death (American Heart Association, 2012).

CHD is also a major chronic disease: Millions of Americans live with the diagnosis and symptoms. Because of its great frequency and the toll it takes on middle-aged and older people, understanding heart disease has been a high priority of health psychology.

### What Is CHD?

**Coronary heart disease (CHD)** is a general term that refers to illnesses caused by atherosclerosis, the narrowing of the coronary arteries, the vessels that supply the heart with blood (see Figure 13.1). As we saw in Chapter 2, when these vessels become narrowed or closed, the flow of oxygen and nourishment to the heart is partially or completely obstructed. Temporary shortages of oxygen and nourishment frequently cause pain, called angina pectoris, that radiates across the chest and arm. When severe deprivation occurs, a

heart attack (myocardial infarction [MI]) can result. Heart failure is a potential consequence of CHD, whereby the heart does not pump blood as well as it should.

Risk factors for CHD include high cholesterol, high blood pressure, elevated levels of inflammation, and diabetes, as well as the behaviors of cigarette smoking, obesity, and little exercise (American Heart Association, 2004b). Identifying people with **metabolic syndrome** also helps predict heart attacks. Metabolic syndrome is diagnosed when a person has three or more of the following problems: obesity centered around the waist; high blood pressure; low levels of HDL, the so-called good cholesterol; difficulty metabolizing blood sugar, an indicator of risk for diabetes; and high levels of triglycerides, which are related to bad cholesterol. African Americans and U.S. Hispanics/Latinos are at particular risk of developing metabolic syndrome (McCurley et al., 2017), and discrimination is thought to play a role (Ikram et al., 2017). Although metabolic syndrome is often thought of as a risk factor, it can itself be modified by lifestyle interventions that target physical activity, diet, and stress (Powell et al., 2018). Depression may play a role in its development as well (Womack et al., 2016). Initiating changes in these health risks in childhood and adolescence is advisable (Ames, Leadbeater, & MacDonald, 2018), because metabolic health disparities begin to emerge in childhood (Hostinar, Ross, Chen, & Miller, 2017).

Risk factors for heart disease begin to cluster by age 14, especially for those low in socioeconomic status (SES) (Goodman, McEwen, Huang, Dolan, & Adler, 2005; Lawlor et al., 2005). However, all known risk factors together account for less than half of all newly diagnosed cases of CHD; accordingly, a number of risk factors remain to be identified.

### Risk Factors for CHD

Risk factors for CHD include being sedentary and getting little exercise, being obese, having a poor diet of too much food and too few vegetables and fruits, having high cholesterol and triglycerides, and having little social support and a family history of heart disease (Savelieva et al., 2017).

**Biological Reactivity to Stress**   Biological reactivity to stress contributes to the development of CHD and **cardiovascular disease (CVD),** specifically the increases and decreases of physiological activity

**FIGURE 13.1 | Atherosclerosis**   The figure shows a normal artery with normal blood flow (figure A) and an artery containing plaque buildup (figure B).    *Source:* National Heart, Lung, and Blood Institute. "What Is Cholesterol?" Last Modified from 2010.

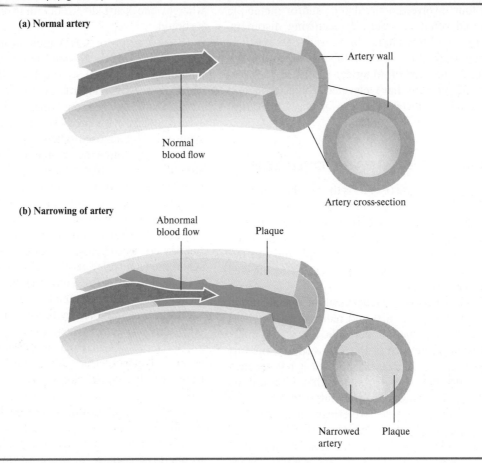

that can accompany stress. The cumulative effects of reactivity damage the endothelial cells that line the coronary vessels: This process enables lipids to deposit plaque, increasing inflammation and leading to the development of lesions.

Reactivity not only is reflected in initial reactions to stress but can also be reflected in a prolonged recovery period; some people recover from sympathetic activity due to parasympathetic counterregulation quite quickly, whereas others do not. That is, as we saw in Chapter 2, following cardiovascular activation due to stress, there is parasympathetic modulation of sympathetic reactivity. This rebound is an important part of the stress process, and diminished vagal rebound during recovery is strongly tied to risk factors for cardiovascular disease as early as childhood (Meghan et al., 2017).

## Stress and CHD

Stress is also an important culprit in the development of CHD and may interact with genetically based weaknesses to increase its likelihood. Extensive research links chronic stress, trauma exposure, and acute stress to CHD and to adverse clinical events (Hendrickson, Neylan, Na, Regan, Zhang, & Cohen, 2013; Phillips, Carroll, Ring, Sweeting, & West, 2005; Vitaliano et al., 2002). Acute stress involving emotional pressure, anger, extreme excitement (Strike & Steptoe, 2005), negative emotions, and sudden bursts of activity can precipitate sudden clinical events, such as a heart attack, angina, or death (Lane et al., 2006; Nicholson, Fuhrer, & Marmot, 2005). The stress reactivity associated with these events can lead to plaque rupture and risk of a clot. This process may explain why stress can trigger acute coronary events such as heart attacks (Strike, Magid,

**FIGURE 13.2 | Annual Rate of First Heart Attacks by Age, Sex, and Race**   *Sources:* Lloyd-Jones, Donald, Robert Adams, Mercedes Carnethon, Giovanni De Simone, T. Bruce Ferguson, Katherine Flegal, Earl Ford, et. al. "Heart Disease and Stroke Statistics—2009 Update." *American Heart Association* 119, no. 3 (2009): 121–181; Roger, V. L., D. M. Lloyd-Jones, E. J. Benjamin, J. D. Berry, W. B. Borden, D. M. Bravata, S. Dai, et. al. "Heart Disease and Stroke Statistics–2012 Update: A Report from the American Heart Association." *American Heart Association* 125, no. 1 (2012): 2–220.

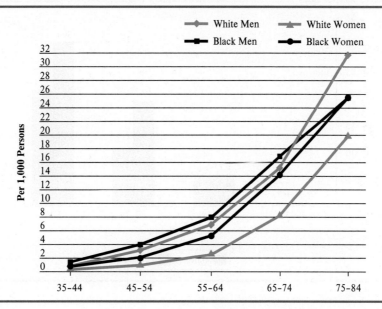

Brydon, Edwards, McEwan, & Steptoe, 2004). Stress has been linked directly to increased inflammatory activity as well (McDade, Hawkley, & Cacioppo, 2006).

Low social status is implicated in the development and course of coronary artery disease. Risk factors for heart disease are more common in individuals low in SES, especially men, and the symptoms of cardiovascular disease develop earlier (Chichlowska et al., 2008; Matthews, Räikkönen, Gallo, & Kuller, 2008) (Figure 13.2). These patterns reflect the greater chronic stress that people experience, the lower they are on the socioeconomic ladder (Adler et al., 1994; Gallo et al., 2014). People who think of themselves as low in social standing are also more likely to have cardiovascular profiles reflecting the metabolic syndrome (Manuck, Phillips, Gianaros, Flory, & Muldoon, 2010). A genetically based predisposition to cardiovascular reactivity, which emerges early in life (Yamada et al., 2002), can be exacerbated by low SES. A harsh (abusive, nonnurturant, neglectful, and/or conflictual) family environment in childhood (Thurston et al., 2017) increases risk in its own right, and the stress and difficulty developing social support that can result from these early harsh circumstances also increase cardiovascular risk (Gallo & Matthews, 2006; Kapuku, Davis, Murdison,

Robinson, & Harshfield, 2012). Poor intimate relationships in adulthood can also exacerbate negative emotions and other risk factors for CHD (Smith & Baucom, 2017). Low SES also predicts a worsened course of illness (Sacker, Head, & Bartley, 2008) and poor prospects for recovery (Ickovics, Viscoli, & Horwitz, 1997).

African Americans are disproportionately exposed to chronic stress and, as a result, are at elevated risk for CHD (Troxel, Matthews, Bromberger, & Sutton-Tyrrell, 2003). Although deaths from CHD among both African Americans and whites have decreased in recent years, the racial gap has actually increased (Zheng, Croft, Labarthe, Williams, & Mensah, 2001). Racial discrimination plays a role in these vulnerabilities (Hill, Sherwood, McNeilly, Anderson, Blumenthal, & Hinderliter, 2018). Risks are rising for Latinos as well (Gallo et al., 2014).

As we saw in Chapter 6, stress in the workplace can lead to the development of coronary heart disease. Job-related risk factors are: job strain, especially the combination of high work demands and low control; a discrepancy between educational level and occupation (e.g., being well educated and having a low-status job); low job security; little social support at work; and high work pressure. Although men with little risk for CHD

**FIGURE 13.3** | **Prevalence of Coronary Heart Disease by Age and Sex (NHANES:2011–2014).**    NHANES indicates National Health and Nutrition Examination Survey.    *Source:* Benjamin, E. J., Salim S. Virani, Clifton W. Callaway, Alanna M. Chamberlain, Alexander R. Chang, Susan Cheng, and Stephanie E. Chiuve. "Heart Disease and Stroke Statistics–2018 Update: A Report from the American Heart Association." *American Heart Association,* 137, no. 12 (2018): 67–492.

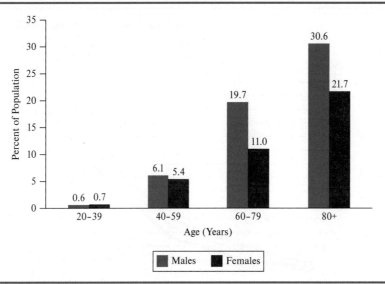

may not develop CHD in response to these factors, among men with high risk, these job factors enhance risk (Ferris, Kline, & Bourdage, 2012; Siegrist, Peter, Runge, Cremer, & Seidel, 1990).

More recently, research has suggested that an imbalance between control and demands in daily life more generally (not only at work) is a risk for atherosclerosis. That is, people whose lives are characterized by high levels of demands coupled with low levels of control both in and outside the workplace are at higher risk for atherosclerosis (Kamarck et al., 2004; Kamarck, Muldoon, Shiffman, & Sutton-Tyrrell, 2007).

Social instability is linked to higher rates of CHD. Migrants have a higher incidence of CHD than do geographically stable individuals, and acculturation to Western society is a risk factor for high blood pressure, possibly due to distress associated with cultural change (Steffen, Smith, Larson, & Butler, 2006). People who are occupationally, residentially, or socially mobile have a higher likelihood of CHD than do people who are less mobile (Kasl & Berkman, 1983). Urban and industrialized countries have a higher incidence of CHD than do underdeveloped countries; people in underdeveloped countries die younger and may not live long enough to die of heart disease or receive the medical care needed to diagnose heart disease.

## Women and CHD

CHD is the leading killer of women in the United States and most other developed countries (American Heart Association, 2012). Although the onset of CHD typically occurs about 10 years later in women than men, more women than men die of heart disease (American Heart Association, 2012).

Because studies of risk factors, diagnosis, prognosis, and rehabilitation have typically focused on men, less is known about women's heart disease (Burell & Granlund, 2002) (Figure 13.3). However, although heart disease typically occurs later for women, it is more dangerous when it does occur. Women have a 50 percent chance of dying from a first heart attack, compared to 30 percent for men. Of those who survive their heart attack, 38 percent will die within a year, compared to 25 percent for men.

Women may be protected against early-onset coronary disease by factors related to estrogen. Estrogen diminishes sympathetic nervous system arousal, and premenopausal women show smaller increases in blood pressure and in neuroendocrine and metabolic responses to stress than do men and older women. Women's risk of coronary heart disease goes up substantially after menopause. Weight gain, increases in blood pressure, elevated cholesterol and triglycerides, and heightened cardiovascular reactivity may explain this rising risk (Hirokawa et al., 2014; Wing, Matthews, Kuller, Meilahn, & Plantinga, 1991). These points might suggest that estrogen replacement following menopause might help keep CHD levels in older women low. Unfortunately, though, if anything, estrogen replacement may increase these risks.

The lack of research on women and CHD leaves women misinformed about their risks. There is less information available to women about CHD in the media, and women are less likely than men to be counseled about heart disease and ways to avoid it by their physicians (Stewart, Abbey, Shnek, Irvine, & Grace, 2004). They are more likely to be misdiagnosed or not to be diagnosed at all, and consequently, are less likely than men to receive and use drugs that can retard the progression of heart disease, including aspirin (Vittinghoff et al., 2003).

What research there is suggests that CHD risk factors for women are similar to those for men. As is true for men, women who are more physically active, who get regular exercise, and who have low body fat, low cholesterol, and low triglyceride levels (Lewis et al., 2009; Owens, Matthews, Wing, & Kuller, 1990) are less likely to develop heart disease. As is also true for men, social support, especially in marriage, is associated with less advanced disease in women (Gallo, Troxel, Kuller, et al., 2003; Whisman & Uebelacker, 2011). Depression, anxiety, hostility, suppression of anger, and stress are all tied to elevated risk for coronary heart disease among women (Low, Thurston, & Matthews, 2010). Sex discrimination also plays a role in women's CHD risk factors (Beatty Moody, Chang, Brown, Bromberger, & Matthews, 2018).

Low SES, including early life low SES (Janicki-Deverts, Cohen, Matthews, & Jacobs, 2012), is associated with greater risk for early-stage atherosclerosis in women, as it is in men (Gallo, Matthews, Kuller, Sutton-Tyrrell, & Edmundowicz, 2001). Some of the same job-related factors that predict CHD in men may do so for women as well (Lallukka et al., 2006). Employment as a clerical worker as opposed to a white-collar worker enhances risk for coronary artery disease in women (Gallo, Troxel, Matthews, et al., 2003).

Personality qualities associated with masculine or feminine construals of the world may be associated with health risks. Research has especially focused on agency, which is a focus on the self, on communion, which is a focus on others, and on unmitigated communion, which is an extreme focus on others to the exclusion of the self. Men typically score higher than women do on agency. Agency has been associated with good physical and mental health outcomes (Helgeson, 1993; Helgeson & Fritz, 1999; Helgeson & Lepore, 1997).

Communion, a focus on other people in relationships, reflects a positive caring orientation to others, and it is typically higher in women than in men. It has few relations to mental and physical health outcomes. Unmitigated communion, however, exemplified in a self-sacrificing individual who fails to focus on her own needs, is tied to poor mental and physical health outcomes (Fritz, 2000; Helgeson & Fritz, 1999). Agonistic striving, that is, seeking to influence or control others, also contributes to CVD risk (Ewart, Elder, Jorgensen, & Fitzgerald, 2016).

Much of what has been learned about women's heart disease has come from long-term clinical studies, such as the Nurses' Health Study. The Nurses' Health Study began in 1976 when more than 120,000 female nurses age 30 to 55 agreed to participate in a long-term study of medical history and lifestyle (Nurses' Health Study, 2004). Over the past 25 years, the expected incidence of heart disease in this sample has not appeared—in large part because more older women have stopped smoking and have changed their diets in healthy directions (Stoney, Owens, Guzick, & Matthews, 1997). Indeed, among women who adhered to recommended guidelines involving diet, exercise, and abstinence from smoking, there is a very low risk of CHD (Stampfer, Hu, Manson, Rimm, & Willett, 2000). As levels of obesity increase in this population, the incidence of heart disease may rise again (Hu et al., 2000), but at present, the study is testimony to the payoffs of good health habits.

## Personality, Cardiovascular Reactivity, and CHD

Negative emotions, including anger and hostility, increase risk for metabolic syndrome (Puustinen, Koponen, Kautiainen, Mäntyselkä, & Vanhala, 2011) and for CHD (Bleil, Gianaros, Jennings, Flory, & Manuck, 2008). Anger not only increases the risk of heart disease (Gallacher et al., 1999) but also predicts poor likelihood of survival (Boyle et al., 2004) and acts as a potential trigger for heart attacks (Moller et al., 1999). As we will see, anger has also been implicated in hypertension and to a lesser degree in stroke and

BOX **13.1** Hostility and Cardiovascular Disease

Research has implicated cynical hostility as a psychological culprit in the development of CHD. Many studies have employed measures of hostility to look at this association. Here are some sample statements of cynical hostility.

1. I don't matter much to other people.
2. People in charge often don't really know what they are doing.
3. Most people lie to get ahead in life.
4. People look at me like I'm incompetent.
5. Many of my friends irritate me with the things they do.
6. People who tell me what to do frequently know less than I do.
7. I trust no one; life is easier that way.
8. People who are happy most of the time rub me the wrong way.
9. I am often dissatisfied with others.
10. People often misinterpret my actions.

diabetes, suggesting that it may be a general risk factor for CHD, cardiovascular disease, and their complications.

A particular type of hostility is especially implicated, namely, cynical hostility, characterized by suspiciousness, resentment, frequent anger, antagonism, and distrust of others. People who have negative beliefs about others, such as the perception that other people are being antagonistic or threatening, are often verbally aggressive and exhibit subtly antagonistic behavior. People who are high in cynical hostility may have difficulty extracting social support from others, and they may fail to make effective use of available social support (Box 13.1). They also have more conflict with others, more negative affect, and more resulting sleep disturbance, which may further contribute to their heightened risk (Brissette & Cohen, 2002). Hostility combined with defensiveness may be particularly problematic (Helmers & Krantz, 1996).

Who's Hostile?    Hostility can be reliably measured at a young age and shows considerable stability among boys but not among girls (Woodall & Matthews, 1993). In adulthood, men show higher hostility, which may partially explain their heightened risk for CHD, relative to women (Matthews, Owens, Allen, & Stoney, 1992). People of lower SES are more hostile (Barefoot, 1992; Siegman, Townsend, Civelek, & Blumenthal, 2000).

Developmental Antecedents    Hostility reflects an oppositional orientation toward people that develops in childhood, stemming from feelings of insecurity about oneself and negative feelings toward others (Houston & Vavak, 1991). Certain child-rearing practices may foster hostility, specifically, parental interference, punitiveness, lack of acceptance, conflict, or abuse. Family environments that are nonsupportive, unaccepting, and filled with conflict promote the development of hostility in sons (Matthews, Woodall, Kenyon, & Jacob, 1996), and early hostility is related to early risk factors for cardiovascular disease (Matthews, Woodall, & Allen, 1993). Hostility runs in families, and both genetic and environmental factors appear to be implicated (Weidner et al., 2000).

Expressing Versus Harboring Hostility    The expression of hostile emotions, such as anger and cynicism, is more reliably tied to higher cardiovascular reactivity than is the state of anger or hostility (Siegman & Snow, 1997). For example, among men low in SES, the overt behavioral expression of anger is related to CHD incidence, but trait anger, or the experience of anger without expressing it, bears no relationship (Mendes de Leon, 1992). Although anger suppression and hostile attitudes have been related to atherosclerosis in women (Matthews, Owen, Kuller, Sutton-Tyrrell, & Jansen-McWilliams, 1998), the relation between hostile style and enhanced cardiovascular reactivity to stress is not as reliable for women as for men (Davidson, Hall, & MacGregor, 1996; Engebretson & Matthews, 1992) or for cultures in which anger is less likely to be widely expressed (Kitayama et al., 2015).

Hostility and Social Relationships    Hostile people have more interpersonal conflict in their lives and less social support, and this fallout may also contribute to their risk for disease. Their reactivity to stress seems especially to be engaged during these episodes of interpersonal conflict. For example, in one study, 60 couples participated in a discussion under conditions of high or low threat of evaluation by others while they were either agreeing or disagreeing with each other. Husbands who were high in hostility showed a greater blood pressure reactivity in response to stressful marital interaction in response to threat; the same relationship was not found for wives (Smith & Gallo, 1999).

Hostile people may even create and seek out more stressful interpersonal encounters in their daily lives and, by doing so, undermine the effectiveness of their social support network (Allen, Markovitz, Jacobs, & Knox, 2001; Holt-Lunstad, Smith, & Uchino, 2008). Hostile people may ruminate on the causes of their anger and thereby turn acutely stressful events into chronic stress (Fernandez et al., 2010). Researchers are uncertain whether the enhanced CHD risk of hostile people is caused by the lack of social support that hostility produces, by the hostile anger itself, or by the underlying cardiovascular reactivity that hostility may reflect.

**Hostility and Reactivity**   Some health psychologists now suspect that hostility is, at least in part, a social manifestation of cardiovascular reactivity. That is, when a hostile person is provoked in interpersonal situations, he or she shows exaggerated cardiovascular reactivity (Suls & Wan, 1993). Chronically hostile people also show more pronounced physiological reactions to interpersonal stressors (Guyll & Contrada, 1998).

Hostile people exhibit a weak antagonistic response to sympathetic activity in response to stress, suggesting that their physiological reactivity not only is greater initially but also may last longer (Fukudo et al., 1992; Nelson et al., 2005). In response to provocation, hostile people have larger and longer-lasting blood pressure responses to anger-arousing situations (Fredrickson et al., 2000). Inflammation is higher among people who are chronically angry and this is especially true of people with little education (Boylan & Ryff, 2013). When coupled with anger and depression, hostility predicts high levels of C-reactive protein, an indicator of inflammation (Suarez, 2004).

Hostile people also are more likely to engage in health behaviors and have risk profiles that enhance their CHD risk, such as greater caffeine consumption, higher weight, higher lipid levels, smoking, greater alcohol consumption, and hypertension (Greene, Houston, & Holleran, 1995; Lipkus, Barefoot, Williams, & Siegler,

1994; Siegler, Peterson, Barefoot, & Williams, 1992). Although there are cognitive–behavioral interventions designed to modify hostility, as will be seen, hostile people show low adherence to these interventions (Christensen, Wiebe, & Lawton, 1997). Hostility may be a step on the way to depression, to which we next turn (Stewart, Fitzgerald, & Kamarck, 2010).

To summarize, then, researchers believe that hostility reflects a genetically based predisposition to physiological reactivity, especially in response to stress. Parents and children predisposed to reactivity may create a family environment that fosters this pattern. Poor health habits and poor social relationships exacerbate this pattern.

## Depression and CHD

Depression affects the development, progression, and mortality from CHD. The relation of depression to CHD risk and to metabolic syndrome (Smith, Eagle, & Proeschold-Bell, 2017) is now so well established that many practitioners believe that all CHD patients should be assessed for possible depression and treated if there are symptoms (Stewart, Perkins, & Callahan, 2014). As one newspaper headline put it, a life of quiet desperation is as dangerous as smoking. Depression is not a psychological by-product of other risk factors for CHD but an independent risk factor, and it appears to be environmentally rather than genetically based

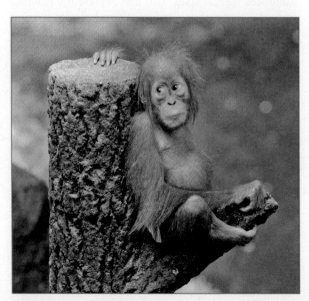

*Depression is a risk factor for CHD, even in some animals.*
G-miner/istock/Getty Images

(Kronish, Rieckmann, Schwartz, Schwartz, & Davidson, 2009). The risk that depression poses for heart disease is greater than that posed by secondhand smoke. Even depressed monkeys have an elevated risk for CHD (Shively et al., 2008).

Depression is also linked to risk factors for coronary heart disease (Polanka, Berntson, Vrany, & Stewart, 2018), metabolic syndrome (Goldbacher, Bromberger, & Matthews, 2009), inflammation (Brummett et al., 2010), poor health habits (Sin, Kumar, Gehi, & Whooley, 2016), the likelihood of a heart attack, heart failure (Garfield et al., 2014), and mortality following coronary artery bypass graft (CABG) surgery (Burg, Benedetto, Rosenberg, & Soufer, 2003). Risk of suicide is higher as well (Chang, Yen, Lee, Chen, Chiu, Fann, & Chen, 2013).

Perhaps the most important way depression is linked to coronary heart disease progression and prognosis is through inflammation (Brummett et al., 2010). Inflammation is typically measured as C-reactive protein, which provides an indication of buildup of plaque on artery walls. Depression may be more closely linked to C-reactive protein in people who are hostile and in African Americans (Deverts et al., 2010). These risks are not explained by health behaviors, social isolation, or work characteristics, and this relation is stronger in men than in women (Stansfeld, Fuhrer, Shipley, & Marmot, 2002). Sometimes an acute coronary event such as a heart attack is preceded by a depressed, exhausted mental state. This may represent a reactivation of latent viruses and resulting inflammation of coronary vessels.

Treatment of depression may reduce the prospects of cardiac events (Lavoie et al., 2018), and improve long-term recovery from heart attack. Depression is typically treated with serotonin reuptake inhibitors, such as Prozac, which help prevent serotonin from attaching to receptors (Bruce & Musselman, 2005). When the receptors in the bloodstream are blocked, it may reduce the formation of clots by preventing the aggregation of platelets in the arteries (Schins, Honig, Crijns, Baur, & Hamulyak, 2003). Essentially, antidepressants may act as blood thinners (Gupta, 2002, August 26). Treatment for depression can also reduce inflammation (Thornton, Andersen, Schuler, & Carson, 2009) but it may somewhat increase risk for diabetes (de Groot et al., 2018). Depression remains an underdiagnosed and largely untreated contributor to CHD morbidity and mortality.

## Other Psychosocial Risk Factors and CHD

Vigilant coping—that is, chronically searching the environment for potential threats—has also been associated with risk factors for heart disease (Gump & Matthews, 1998). Anxiety predicts a worsened course of illness (Roest, Martens, Denollet, & de Jonge, 2010) and sudden cardiac death (Moser et al., 2011), perhaps because anxiety may reduce parasympathetic control of heart rate (Phillips et al., 2009). A composite of depression, anxiety, hostility, and anger may predict CHD better than each factor in isolation (Boyle, Michalek, & Suarez, 2006), suggesting that negative affectivity (see Chapter 7) is a broad general risk factor for CHD (Suls & Bunde, 2005).

Investigators have related vital exhaustion, a mental state characterized by extreme fatigue, feelings of being dejected or defeated, and enhanced irritability to cardiovascular disease (Cheung et al., 2009). Vital exhaustion may be a bodily expression of depression (Balog, Falger, Szabó, Rafael, Székely, & Thege, 2017). In combination with other risk factors, vital exhaustion predicts disease progression, the likelihood of a heart attack, and of a second heart attack after initial recovery (Frestad & Prescott, 2017). It also predicts mortality (Ekmann, Osler, & Avlund, 2012).

As we saw earlier, hostility can interfere with the ability to get social support. Social isolation in its own right confers increased risk for CHD, as does chronic interpersonal conflict (Smith & Ruiz, 2002). Unchecked inflammatory processes may account for these findings (Wirtz et al., 2003). The tendency to experience negative emotions and to inhibit their expression in interpersonal situations (sometimes referred to as Type D [distressed] personality) may be a risk factor for CHD and for cardiovascular events (Denollet, Pedersen, Vrints, & Conraads, 2013; Pedersen, Herrmann-Lingen, de Jonge, & Scherer, 2010; Williams, O'Carroll, & O'Connor, 2008), that can begin early in life (Winning, McCormick, Glymour, Gilsanz & Kubzansky, 2018); however, the evidence is mixed (Coyne et al., 2011; Grande et al., 2011). These effects may be explained by multiple factors, including poor regulation of the HPA axis (Molloy, Perkins-Porras, Strike, & Steptoe, 2008) and by poor health behaviors (Williams, O'Carroll, et al., 2008).

On the protective side, positive emotions, emotional vitality, conscientiousness, mastery, optimism, and general well-being protect against depressive symptoms in heart disease (Kubzansky, Sparrow, Vokonas, & Kawachi, 2001), risk factors for CHD (Roepke & Grant, 2011), recovery following surgery (Tindle et al., 2012), and the course of CHD itself (Boehm & Kubzansky, 2012; Terracciano et al., 2014).

## Management of Heart Disease

In Chapters 3, 4, and 5, we focused on how to modify some of the risk factors for heart disease, such as diet, smoking, and low exercise. In this chapter, we focus primarily on the management of heart disease in people already diagnosed with the disease. Over 1 million individuals suffer a heart attack each year in the United States (American Heart Association, 2018). Of these, more than 140,000 die before reaching the hospital or while in the emergency room (American Heart Association, 2012). Despite these dire statistics, hospital admissions for myocardial infarction have declined (American Heart Association, 2012), and quality of care has improved steadily (Williams, Schmaltz, Morton, Koss, & Loeb, 2005), with the result that the number of heart attack deaths has been sharply lower in recent decades (American Heart Association, 2012).

The Role of Delay   One reason for high rates of mortality and disability following heart attacks is that patients often delay several hours or even days before seeking treatment. Some people interpret the symptoms as more mild disorders, such as gastric distress, and treat themselves. People who believe their symptoms are caused by stress delay longer (Perkins-Porras, Whitehead, Strike, & Steptoe, 2008). Depression promotes delay as well (Bunde & Martin, 2006).

Older patients and African American heart attack victims delay longer, as do patients who have consulted with a physician or engaged in self-treatment for their symptoms. Experiencing the attack during the daytime, as well as having a family member present, enhances delay, perhaps because the environment is more distracting under these circumstances. Surprisingly, too, a history of angina or diabetes actually increases, rather than decreases, delay (Dracup & Moser, 1991).

One of the psychosocial issues raised by heart attack, then, is how to improve treatment-seeking behavior and reduce these long delays. At minimum, people at high risk for an acute coronary event and their family members need to be trained to recognize the signs of an impending or actual acute event.

Initial Treatment   Depending on the clinical symptoms, the diagnosis of CHD may be managed in any of several ways. Some people have CABG surgery to treat blockage of major arteries. Following MI, the patient is typically hospitalized in a coronary care unit in which cardiac functioning is continually monitored. Many MI patients experience anxiety in the aftermath of an event (Roest, Heideveld, Martens, de Jonge, & Denollet, 2014). Anxiety predicts complications such as reinfarction and recurrent **ischemia** during the hospital phase. Sometimes, though, MI patients in the acute phase of the disease cope by using denial and thus may be relatively anxiety-free during this period. Depression, a diagnosis of posttraumatic stress disorder (PTSD), anger, and poor social support predict longer hospital stays (Contrada et al., 2008; Oxlad, Stubberfield, Stuklis, Edwards, & Wade, 2006). Good cognitive functioning predicts better recovery from surgery (Poole et al., 2016).

Once the acute phase of illness has passed, a program of education and intervention begins. **Cardiac rehabilitation** is the active and progressive process by which people with heart disease attain their optimal physical, medical, psychological, social, emotional, vocational, and economic status. The goals of rehabilitation are to produce relief from symptoms, reduce the severity of the disease, limit further progression of disease, and promote psychological and social adjustment. Underlying the philosophy of cardiac rehabilitation is the belief that such efforts can stem advancing disease, reduce the likelihood of a repeat MI, and reduce the risk of sudden death.

Successful cardiac rehabilitation depends critically on the patient's active participation and commitment (see Box 13.2). An underlying goal of such programs is to restore a sense of mastery or self-efficacy; in its absence, adherence to rehabilitation and course of illness are poor (Sarkar, Ali, & Whooley, 2009).

Treatment by Medication   An important component of cardiac rehabilitation involves medication. Such a regimen often includes self-administration of beta-adrenergic blocking agents. These are drugs that resist the effects of sympathetic nervous system stimulation. Unfortunately, these drugs can have negative side effects including fatigue and impotence, and so targeting adherence is important. Aspirin is commonly prescribed for people recovering from, or at risk for, heart attacks. Aspirin helps prevent blood clots by blocking one of the enzymes that causes platelets to

Do heart attack patients have knowledge about the damage that has been done to their hearts? And does that knowledge predict subsequent functioning? In an ingenious study, Elizabeth Broadbent, Keith Petrie, and colleagues (2004) examined whether myocardial infarction patients' drawings of their hearts predicted return to work, the amount of exercise they did, their distress about symptoms, and perceived recovery at 3 months.

Seventy-four middle-aged patients were asked to draw pictures of their hearts (Figure 13.4). Three months later, their functioning was assessed. Patients who drew damage to their hearts had recovered less 3 months later,

believed their heart condition would last longer, believed that they had less control over their condition, and were slower returning to work. Moreover, patients' drawings of the damage to their heart predicted recovery better than did medical indicators of damage.

In a subsequent study, Broadbent and colleagues (Broadbent, Ellis, Gamble, & Petrie, 2006) found that drawings of damage to the heart predicted long-term anxiety and more use of health services. Thus, a simple drawing of the heart may offer a good basis for doctors to assess patients' beliefs and follow-up problems when discussing their heart conditions.

**FIGURE 13.4 | Patients' Drawings of Their Hearts Reflect Damage**

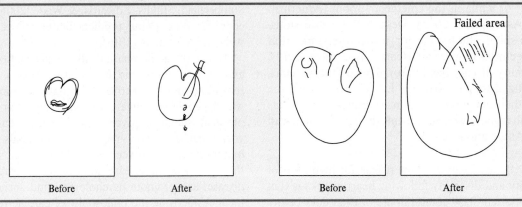

Before        After              Before        After

---

aggregate. Drugs called statins are now frequently prescribed for patients following an acute coronary event, particularly if they have elevated lipids (*Facts of Life*, February 2007). Adherence is sometimes poor, however (Gathright et al., 2017; Shen & Maeda, 2018), especially in minority groups, because of cost, negative beliefs about medications and the rest of life's demands just getting in the way (Cornelius, Voils, Birk, Romero, Edmonson, & Kronish, 2018).

Diet and Activity Level    Most people involved in cardiac rehabilitation are given dietary instructions and put on an exercise program involving walking, jogging, bicycling, or other exercises at least three times a week for 30 to 45 minutes. Exercise improves prognosis and may be especially important for people low in SES with or at risk for coronary heart disease (Puterman, Adler, Matthews, & Epel, 2012; Sweet, Tulloch, Fortier, Pipe, &

Reid, 2011). As in all lifestyle interventions, adherence can be low, and so the significance of dietary and activity level changes to recovery must be made clear to patients.

Stress Management    Stress management is an important ingredient in cardiac rehabilitation because stress can trigger fatal cardiac events (Donahue, Lampert, Dornelas, Clemow, & Burg, 2010). Younger patients, women, and people with little social support, high social conflict, and negative coping styles are most at risk for high stress, and therefore might be especially targeted for stress management interventions (Xu et al., 2017).

Yet, at present, stress management with coronary artery disease patients is hit or miss and often haphazard. Patients are urged to avoid stressful situations at work and at home, but these comments are often presented as vague treatment goals. Moreover, as many as 50 percent of patients say that they are unable to modify the stress in their lives.

These problems can be solved by employing methods such as those outlined in Chapter 6, namely, stress management programs. The patient is taught how to recognize stressful events, how to avoid stress when possible, and what to do about stress if it is unavoidable. Training in specific techniques, such as relaxation and mindfulness, improves the ability to manage stress (Cole, Pomerleau, & Harris, 1992).

Some stress management interventions target hostility. Declines in hostility in midlife are associated with lower risk (Siegler et al., 2003). Accordingly, eight weekly sessions designed to alter antagonism, cynicism, and anger were somewhat successful in reducing hostility levels (Gidron & Davidson, 1996; Gidron, Davidson, & Bata, 1999). Because anger is a risk factor both for heart disease initially and for a second heart attack (Mendes de Leon, Kop, de Swart, Bar, & Appels, 1996), interventions targeting anger have been implemented. However, because hostility can be a reflection rather than a cause of cardiovascular reactivity, modifying hostility may not modify cardiovascular risk factors very much (Hajjari et al., 2016).

**Targeting Depression**   Cardiovascular risk factors can predict depression in their own right (Herrmann-Lingen & al'Absi, 2018; Patel et al., 2018), and depression continues to be a significant problem during cardiac rehabilitation. Depression is tied to more inflammation, myocardial strain, and other indicators of heart functioning (Celano et al., 2017), and it compromises treatment and adherence (Spatola et al., 2018). It is also one of the chief risk factors for rehospitalization following cardiac surgery and for death (Ossola, Gerra, Panfilis, Tonna, & Marchesi, 2018). Cognitive–behavioral therapy (CBT) for depression can have beneficial effects on risk factors for advancing disease, although benefits can be modest (Hundt et al., 2018). Even brief telephone counseling interventions to reduce depression show benefits (Bambauer et al., 2005). Interventions to increase positive affect have also been developed and show promise (Celano et al., 2018). It is not clear that children who have CHD will benefit from psychological interventions, however (Tesson, Butow, Sholler, Sharpe, Kovacs, & Kasparian, 2019).

**Problems of Social Support**   As is true for other diseases, social support and marriage can help heart patients recover (Idler, Boulifard, & Contrada,

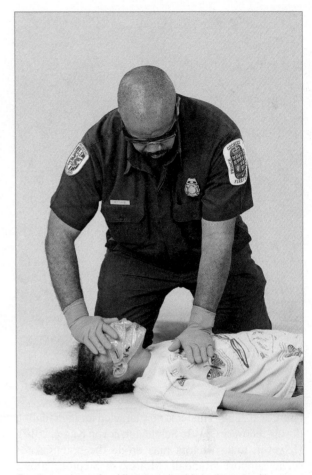

*Family members of an MI patient should also be trained in cardiopulmonary resuscitation (CPR). Approximately 70 percent of sudden deaths from heart attacks occur in the home rather than the workplace, but relatively few programs train family members in CPR. More such training programs should be made available.*
Rick Brady/McGraw-Hill Education

2012). Heart patients who are socially isolated (Shankar et al., 2011) and who are without a spouse or a confidant do more poorly (Kreibig, Whooley, & Gross, 2014). Lack of social support during hospitalization predicts depression during recovery (Brummett et al., 1998), and a supportive marriage predicts long-term survival following coronary artery bypass graft surgery, a common treatment for cardiac patients (King & Reis, 2012). Social support predicts a lower likelihood of smoking (Kreibig et al., 2014) and exercise tolerance during cardiac rehabilitation, and so is vital to the rehabilitation process (Fraser & Rodgers, 2010). So important is social support for long-term prognosis

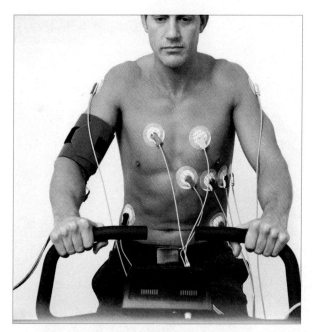

*The treadmill test provides a useful indicator of the functional capacity of recovering myocardial infarction patients.*

Digital Vision/Punchstock/Getty Images

(Burg et al., 2005) that it is now targeted for intervention during recovery (Barth, Schneider, & von Känel, 2010). However, many factors may erode the potential for social support (Randall, Molloy, & Steptoe, 2009). For example, many patients live alone or have small social networks (Rutledge et al., 2004). In other cases, primary relationships are threatened.

Partners of recovering heart attack patients may see the patient as dependent and irritable, whereas the recovering patient may regard the spouse as meddlesome and overprotective. Conflict over changes in lifestyle can increase marital strife (Croog & Fitzgerald, 1978; Michela, 1987), and ambivalent relationships can actually increase risks (Uchino et al., 2013). The patient may find it difficult to adhere to dietary restrictions and exercise, whereas the spouse may push the patient to comply. An overly solicitous partner can also aggregate symptoms, disability, and depression (Itkowitz, Kerns, & Otis, 2003). Unfortunately, too, spouses of heart attack victims often show severe distress in response to the MI, including depression, nightmares, and chronic anxiety over the patient's survival (Moser & Dracup, 2004). Although there is no evidence that a heart attack drives married couples apart, neither does it bring them closer together. It is a difficult situation for

everyone, and marital counseling or family therapy may be needed to deal with marital strain.

**Cardiac invalidism** can be one consequence of MI: Patients and their spouses see the patient's abilities as lower than they actually are (Itkowitz et al., 2003). In a study designed to reduce this problem (Taylor, Bandura, Ewart, Miller, & DeBusk, 1985), wives of recovering MI patients were provided with information about their husbands' cardiovascular capabilities, they observed their husbands' performance on a treadmill task, or they took part in the treadmill activity personally. Wives who personally experienced the treadmill task increased their perceptions of their husbands' physical and cardiac efficiency after observing their husbands' treadmill attainments. Wives who were simply informed about their husbands' performance or who observed treadmill activity continued to regard their husbands as impaired.

The family has an important role in follow-up care. Both patients and family members should be taught how to recognize the symptoms of an impending heart attack; how to differentiate them from more minor physical complaints, such as heartburn; and how to activate the emergency response system. In this way, delay behavior can be reduced and treatment can be improved in the event of a repeat event.

**Evaluation of Cardiac Rehabilitation**    Cardiac rehabilitation is now a standard part of the aftercare of patients who have had heart attacks or who have been hospitalized for heart disease. Several hundred published studies have evaluated cardiovascular disease management programs, and most find that interventions that target weight, exercise, blood pressure, smoking, and, increasingly, quality of life are successful in reducing patients' risk factors for heart disease and, in some cases, the risk of death from cardiovascular disease (Center for the Advancement of Health, 2000b; Pischke, Scherwitz, Weidner, & Ornish, 2008). Motivation and self-efficacy are critical to success (Slovinec D'Angelo, Pelletier, Reid, & Huta, 2014). Although adherence is variable (Leung, Ceccato, Stewart, & Grace, 2007), evaluations show that the addition of psychosocial treatments for depression, social support, and other psychosocial issues to standard cardiac rehabilitation programs can reduce psychological distress and lower the likelihood that cardiac patients will experience cardiac symptoms, suffer a recurrence, or die following an acute cardiac event (Dornelas & Sears, 2018; Rutledge, Redwine, Linke, & Mills, 2013).

## Prevention of Heart Disease

Many components of the interventions just described are now also used to try to prevent heart disease before it takes a toll on health. Because the risk factors are well known, interventions can target elevated blood pressure and high cholesterol and triglycerides, which are widely screened for, at least in the United States (Carroll, Kit, Lacher, & Yoon, 2013). Changes in diet and activity level are encouraged, and some interventions include stress management to help people deal with work strain, stress at home, and the strain of multiple roles. Many people are making these heart-healthy life changes on their own, most commonly by increasing their exercise and improving diet. As a result, early-onset heart disease is not as prevalent as it once was. Taking a step even farther back can be helpful. Because risk factors for CHD can show up in children and adolescents and predict adult disorders (Ehrlich, Hoyt, Sumner, McDade, & Adam, 2015), interventions should target young people's abilities to cultivate psychosocial resources, such as social support (Wickrama, O'Neal, Lee, & Wickrama, 2015) and their risk of depression. This is especially important for youths exposed to socioeconomic adversity (Wickrama et al., 2015).

## ■ HYPERTENSION

**Hypertension,** also known as high blood pressure, occurs when the supply of blood through the vessels is excessive. It can occur when cardiac output is too high, which puts pressure on the arterial walls as blood flow increases. It also occurs in response to peripheral resistance—that is, the resistance to blood flow in the small arteries of the body.

Hypertension is a serious medical problem. According to recent estimates, over 29 percent of U.S. adults have high blood pressure (Nwankwo, Yoon, Burt, & Gu, 2013), but because there are no symptoms, nearly one-third of these people don't know they have it (Yoon, Burt, Louis, & Carroll, 2012). Moreover, about 47 percent of adults in the United States may be at risk for hypertension (Fryar, Chen, & Li, 2012). Hypertension is a risk factor for other disorders, such as heart disease and kidney failure.

Untreated hypertension can affect cognitive functioning, producing problems in learning, memory, attention, abstract reasoning, mental flexibility, and other cognitive skills (Blumenthal et al., 2017). These problems are particularly significant among young people with hypertension (Waldstein et al., 1996). Given the

risks and scope of hypertension, early diagnosis and treatment are essential.

## How Is Hypertension Measured?

Hypertension is assessed by the levels of systolic and diastolic blood pressure as measured by a sphygmomanometer. As noted in Chapter 2, systolic blood pressure is the greatest force developed during contraction of the heart's ventricles. Diastolic pressure is the pressure in the arteries when the heart is relaxed; it is related to resistance of the blood vessels to blood flow.

Of the two, systolic pressure has somewhat greater value in diagnosing hypertension, and keeping systolic blood pressure under 120 is best. Mild hypertension is defined by a systolic pressure consistently between 140 and 159; moderate hypertension involves a systolic pressure consistently between 160 and 179; and severe hypertension means a systolic pressure consistently above 180.

## What Causes Hypertension?

Approximately five percent of hypertension is caused by failure of the kidneys to regulate blood pressure. However, almost 90 percent of all hypertension is *essential*—that is, of unknown origin.

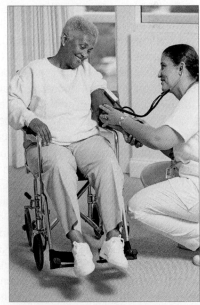

*Hypertension is a symptomless disease. As a result, unless they obtain regular physical checkups or participate in hypertension screening programs, many adults are unaware that they have this disorder.*
Rolf Bruderer/Getty Images

Some risk factors have been identified. Hypertension runs in families (Savelieva et al., 2017). Childhood temperament (emotional excitability) promotes central weight gain in adolescence (Pulkki-Råback, Elovainio, Kivimäki, Raitakari, & Keltikangas-Järvinen, 2005), which, in turn predicts CVD (Goldbacher, Matthews, & Salomon, 2005). Blood pressure reactivity in childhood and adolescence predicts later development of hypertension (Ingelfinger, 2004; Matthews, Salomon, Brady, & Allen, 2003). Gender predicts hypertension prior to age 45, with males at greater risk than females; from age 55 to 64, men and women in the United States face a similar chance of developing hypertension; after age 65, a higher percentage of women have hypertension than men. CVD risk is especially high among minorities, and this increased risk is due in part to factors related to low SES (Ruiz & Brondolo, 2016). PTSD is also tied to a higher risk of hypertension (Burg et al., 2017).

Genetic factors play a role (Wu, Treiber, & Snieder, 2013). If one parent has high blood pressure, the offspring has a 45 percent chance of developing it; if two parents have high blood pressure, the probability increases to 95 percent. As is true for coronary heart disease, the genetic factor in hypertension may be reactivity, a predisposition toward elevated sympathetic nervous system activity especially in response to stressful events (Everson, Lovallo, Sausen, & Wilson, 1992). Reactivity predicts higher future blood pressure (Carroll, Phillips, Der, Hunt, & Benzeval, 2011).

Emotional factors are also implicated in this constellation of risk. Depression, even in childhood, hostility, and frequent experiences of intense arousal predict increases in blood pressure over time (Betensky & Contrada, 2010; Rottenberg et al, 2014). The importance of pre existing depression in cardiovascular disease is so clear that some researchers recommend treatment for people who are depressed as soon as CVD risk factors are identified (Stewart, Perkins, & Callahan, 2014). Anger (Harburg, Julius, Kacirotti, Gleiberman, & Schork, 2003), cynical distrust (Williams, 1984), hostility (Mezick et al., 2010), and excessive striving in the face of significant odds (James, Hartnett, & Kalsbeek, 1983) have all been implicated in the development of hypertension. Discrimination has also been tied to hypertension risk (Rodriguez et al., 2016). Rumination following stressful events may prolong cardiovascular reactivity and contribute to the development of CVD (Key, Campbell, Bacon, & Gerin, 2008). Repressive coping may also be a significant contributor (Mund & Mitte, 2012).

A meta-analysis found that childhood adversity is tied to CVD (Jakubowski, Cundiff, & Matthews, 2018), and family conflict increases CVD risk in part by shaping the negative quality of adult social interactions (John-Henderson, Kamarck, Muldoon, & Manuck, 2016). A family environment that fosters chronic anger is also implicated (Ewart, 1991). In contrast, children and adolescents who develop social competence skills have a reduced risk for CVD (Chen, Matthews, Salomon, & Ewart, 2002; Ewart & Jorgensen, 2004). Positive parenting, especially during adolescence, may benefit adult cardiovascular health (Matthews et al., 2017). Such observations suggest the importance of intervening early in the family environment to modify communication patterns.

Stress has been suspected as a contributor to hypertension for many years (Henry & Cassel, 1969). High numbers of stressful life events, chronic social conflict, job strain, namely, the combination of high demands with little control and crowded, high-stress, and noisy locales all produce higher rates of hypertension (Feeney, Dooley, Finucane, & Kenny, 2015). People who ultimately develop hypertension often show a prior pattern of heightened cardiovascular and inflammatory responses to stress. Low SES in childhood and in adulthood both predict risk for cardiovascular disease (Appleton et al., 2012; Hagger-Johnson, Mõttus, Craig, Starr, & Deary, 2012). Groups that have migrated from rural to urban areas have high rates of hypertension. In women, elevated blood pressure has been related to having extensive family responsibilities, and among women in white-collar occupations, the combined impact of family responsibilities and job strain. Negative social interactions increase hypertension risk, especially among women (Sneed & Cohen, 2014). These risks may occur, in part, because CVD recovery from acute stress is poor (Boylan, Cundiff, & Matthews, 2018).

### Stress and Hypertension Among African Americans

Hypertension is a common medical problem in African American communities. Its high prevalence is tied to stress and low SES (Hong, Nelesen, Krohn, Mills, & Dimsdale, 2006). Hostility and anger may also contribute to this ethnic difference (Thomas, Nelesen, & Dimsdale, 2004). Hereditary factors may be implicated as well: Racial differences in neuropeptide and cardiovascular responses to stressors appear to influence the development of hypertension (Saab et al., 1997).

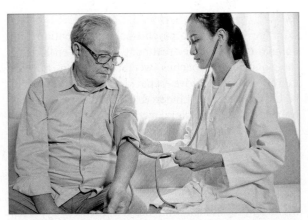

*Many people have "white coat hypertension," that is, elevations in blood pressure during medical visits but not otherwise. White coat hypertension is sometimes misdiagnosed and medicated as hypertension.*

Dinis Tolipov/123RF

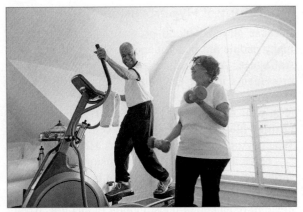

*Hypertension is a particular problem in African American communities. Practicing healthy behaviors, including exercise, is widely recommended.*

LWA/Dann Tardif/Blend Images LLC

Low-income Blacks are especially vulnerable. They are likely to live in stressful neighborhoods (Fleming, Baum, Davidson, Rectanus, & McArdle, 1987); they report more psychological distress than do higher-income whites and Blacks; and chronic life stress may interfere with sympathetic nervous system recovery in response to stress (Pardine & Napoli, 1983). Exposure to discrimination and racism can contribute to high blood pressure among Blacks (Beatty, Moody-Waldstein, Tobin, Cassels, Schwartz, & Brondolo, 2016; Dolezsar, McGrath, Herzig, & Miller, 2014), possibly by interfering with the normal decline in blood pressure at night (Euteneuer, Mills, Pung, Rief, & Dimsdale, 2014), by undermining adherence to treatment (Forsyth, Schoenthaler, Chaplin, Ogedegbe, & Ravenell, 2014), and by rejecting treatment from providers who are perceived to be racially biased (Greer, Brondolo, & Brown, 2014).

African Americans have an elevated risk of obesity, which is tied to hypertension. Dietary factors (Myers, 1996) and salt intake may play a causal role. Cigarette smoking and low exercise are also implicated (Kershaw, Mezuk, Abdou, Rafferty, & Jackson, 2010).

Cardiovascular reactivity among African Americans, especially older African Americans, may be part of a more general syndrome that implicates multiple risk factors for CVD, including greater heart rate reactivity, higher fasting insulin levels, lower high-density lipoprotein cholesterol levels, a higher waist-to-hip ratio, and greater body mass overall (Waldstein, Burns, Toth, & Poehlman, 1999). This clustering of metabolic factors, namely, metabolic syndrome, may predispose older African Americans to a higher risk for CVD and metabolic disorders, such as diabetes. Latinos in the United States are also at risk for developing hypertension, and worry about deportation may be a significant risk factor for CVD (Torres, 2018).

**John Henryism**   Because hypertension is a particular risk for Blacks, research has examined a phenomenon known as **John Henryism.** John Henry, the "steel-driving" man, was an uneducated black laborer who allegedly defeated a mechanical steam drill in a contest to see who could complete the most work in the shortest period of time. However, after winning the battle, John Henry reportedly dropped dead.

James and colleagues (James, Hartnett, & Kalsbeek, 1983) coined the term "John Henryism" to refer to a personality predisposition to cope actively with psychosocial stressors. It becomes a lethal predisposition when active coping efforts are likely to be unsuccessful. The person scoring high on John Henryism would try harder and harder against ultimately insurmountable odds. Consequently, one would expect to find John Henryism to be especially lethal among the disadvantaged, especially low-income and poorly educated Blacks. Research tends to confirm these relations (James, Keenan, Strogatz, Browning, & Garrett, 1992). The specific factors tying John Henryism to the increased risk for hypertension are greater cardiovascular reactivity to stress and less rapid recovery from stress (Merritt, Bennett, Williams, Sollers, & Thayer, 2004).

## Treatment of Hypertension

Because elevated blood pressure is easily detected, many people are being identified at the prehypertension stage. At this stage, goals are weight loss, improvements in diet (including lowering salt intake), and increased physical activity, as through exercise (National Academy of Medicine, 2013). A long-term healthy lifestyle is the best prevention (Dorough, Winett, Anderson, Davy, Martin, & Hedrick, 2014).

Once it is diagnosed, hypertension is treated in a variety of ways. Most commonly, it is treated through drugs. Patients are also put on low-sodium diets and urged to reduce their consumption of alcohol. Weight reduction in overweight patients is strongly urged, and exercise is recommended for all hypertensive patients. Caffeine restriction is often included as part of the dietary treatment of hypertension, because caffeine, in conjunction with stress, elevates blood pressure responses among those at risk for or already diagnosed with hypertension (Lovallo et al., 2000). Medications can be effective, but adherence can be poor, especially among people who are depressed; building a sense of self-efficacy can help offset the risks of nonadherence (Bosworth, Blalock, Hoyle, & Czajkowski, Voils, 2018; Schoenthaler, Butler, Chaplin, Tobin, & Ogedegbe, 2016).

**Cognitive–Behavioral Treatments**    A variety of cognitive–behavioral methods have been used to treat high blood pressure. These include biofeedback, progressive muscle relaxation, hypnosis, and meditation, all of which reduce blood pressure via the induction of a state of low arousal. Deep breathing and imagery are often added to accomplish this task. Evaluations of these treatments suggest modestly positive effects (Davison, Williams, Nezami, Bice, & DeQuattro, 1991), although adherence levels are modest (Hoelscher, Lichstein, & Rosenthal, 1986).

The fact that anger has been linked to hypertension implies that teaching people how to manage their anger might be useful. In fact, training hypertensive patients how to manage confrontational encounters through such behavioral techniques as role-playing can produce better skills for managing such situations and can lower blood pressure reactivity (Davidson, MacGregor, Stuhr, & Gidron, 1999; Larkin & Zayfert, 1996). Depression is also an important treatment target and may affect adherence as well as well-being (Krousel-Wood et al., 2010).

**Evaluation of Cognitive–Behavioral Interventions**    How do psychosocial interventions fare comparatively in the treatment of hypertension? Of the nondrug approaches, weight reduction, physical exercise, and cognitive–behavioral therapy appear to be quite successful (Linden & Chambers, 1994). Moreover, cognitive–behavioral methods are inexpensive and easy to implement: They can be used without supervision, and they have no side effects. Lifestyle interventions that focus on increasing physical activity and improving diet are essential (Blumenthal et al., 2017).

Cognitive-behavioral interventions may reduce the drug requirements for the treatment of hypertension (Shapiro, Hui, Oakley, Pasic, & Jamner, 1997), and accordingly be especially helpful to those people who do not tolerate the drugs well (Kristal-Boneh, Melamed, Bernheim, Peled, & Green, 1995). CBT appears to be especially successful with mild or borderline hypertensives and, with these groups, may actually substitute for drug control.

However, rates of adherence to cognitive–behavioral interventions are not particularly high (Langford, Solid, Gann, Rabinowitz, Williams, & Seixas, 2018). One reason is people's "commonsense" understanding of hypertension (Hekler et al., 2008). For example, some people take the concept of "hyper-tension" quite literally and assume that relaxing and reducing their level of stress is sufficient and that medication is not required (Frosch, Kimmel, & Volpp, 2008). Moreover, as hypertension is symptomless, many people believe that they are vulnerable only when they are cranked up. They are wrong. At present, the combination of drugs and cognitive–behavioral treatments appears to be the best approach to the management of hypertension.

## The Hidden Disease

One of the biggest problems in the treatment of hypertension is that so many people who are hypertensive do not know that they are. Hypertension is largely a symptomless disease, and many thousands of people who do not get regular physicals suffer from hypertension without realizing it. Yet they experience the costs of a lower quality of life, compromised cognitive functioning, and fewer social activities, nonetheless (Saxby, Harrington, McKeith, Wesnes, & Ford, 2003).

National campaigns to educate the public about hypertension have had some success in getting people diagnosed (Horan & Roccella, 1988). Worksite screening programs have been successful in identifying people with hypertension (Alderman & Lamport, 1988).

Increasingly, community interventions enable people to have their blood pressure checked by going to mobile units, churches or community centers, or even the local drugstore. The widespread availability of these screening programs has helped with early identification of people with hypertension.

Once prehypertension or hypertension is diagnosed, it can be managed through lifestyle change and, if needed, medication. The current push is to try to get people to change their behavior as early as possible, using lifestyle intervention programs that can be delivered efficiently, including electronically (Dorough et al., 2014).

## ■ STROKE

Lee Phillips, 62, was shopping at a San Diego mall with her husband, Eric, when she felt an odd tugging on the right side of her face. Her mouth twisted into a lurid grimace. Suddenly she felt weak. "What kind of game are you playing?" asked Eric. "I'm not," Lee tried to respond—but her words came out in a jumble. "Let's go to the hospital," Eric urged her. All Lee wanted to do was go home and lie down. Fortunately, her husband summoned an ambulance instead. Lee was suffering a stroke (Gorman, 1996, September 19).

Lee was fortunate for two reasons. First, she got medical attention quickly, which is vital to minimizing damage and its consequences. Second, her husband was with her. Research shows that people who arrive at the emergency room with a companion are treated more promptly than those who do not (Ashkenazi et al., 2015).

**Stroke,** the fifth major cause of death in the United States, results from a disturbance in blood flow to the brain (American Heart Association, 2018). Some strokes occur when blood flow to localized areas of the brain is interrupted, which can result from arteriosclerosis or hypertension. For example, when arteriosclerotic plaques damage the cerebral blood vessels, the damaged area may trap blood clots (thrombi) or produce circulating blood clots (emboli) that block the flow of blood (see Figure 13.5). Stroke can also be caused by cerebral hemorrhage (bleeding caused by the rupture of a blood vessel in the brain). When blood leaks into the brain, large areas of nervous tissue may be compressed against the skull, producing widespread or fatal damage.

Strokes caused approximately 1 of every 19 deaths in the United States in 2016 (Benjamin et al., 2019), whereby it is estimated that every 4 minutes someone dies of stroke (Centers for Disease Control and Prevention, 2015, November). In the United States, approximately

**FIGURE 13.5 | Stroke**   Stroke is a condition that results from a disturbance in blood flow to the brain.
*Source:* National Heart, Lung, and Blood Institute. "What Are the Signs and Symptoms of Atrial Fibrillation?" Last modified from June 6, 2010.

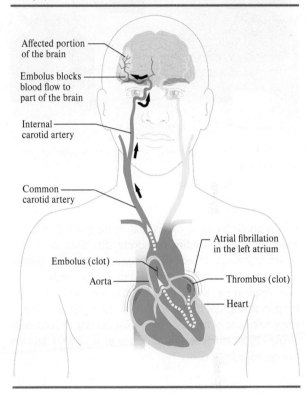

800,000 individuals experience a stroke every year (Centers for Disease Control and Prevention, 2015, November). And stroke compromises mobility in half of elderly survivors (Centers for Disease Control and Prevention, 2015, November). The warning signs of stroke are listed in Table 13.1.

**TABLE 13.1 | Stroke Warning Signs**

| The American Stroke Association says these are the warning signs of stroke: |
| --- |
| • Sudden numbness or weakness of the face, arm, or leg, especially on one side of the body |
| • Sudden confusion, trouble speaking or understanding |
| • Sudden trouble seeing in one or both eyes |
| • Sudden trouble walking, dizziness, loss of balance or coordination |
| • Sudden, severe headache with no known cause |

*Source:* Thom, Thomas, Nancy Haase, Wayne Rosamond, Virginia J. Howard, John Rumsfeld, Teri Manolio, and Zhi-Jie Zheng. "Heart Disease and Stroke Statistics—2006 Update." *American Heart Association* 113, no. 6 (2004): 85–151.

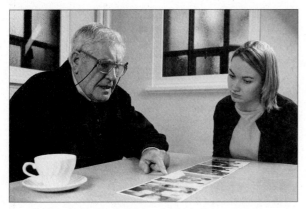

*People who have had strokes often must relearn some aspects of cognitive functioning.*

Colin Cuthbert/SPL/Science Source

A chief risk of stroke is that more will follow in its wake, ultimately leading to severe disability or death. Researchers have recently discovered that a simple intervention, namely, aspirin, can greatly reduce this risk. Aspirin has immediate benefits for stroke patients by preventing coagulation. Following a stroke, even a few weeks' use of aspirin can reduce the risk of recurrent strokes by as much as a third (Chen et al., 2000). Statins appear to help, too.

## Risk Factors for Stroke

Risk factors for stroke overlap heavily with those for heart disease. They include high blood pressure, heart disease, cigarette smoking, a high red blood cell count, and transient ischemic attacks. TIAs are little strokes that produce temporary weakness, clumsiness, or loss of feeling in one side or limb; a temporary dimness or loss of vision; or a temporary loss of speech or difficulty understanding speech (American Heart Association, 2000).

The likelihood of a stroke increases with age, occurs more often in men than in women, and occurs more often in African Americans and among those who have diabetes. A prior stroke or a family history of stroke also increases the likelihood. Acute triggers for stroke include negative emotions, anger, and sudden change in posture in response to a startling event (Koton, Tanne, Bornstein, & Green, 2004). Anger expression also appears to be related to stroke, as it is for coronary heart disease and hypertension; low levels of anger expression appear to be mildly protective (Eng, Fitzmaurice, Kubzansky, Rimm, & Kawachi, 2003).

Stress increases the risk of stroke, as does job strain, especially among women (Kaplan, 2015). Discrimination may also play a role (Beatty Moody et al., 2019). Psychological health is protective against stroke (Lambiase, Kubzansky, & Thurston, 2015).

Depression and anxiety are predictive of stroke (Neu, Schlattmann, Schilling, & Hartmann, 2004) and are especially strong predictors for white women and for African Americans (Jonas & Mussolino, 2000). The incidence of first stroke by race is shown in Figure 13.6. The group at highest risk for stroke is Black men age 45 to 64. Strokes kill Black men at about three times the rate for white men (Villarosa, 2002, September 23).

## Consequences of Stroke

Stroke affects all aspects of one's life: personal, social, vocational, and physical.

**Motor Problems**    Immediately after a stroke, motor difficulties are common. Because the right side of the brain controls movement in the left half of the body and the left side of the brain controls movement in the right half of the body, motor impairments occur on the side opposite to the stroke side. It is usually difficult or impossible for the patient to move the arm and leg on the affected side; therefore, he or she usually requires help walking, dressing, and performing other physical activities. Stroke almost inevitably leads to increased dependence on others, at least for a while; as a consequence, family and other social relationships may be profoundly affected. With physical therapy, some of these problems are diminished (Gordon & Diller, 1983).

**FIGURE 13.6 | First Stroke Rates by Race**

Source: Roger, V. L., D. M. Lloyd-Jones, E. J. Benjamin, J. D. Berry, W. B. Borden, D. M. Bravata, S. Dai, et al. "Heart Disease and Stroke Statistics–2012 Update: A Report from the American Heart Association." *American Heart Association* 125, no. 1 (2012): 2–220.

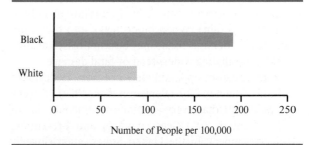

Number of People per 100,000

Cognitive Problems   The cognitive difficulties that the stroke victim faces depend on which side of the brain was damaged. Patients with left-brain damage may have communication disorders, such as aphasia, which involves difficulty in understanding others and expressing oneself, and problems with short-term memory. A stroke patient described a relevant incident:

> One of my first shopping expeditions was to a hardware store, but when I got there I couldn't think of the words "electric plug," and it took me a while to get the message across. Naturally, I was humiliated and frustrated. I was close to tears at the store, and let them out to Jane [the patient's wife] at home. I was learning day by day the frustrations of a body and mind I could not command. (Dahlberg, 1977, p. 124)

Patients with right-brain damage may be unable to process or make use of certain kinds of visual feedback. As a result, such a patient may shave only one side of his face or put makeup on only half her face. These patients also may have difficulty perceiving distances accurately and may bump into objects or walls or have trouble reading a clock, dialing a phone, or making change.

In addition, patients with right-brain damage may feel that they are going crazy because they cannot understand the words they read or can perceive only the last part of each word. They may also think they are hearing voices if a speaker is physically positioned on the impaired side and can thus be heard but not seen (Gordon & Diller, 1983). Cognitive compromise can also interfere with stroke patients' adherence to medication (O'Carroll et al., 2011).

Emotional Problems   Emotional problems after a stroke are common. Patients with left-brain damage often react to their disorder with anxiety and depression; patients with right-brain damage more commonly may seem indifferent to their situation, a condition known as alexithymia.

## Rehabilitative Interventions

Interventions with stroke patients typically take five approaches: medication; psychotherapy, including treatment for depression; cognitive remedial training to restore intellectual functioning; movement therapies, which include training in specific skills development; and the use of structured, stimulating environments to challenge the stroke patient's capabilities. Post stroke medications are effective, but adherence can be poor,

especially among people high in negative affect (Crayton et al., 2017).

Movement-based therapies can help restore functioning following stroke. Although conventional physical therapy is not beneficial to stroke patients, a form of physical therapy called constraint-induced movement therapy, which is targeted to the upper extremities, is effective (Taub et al., 2006; Wolf et al., 2010). Basically, it requires patients to use a more affected limb (such as the left arm) to the relative exclusion of a less affected limb (such as the right arm) for several hours each day. Patients so trained show improved functioning in the affected limbs (Taub et al., 2006).

Interventions designed to deal with cognitive problems after stroke have several goals (Gordon & Diller, 1983). First, patients must be made aware that they have problems. Often, the stroke patient thinks he or she is performing adequately when this is not the case. A risk of making patients aware of these problems is the sense of discouragement or failure that may arise, and so, it is important for patients to see that these deficits are correctable.

Several techniques help right-brain-damaged stroke patients regain a full visual field (Gordon & Diller, 1983). One method involves spreading out an array of money before a patient and asking him or her to pick all of it up. The right-brain-damaged patient will pick up only the money on the right side, ignoring that on the left. When the patient is induced to turn his or her head toward the impaired side, he or she will see the remaining money and can then pick it up as well. A scanning machine can improve this process further.

Cognitive remediation is a slow process, and skills retraining needs to proceed in an orderly fashion, beginning with easy problems and moving to more difficult ones. As each skill is acquired, practice is essential (Gordon & Hibbard, 1991).

A relatively recent approach to therapy with stroke patients, called neurorehabilitation, relies on the brain's ability to rebuild itself and learn new tasks (Bryck & Fisher, 2012). Essentially, the idea is to rewire the brain so that areas of the brain other than the one affected by the stroke can come to take on those functions, thus improving patients' ability to move, speak, and articulate.

Whereas it was once believed that stroke patients would achieve their maximum recovery within the first 6 months after stroke, it now appears that additional gains can occur over subsequent years (Allen, 2003, April 7).

# ■ TYPE 2 DIABETES

**Type 2 diabetes** is one of the most common chronic diseases in this country and the leading cause of kidney failure in adults (Centers for Disease Control and Prevention, 2017). In 2015, over 9 percent of the U.S. population had diabetes, and of the roughly 29 million individuals who had it, an estimated 8 million cases remained undiagnosed (Centers for Disease Control and Prevention, 2017). Diabetes costs the United States more than $327 billion a year in medical costs (American Diabetes Association, 2018). Diabetes is not just a problem in the United States; as Figure 13.7 shows, diabetes cases are projected to increase dramatically throughout the world.

In the past 30 years in the United States, the incidence of diabetes has doubled (Centers for Disease Control and Prevention, 2017). Altogether, diabetes contributed to over 80,000 deaths in 2015 alone (Centers for Disease Control and Prevention, 2017).

Together with type 1 diabetes, an autoimmune disorder covered in the next chapter, type 2 diabetes is estimated to cause approximately 48,400 cases of kidney failure, 24,000 cases of blindness, and 65,700 amputations yearly. About 68 percent of deaths among people with diabetes are due to heart disease and stroke (Centers for Disease Control and Prevention, 2011, January). The incidence of cases of type 2 diabetes is increasing so rapidly that it is considered a pandemic (Taylor, 2004). The complications of diabetes are pictured in Figure 13.8.

Until recently, type 2 (or non-insulin-dependent) diabetes was typically a disorder of middle and old age. As obesity has become rampant and the consumption of sugary foods and drinks has increased, type 2 diabetes, to which these factors are contributors, has become more prevalent at earlier ages (Malik et al., 2010). Children and adolescents are now at risk for type 2 diabetes, and moreover, the disease progresses more rapidly and is harder to treat in younger people

**FIGURE 13.7 | Diabetes Worldwide, Present and Projected**    *Source:* World Health Organization. Diabetes Programme. Retrieved July 22, 2010, from http://www.who.int/diabetes/actionnow/en/mapdiabprev.pdf.

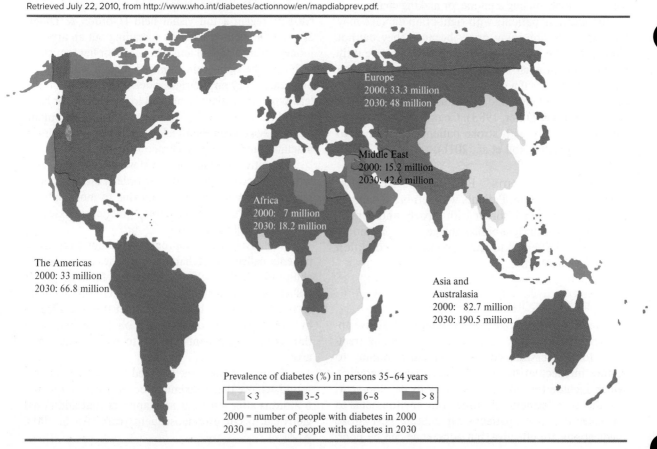

Europe
2000: 33.3 million
2030: 48 million

Middle East
2000: 15.2 million
2030: 42.6 million

Africa
2000:  7 million
2030: 18.2 million

The Americas
2000: 33 million
2030: 66.8 million

Asia and
Australasia
2000:  82.7 million
2030: 190.5 million

Prevalence of diabetes (%) in persons 35–64 years

| < 3 | 3–5 | 6–8 | > 8 |

2000 = number of people with diabetes in 2000
2030 = number of people with diabetes in 2030

**FIGURE 13.8  |  The Potential Health Complications of Diabetes Are Extensive, Life-Threatening, and Costly**

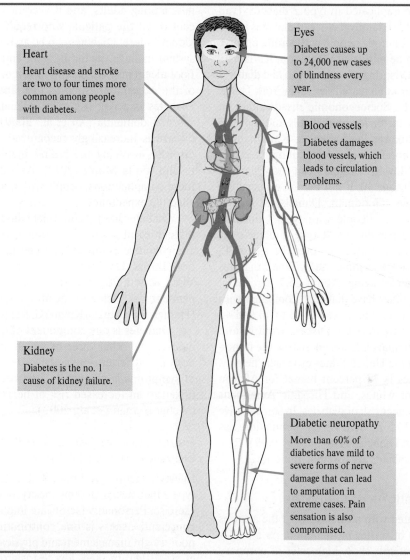

**Heart**

Heart disease and stroke are two to four times more common among people with diabetes.

**Eyes**

Diabetes causes up to 24,000 new cases of blindness every year.

**Blood vessels**

Diabetes damages blood vessels, which leads to circulation problems.

**Kidney**

Diabetes is the no. 1 cause of kidney failure.

**Diabetic neuropathy**

More than 60% of diabetics have mild to severe forms of nerve damage that can lead to amputation in extreme cases. Pain sensation is also compromised.

(Grady, 2012, April 30). As a result, type 2 diabetes is a major and growing health problem.

A good deal is known about the mechanisms that trigger type 2 diabetes (Kiberstis, 2005). Glucose metabolism involves a delicate balance between insulin production and insulin responsiveness. As food is digested, carbohydrates are broken down into glucose. Glucose is absorbed from the intestines into the blood, where it travels to the liver and other organs. Rising levels of glucose in the blood trigger the pancreas to secrete insulin into the bloodstream.

When this balance goes awry, it sets the stage for type 2 diabetes. First, cells in muscle, fat, and the liver lose some of their ability to respond fully to insulin, a condition known as insulin resistance. In response to insulin resistance, the pancreas temporarily increases its production of insulin. At this point, insulin-producing cells may give out, with the result that insulin production falls, and the balance between insulin action and insulin secretion becomes disregulated, resulting in type 2 diabetes (Alper, 2000). The symptoms include frequent urination; fatigue; dryness of the mouth; impotence; irregular menstruation; loss of sensation; frequent infection of the skin, gums, or urinary system; pain or cramps in legs, feet, or fingers; slow healing of cuts and bruises; and intense itching and drowsiness.

Precursors for type 2 diabetes can begin early. Genetic factors are implicated in type 2 diabetes (van Zon et al., 2018) and so family history of diabetes is one risk factor; however, among people with strong positive affect, this risk can be mitigated (Tsenkova, Karlamangla, & Ryff, 2016). Offspring of women who had diabetes during pregnancy are at increased risk (New York Times, September 9, 2014). Socioeconomic disadvantage in childhood is a risk factor for prediabetes and diabetes in adulthood (Tsenkova, Pudrovska, & Karlamangla, 2014), as is childhood adversity (Jakubowski et al., 2018). Children of low-SES parents can show signs of insulin resistance by age 10, if not before, especially if they are also obese (Goodman, Daniels, & Dolan, 2007). The majority of people with type 2 diabetes are overweight (90 percent), and type 2 diabetes is more common in men and people over the age of 45 (American Diabetes Association, 2012). Type 2 diabetes is heavily a disorder of aging. About 25.2 percent of people aged 65 or older have diabetes, compared with 4.6 and 14.3 percent among those age 18 to 44 and 45 to 64, respectively (Centers for Disease Control and Prevention, 2017, January). Diabetes strikes the minority communities in the United States especially heavily. The risk of diabetes is 77 percent higher for African Americans than for whites, and Hispanic Americans have a 66 percent higher risk of diabetes. In some Native American tribes, 33.5 percent of the population has diabetes (American Diabetes Association, 1999). Risk factors for type 2 diabetes are listed in Table 13.2.

## Health Implications of Diabetes

Diabetes is associated with a thickening of the arteries due to the buildup of wastes in the blood. As a consequence, diabetic patients show high rates of coronary heart disease. Diabetes is the leading cause of blindness among adults, and it accounts for nearly 50 percent of all the patients who require renal dialysis for kidney failure. Diabetes can be associated with nervous system damage, including pain and loss of sensation. Foot ulcers may result, and in severe cases, amputation of the extremities, such as toes and feet, is required. Diabetes is a risk factor for Alzheimer's disease and vascular dementia (Xu et al., 2009), and Alzheimer's disease is increasingly recognized to be a metabolic disorder involving the brain's inability to respond to insulin (de la Monte, 2012). As a consequence of all these complications, people with diabetes have a shortened life expectancy.

Diabetes has psychosocial fallout as well, including difficulties in sexual functioning, risk for depression, and cognitive dysfunction, especially concerning memory (Burns, Deschênes, & Schmitz, 2016; Chiu, Hu, Wray, & Wu, 2016). Psychological distress is an independent risk factor for death among diabetic patients (Hamer, Stamatakis, Kivimäki, Kengne, & Batty, 2010).

Diabetes is one component of the so-called deadly quartet, the other three of which are intra-abdominal body fat, hypertension, and elevated lipids. This cluster of symptoms is potentially fatal because it is strongly linked to an increased risk of heart attack and stroke (Weber-Hamann et al., 2002).

## Psychosocial Factors in the Development of Diabetes

Lifestyle factors are implicated in the development of type 2 diabetes, including obesity, poor diet, and lack of exercise. Personality factors are implicated as well. Low conscientiousness is one contributing factor, through poor weight management and physical inactivity (Jokela et al., 2014). In men, low testosterone and higher depression predict type 2 diabetes risk (Tully et al., 2016). Maladaptive coping may also be implicated (Burns, Deschênes, & Schmitz, 2016). Job strain has been related to an increased risk (Huth et al., 2014), as has poor marital quality (Whisman, Li, Sbarra, & Raison, 2014). Depression is a risk factor too, in part through its relation to increasing weight (Shomaker et al., 2016). Psychological well-being and purpose in life are protective against diabetes (Boehm, Trudel-Fitzgerald, Kivimaki, & Kubzansky, 2015; Hafez et al., 2018).

**Stress and Diabetes**    People with type 2 diabetes are sensitive to the effects of stress (Gonder-Frederick, Carter, Cox, & Clarke, 1990; Halford, Cuddihy, &

**TABLE 13.2 | Risk Factors for Type 2 Diabetes**

You are at risk if:
- You are overweight.
- You get little exercise.
- You have high blood pressure.
- You have a sibling or parent with diabetes.
- You had a baby weighing over 9 pounds at birth.
- You are a member of a high-risk ethnic group, which includes African Americans, Latinos, Native Americans, Asian Americans, and Pacific Islanders.

*Source:* American Diabetes Association. "Are You at Risk?" Last modified 2012. http://www.diabetes.org/are-you-at-risk/.

Mrs. Goldberg had had type 2 diabetes for some time. Her doctor had made the diagnosis 10 years earlier, just after her 40th birthday. She watched her diet, got sufficient exercise, and was able to control her blood glucose with oral medication. During the past several months, however, Mrs. Goldberg's diabetes control had begun to deteriorate. Despite the fact that she continued to follow her diet and exercise regimen, her blood glucose levels became elevated more frequently.

Mrs. Goldberg consulted her physician, who asked if her lifestyle had changed in any way over the past several months. She told him that her boss had added several new responsibilities to her job and that they made her workday much more stressful. Things were so bad that she was having trouble sleeping at night and dreaded going to work in the morning. Mrs. Goldberg's physician told her that this additional stress might be responsible for her poor diabetes control. Rather than

initially changing her medications, he suggested that she first speak with her boss to see if some of the stress of her job might be relieved. Fortunately, her boss was understanding and allowed Mrs. Goldberg to share her responsibilities with another employee. Within several weeks, she no longer dreaded going to work, and her diabetes control improved significantly.

This case illustrates how a relatively simple change in a patient's environment may have a clinically significant impact on blood glucose control. It underscores the need for the physician to be aware of what is happening in the patient's life in order to determine requirements for treatment. Under the circumstances, it would have been inappropriate to have altered this patient's medication.

*Source:* Feinglos, M. N., and R. S. Surwit. *Behavior and Diabetes Mellitus.* Kalamazoo, MI: Upjohn.

---

Mortimer, 1990). People at high risk for diabetes show abnormal glycemic responsiveness to stress, which may foster the disease (Esposito-Del Puente et al., 1994). Stress also aggravates type 2 diabetes after the disease is diagnosed (Surwit & Schneider, 1993; Surwit & Williams, 1996), as explained in Box 13.3. Just as sympathetic nervous system reactivity is implicated in the development of CHD and hypertension, it is involved in the pathophysiology of type 2 diabetes.

## The Management of Diabetes

The key to the successful control of diabetes is active self-management (Auerbach et al., 2001). Indeed, type 2 diabetes can be completely prevented by changes in the lifestyle of high-risk individuals (Tuomilehto et al., 2001). Support from health providers for self-management improves outcomes (Lee, Piette, Heisler, Janevic, & Rosland, 2019). Exercise, weight loss among those who are overweight, stress management, and dietary control are encouraged (Wing, Blair, Marcus, Epstein, & Harvey, 1994; Wing, Epstein, et al., 1986). Dietary intervention involves reducing sugar and carbohydrate intake. Obesity especially seems to tax the insulin system, so patients are encouraged to achieve a normal weight. Exercise is especially important (Von Korff et al., 2005) because it helps use up glucose in the blood and helps reduce weight.

However, adherence to lifestyle change is problematic. People with type 2 diabetes are often unaware of the health risks they face. One survey found that only one-third of diagnosed diabetic patients realized that heart disease was among their most serious potential complications (*New York Times,* 2001, May 22). Many diabetic patients do not have enough information about glucose utilization and metabolic control of insulin. A patient may be told what to do without understanding the rationale for it. Many patients fail to recognize that they have a chronic health condition that requires sustained commitment to medications and behavior change, and so ensuring that these patients have the correct beliefs about their illness is critical to adherence (Mann, Ponieman, Leventhal, & Halm, 2009). Clearly, education is an important component of intervention.

Several additional factors are critical to adherence. People with good self-control skills do a better job of achieving glycemic control by virtue of their greater adherence to a treatment regimen (Peyrot, McMurry, & Kruger, 1999). The belief that one can control one's diabetes is also important (Gonzales, Shreck, Psaros, & Safren, 2015). Generally, social support improves adherence, but this is not true for diabetes. Social contact can lead to temptations to eat that compromise diabetic functioning (Littlefield, Rodin, Murray, & Craven, 1990). However, spousal support for exercise improves adherence (Khan, Stephens, Franks, Rook, & Salem, 2013) and can affect dietary adherence as well (Stephens, Franks, Rook, Iida, Hemphill, & Salem, 2013).

Cognitive–behavioral interventions have been undertaken with type 2 diabetics to improve adherence to aspects of their regimen. Much nonadherence results from running out of medications or forgetting to take them, and so these are obvious targets for intervention (Hill-Briggs et al., 2005). Programs have also focused on training patients to monitor blood sugar levels effectively (Wing, Epstein et al., 1986). Even very brief interventions via telephone can improve self-care among type 2 diabetics (Sacco, Malone, Morrison, Friedman, & Wells, 2009). Training in self-management and problem-solving skills is a vital part of many interventions with diabetes (Hill-Briggs, 2003). Recently too, personal digital assistants that prompt people about aspects of their self-care have been used (Sevick et al., 2010).

Depression complicates prognosis and also interferes with the active self-management role that diabetes patients must play (Katon et al., 2009). Interventions that target depression, a sense of self-efficacy, physical activity, and quality of life (Corathers et al., 2017) improve satisfaction with health care, adherence, and the ability to achieve control over blood sugar levels (Cherrington, Wallston, & Rothman, 2010). Anger may undermine glycemic control (Yi, Yi, Vitaliano, & Weinger, 2008). Moreover, diabetes itself can lead to higher levels of negative affect and emotional reactivity (Wolf, Tsenkova, Ryff, Davidson, & Willette, 2018). Consequently, therapeutic interventions focus on these emotional consequences as well. As a result of ties between stress and diabetes (Herschbach et al., 1997), behavioral investigators have examined the effect of stress management programs on diabetes control.

Because the diabetes regimen is complex, involves lifestyle change, and implicates multiple risk factors, multifactor lifestyle interventions have been used to approach this regimen (Moncrieft et al., 2016). However, at present, the evidence base for multifactor lifestyle interventions is mixed (Angermayr, Melchart, & Linde, 2010; Kolata, 2012).

Because of problems involving adherence, a focus on maintenance and relapse prevention is also essential. The fact that stress and social pressure to eat reduce adherence has led researchers to focus on social skills and problem-solving skills so that people with diabetes can manage high-risk situations (Glasgow, Toobert, Hampson, & Wilson, 1995).

Diabetes Prevention   Because diabetes is such a major and growing public health problem, increasingly, health psychologists and policy makers are focusing on prevention. One study guided by this focus (Diabetes Prevention Program Research Group, 2002) enrolled 3,000 adults whose blood sugar levels were high but not yet high enough to be diagnosed with diabetes. These high-risk individuals were then assigned to one of three groups. One group received a placebo medication and lifestyle recommendations; the second group received lifestyle recommendations and a medication that lowers blood sugar; the third group received an intensive lifestyle intervention focused on weight loss, physical activity, and diet change. After only 4 years, the incidence of diabetes was decreased by 58 percent in the lifestyle intervention group and by 31 percent in the medication group when compared to the placebo group. The fact that only modest weight loss and small increases in physical activity were needed to achieve these results suggests that intervening with high-risk individuals to modify a lifestyle can be successful in reducing the incidence of diabetes.

As is the case for all chronic diseases, researchers are constantly seeking the most effective and cost-effective methods for bringing self-management skills to patient groups, and this is true for type 2 diabetes patients as well. Internet-based diabetes self-management programs, for example, may be a way of the future (Glasgow et al., 2010), and mobile phones have been used to assess adherence (Mulvaney et al., 2012). •

## SUMMARY

1. Coronary heart disease (CHD) is the leading cause of death in developed countries. It is a disease of lifestyle, and risk factors include cigarette smoking, obesity, high cholesterol, low levels of physical activity, chronic stress, and hostility.

2. Coronary proneness is associated with hostility, depression, and hyperreactivity to stressful situations, including a slow return to baseline. These exaggerated cardiovascular responses to stress may be partly genetically based, and may be aggravated by a conflict-ridden social environment, especially in the early family.

3. Efforts to modify excessive reactivity to stress and hostility through training in relaxation and stress management may have promise for reducing morbidity and mortality due to CHD.

4. Cardiac rehabilitation helps CHD patients obtain their optimal physical, medical, psychological, social, emotional, vocational, and economic status. Components of these programs typically include education about CHD, drug treatments, nutritional counseling, supervised exercise, stress management, and, under some circumstances, psychological counseling and/or social support group participation.

5. People who have had heart attacks (MI) often have difficulty managing the stress reduction aspects of their regimens, and sometimes marital relations can be strained as a result of the changes forced on patient and spouse by the post-MI rehabilitative regimen.

6. Hypertension, or high blood pressure, affects one in four Americans. Most hypertension is of unknown origin, although risk factors include family history of hypertension. Low-SES Blacks are particularly vulnerable.

7. Hypertensives show heightened reactivity to stressful events. Hostility is also implicated.

8. Hypertension is typically treated by diuretics or beta-blocking drugs, which may have adverse side effects. Cognitive–behavioral treatments, including stress management, have been used to control the disorder and to reduce drug dosages.

9. The biggest problems related to the control of hypertension concern high rates of nondiagnosis and nonadherence to therapy. The fact that the disease is symptomless helps explain both problems. Low rates of adherence are also explained by the adverse side effects of drugs.

10. Stroke results from a disturbance in blood flow to the brain. It may disrupt all aspects of life. Motor difficulties, cognitive impairments, and depression are particular problems associated with stroke.

11. Interventions for stroke patients have typically involved psychotherapy, including treatment for depression; cognitive remedial training to restore intellectual functioning; movement therapy; skill building; and structured, stimulating environments to challenge the stroke patient's capabilities.

12. Type 2 diabetes is one of the most common chronic diseases in the United States. It typically develops after age 40.

13. The diabetes self-care regimen chiefly involves exercise, controlling diet, and stress reduction. Adherence to this regimen is often poor.

14. Interventions can improve adherence, especially if the different components of the regimen are logically linked to each other in a programmatic effort toward effective self-care. Training in diabetes-specific skills is important, as is treatment for depression, if relevant.

## KEY TERMS

cardiac invalidism
cardiac rehabilitation
cardiovascular disease (CVD)
coronary heart disease (CHD)

hypertension
ischemia
John Henryism
metabolic syndrome

stroke
Type 2 diabetes

# 14

# Psychoneuroimmunology and Immune-Related Disorders

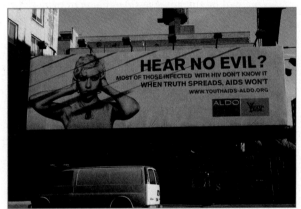

Lars Niki

The immune system is implicated in many acute and chronic diseases. In this chapter, we focus on a set of disorders in which immune functioning is especially implicated, specifically, HIV infection, cancer, arthritis, and type 1 diabetes. We begin with a general discussion of psychoneuroimmunology. **Psychoneuroimmunology** refers to the interactions among behavioral, neuroendocrine, and immunological processes of adaptation.

## ■ PSYCHONEUROIMMUNOLOGY

### The Immune System

As noted in Chapter 2, the immune system is the surveillance system of the body. It is implicated in infection, allergies, cancer, and autoimmune diseases, among other disorders. The primary function of the immune system is to distinguish between what is "self" and what is foreign and then to attack and rid the body of foreign invaders. It does so through natural immunity, a generalized defense against pathogens, and specific immunity, which responds to only one invader. Natural and specific immunity work together, such that natural immunity contains infection and wounds rapidly, whereas specific immunity is a response to a specific pathogen.

### Assessing Immune Functioning

Many indicators of immune functioning have been used in research. Some approaches have been:

1. Assessing the functioning of immune cells
2. Assessing the production of antibodies to latent viruses
3. Assessing levels of immune system products, such as proinflammatory cytokines
4. Using indirect measures, such as how quickly wounds heal

Assessing the functioning of cells involves examining the activation, proliferation, transformation, and cytotoxicity of cells. One might assess the ability of lymphocytes to kill invading cells (lymphocyte cytotoxicity), the ability of lymphocytes to reproduce when artificially stimulated by a chemical (mitogen), or the ability of certain white blood cells to ingest foreign particles (phagocytotic activity).

Researchers also assess a person's ability to produce antibodies to a latent virus. All of us carry around viruses that are inactive. If our bodies begin to produce

antibodies to these inactive viruses (such as Epstein–Barr virus or herpes simplex virus), this is a sign that the immune system is not working well enough to control these latent viruses. Consequently, levels of antibodies to these latent viruses constitute a measure of how well the immune system is functioning.

Producing antibodies to a vaccine is also a measure of immune functioning. When people have received a vaccination for a particular disorder, the degree to which the body produces antibodies to the vaccine is a sign of good immune functioning.

Researchers can also measure immune-related products in the blood, such as proinflammatory cytokines. Cytokine levels are indicative of inflammatory activity and may increase in response to stress. For example, one study (Moons, Eisenberger, & Taylor, 2010) found elevations in IL-6, a proinflammatory cytokine, following exposure to laboratory stressors, especially among people who responded to those stressors with fear.

Researchers also use wound healing as a method to study immune functioning. Wounds heal faster when the immune system is functioning vigorously. Using this method, researchers make a small puncture, usually in the forearm, and then examine how quickly the wound heals over and shrinks in people who are, for example, under stress or not. Psychological distress impairs the inflammatory response that initiates wound repair (Broadbent, Petrie, Alley, & Booth, 2003). Tape stripping, a less invasive procedure, involves applying an adhesive strip to the skin and pulling it off and assessing how quickly skin barrier function recovers (Robles, 2007). Although these methods only indirectly assess functioning of the immune system, they are important because they involve a specific health outcome. For example, stress impairs wound repair due to surgery and thus may prolong the recovery period (Broadbent et al., 2003).

### Stress and Immune Functioning

Many common stressors can adversely affect the immune system. Early studies, for example, showed compromised immune functioning among people who had been bereaved, under stress, or awaiting examinations (Bartrop, Lockhurst, Lazarus, Kiloh, & Penny, 1977; Zisook et al., 1994).

**Stress and Immunity in Humans**   More than 300 studies examine the relation of stress to immune functioning in humans (Segerstrom & Miller, 2004).

Different kinds of stressors create different demands on the body, so they show different effects on the immune system.

Two basic principles are important for understanding the relation of stress and immunity. The first is that different kinds of stressors require different kinds of defenses, and so a particular immune response may be favored over another in response to certain stressors. For example, short-term stressors raise the risk of injury, and so immune system changes involved in wound repair are very likely in response to short-term stress. A second important principle is that a maximally efficient immune response to any situation entails costs, and so some aspects of immunity may be adaptively suppressed as others are actively engaged (Segerstrom, 2010). These are useful principles to keep in mind as we look at the relation of immune functioning to different sorts of stressors.

Human beings evolved so that, in response to sudden stress, changes in the immune system could take place quickly, leading to wound repair and infection prevention. Thus, short-term stressors (of a few minutes' duration) elicit immune responses that anticipate risk of injury and possible entry of infectious agents into the bloodstream. Although short-term stressors now rarely involve wounds and the threat of infection, the system that evolved to deal with these threats remains a part of human physiology and so is mobilized in response to short-term stressors, such as being called on to speak in class. In contrast, specific immunity decreases in response to acute short-term stressors. Specific immunity is slow to develop, so specific immunity would be of little if any help in combating short-term stressors. Thus, immediate short-term stressors produce a pattern of immune responses involving up regulation of natural immunity accompanied by down regulation of specific immunity (Segerstrom & Miller, 2004).

Brief stressors of several days' duration, such as preparing for examinations, show a different pattern. Rather than altering the number or percentage of cells in the blood, brief stressors lead to changes in cytokine production, indicating a shift away from cellular immunity and toward humoral immunity (see Chapter 2) (Segerstrom & Miller, 2004).

Chronically stressful events, such as being unemployed or engaging in long-term caregiving, are linked to adverse effects on almost all functional measures of the immune system. These effects are stronger among people with preexisting vulnerabilities, such as old age or disease. Chronic low-level inflammation, which can occur in response to chronically stressful conditions (Rohleder, 2014), contributes to a broad range of disorders, including heart disease (Miller & Blackwell, 2006) and declines in cognitive performance (Marsland Petersen, et al., 2006).

Thus, different types of stressful events (short term versus a few days versus long term) make different demands on the body that are reflected in different patterns of immune activity. The body's stress systems appear to partially regulate these effects. As we saw in Chapter 6, stress engages the sympathetic nervous system and the HPA axis, both of which influence immune functioning. Sympathetic activation in response to stress has immediate effects of increasing immune activity, especially natural killer (NK) cell activity. Stress-related changes in hypothalamic adrenocortical functioning have immunosuppressive effects (Miller, Chen, & Zhou, 2007). That is, activation of the HPA axis, as happens when people are under stress, leads to the release of glucocorticoids such as cortisol; cortisol reduces the number of white blood cells, affects the functioning of lymphocytes, and reduces the release of cytokines, which can reduce the ability of these substances to signal and communicate with other aspects of the immune system.

Examples of Stress Studies    Studies showing the relation of stress to immune functioning have considered a variety of naturalistic stressors. For example, 11 astronauts who flew five different space shuttle flights ranging in length from 4 to 16 days were studied before launch and after landing (Mills, Meck, Waters, D'Aunno, & Ziegler, 2001). As expected, space flight was associated with a significant increase in the number of circulating white blood cells, and natural killer cells decreased. At landing, sympathetic activation increased substantially, as did numbers of circulating white blood cells.

Some studies of stress involve the effects of natural disasters and other traumas on immune functioning. A study of community responses to Hurricane Andrew damage in 1992, for example, revealed substantial changes in the immune systems of people directly affected, changes that appeared to be due primarily to sleep problems that occurred in the wake of the hurricane (Ironson et al., 1997). Chronic stressors, such as living in a disadvantaged neighborhood (Miller & Chen, 2007) and adapting to a new culture (Fang, Ross, Pathak, Godwin, & Tseng, 2014), also compromise immune functioning.

In autoimmune diseases, the immune system attacks the body's own tissues, falsely identifying them as invaders. Autoimmune diseases include more than 80 conditions, and virtually every organ is potentially vulnerable. Some of the most common disorders include type 1 diabetes; Graves' disease, involving excessive production of thyroid hormones; chronic active hepatitis, involving the chronic inflammation of the liver; lupus, which is chronic inflammation of the connective tissue and which can affect multiple organ systems; multiple sclerosis, which involves the destruction of the myelin sheath that surrounds nerves; and rheumatoid arthritis, in which the immune system attacks and inflames the tissue lining the joints. The conditions range from mildly annoying to severe, progressive, and fatal.

Nearly 80 percent of people who have these and other autoimmune disorders are women. Exactly why women are so vulnerable is not yet completely understood. One possibility is that hormonal changes related to estrogen are implicated. Consistent with this point, many women first develop symptoms of an autoimmune disorder in their 20s, when estrogen levels are high. Another theory is that testosterone, a hormone that women have in short supply, may help protect against autoimmune disorders (Angier, June 19, 2001). A third theory is that during pregnancy, mother and fetus exchange bodily cells, which can remain in the mother's body for years. Although these cells are very similar to the mother's own, they are not identical, and so, the theory suggests, the immune system may get confused and attack both the leftover fetal cells and the maternal cells that look similar.

Because autoimmune disorders are a related group of conditions, the likelihood of suffering from one and then contracting another is fairly high. Genetic factors are implicated in autoimmunity (Ueda et al., 2003); one family member may develop lupus, another rheumatoid arthritis, and a third Graves' disease. Immune-related disorders are implicated in atherosclerosis and diabetes, which are common and often fatal disorders, lending urgency to the search for treatments and cures. For example, people with lupus are at risk for early-onset atherosclerosis (Asanuma et al., 2003) and accelerated atherosclerosis (Ham, 2003; Roman et al., 2003).

Autoimmune conditions appear to be on the rise, and consequently, understanding their causes and effective management is a high priority for both scientists and health care practitioners.

---

Stress involving threats to the self is especially likely to produce changes in immune functioning. A study by Dickerson and colleagues (Dickerson, Kemeny, Aziz, Kim, & Fahey, 2004) had healthy participants write about neutral experiences or about traumatic experiences for which they blamed themselves. Those who wrote about traumas for which they blamed themselves showed an increase in shame and guilt, coupled with elevations in proinflammatory cytokine activity. These findings indicate that self-related emotions can cause increases in inflammatory processes (Gruenewald, Kemeny, Aziz, & Fahey, 2004).

Even children experience stress-related changes in immune functioning. Boyce and colleagues (Boyce et al., 1993) conducted a study with children who had recently begun kindergarten and who experienced a mild earthquake about 6 weeks into the school year. Those who had shown significant alterations in immune functioning in response to beginning kindergarten were more likely to experience a respiratory infection, such as a cold, following the earthquake (Boyce et al., 1993). More generally, children whose stress systems are highly reactive are most vulnerable to challenging social contexts (Thomas, Wara, Saxton, Truskier, Chesney, & Boyce, 2013).

Health Risks   Is the immune modulation that occurs in response to psychological stressors sufficient to lead to actual effects on health? The answer seems to be yes. Both children and adults under stress show increased vulnerability to infectious disease, including colds, flus, herpes virus infections (such as cold sores or genital lesions), chicken pox, mononucleosis, and Epstein–Barr virus (Cohen & Herbert, 1996; Cohen, Tyrrell, & Smith, 1993; Kiecolt-Glaser & Glaser, 1987). Among people who are already ill, stress predicts more severe illness and higher production of cytokines (Cohen, Doyle, & Skoner, 1999). Autoimmune disorders, which are described in Box 14.1, are also affected by stress.

### Negative Affect and Immune Functioning

Stress may compromise immune functioning, in part, because it increases negative emotions that accompany depression or anxiety. Depression is associated with several alterations in cellular immunity and with inflammation (Duivis et al., 2015). In one study, these immune effects were stronger among older people and people who were hospitalized, suggesting that already vulnerable people are at special risk (Miller, Cohen, & Herbert, 1999).

Depression and inflammation promote each other (Kiecolt-Glaser, Derry, & Fagundes, 2015). Depression is tied to delayed wound healing (Bosch, Engeland, Cacioppo, & Marucha, 2007). The adverse effects of depression on immunity may result in part from the sleep disturbance involved in depression (Cover & Irwin, 1994). By contrast, positive affect has been tied to more rapid wound healing (Robles, Brooks, & Pressman, 2009), an indicator of immune functioning. Suppressing emotion is tied to greater inflammation and reappraising emotion-eliciting situations is associated with lower levels of inflammation (Appleton, Buka, Loucks, Gilman, & Kubzansky, 2013).

## Stress, Immune Functioning, and Interpersonal Relationships

Both human and animal research suggest the importance of personal relationships to immune functioning (Cohen & Herbert, 1996). Bereavement is tied to immunocompromise (Knowles, Ruiz, & O'Connor, 2019), and lonely people have poorer health and immunocompromise than people who are not lonely (Glaser, Kiecolt-Glaser, Speicher, & Holliday, 1985; Pressman et al., 2005). People with insecure attachments to others show lower NK cell cytotoxicity, suggesting potential health risks as well (Picardi et al., 2007). Chronic interpersonal stress as early as adolescence predicts inflammatory activity over time; this pathway may underlie the relation of social stress to such disorders as depression and atherosclerosis (Miller, Rohleder, & Cole, 2009).

**Marital Disruption and Conflict**    Marital disruption and conflict have also been tied to adverse changes in immunity. In a study by Kiecolt-Glaser and colleagues (Kiecolt-Glaser et al., 1987), women who had been separated from their husbands for 1 year or less showed poorer functioning on some immune parameters than did their matched married counterparts. Among separated and divorced women, recent separation and continued attachment to or preoccupation with the ex-husband were associated with poorer immune functioning and

with more depression and loneliness. Similar results have been found for men facing separation or divorce (Kiecolt-Glaser & Newton, 2001).

Not surprisingly, partner violence has been tied to adverse changes in immune functioning as well (Garcia-Linares, Sanchez-Lorente, Coe, & Martinez, 2004; Kiecolt-Glaser et al., 2005). Even short-term marital conflict can have a discernible effect on the immune system. Notably, these changes are evident both in newlyweds for whom marital adjustment is generally very high (Kiecolt-Glaser et al., 1993) as well as people in long-term marriages (Kiecolt-Glaser et al., 1997). These risks appear to fall more heavily on women than on men (Kiecolt-Glaser & Newton, 2001).

**Caregiving**    In Chapter 11, we saw how stressful caregiving can be for people who provide care for a friend or family member with a long-term illness, such as AIDS or Alzheimer's disease. Intensive, stressful caregiving has an adverse effect on the immune system (Kiecolt-Glaser, Glaser, Gravenstein, Malarkey, & Sheridan, 1996). In one study, caregivers for Alzheimer's patients were more depressed and showed lower life satisfaction than did a comparison sample. The caregivers also had higher EBV antibody titers (an indication of poor immune control of latent virus reactivation) and lower percentages of T cells.

Other studies demonstrate that the stress of caregiving has adverse effects on wound repair (Kiecolt-Glaser, Marucha, Malarkey, Mercado, & Glaser, 1995), on defects in natural killer cell function (Esterling, Kiecolt-Glaser, & Glaser, 1996), and on reactions to flu vaccine (Kiecolt-Glaser et al., 1996). Caregivers who experience emotional distress, such as anger or depression, may be at particular risk for adverse effects on the immune system (Scanlan, Vitaliano, Zhang, Savage, & Ochs, 2001).

These stressors leave caregivers vulnerable to a range of health-related problems, which can persist well beyond the end of the stressful situation—that is, after caregiving activities have ceased (Esterling, Kiecolt-Glaser, Bodnar, & Glaser, 1994).

## Psychosocial Resources and Immune Functioning

Evidence indicates that coping resources can influence immune function, and vice versa (Dantzer, Cohen, Russo, & Dinan, 2018). Coping resources also affect the relation between stress and immune functioning.

## Protective Effects of Psychosocial Resources

Social support can buffer people against adverse immune change in response to stress. For example, in a study of breast cancer patients, Levy and colleagues (Levy et al., 1990) found that receiving emotional support from one's spouse or partner or from a physician were associated with high NK cell activity. Other resources, including having money, can also limit deterioration in immune functioning (Segerstrom, Al-Attar, & Lutz, 2012).

### Optimism
Segerstrom and colleagues (Segerstrom, Taylor, Kemeny, & Fahey, 1998) found that optimism and active coping strategies protect against stress. In this study, 90 first-year law students, tested at the beginning of law school and again halfway through the first semester, completed questionnaires measuring how they coped with the stress of law school, and they had blood drawn for an assessment of immune measures. The optimistic law students and students who used fewer avoidant coping methods showed less distress across the quarter. Pessimism, avoidance coping, and mood disturbance were tied to lower natural killer cell cytotoxicity and fewer T cells, suggesting that optimism and coping can be important influences on stress-related distress and immune changes.

### Personal Control/Benefit Finding
People who regard stressors they are undergoing as uncontrollable are more likely to show adverse immune effects (Sieber et al., 1992). For example, a study of women with rheumatoid arthritis (Zautra, Okun, Roth, & Emmanual, 1989) found that those who perceived themselves as unable to cope with stressful events had lower levels of circulating B cells.

Finding benefits in stressful events may improve immune functioning or at least undercut the potential damage that stress may otherwise do. Bower and colleagues (Bower, Kemeny, Taylor, & Fahey, 2003) found that women who wrote about positive changes in important personal goals over a monthlong period showed increases in natural killer cell cytotoxicity. Potentially, then, prioritizing goals and emphasizing relationships, personal growth, and meaning in life may have beneficial biological effects on immune functioning.

## Interventions to Improve Immune Functioning

Can stress management interventions mute the impact of stressful events on the immune system? In Chapter 7,

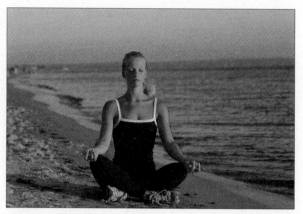

*Training in relaxation may help people learn how to mute the adverse effects of stress on the immune system.*
Colin Anderson/Brand X Pictures/Getty Images

we saw that emotional disclosure enhances health and mood in people who have suffered a traumatic event. These results may be due to improved immune functioning. In one study (Pennebaker, Kiecolt-Glaser, & Glaser, 1988), 50 undergraduates wrote about either traumatic experiences or superficial topics for 20 minutes on each of 4 consecutive days. Those students who wrote about traumatic or upsetting events demonstrated a stronger immune response than did students who wrote about superficial topics.

### Relaxation
Relaxation may mute the effects of stress on the immune system. In a study with elderly adults (a group at risk for illness because of age-related declines in immune functioning), participants were assigned to relaxation training, social contact, or no intervention (Kiecolt-Glaser et al., 1985). Participants in the relaxation condition had significantly higher levels of NK cell activity after the intervention than at baseline and significantly lower antibody titres to herpes simplex virus 1. This pattern suggests some enhancement of cellular immunity associated with relaxation. Training in mindfulness meditation can affect immune functioning (Davidson et al., 2003). Relaxation interventions also appear to promote wound healing (Robinson, Norton, Jarrett, & Broadbent, 2017). A study in which older adults were trained in tai chi chih (TCC), which involves mindful movement meditation, showed reduced intensity and severity of herpes zoster (shingles), suggesting that this may be a useful intervention as well (Irwin, Pike, Cole, & Oxman, 2003).

Overall, the evidence suggests that interventions can have significant effects on the immune system and on health outcomes (Miller & Cohen, 2001; O'Toole et al., 2018). Stress management interventions including relaxation show the most consistent benefits (Miller & Cohen, 2001).

## ■ HIV INFECTION AND AIDS

### A Brief History of HIV Infection and AIDS

**Acquired immune deficiency syndrome (AIDS)** seems to have begun in central Africa, perhaps in the 1920s. Transportation links promoted its spread in Africa in the 1960s (Faria et al., 2014). A high rate of extramarital sex, a lack of condom use, and a high rate of gonorrhea facilitated the spread of the AIDS virus in the heterosexual population. Medical clinics inadvertently promoted the spread of AIDS because, in attempting to vaccinate as many people as possible against common diseases in the area, needles were used over and over again, promoting the exchange of fluids. From Africa, the disease made its way to Europe and to Haiti, and from Haiti into the United States in the 1970s (Worobey et al., 2016). The prevalence of HIV infection is shown in Figure 14.1.

Currently, an estimated 36.9 million people worldwide—35.1 million adults and 1.8 million children

**TABLE 14.1 | How We Get HIV: Cases by Mode of Transmission (2017)**

|  | World | United States |
|---|---|---|
| Heterosexual contact | 70–75% | 24% |
| Male-to-male contact | 18 | 67 |
| Male-to-male contact coupled with intravenous drug use | Unknown | 3 |
| Injection drug use | 9 | 6 |
| Other | Unknown | 1 |

*Source:* Joint United Nations Programme on HIV/AIDS. "HIV Modes of Transmission Model." Accessed July 09, 2019. http://files.unaids.org/en/media/unaids/contentassets/documents/countryreport/2010/

younger than 15 years—are living with HIV/AIDS, 18.2 million of whom are women (UNAIDS, 2018). Approximately two-thirds of these people (25.7 million) live in Africa; the next largest population (3.5 million) live in Asia and the Pacific (UNAIDS, 2018). Approximately 1 million U.S. residents are living with HIV (UNAIDS, 2018). Table 14.1 shows how HIV is transmitted.

Since the start of the HIV epidemic, approximately 35 million people have died, including 940,000 in 2017. Although that figure represents 52 percent

**FIGURE 14.1 | Adults and children estimated to be living with HIV, 2017**    *Source:* World Health Organization, 2019.

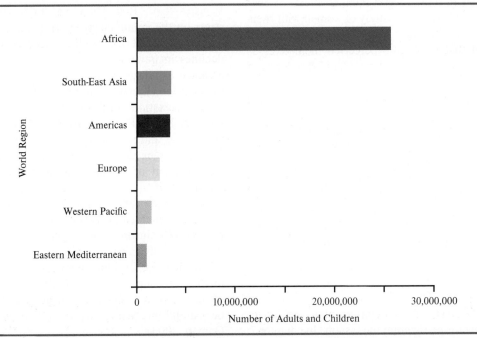

fewer people since the 2004 peak in mortality, continuing efforts toward primary prevention and treatment development are essential (World Health Organization, 2019). In 2016, HIV/AIDS was the fourth leading cause of death in low-income countries (World Health Organization, 2019).

## HIV Infection and AIDS in the United States

The first case of AIDS in the United States was diagnosed in 1981. The viral agent is a retrovirus, the **human immunodeficiency virus (HIV)**, and it attacks the helper T cells and macrophages of the immune system. The virus appears to be transmitted exclusively by the exchange of cell-containing bodily fluids, especially semen and blood.

The period between contracting the virus and developing symptoms of AIDS is variable, with some people developing symptoms quite quickly and others free of symptoms for years. Thus, a person may test HIV-seropositive (HIV+) but be free of AIDS and, during the asymptomatic period, pass on the virus to many other people.

How is HIV transmitted? Among drug users, needle sharing leads to the exchange of bodily fluids, thereby spreading the virus. Among men who have sex with men, exchange of the virus has been tied to sexual practices, especially anal-receptive sex involving the exchange of semen without a condom. In the heterosexual population, vaginal intercourse is associated with the transmission of AIDS, with women more at risk than men. The likelihood of developing AIDS increases with the number of sexual partners a person has had and with the number of anonymous sexual partners. Consequently, women working in the sex trade, child and adolescent runaways, and homeless youths are especially vulnerable (Slesnick & Kang, 2008), and rates of infection among the poor have increased substantially (Pellowski, Kalichman, Matthews, & Adler, 2013).

**How HIV Infection Progresses**  Following transmission, HIV grows very rapidly within the first few weeks of infection and spreads throughout the body. Early symptoms are mild, with swollen glands and mild, flulike symptoms predominating. After 3 to 6 weeks, the infection may abate, leading to a long asymptomatic period, during which viral growth is slow and gradual, eventually severely compromising

the immune system by killing the helper T cells and producing a vulnerability to opportunistic infections that leads to the diagnosis of AIDS.

Some of the more common opportunistic infections that result from the impaired immune system include pneumonia and unusual cancers, such as Kaposi's sarcoma or non-Hodgkin's lymphoma. Early in the disease process, people infected with HIV also begin to show abnormalities in their neuroendocrine and cardiovascular responses to stress (Starr et al., 1996). Chronic diarrhea, wasting, skeletal pain, and blindness are later complications. AIDS eventually leads to neurological involvement. Early symptoms of central nervous system impairment are similar to those of depression and include forgetfulness, inability to concentrate, psychomotor retardation, decreased alertness, apathy, withdrawal, diminished interest in work, and loss of sexual desire. In more advanced stages, patients may experience confusion, disorientation, seizures, profound dementia, and coma. A common symptom for women with AIDS is gynecologic infection, but because it was not considered an AIDS-related condition until 1993, often women were diagnosed very late.

The rate at which these changes take place can differ widely. Low-income Blacks and Hispanics are somewhat less likely to get tested than people in higher income groups (McGarrity & Huebner, 2014). Those who do test positive for HIV go on to develop AIDS faster than do whites. Possible reasons include the greater prevalence of intravenous (IV) drug use, higher levels of stress, low SES, and discrimination or racism (Bogart, Wagner, Galvan, & Klein, 2010; Stock, Gibbons, Peterson, & Gerrard, 2013). Perceived discrimination and experiences with racism may undermine commitment to risk reduction behavior (Huebner et al., 2014; Stock, Gibbons, Peterson, & Gerrard, 2013). In addition, low-income Blacks and Hispanics do not get new medications as quickly as whites do, so at any given time, they are less likely to have state-of-the-art treatment or access to clinics (Lynch et al., 2012). Consequently, people from higher socioeconomic status (SES) groups have a much greater chance of survival over the long term.

**Antiretroviral Therapy**  Antiretroviral therapy (ART) has made what was once a virtual death sentence a chronic disease instead. ART is a combination of antiretroviral medications (e.g., protease inhibitors), and in some patients, HIV can no longer be discerned in the bloodstream. The earlier ART is initiated, the better for reducing sexual transmission (Cohen et al., 2011). However, people on ART must take these drugs faithfully, up to several times a day, or the drugs will fail to work.

Pre-exposure prophylaxis (PrEP) and post-exposure prophylaxis (PEP) both reduce the risk of HIV infection dramatically. In PrEP, people at very high risk of infection, for example, those whose partner has HIV, can take HIV medicines daily. PEP requires taking HIV medicine for 28 days, starting within 72 hours of HIV exposure. Again, If adherence is not perfect, the effect drops substantially.

## The Psychosocial Impact of HIV Infection

Depression commonly accompanies an HIV diagnosis, especially for people with little social support, who feel stigmatized by their sexual preference or race (Hatzenbuehler, Nolen-Hoeksema, & Erickson, 2008), who engage in avoidant coping, and/or who have more severe HIV symptoms (Heckman et al., 2004). Depression can reduce receptivity to interventions, as well as lowering quality of life (Safren, O'Cleirigh, Skeer, Elsesser, & Mayer, 2013). Depression may also prompt self-medication through alcohol, methamphetamine use, and other drug use, which in turn can increase the likelihood of risky sexual behavior (Fletcher & Reback, 2015). A meta-analysis of 45 studies showed that mental health problems, and specifically depression, contributed to patients not staying in HIV medical care. When patients used mental health services, however, they were more likely to stick with HIV care (Rooks-Peck et al., 2018). Interventions that reduce depression are, thus, useful in the fight against AIDS (Motivala et al., 2003; Safren et al., 2010).

Nonetheless, over the long term, most people cope with HIV infection fairly well. For example, young sexual minority men who have HIV report similar or fewer worries about self-esteem and loneliness than HIV men (Halkitis et al., 2018). The majority of people who are HIV seropositive make positive changes in their health behaviors almost immediately after diagnosis, including changing diet in a healthier direction, getting more exercise, quitting or reducing smoking, and reducing or eliminating drug use (Collins et al., 2001). They also use various complementary and alternative medicine (CAM) strategies, which do not seem to compromise adherence to ART (Littlewood & Vanable, 2014). Coping skills training

and the practice of meditation may also improve adjustment (SeyedAlinaghi et al., 2012). Many of these changes also improve psychological well-being, and they may affect the course of infection as well.

**Disclosure**    Not disclosing HIV status or simply lying about risk factors, such as the number of partners one has had, is a major barrier to controlling the spread of HIV infection (Kalichman, DiMarco, Austin, Luke, & DiFonzo, 2003). Moreover, those less likely to disclose their HIV+ status to sex partners also are less likely to use condoms during intercourse (DeRosa & Marks, 1998).

People with strong social support networks are more likely to disclose and are, in turn, more likely to receive social support (Kalichman et al., 2003). Thus, disclosure appears to have psychosocial benefits. In addition, disclosure can have health benefits. In one study, those who had disclosed their HIV+ status to

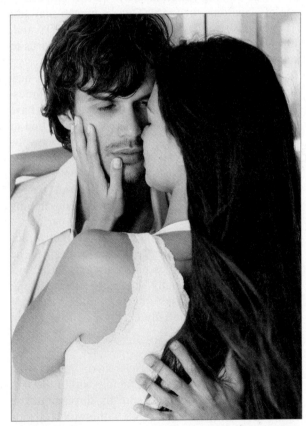

The possibility that HIV may move into the adolescent population is substantial, but as yet there are few signs that adolescents have changed their sexual practices in response to the threat of AIDS.
Stockbyte/Getty Images

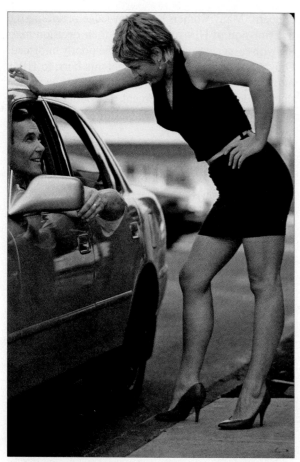

*Prostitution is one source of the increasing numbers of women who are infected with HIV.*

Ingram Publishing/SuperStock

their friends had significantly higher levels of CD4 and helper cells than those who had not (Strachan, Bennett, Russo, & Roy-Byrne, 2007).

**Women and HIV**   The lives of HIV-infected women, particularly those with symptoms, are often chaotic and unstable (Mitrani, McCabe, Burns, & Feaster, 2012). Many of these women have no partners, they may not hold jobs, and many depend on social services and Medicaid to survive. Some have problems with drugs, and many have experienced trauma from sexual or physical abuse (Simoni & Ng, 2002). Discrimination due to race or ethnicity complicates their situation further (Wyatt, Gómez, Hamilton, Valencia-Garcia, Grant, & Graham, 2013). To an outsider, being HIV+ would seem to be their biggest problem, but in fact, getting food and shelter for the family is often more difficult (Updegraff, Taylor, Kemeny, & Wyatt, 2002).

Poverty acts as a barrier to adherence, and unless food insufficiency is addressed, other interventions may not be successful (Kalichman & Grebler, 2010). Low-income women who are HIV+ especially experience stress related to family issues (Schrimshaw, 2003), and any resulting depression can exacerbate the disease (Jones, Beach, Forehand, & Foster, 2003). Suicide attempts are not uncommon (Cooperman & Simoni, 2005).

Nonetheless, many women are able to find meaning in their lives, often prompted by the shock of testing positive. A study of low-income, HIV+ women (Updegraff et al., 2002) found that the majority reported positive (as well as negative) changes in their lives, including the fact that the HIV diagnosis had gotten them off drugs, gotten them off the street, and enabled them to feel better about themselves (see also Littlewood, Vanable, Carey, & Blair, 2008).

## Interventions to Reduce the Spread of HIV Infection

Interventions to reduce risk-related behavior loom large as the best way to control the spread of HIV infection. These interventions center around getting tested, refraining from high-risk sex, using a condom, and not sharing needles. Given the diversity of groups at special risk for AIDS—adolescents, homosexuals, low-income women, minorities—intensive, community-based interventions tailored to particular at-risk groups are most effective. The Centers for Disease Control and Prevention recommend that HIV testing be a standard part of medical care, as 15 percent of people who are HIV positive do not know it. However, even brief educational or stages-of-change based interventions can increase the willingness to be tested (Carey, Coury-Doniger, Senn, Vanable, & Urban, 2008). Interventions to promote and provide testing in churches increase testing in African Americans (Berkley-Patton et al., 2019).

**Education**   Most interventions begin by educating the target population about risky activity, providing information about HIV infection and modes of transmission. Studies suggest a high degree of "magical thinking" about HIV, with people overreacting to casual contact with HIV+ individuals but underreacting to their own health risks resulting from casual sex and failure to use a condom. Beliefs that HIV infection is now a manageable disease and that people under treatment will not pass on an infection have contributed to a resurgence of new infections

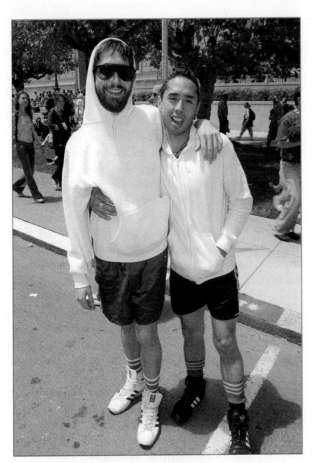

*The overwhelming majority of early AIDS cases in the United States occurred among gay men. The gay community responded with dramatic and impressive efforts to reduce risk-related behaviors.*

Christopher Kerrigan/McGraw-Hill Education

concern. Many women lack knowledge regarding the transmission of HIV to infants, so their decision making with respect to pregnancy may be poorly informed. Only about 15 to 30 percent of infants born to HIV+ mothers will be seropositive, and treatment can reduce that incidence to 4 to 8 percent. Providing education with respect to HIV and pregnancy, then, is an important educational priority.

How successful are educational interventions? A review of 27 published studies that provided HIV counseling and testing information found that this type of education was an effective means of secondary prevention for HIV+ individuals, reducing behaviors that might infect others. However, it was not an effective primary prevention strategy for uninfected people (Weinhardt, Carey, Johnson, & Bickman, 1999).

Culturally sensitive interventions pitched to a specific target group may fare somewhat better (Jemmott et al., 2015). A study of African American, male, inner-city adolescents revealed that providing information can be an effective agent of behavior change when knowledge is low (Jemmott, Jemmott, & Fong, 1992). The young men in this study were randomly assigned to an AIDS risk-reduction intervention aimed at increasing their knowledge about AIDS and risky sexual behavior or to a control group. The materials were developed so as to be especially interesting to inner-city African American adolescents. This culturally sensitive intervention was successful over a 3-month period. The adolescents exposed to the intervention reported fewer instances of intercourse, fewer partners, greater use of condoms, and less anal intercourse, compared with adolescents not exposed to the intervention.

(Kalichman et al., 2007). These false beliefs need to be addressed in interventions (Kalichman, 2008).

On the whole, gay men are well informed about HIV, heterosexual adolescents are considerably less so, and some at-risk groups are very poorly informed. A study of urban adolescent girls revealed that about half of the girls underestimated the risks involved in their sexual behavior (Kershaw, Ethier, Niccolai, Lewis, & Ickovics, 2003). Studies of single, pregnant, inner-city women likewise reveal poor knowledge about AIDS, little practice of safe sex, and little knowledge of their partner's current or past behavior and the ways in which it might place them at risk (Hobfoll, Jackson, Lavin, Britton, & Shepherd, 1993).

As more women have become infected with HIV, issues around pregnancy have assumed increasing

**Targeting Sexual Activity**    Sexual activity is a very personal aspect of life. Consequently, knowledge of how to practice safe sex may not translate into behavior change if spontaneous sexuality is seen as an inherent part of one's identity.

For example, adolescents and young adults are a population that is difficult to reach. Beliefs and sexual behavior can be very hard to modify because sex is highly valued. One study found that simply imagining a new lover reduced perceptions of risk (Blanton & Gerrard, 1997; Corbin & Fromme, 2002). Complicating the picture still further, attitudes toward condom use can be quite negative and condom use can be highly variable (Kiene, Tennen & Armeli, 2008). Beliefs about relationships also might need to be addressed. In one study, young black men who reported being neglected while they were growing up had more negative beliefs about relationships, which in turn were linked to riskier sexual behaviors (Kogan, Cho, & Oshri, 2016).

Past sexual practice predicts AIDS risk-related behavior (Guilamo-Ramos et al., 2005). People who have had a large number of partners (especially anonymous partners), who have not used condoms in the past, and who meet their partners in bars or through the Internet may continue to expose themselves to risk, perhaps because those behaviors are well integrated into their sexual style (Horvath, Bowen, & Williams, 2006).

Sexual encounters, particularly with a new partner, are often rushed, nonverbal, and passionate, conditions not very conducive to a rational discussion of safe-sex practices. To address these issues, health psychologists have developed interventions that involve practice in sexual negotiation skills. For example, in a cognitive–behavioral intervention (Kelly, Lawrence, Hood, & Brasfield, 1989), gay men were taught through modeling, role-playing, and feedback how to exercise self-control in sexual relationships and how to resist pressure to engage in high-risk sexual activity. With this training, the men became somewhat more skillful in handling sexual situations and were able to reduce their risky sexual behaviors and increase their use of condoms.

Sexual compulsivity is an issue among sexually active gay men that has implications for the spread of HIV (Starks, Grov, & Parsons, 2013). Internalized homo-negativity and problems with effectively managing emotions are possible targets for reducing this behavior, unsafe sex practices, and the depression and anxiety that can accompany having HIV (Rendina et al., 2017).

Condom negotiation skills are especially important in interventions with high-risk groups, such as minorities, women, and adolescents (Widman, Noar, Choukas-Bradley, & Francis, 2014). One of the reasons that young women engage in unsafe sex is the coercive sexual behavior of their young male partners (VanderDrift, Agnew, Harvey, & Warren, 2013). Teaching young women how to resist coercion is therefore important (Walsh, Senn, Scott-Sheldon, Vanable, & Carey, 2011). Interventions also need to be focused on building self-efficacy for practicing safe sex (Mausbach, Semple, Strathdee, Zians, & Patterson, 2007; O'Leary, Jemmott, & Jemmott, 2008; Safren et al., 2018).

Many people don't like to use condoms, and changing these feelings has been a target of some interventions (Ellis, Homish, Parks, Collins, & Kiviniemi, 2015). Some programs have built in a motivational component to try to increase the motivation for at-risk groups to change their risk-related behavior. Recall that "motivation training" induces a state of readiness to change, by helping people develop behavior-change goals, recognize the discrepancy between their goals and their current behavior, and develop a sense of self-efficacy that they can change. Self-reevaluation involves cognitively reappraising one's behavior changes as now part of one's identity, and this process plays an important role in sustained behavior change as well (Longmire-Avital, Golub, & Parsons, 2010). Addressing perceived barriers to condom use is recommended (Protogerou, Johnson, & Hagger, 2018). Adding a motivational component to education and skills training can enhance the effectiveness of interventions designed to reduce HIV risk-related behavior (Kalichman et al., 2005). The information–motivation–behavioral skills model (Fisher & Fisher, 1993) incorporates all these components and provides a conceptual framework for effective intervention to reduce risky sexual behaviors (Cruess et al., 2018).

In a major review of behavioral interventions conducted with adolescents, gay and bisexual men, inner-city women, college students, and mentally ill adults—all groups at significant risk for AIDS—interventions oriented toward reducing their sexual activity and enhancing their abilities to negotiate condom use with partners reduced risk-related behavior (Kalichman, Carey, & Johnson, 1996; Widman, Noar, Choukas-Bradley, & Francis, 2014). Even brief but intensive interventions addressing risk factors, motivation, self-efficacy, social support, and sexual negotiation skills may have these beneficial effects (Kalichman et al., 2005; Naar-King et al., 2006). Also indicating the promise of interventions that can be widely disseminated to the public, a meta-analysis showed that single-session behavioral interventions can reduce unprotected sex (Sagherian, Huedo-Medina, Pellowski, Eaton, & Johnson, 2016). Addressing identity issues and mental health needs have particular priority for young men of color who have sex with men (Lelutiu-Weinberger, Gamarel, Golub, & Parsons, 2015); they may be coping both with the stigma of HIV and with race or ethnicity-related discrimination (Earnshaw, Bogart, Dovidio, & Williams, 2013).

HIV Prevention Programs  Prevention programs have been developed for U.S. public schools to warn adolescents about the risks of unprotected sexual intercourse and to help instill safe-sex practices

(DiClemente et al., 2008). Teenagers who are HIV+ sometimes pitch these programs, making the risk graphically clear to the audience. However, adolescents may try to distance themselves from peers who have HIV in an effort to reduce the threat. Interventions that stress information, motivation, and sexual negotiation skills may be more successful in changing adolescent behavior (Fisher, Fisher, Bryan, & Misovich, 2002). Research is still exploring which elements of school-based prevention programs are most successful.

The stage model of behavior change (Chapter 3) may be helpful in guiding interventions to increase condom use. Some people have gaps in their knowledge about HIV or about their own or their partners' behaviors that may put them at risk (Hobfoll et al., 1993). Therefore, they may profit from information-based interventions that move them from a precontemplation to a contemplation phase with regard to safe-sex practices. In contrast, moving from contemplation to preparation, or from preparation to action, may require specific training in condom negotiation skills (Catania, Kegeles, & Coates, 1990).

Interventions that address the norms surrounding sexual activity are needed as well. Any intervention that supports norms favoring more long-term relationships or decreasing the number of short-term sexual relationships an individual has is a reasonable approach to prevention (Tucker, Elliott, Wenzel, & Hambarsoomian, 2007). Perceived norms about condom use also influence one's own choices and accordingly need to be targeted (van den Boom, Stolte, Roggen, Sandfort, Prins, & Davidovich, 2015).

A large meta-analysis of 354 interventions to prevent HIV revealed that the most effective ones provided education, arguments in favor of attitudinal and behavioral change, and behavioral skills training (Albarracín et al., 2005). Interventions did not have a "one-size-fits-all" impact, however. For example, behavioral skills arguments were effective for males but not for females, suggesting a need for targeted interventions.

Cognitive–Behavioral Interventions  CBT is a guiding framework for many interventions with people who are HIV+. Many of these include a stress management component. Stress management interventions improve quality of life and mental health (Brown & Vanable, 2008), but stress management may not affect immunologic functioning related to the course of illness (Scott-Sheldon, Kalichman, Carey, & Fielder, 2008).

CBT interventions may need to be directed not only to stress management, but also to health behaviors. Smoking, excessive alcohol use, and drug use commonly compromise health and adherence among people who are HIV seropositive (Webb, Vanable, Carey, & Blair, 2007). Cognitive–behavioral interventions can help reduce risk-related sexual behavior (Scott-Sheldon, Fielder, & Carey, 2010), maintain adherence, and reduce viral load (Safren et al., 2009). CBT specifically addressing body image and self-care substantially improved both depressive symptoms and ART adherence in sexual minority men with HIV (Blashill et al., 2017).

Targeting Adherence  Because maintaining good health for people with AIDS depends so critically on adhering to ART, adherence is fairly high. However, stress can impede adherence (Mugavero et al., 2009), as can alcohol use (Parsons, Rosof, & Mustanski, 2008). Some people who are HIV+ have difficulty getting ART, and using it may be a poor fit with their lifestyle. Homeless people, IV drug users, and alcoholics show poor adherence rates (Tucker et al., 2004). For example, most of the drugs used to fight HIV infection must be refrigerated, and homeless people, by definition, do not have refrigerators. Practical problems related to poverty account for some adherence problems (Kalichman & Grebler, 2010).

Psychosocial resources contribute to adherence (Gore-Felton & Koopman, 2008). Those who adhere to ART are more likely to have social support, low levels of depression, and a sense of self-efficacy (Johnson et al., 2007; Lee, Milloy, Walsh, Nguyen, Wood, & Kerr, 2016). Those who fail to adhere have more psychological distress, lower social support, more avoidant coping strategies, and more use of stimulants and alcohol (Carrico et al., 2007; Davis et al., 2016).

As is true for risk-related behavior, adherence to ART is affected by motivational training. Having the right information, the motivation to adhere, and skills to do so significantly improves adherence to treatment (Starace, Massa, Amico, & Fisher, 2006). Overcoming cultural barriers can improve adherence. In a randomized controlled trial when a trained peer counselor addressed such barriers as mistrust of the medical system, HIV stigma, and lack of links to supportive services, Black men's and women's electronically measured adherence to their HIV medication was substantially higher 6 months later, compared to participants who did not receive the counseling (Bogart et al., 2017). Interventions that enhance social support have also shown some success in improving adherence (Koenig et al., 2008).

Targeting IV Drug Use    Interventions with IV drug users need to be targeted toward both reducing contact with infected needles and changing sexual activity. Information about AIDS transmission, needle exchange programs, and instruction on how to sterilize needles can reduce risky injection practices among IV drug users (Des Jarlais & Semaan, 2008). Methadone maintenance treatments, coupled with HIV-related education, may help reduce the spread of AIDS by reducing the frequency of injections and shared needle contacts, by reducing health-risk behaviors, by increasing the use of condoms, and by reducing the number of sexual partners (Margolin, Avants, Warburton, Hawkins, & Shi, 2003). However, the cognitive–behavioral intervention programs that work with other at-risk populations may not work as well with IV drug users because they often lack impulse control.

## Coping with HIV+ Status and AIDS

Coping with a life-threatening illness is always challenging and may be especially so for people with HIV infection. They are more likely to have a history of traumas and coexisting mental health problems, such as anxiety disorders, depression, and substance abuse disorders (Gaynes, Pence, Eron, & Miller, 2008; Whetten, Reif, Whetten, & Murphy-McMillan, 2008). Consequently, they may not have particularly good coping skills to draw on.

Moreover, people with HIV infection face particular challenges. Now that HIV infection is a chronic rather than an acute condition, psychosocial issues raised by chronic illness come to the fore. One such issue is employment. Interventions may be needed to help those who can return to work do so (Rabkin, McElhiney, Ferrando, Van Gorp, & Lin, 2004). People with HIV must continually cope with the fear, prejudice, and stigma that they encounter from the general community, which can increase psychological distress (Hatzenbuehler, O'Cleirigh, Mayer, Mimiaga, & Safren, 2011).

Coping Skills    Stress and its neuroendocrine consequences foster a more rapid course of illness in people who are infected with HIV and lead to more opportunistic or more aggressive symptoms (Cole, 2008; Pereira et al., 2003). Thus, good coping skills are essential (Temoshok, Wald, Synowski, & Garzino-Demo,

2008). Coping effectiveness training and mindfulness-based stress reduction are helpful in managing the psychological distress that can be associated with HIV+ status (Chesney, Chambers, Taylor, Johnson, & Folkman, 2003; Riley & Kalichman, 2015). Perceiving that one has control over a stressor is usually associated with better adjustment to that stressor, and this is also true of HIV (Benight et al., 1997; Rotheram-Borus, Murphy, Reid, & Coleman, 1996). Positive affect promotes good HIV care and adherence to ART (Carrico & Moskowitz, 2014). It also predicts low likelihood of risky sexual episodes (Wilson, Stadler, Boone, & Bolger, 2014), making positive affect an important target for coping interventions.

Written disclosure is a successful coping intervention (see Chapter 7), and it appears to be so for people with HIV as well. A study by Petrie and associates (Petrie, Fontanilla, Thomas, Booth, & Pennebaker, 2004) found that writing about emotional topics led to higher CD4 lymphocyte counts, compared to writing about neutral topics, among HIV-infected patients.

Social Support    Social support is very important to people with HIV infection or AIDS. Social support has been tied to greater adherence and lower viral load, for example (Simoni, Frick, & Huang, 2006). Thus, addressing social support needs can have multiple positive repercussions (Mitrani et al., 2012). Gay men infected with HIV who have emotional, practical, and informational support are less depressed (Turner-Cobb et al., 2002), and men with strong partner support are less likely to practice risky sex (Darbes & Lewis, 2005). Intervention programs that include a family member or address the interpersonal context can reduce depressive symptoms (Heckman et al., 2018; Li et al., 2017).

Support from family appears to be especially important for preventing depression (Schrimshaw, 2003). Not all families are helpful, however, and so other sources of support are vital. The Internet represents an important resource for people infected with HIV (Bowen, Williams, Daniel, & Clayton, 2008). Those who use the Internet to help manage their HIV+ status typically are more knowledgeable about HIV, have more active coping skills, and have more social support than those not using the Internet (Kalichman et al., 2003).

## Psychosocial Factors That Affect the Course of HIV Infection

Psychosocial factors can influence not only coping, but also the rate of immune system decline from HIV infection (Ironson et al., 2005). Depression is a common intermittent experience of HIV-infected individuals and is an important target for intervention, not only to improve quality of life but also because depression predicts nonadherence (Gonzalez et al., 2011) and higher mortality, particularly in some groups (e.g., highly educated; Ironson, Fitch, & Stuetzle, 2017). Negative expectations about the course of illness can lead to an accelerated course of disease (Ironson et al., 2005; Reed, Kemeny, Taylor, & Visscher, 1999; Reed, Kemeny, Taylor, Wang, & Visscher, 1994). Depression, stress, and trauma all adversely affect disease progression (Leserman, 2008).

Psychological inhibition may promote a more rapid course of illness. In one investigation, HIV infection advanced more rapidly in men who concealed their homosexual identity relative to men who were openly gay (Cole, Kemeny, Taylor, Visscher, & Fahey, 1996). Psychological inhibition leads to alterations in sympathetic nervous system activation and immune system function, which may largely account for these effects on physical health (Cole et al., 2003).

On the positive side, optimism, active coping, extraversion, conscientiousness, and spirituality all predict slower disease progression (Ironson & Hayward, 2008; Ironson, O'Cleirigh, Weiss, Schneiderman, & Costa, 2008). The ability to find meaning in one's experiences slows declines in CD4+ cell levels and has been related to a lower risk of death (Bower et al., 1997).

Positive affect predicts better HIV control when negative affect is relatively low (Wilson et al., 2017), and positive affect can lower the risk of AIDS mortality (Moskowitz, 2003). In one intervention study, treating depression via cognitive–behavioral stress management (coupled with medication adherence training) not only alleviated depressed mood, but enhanced the effects of ART on suppression of HIV viral load (Antoni et al., 2006). Antidepressants can help as well (Repetto & Petitto, 2008). Thus, the successful management of depression may also affect the course of disease.

The research that ties psychosocial factors to the course of illness—such as beliefs about one's illness, coping strategies, and social support—is especially exciting. It not only clarifies the factors that may promote long-term survival in people with HIV infection but also provides more general hypotheses for understanding how psychological and social factors affect the course of illness.

## ■ CANCER

Cancer is a set of more than 100 diseases that have several factors in common. All cancers result from a dysfunction in DNA—that part of the cellular programming that controls cell growth and reproduction. Instead of ensuring the regular, slow production of new cells, this malfunctioning DNA causes uncontrolled growth and proliferation of abnormal cells. Unlike other cells, cancerous cells provide no benefit to the body. They merely sap it of resources.

Cancer is second only to heart disease in causes of death in the United States and most developed countries (American Cancer Society, 2019) (Figure 14.2). From 1900 until 1990, death rates from cancer progressively climbed. Since 1991, however, the U.S. cancer death rate has dropped by 27 percent, due primarily to declines in smoking and improvements in early detection and treatment (American Cancer Society, 2019).

Many specialists often are involved in the treatment of the person with cancer, and coordinated care, which involves, for example, a navigator to help patients negotiate the diagnostic and treatment system, telehealth, or coordinated case management, results in more appropriate health care utilization (Sheinfeld Gorin, Haggstrom, Han, Fairfield, Krebs, & Clauser et al., 2017).

In addition to surgery, chemotherapy, and radiation therapy, effective treatments now include targeted therapy, which interferes with specific molecules to block the growth and spread of cancer, and immunotherapy, which helps the body's immune system fight cancer. Although side effects can be arduous and many patients do not respond to treatment, immunotherapy has received tremendous public attention for its effectiveness in treating stubborn cancers (e.g., lung cancer; Grady, November 2018). It is important to know that when people elect alternative, non-evidence-based treatments, their chance of dying is more than twice as high as patients who choose conventional cancer treatments (Johnson, Park, Gross, & Yu, 2018). More than 600,000 people die of cancer each year in the United States (American Cancer Society, 2019). However, many hundreds of thousands more people live long lives after having had cancer. In 2019, more than 16.9 million cancer survivors were living in the United States, a figure that is projected to rise to 21.7 million by 2029 (National Cancer Institute, February 2019).

Because psychosocial factors are implicated in the causes and course of cancer, the health psychologist

**FIGURE 14.2 | Leading Sites of New Cancer Cases and Deaths, 2019 Estimates** *Source:* ©2019, American Cancer Society, Inc., Surveillance Research.

**Estimated New Cases**

| Males | | | Females | | |
|---|---|---|---|---|---|
| Prostate | 174,650 | 20% | Breast | 268,600 | 30% |
| Lung & bronchus | 116,440 | 13% | Lung & bronchus | 111,710 | 13% |
| Colon & rectum | 78,500 | 9% | Colon & rectum | 67,100 | 8% |
| Urinary bladder | 61,700 | 7% | Uterine corpus | 61,880 | 7% |
| Melanoma of the skin | 57,220 | 7% | Melanoma of the skin | 39,260 | 4% |
| Kidney & renal pelvis | 44,120 | 5% | Thyroid | 37,810 | 4% |
| Non-Hodgkin lymphoma | 41,090 | 5% | Non-Hodgkin lymphoma | 33,110 | 4% |
| Oral cavity & pharynx | 38,140 | 4% | Kidney & renal pelvis | 29,700 | 3% |
| Leukemia | 35,920 | 4% | Pancreas | 26,830 | 3% |
| Pancreas | 29,940 | 3% | Leukemia | 25,860 | 3% |
| All sites | 870,970 | 100% | All sites | 891,480 | 100% |

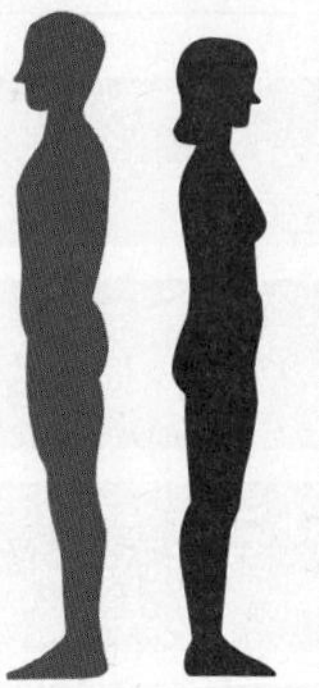

**Estimated Deaths**

| Males | | | Females | | |
|---|---|---|---|---|---|
| Lung & bronchus | 76,650 | 24% | Lung & bronchus | 66,020 | 23% |
| Prostate | 31,620 | 10% | Breast | 41,760 | 15% |
| Colon & rectum | 27,640 | 9% | Colon & rectum | 23,380 | 8% |
| Pancreas | 23,800 | 7% | Pancreas | 21,950 | 8% |
| Liver & intrahepatic bile duct | 21,600 | 7% | Ovary | 13,980 | 5% |
| Leukemia | 13,150 | 4% | Uterine corpus | 12,160 | 4% |
| Esophagus | 13,020 | 4% | Liver & intrahepatic bile duct | 10,180 | 4% |
| Urinary bladder | 12,870 | 4% | Leukemia | 9,690 | 3% |
| Non-Hodgkin lymphoma | 11,510 | 4% | Non-Hodgkin lymphoma | 8,460 | 3% |
| Brain & other nervous system | 9,910 | 3% | Brain & other nervous system | 7,850 | 3% |
| All sites | 321,670 | 100% | All sites | 285,210 | 100% |

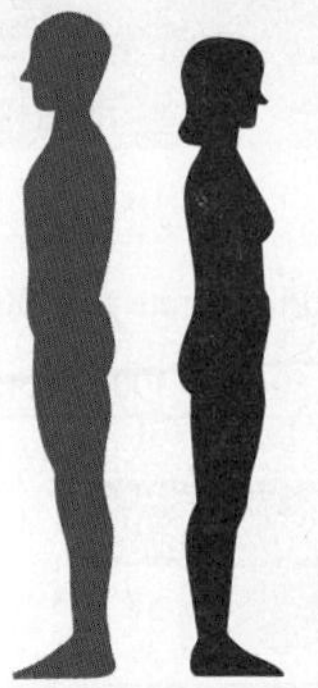

has an important role in addressing these issues. Moreover, because cancer is a disease with which people often live for many years, interventions to reduce risk factors and to improve coping with it are essential.

## Why Is Cancer Hard to Study?

Cancer has been hard to study for a number of reasons. The causes, symptoms, and treatment for each cancer vary. Many cancers have long or irregular growth cycles. It may be difficult to identify precipitating or co-occurring risk factors: Of three people exposed to a carcinogen, one might go on to develop cancer and the others, not.

## Who Gets Cancer? A Complex Profile

Many cancers run in families, in part because of genetic factors. However, family history does not always imply a genetically inherited predisposition to cancer. Many things run in families besides genes, including diet and other lifestyle factors. Infectious agents are implicated in some cancers. For example, the human papillomavirus (HPV) is the main cause of cervical cancer, and *Helicobacter pylori* is implicated in some types of gastric cancer. Although 70 percent of Americans are unaware of the relationship between cancer and age (Taber, Klein, Suls, & Ferrer, 2017), advancing age is the primary risk factor for cancer. Eighty percent of cancers are diagnosed in adults age 55 and older. More than 40 percent of new cancer diagnoses in the United States could be prevented through behaviors such as not smoking or drinking heavily, staying physically active, limiting sun exposure, getting relevant vaccinations, eating healthfully, and engaging in recommended cancer screening (American Cancer Society, 2019).

**FIGURE 14.3** | **Average Yearly Incidence and Mortality Rates of All Types of Cancer in the United States by Ethnicity**    Source: U.S. Department of Health and Human Services. National Cancer Institute. "Cancer Statistics." Accessed July 9, 2019. https://www.cancer.gov/about-cancer/understanding/statistics.

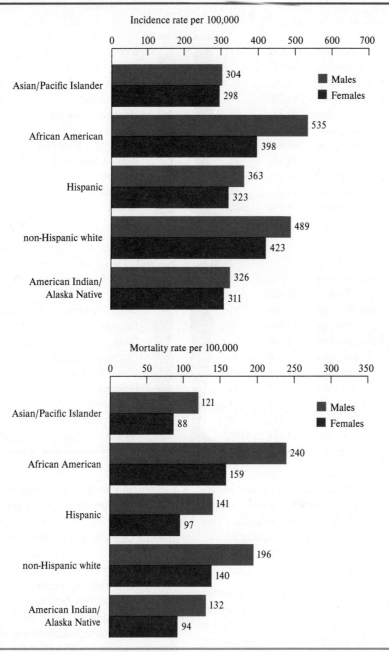

A **cancer disparity** exists when a disproportionate burden of cancer is carried by some group(s) in comparison to others. Socioeconomic and cultural factors, diet and other lifestyle behaviors, environmental factors, stress, and biology all contribute to cancer disparities (American Cancer Society, 2019; National Cancer Institute, March 2019). Figure 14.3 shows cancers of all types broken down by different ethnic groups in the United States, both by incidence and by mortality.

Low socioeconomic status is a primary culprit in creating cancer disparities (American Cancer Society, 2019; National Cancer Institute, March 2019). In comparison to people with more educational and financial resources, poor people often lack access and referral to cancer screening, are recipients of targeted marketing to encourage cigarette smoking and other unhealthy behaviors, and are exposed to more environmental carcinogens such as air pollution. Barriers to getting physical exercise and fruits and vegetables also exist in impoverished urban communities.

Several cancer disparities associated with race, ethnicity, and culture can be traced to socioeconomic burden. In addition, discrimination can contribute to getting poorer-quality health care and not trusting the medical system. Language barriers impede communication between patients and medical professionals. Recent immigrants can have contracted infections in their countries of origin that increase risk for stomach and cervical cancers. African Americans might be prone to breast, prostate, and colorectal cancers that have unique biological signatures, contributing to those cancers' higher incidence or greater aggressiveness (American Cancer Society, 2019; National Cancer Institute, March 2019). Protective cultural factors also exist; for example, low smoking prevalence contributes to relative protection from lung cancer in Hispanic and most Asian groups, compared to non-Hispanic whites. Because cancer disparities have multiple contributors, multilevel interventions are needed to eliminate them.

## Psychosocial Factors and Cancer

We have already considered many risk factors for cancer initiation and progression, including smoking, alcohol consumption, and poor diet (Chapters 4 and 5). In this chapter, we focus more heavily on the evidence regarding psychosocial factors in the initiation and progression of cancer.

As Woody Allen remarked in the film *Manhattan,* "I can't express anger. That's one of the problems I have. I grow a tumor instead." For decades, there has been a stereotype of a cancer-prone personality as a person who is easygoing and acquiescent, repressing emotions that might interfere with smooth social and emotional functioning. In fact, there is little evidence for such a stereotype (Lemogne et al., 2013).

### Stress and Cancer   Do stress and other psychosocial factors contribute to cancer onset? Social isolation, trauma and chronic stress (e.g., adverse childhood experiences), and depression have received the most empirical support. At best, however, the findings are mixed (Fagundes, Murdock, Chirinos, & Green, 2017; Lutgendorf & Andersen, 2015). Several pathways might account for any links that do exist between psychosocial factors and cancer onset. For example, depression is related to poorer immune functioning, and depressed people are more likely to smoke cigarettes (Fluharty, Taylor, Grabski, & Munafò, 2017). Both of these factors could contribute to a link between depression and cancer onset. Early life adversity can influence the developing brain, with subsequent consequences for engagement in unhealthy behaviors linked to cancer (Duffy, McLaughlin, & Green, 2018).

## Psychosocial Factors and the Course of Cancer

Greater research support exists for the role of psychosocial factors in cancer progression than for its onset (Lutgendorf & Andersen, 2015). Controlled experiments definitively show the effect of stress and social isolation on cancer progression in nonhuman animals (Antoni & Dhabhar, 2019; Cole, Nagaraja, Lutgendorf, Green, & Sood, 2015). In humans, evidence is mounting that psychosocial factors are relevant to cancer growth and **metastasis** (i.e., spread of cancer from the original site to other parts of the body). Again, trauma, chronic stress, depression, social isolation, and lack of social support have the strongest research support (Lutgendorf & Andersen, 2015). Depression is implicated in the progression of cancer, both by itself (Brown, Levy, Rosberger, & Edgar, 2003) and in conjunction with other risk factors (Schofield et al., 2016). Depression can also exacerbate the impact of other risk factors. Research has found an 18.5-fold increase in risk for smoking-related cancers among smokers who were depressed, as well as a 2.9-fold increase for non-smoking-associated cancers (Linkins & Comstock, 1990). People who were depressed or anxious prior to having cancer may be especially benefitted by interventions to reduce these mental health problems (Schneider et al., 2010).

Cancer progression also is related to attempts to avoid thoughts and feelings about the disease (Epping-Jordan, Compas, & Howell, 1994). Avoidant or passive coping is also a risk factor for psychological distress, depression, poor sleep, and other risk-related factors, which may represent additional influences on the course of cancer (Hoyt, Thomas, Epstein, & Dirksen, 2009; Kim, Valdimarsdottir, & Bovbjerg, 2003).

## Adjusting to Cancer

Two out of every three families will have a family member who develops cancer, and virtually every member of these families will be affected by the disease. The good news is that 67 percent of cancer survivors live at least 5 years, and 18 percent live at least 20 years (National Cancer Institute, February 2019). Sixty-four percent of cancer patients are at least age 65, and many ultimately die of causes unrelated to their cancer. Nonetheless, many of the issues that we explored in Chapters 11 and 12 in the context of chronic, advancing, and terminal illness are relevant to the cancer experience. We highlight a few additional issues in this section.

**Coping with Physical Limitations**    Physical difficulties usually stem from the pain and discomfort cancer can produce, particularly in the advancing and terminal phases of illness. Sleep disturbance, fatigue, and depression are especially common and debilitating symptoms (Bower, 2019; Jacobsen & Andrykowski, 2015; Stanton, Rowland, & Ganz, 2015). Risk factors for cancer-related fatigue include the experience of childhood adversity, lack of physical activity, ruminating about fatigue in ways that magnify its threat (i.e., catastrophizing), and depression (Bower, 2019). In a daily diary study, on days when a partner encouraged being active, cancer patients' fatigue interfered less and they felt more satisfied with their relationship (Müller et al., 2018). Nutrition can be compromised by cancer and its treatments, and so nutrition therapy is often recommended (Laviano et al., 2011).

**Treatment-Related Problems**    Difficulties also arise as a consequence of treatment. In some cases, organs that are vital to bodily functions must be taken over by a prosthesis. For example, a patient whose larynx has been removed must learn to speak with the help of a prosthetic speech device. Men with prostate cancer often go through treatments that compromise sexual functioning (Steginga & Occhipinti, 2006).

Cancer patients may receive debilitating follow-up treatments. Patients undergoing chemotherapy may experience nausea and vomiting, and then can develop anticipatory nausea and vomiting that occur before the chemotherapy session begins (Montgomery & Bovbjerg, 2004). Expectations that post chemotherapy nausea will occur can increase its likelihood, and so targeting these beliefs can be a valuable addition to interventions (Colagiuri & Zachariae, 2010). Many people whose cancers are treated with chemotherapy report cognitive impairment or chemo-brain, which is diffuse mental cloudiness that can compromise work, social activities, and sense of self (Ahles & Root, 2018; Nelson, Suls, & Padgett, 2014). Memory, concentration, the ability to multitask, and other cognitive skills can be affected. Cognitive rehabilitation has promising effects (Fernandes, Richard, & Edelstein, 2019). Fortunately, in recent years, chemotherapies with less virulent side effects have been developed.

## Psychosocial Issues and Cancer

Many people who are diagnosed with cancer live long and fulfilling lives free of disease. Others may have recurrences but nonetheless maintain a high quality of life for 15 to 20 years or more. Still others live with active cancers over the long term, knowing that the disease will ultimately be fatal. All of these trajectories indicate that cancer is now a chronic disease.

Depression is among the most common difficulties experienced as a result of cancer and its treatment (Kuba et al., 2019; Stommel, Kurtz, Kurtz, Given, & Given, 2004). Depression not only is painful in its own right but also can have adverse effects on physical health outcomes (Wang et al., 2012) and on responses to treatment (Hopko, Clark, Cannity, & Bell, 2016). In one study, women who were more depressed or anxious after a diagnosis of colorectal cancer engaged in fewer healthy lifestyle behaviors over the next decade (Trudel-Fitzgerald et al., 2018). Depression, pain, and fatigue often co-occur among cancer patients, and this complex of symptoms is associated with stress hormones (Thornton, Andersen, & Blakely, 2010). Problems appear to be greatest among people who cope through avoiding the cancer experience and make little use of active, approach-oriented coping strategies, as well as who have chronic stress, a diagnosis of PTSD, or a lack of social support (Bower, 2019; Butler, Koopman, Classen, & Spiegel, 1999; Golden-Kreutz et al., 2005; Langford et al., 2017; Stanton, Wiley, Krull, Crespi, & Weihs, 2018).

**Interventions Involving Stress**    Stress aggravates virtually all illnesses and cancer is no exception. For the most part, cancer survivors respond to day-to-day stressors much as other people do. Nonetheless, stress can increase the likelihood of depression and exacerbate physical symptoms, and thus, interventions directed to stress management can be helpful (Costanzo, Stawski, Ryff, Coe, & Almeida, 2012).

Fear of recurrence is a major source of anxiety for cancer patients (Van Liew, Christensen, Howren, Hynds Karnell, & Funk, 2014). It can especially increase at the time of follow-up visits (McGinty, Small, Laronga, & Jacobsen, 2016) and so should be one target of interventions (McGinty, Small, Laronga, & Jacobsen, 2016), especially for young women who may have more such fears (Lebel, Beattie, Ares, & Bielajew, 2013). Intrusive thoughts impair quality of life and predict symptoms (Dupont, Bower, Stanton, & Ganz, 2014). Cognitive–behavioral therapy can help keep these fears from being debilitating.

### Issues Involving Social Support

Social support is important for cancer patients' recovery (Carpenter, Fowler, Maxwell, & Andersen, 2010) for several reasons. It improves psychological adjustment to cancer, it can help patients deal with intrusive thoughts and ruminations about the cancer (Lewis et al., 2001), and it may improve immunologic responses to cancer as well. One investigation (Lai et al., 1999) found that married patients with cancers have significantly better survival rates than single, separated, divorced, or widowed patients. Socially isolated cancer patients fare very poorly and have an elevated risk of mortality (Kroenke, Kubzansky, Schernhammer, Holmes, & Kawachi, 2006). Intervening to improve social support early on, at the time of diagnosis and treatment, is recommended (Thompson, Rodebaugh, Pérez, Schootmann, & Jeffe, 2013).

A strong partner relationship is important, even if, in the short term, the partner is not especially responsive to the patient's needs (Hagedoorn et al., 2011). Unfortunately, disturbances in relationships after a diagnosis of cancer are fairly common (Ybema, Kuijer, Buunk, DeJong, & Sanderman, 2001). Sexual functioning is particularly vulnerable and can be affected by treatments, such as surgery or chemotherapy, and indirectly affected by anxiety or depression, which reduces sexual desire (Loaring, Larkin, Shaw, & Flowers, 2015). These problems are especially common in gynecologic cancers and prostate cancer. Discussion and evidence-based treatment of sexual problems is important (Carter et al., 2018).

Problems concerning a cancer patient's children are relatively common. Young children may show fear or distress over the parent's prognosis (Compas et al., 1994), whereas older children may find new responsibilities thrust on them and in response may rebel. If the cancer has a hereditary component, the children may be distressed by their increased risk (Lichtman et al., 1984).

### Post Traumatic Growth

Nonetheless, some cancer patients report that their lives have been made better in important ways by the cancer experience, permitting them to experience growth (Arpawong, Richeimer, Wenstein, Elghamrawy, & Milam, 2013; Katz, Flasher, Cacciapaglia, & Nelson, 2001; Taylor, 1983). These effects have been reported in many cultures, so growth in response to cancer appears to be a reliable outcome (Gonzales, Nuñez, Wang-Letzkus, Lim, Flores, & Nápoles, 2016; Wang et al., 2017). Such growth experiences may improve psychological adjustment (Gonzalez et al., 2016; Wang et al., 2017; Zhu et al., 2018) and mute neuroendocrine stress responses, which may, in turn, have a beneficial effect on the immune system (Cruess et al., 2000).

### Interventions

Prior to treatment, educational interventions are vital (Zimmermann, Heinrichs, & Baucom, 2007). During or following treatment, cognitive–behavioral approaches to cancer-related problems are typically employed, focusing on depression, stress, fatigue, pain, appetite control, and side effects associated with chemotherapy, radiation therapy, and other cancer treatments (Montgomery et al., 2009; Phillips et al., 2008; Stagl et al., 2015). These interventions can significantly improve quality of life. Treatment of depression in people with cancer also is linked to lower annual health care costs (Mausbach, Bos, & Irwin, 2018).

Mindfulness-based stress-reduction interventions hold promise as well (Bränström, Kvillemo, Brandberg, & Moskowitz, 2010). For example, a mindfulness intervention with breast and prostate cancer patients involving the active cultivation of conscious awareness through relaxation, meditation, and yoga not only enhanced quality of life and decreased stress symptoms but also produced a beneficial shift in immune functioning. Mindfulness interventions can even be effective when provided online (Zernicke et al., 2014).

Improving health behaviors is a major target of interventions with cancer survivors (Rabin, 2011). Exercise can improve quality of life following cancer (Basen-Engquist et al., 2013; Courneya et al., 2010; Floyd & Moyer, 2010). A review of 24 research studies found that physical exercise had a positive effect on quality of life following cancer diagnosis, including a heightened sense of self-efficacy, better physical functioning, and improved emotional well-being (McAuley,

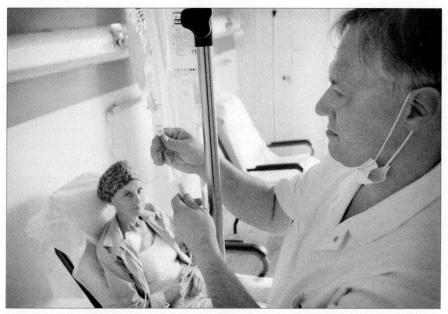

*Some cancer patients who receive intravenously administered chemotherapy experience intense nausea and vomiting. Interventions using relaxation and guided imagery can substantially improve these problems.*
BSIP SA/Alamy Stock Photo

White, Rogers, Motl, & Courneya, 2010; Milne, Wallman, Gordon, & Courneya, 2008). Exercise adherence, though, can be a problem (Courneya et al., 2008). Interventions that draw on the theory of planned behavior or the stages of change model to promote exercise have shown some success with cancer patients (Park & Gaffey, 2007; Vallance, Courneya, Plotnikoff, & Mackey, 2008) and increasing self-efficacy to exercise predicts maintenance (Cox et al., 2015). Telephone prompts may also help with exercise adherence (Pinto, Papandonatos, & Goldstein, 2013). Exercise also improves fitness and well-being in caregivers (Cuthbert et al., 2018).

Pain is a relatively common problem among cancer patients, particularly those with advancing disease. Although painkillers remain the primary method of treating cancer-related pain, behavioral interventions including relaxation therapy, hypnosis, cognitive-reappraisal techniques, visual imaging, and self-hypnosis also improve the management of cancer pain (Sheinfeld Gorin et al., 2012; Ward et al., 2008).

Writing interventions involving expressive disclosure or writing about benefits derived from cancer have been tied to fewer symptoms and fewer medical appointments for cancer-related problems (Low et al., 2006). The opportunity to affirm important personal values and the use of emotional approach coping appear to account for these benefits (Creswell et al., 2007).

### Therapies with Cancer Patients

**Cognitive–Behavioral Therapy (CBT)**    Some people who are diagnosed with cancer participate in CBT interventions, individually, in groups, or through the Internet. Such interventions often focus on reducing depression, managing stress, controlling fear of recurrence, and developing good coping skills (Stagl et al., 2015).

**Family Therapy**    Because emotional support from family is beneficial to cancer patients, family therapy is often employed (Helgeson & Cohen, 1996; Northouse, Templin, & Mood, 2001). Not all families are able to communicate freely with each other, though. When there is a mismatch in the social support wanted and received by cancer patients, psychological distress may increase (Reynolds & Perrin, 2004). Dyadic coping affects a cancer survivor's quality of life (Rottmann et al., 2015) and so couples coping with cancer may benefit from dyadic coping intervention (Badr & Krebs, 2013).

**Support Groups**   Groups in which patients share emotional concerns are available and helpful to many cancer patients (Helgeson & Cohen, 1996), especially those who have few other personal or social resources (Helgeson, Cohen, Schulz, & Yasko, 2000). A possible reason for the success of support groups is that the self-help format presents patients with an array of potential coping techniques from which they can draw the ones that fit in with their particular styles and problems (Taylor, Falke, Shoptaw, & Lichtman, 1986). However, only a small percent of people take advantage of support group opportunities (Sherman et al., 2008). However, the Internet is now used extensively by cancer patients for social support from other cancer patients (Owen, Klapow, Roth, & Tucker, 2004).

**Internet Interventions**   As just noted, the Internet provides opportunities to intervene with cancer patients. Coping skills, and ways to enhance mood and social support can all be targeted (Cleary & Stanton, 2015).

## ■ ARTHRITIS

Chapter 2 described a set of diseases known as autoimmune diseases, in which the body falsely identifies its own tissue as foreign matter and attacks it. The most prevalent of these autoimmune diseases is arthritis, and it is also one of the most common causes of disability.

Arthritis has been with humankind since the beginning of recorded history. Ancient drawings of people with arthritic joints have been found in caves, and early Greek and Roman writers described the pain of arthritis. *Arthritis* means "inflammation of a joint"; it refers to more than 100 diseases that attack the joints or other connective tissues. About 54 million people in the United States are afflicted with arthritis severe enough to require medical care, a figure that is projected to rise to 78 million by 2040, due to the aging of the population (Centers for Disease Control and Prevention, 2018, July). Although it is rarely fatal, arthritis is a leading cause of disability. Arthritis costs the U.S. economy more than $304 billion per year in medical care and indirect expenses such as lost wages and production (Centers for Disease Control and Prevention, July 2018).

### Rheumatoid Arthritis

**Rheumatoid arthritis (RA)** affects 1.5 million Americans, mostly women (Centers for Disease Control and Prevention, October 2015), and is the most crippling

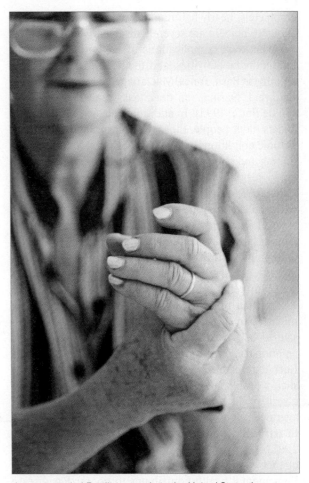

*Approximately 1.5 million people in the United States have rheumatoid arthritis, and it is especially common among older women.*

Pixtal/age fotostock

form of arthritis. The disease strikes primarily the 40 to 60 age group, although it can attack people of any age group, including children. It usually affects the small joints of the hands and feet, as well as the wrists, knees, ankles, and neck. In mild cases, only one or two joints are involved, but in severe cases, there may be inflammation of the heart muscle, blood vessels, and tissues just beneath the skin.

RA is brought on by an autoimmune process (Firestein, 2003): Agents of the immune system that are supposed to protect the body instead attack the thin membranes surrounding the joints. This attack leads to inflammation, stiffness, and pain. If not controlled, the bone and surrounding muscle tissue of the joint may be destroyed. Almost half of RA patients recover completely, nearly half remain somewhat arthritic, and about 10 percent are severely disabled.

The main complications of RA are pain, fatigue, limitations in activities, and the need to be dependent on others (Basu, Jones, Macfarlane, & Druce, 2017; van Lankveld, Naring, van der Staak, van't Pad Bosch, & van de Putte, 1993). In addition, because RA primarily affects older people, those who have it may have other chronic conditions as well, such as poor cognitive functioning and poor vision, which may interact with arthritis to produce disability (Shifren, Park, Bennett, & Morrell, 1999; Verbrugge, 1995). Not surprisingly, one of the most common complications of RA is depression (Dickens, McGowan, Clark-Carter, & Creed, 2002). Depression may feed back into the pain process, enhancing pain (Zautra & Smith, 2001), and may increase arthritis disease activity, setting a vicious spiral into effect (Smith & Zautra, 2002).

At one time, psychologists speculated that there might be an "RA personality." This personality type was said to be perfectionistic, depressed, and restricted in emotional expression, especially the expression of anger. Recent research now casts doubt on the accuracy of such a profile, at least as a cause of arthritis. However, cognitive distortions and feelings of helplessness can aggravate depression and other emotional responses to arthritis (Clemmey & Nicassio, 1997; Fifield et al., 2001). Gaps in social support may also be a consequence (Fyrand, Moum, Finset, & Glennas, 2002). Poor mental health contributes to poorer RA disease outcomes across time, and pain in turn predicts poorer mental health (Euesden et al., 2017).

**Stress and RA**     Stress may play a role both in the development of RA and in its course. Social relationship distress may especially contribute to the development of the disease (Anderson, Bradley, Young, McDaniel, & Wise, 1985) and/or its course (Parrish, Zautra, & Davis, 2008). The spouse appears to play a critical role in the RA experience, and accurate perceptions of fatigue, pain, and physical limitations by the spouse are critical to successful disease management (Lehman et al., 2011). So problematic is miscarried spousal support for managing arthritis that couple-oriented interventions play an important role in its management (Martire, Stephens, & Schulz, 2011).

**Treatment of RA**     Treatments to arrest or control the problems of RA include aspirin, steroids, and disease-modifying antirheumatic drugs (which relieve both pain and inflammation), rest, and supervised exercise. Unfortunately, adherence is often low. Self-management can be improved with strong support from a partner (Strating, van Schuur, & Suurmeijer, 2006).

Increasingly, psychologists have used cognitive-behavioral interventions in the treatment of RA (McCracken, 1991), including biofeedback, relaxation training, problem-solving skills training, a focus on reducing negative expectations, and pain-coping skills training (Dixon, Keefe, Scipio, Perri, & Abernethy, 2007; Zautra et al., 2008). Targeting catastrophizing thoughts and improving self-efficacy may be particularly beneficial (McKnight, Afram, Kashdan, Kasle, & Zautra, 2010). As one patient in such an intervention put it, "I went from thinking about arthritis as a terrible burden that had been thrust upon me to something I could control and manage. I redefined it for myself. It's no longer a tragedy, it's an inconvenience." As this comment implies, an enhanced sense of self-efficacy that one can manage the disease may be largely responsible for the success of CBT interventions with RA.

Recently, mindfulness interventions have been used with RA patients, and patients with depression appear to be especially benefitted (Zautra et al., 2008). Coordinating these behavioral interventions with the use of drug therapies to control pain provides the most comprehensive approach (Zautra & Manne, 1992).

## Osteoarthritis

**Osteoarthritis** affects more than 30 million Americans, mostly after age 50. Women are more commonly affected than men (Centers for Disease Control and Prevention, January 2019). The disorder develops when the smooth lining of a joint, known as the articular cartilage, begins to crack or wear away because of overuse, injury, or other causes. Thus, the disease tends to affect the weight-bearing joints: the hips, knees, and spine. As the cartilage deteriorates, the joint may become inflamed, stiff, and painful. The disease afflicts many elderly people and some athletes. As is true for other forms of arthritis, more serious and extensive symptoms require more aggressive treatment and lead to a poorer quality of life (Hampson, Glasgow, & Zeiss, 1994). Depression may result, and depressive symptoms may, in turn, elevate pain and distress (Zautra & Smith, 2001). Being skilled at handling negative emotions can decrease the relationship between osteoarthritis pain and depressive symptoms (Parmelee, Scicolone, Cox,

DeCaro, Keefe, & Smith, 2018). Psychosocial interventions to reduce distress and improve coping can reduce pain significantly (Zautra et al., 2008). Interventions that target both catastrophizing pain and increasing a sense of self-efficacy may be especially effective (McKnight et al., 2010).

With proper treatment, osteoarthritis can be managed through self-care. Treatment includes being physically active, keeping one's weight down and taking aspirin and other pain killers. People who manage the pain of osteoarthritis through active coping efforts and spontaneous pain control efforts appear to cope better with the disease (Keefe et al., 1987).

## ■ TYPE 1 DIABETES

**Type 1 diabetes** is an autoimmune disorder characterized by the abrupt onset of symptoms, which result from lack of insulin production by the beta cells of the pancreas. Affecting nearly half a million people in the United States, type 1 diabetes accounts for 5 percent of all diabetes (Centers for Disease Control and Prevention, 2017). The disorder may appear following viral infection and probably has a genetic contribution. Stress may precipitate type 1 diabetes in individuals with a genetic risk (Lehman, Rodin, McEwen, & Brinton, 1991), and rates of this disorder are on the rise, jumping more than 1 percent each year from 2002 to 2012 in youth. The increase in type 1 diagnoses in Hispanic youth is especially high, exceeding 4 percent annually (Mayer-Davis et al., 2017). In type 1 diabetes, the immune system falsely identifies cells in the pancreas as invaders and, accordingly, destroys these cells, compromising or eliminating their ability to produce insulin. Type 1 diabetes usually develops relatively early in life, earlier for girls than for boys. There are two common time periods when the disorder arises: between the ages of 5 and 6 or between 10 and 13.

The most common early symptoms are frequent urination, unusual thirst, excessive fluid consumption, weight loss, fatigue, weakness, irritability, nausea, uncontrollable craving for food (especially sweets), and fainting. These symptoms are due to the body's attempt to find sources of energy, which prompts it to feed off its own fats and proteins. By-products of these fats then build up in the body, producing symptoms; if the condition is untreated, a coma can result.

Type 1 diabetes is a life-threatening illness. It is managed primarily through direct injections of

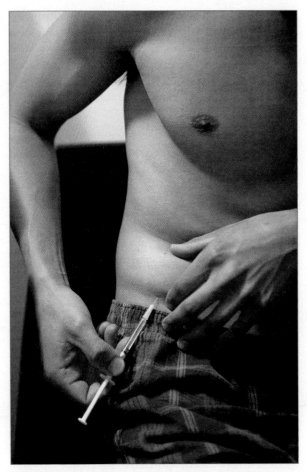

*The management of type 1 diabetes critically depends on proper monitoring of blood glucose levels and regular injections of insulin, yet many adolescents and adults fail to adhere properly to the treatment regimen.*
Keith Brofsky/Getty Images

insulin—hence the name insulin-dependent diabetes. The type 1 diabetic is especially vulnerable to hyperglycemia, namely high blood sugar, and if left untreated, it can lead to coma and death.

Stress aggravates type 1 diabetes. At least 15 studies have reported direct links between stress and poor diabetic control (see Helgeson, Escobar, Siminerio, & Becker, 2010). This relationship is not caused by differences in adherence to medications (Hanson, Henggeler, & Burghen, 1987), coping efforts (Frenzel et al., 1988), insulin regimen, diet, or exercise (Hanson & Pichert, 1986), although stress can adversely affect adherence and diet as well (Balfour, White, Schiffrin, Dougherty, & Dufresne, 1993). The changes imposed by diabetes often lead to risk for psychological difficulties including depression, anxiety, and behavior problems (Reynolds & Helgeson, 2011). Screening for depression is recommended because depression can complicate adherence and glycemic control and potentially affect the course of disease (Baucom, Turner, Tracy, Berg, & Wiebe, 2018).

Managing Type 1 Diabetes   Because very tight control of glucose levels can make a big difference in the progression of this disease, patients with type 1 diabetes need to monitor their glucose levels throughout each day and take immediate action when it is needed. Active involvement of the patient as a co-manager in the disease treatment process is essential to success. This management typically involves regular insulin injections, dietary control, weight control, and exercise. The number of calories taken in each day must be relatively constant. Food intake must be controlled by a meal plan and not by temptation or appetite. When blood glucose levels are actively controlled through such methods, the likelihood and progression of diabetes-related disorders, including eye disease, kidney disease, and nerve disorders, can be reduced by more than 50 percent (National Institute on Diabetes and Digestive and Kidney Disorders, 1999).

Adherence   Unfortunately, adherence to self-management programs appears to be low. Overall, only about 15 percent of patients appear to adhere to all their treatment recommendations.

Because many of the severe complications of diabetes are not evident until 15 to 20 years after its onset, these risks do not frighten people into being adherent. They may feel no symptoms, and so fail to adhere to their treatment regimen. Many of the errors made by diabetic patients in adhering to their treatment regimen, then, are errors of omission rather than commission.

Diabetic patients often fail to self-monitor their blood glucose level (Wysocki, Green, & Huxtable, 1989). Instead, like hypertensive patients, they rely on what their blood glucose level "feels like" (Hampson, Glasgow, & Toobert, 1990), and they rely strongly on their mood for making this judgment (Gonder-Frederick, Cox, Bobbitt, & Pennebaker, 1986). And, as is also the case in hypertension, even training in glucose level awareness fails to produce accurate estimates of blood sugar levels (Diamond, Massey, & Covey, 1989).

Patients do better managing their illness and their diabetes regimen when they use active coping strategies, as opposed to passive or avoidant ones (Luyckx, Vanhalst, Seiffge-Krenke, & Wheets, 2010). Adherence is improved when patients and their physicians share treatment goals. One study found that parents of type 1 diabetics and physicians had quite different goals. The parents' efforts to control diet were designed to avoid hypoglycemia, which is a short-term threat. In contrast, the physicians' goals were centered on the long-term threat of diabetes complications and the need to keep blood glucose levels steady. These differences in goals accounted for many of the departures from the prescribed regimen (Marteau, Johnston, Baum, & Bloch, 1987).

Special Problems of Adolescent Diabetics

The management of diabetes is a particular problem with adolescents (Johnson, Freund, Silverstein, Hansen, & Malone, 1990). They are entangled in issues of independence and a developing self-concept; diabetes and the restrictions that it imposes are inconsistent with these developmental tasks. The common stressors of adolescence aggravate metabolic control (Helgeson et al., 2010). Adolescents may see their parents' limitations on food as efforts to control them. Within the adolescent peer culture, those who are different are often stigmatized. Thus, the adolescent with diabetes may neglect proper care to avoid rejection. Emotionally stable and conscientious adolescents who are able to find benefit in their experiences are more likely to follow the complex regimen that diabetes requires (Tran, Wiebe, Fortenberry, Butler, & Berg, 2011). Depression and stress undermine good self-care (Baucom et al., 2015).

Relations with Family   Parents are critical to the successful management of the treatment regimen (Helgeson, Palladino, Reynolds, Becker, Escobar, & Siminerio, 2014). But they may react in ways that undermine management efforts. Parents, for example, may treat their adolescent daughter or son newly diagnosed with diabetes as a child and restrict activities beyond what is necessary, infantilizing the adolescent and increasing dependence (Berg, Butner, Butler, King, Hughes, & Wiebe, 2013). Alternatively, the parents may try to convince the child that he or she is normal. Unfortunately, family conflict and poor monitoring by parents are both risk factors for poor glycemic control and self-care (Hilliard et al., 2013). A parent may have problems of his or her own, such as depression, which can undermine effective treatment and medical care (Mackey, Struemph, Powell, Chen, Streisand, & Holmes, 2014). Autonomy support for the adolescent, by which he or she gradually assumes responsibility for the treatment regimen, may best maintain it at a time when adherence may start to fall off (Rohan et al., 2014; Wu et al., 2014).

The health psychologist, then, has an important role to play in the management of type 1 diabetes, by developing the best ways of teaching the complex treatment regimen. Ensuring adherence, developing effective means for coping with stress, helping the diabetic patient develop the self-regulatory skills needed to manage the treatment program, and helping the family coordinate their efforts with a minimum of strain (Sood et al., 2012) are primary treatment goals. •

## S U M M A R Y

1. The immune system is the surveillance system of the body that guards against foreign invaders.

2. Stressors, such as academic exams and stressful interpersonal relationships, can compromise immune functioning. Negative emotions, such as depression or anxiety, also compromise immune functioning.

3. Active coping methods may buffer the immune system against adverse changes due to stress. Relaxation and stress management can be successful clinical efforts to augment immune system functioning in the face of stress.

4. Acquired immune deficiency syndrome (AIDS) was first identified in the United States in 1981. It results from the human immunodeficiency virus (HIV) and is marked by the presence of unusual opportunistic infectious diseases.

5. Men who have sex with men and intravenous needle-sharing drug users have been the primary risk groups for AIDS in the United States. More recently, AIDS has spread rapidly in minority populations, especially minority women. Heterosexually active adolescents and young adults are also at risk.

6. Primary prevention, through condom use and control of the number of partners, is the main approach to controlling the spread of HIV. Such interventions focus on providing knowledge, increasing perceived self-efficacy to engage in protective behavior, changing peer norms about sexual practices, and developing sexual negotiation strategies.

7. Many people live with asymptomatic HIV-seropositivity for years. Exercise and active coping may help prolong this state. Drugs such as ART enable people with HIV infection to live longer, healthier lives, making HIV infection a chronic disease.

8. Cancer is a set of more than 100 diseases marked by malfunctioning DNA and rapid cell growth and proliferation. Psychosocial factors appear to be related to the onset and progression of cancer, including stress, depression, and avoidance coping.

9. Cancer can produce physical and psychosocial problems, including debilitating responses to chemotherapy, strain in the social network, job stress, and adverse psychological responses such as depression. CBT, family therapy, and support groups are among the tools to manage these problems.

10. Arthritis, involving inflammation of the joints, affects more than 50 million people in the United States. Rheumatoid arthritis is the most crippling form, but there are more than 100 disorders that account for this highly prevalent set of diseases. Stress exacerbates these disorders.

11. Interventions involving cognitive–behavioral techniques to help people manage pain effectively and increase self-efficacy are helpful for alleviating discomfort and psychosocial difficulties associated with arthritis.

12. Type 1 diabetes is an autoimmune disorder that often strikes in childhood or early adolescence. Its management involves monitoring blood sugar levels and controlling diet, among other health habits. Unfortunately, especially with young type 1 diabetes patients, adherence can be poor. Health psychologists can help in the design of interventions to improve self-management.

## K E Y   T E R M S

acquired immune deficiency syndrome (AIDS)
cancer disparity
cancer metastasis

human immunodeficiency virus (HIV)
osteoarthritis
psychoneuroimmunology

rheumatoid arthritis (RA)
type 1 diabetes

# PART 6

# Toward the Future

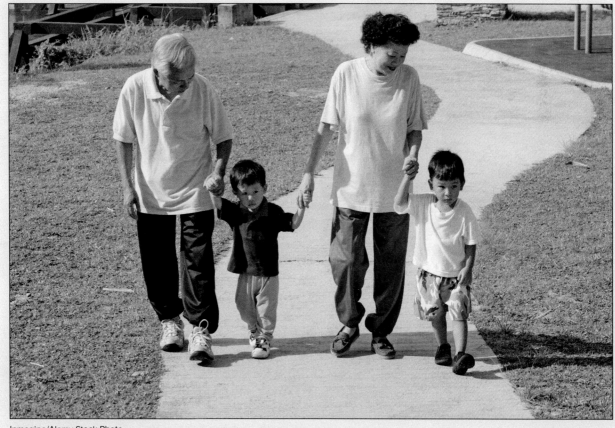

Inmagine/Alamy Stock Photo

CHAPTER 15

# Health Psychology: Challenges for the Future

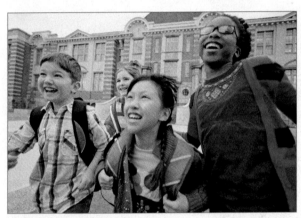

Hero/Corbis/Glow Images

When we focus on all the health-related problems that need to be solved, we forget how much progress in improving health outcomes has already been achieved. Consider the following trends:

* Worldwide, life expectancy has risen to an all-time high of 72 (World Health Organization, 2018).

* Death rates for the two leading causes of death in the United States—heart disease and cancer—have declined since the 1990s (Weir et al., 2016).

* The number of adults in the United States who have high cholesterol—a key risk for heart disease—has declined significantly over the past decade (Centers for Disease Control and Prevention, 2017).

* Fatal car crashes in the United States have declined by more than one-third (Institute of Highway Safety, 2017).

* The percentage of smokers in the United States has dropped from 23.2 percent in 2000 to 15 percent as of 2015 (Centers for Disease Control and Prevention, 2017).

This is an exciting time to be in health psychology for many reasons. A first reason concerns the substantial improvements in health behaviors to which health psychologists have made important contributions. A second reason stems from the extraordinary developments in biopsychosocial bases of behavior that health psychologists have discovered in just the last decade. We have decisive proof that psychological and biological states influence each other (Herrmann-Lingen, 2017). Health psychologists have been instrumental, for example, in the discovery that low-grade inflammation affects the development of numerous physical and mental health disorders, including coronary heart disease, hypertension, some cancers, and depression. As the pathways linking psychological and social factors to illness risk generally and to specific disorders become clear, the potential to intervene at steps along the way becomes more clear.

The health care system itself is changing in the United States. The Patient Protection and Affordable Care Act (ACA) initiated by President Obama brought health insurance to many of the previously uninsured, with the result that less than 9 percent of the population lacked health insurance in 2016 (Centers for Disease Control and Prevention, 2016). However, as of mid-2018, that trend has reversed, with 15.5 percent of the population currently lacking health insurance (Forbes, 2018); as a result, adverse health conditions may be diagnosed later, with resulting poorer prospects for treatment and recovery. Consequently, health psychologists have an increasingly important role to play, both in ensuring that behavioral treatments are included in basic health care and in designing interventions that enable people to be intelligent, effective consumers of the health care they do have.

With the obesity crisis in full view, and the costs of smoking ever more evident, and deaths from opioid abuse continuing to rise, concerns about effective prevention have gained traction. In addition to the implementation of behavioral interventions, helping to draft legislative initiatives and working with legislatures at the state and federal levels to attack health problems represent an increasing role for health psychology.

Technological changes, especially in the form of smartphones and use of the Internet, have an important role to play in the management of health care. Although the benefits of these technologies are still being explored (Kaplan & Stone, 2013), interventions currently range from sending people electronic reminders to take medications at the appropriate time to individually tailoring health interventions to help people control weight gain, exercise routines, and calorie counts for meals, among others. All these interventions can be implemented easily through cell phones. Technology can tell us things about health we don't know. For example, language used on Twitter reflects county-level heart disease deaths: In those counties where Twitter language reflected negative relationships, negative emotions, and disengagement, heart disease deaths were higher (Eichstaedt et al., 2015).

Technology is changing the face of medical practice (Topol, 2015). Through telemedicine, physicians can see patients online. Online visits and texts can substitute for routine office visits (*The Economist*, May 30, 2015) and uncomplicated follow-up appointments. In Wisconsin, a state with a large rural population that has difficulty getting to a medical center, patients have been taught to take pictures of their postsurgical wounds on their cellphones so their physician can see how healing is progressing (Gunter et al., 2016). Robots are likely to play an increasingly important role in health care, by providing social support (think fluffy animal) and assisting in fulfilling basic needs, such as taking medication (Broadbent, 2017).

Advances in neuroscience over the last 20 years have been breathtaking and helped to inform how behavioral and psychosocial factors affect health (Gianaros & Hackman, 2013). As neuroscience advances, so does health psychology.

These exciting times also present challenges. Many of the lifestyle issues that affect health, such as lack of exercise and the increasing obesity of the population, are very difficult to change, and overcoming sources of resistance to intervention is essential. The substantial importance of socioeconomic status (SES) to patterns of illness and disease, availability of treatment, and presence of risk factors suggests that effective interventions need to go hand in hand with policy interventions to reduce the gaps related to SES and income inequality.

Once we believed that all health problems would be solved by education. The philosophy was "tell them and they will change" (Emmons, 2012). We now know that education is only the first step. Even educating physicians as well as patients has not achieved the change we might desire. It is essential to focus on the health care system itself (Emmons, 2012). Nonetheless, many health care providers are still unfamiliar with the skills and interventions that psychologists have to offer, and so a continued collaboration with the medical community to wed psychological and medical treatments in a patient-centered approach to care is vital (Johnson, 2012).

# ■ HEALTH PROMOTION

In recent years, many people have made substantial gains in altering their poor health habits. Some have stopped smoking, and others have reduced their consumption of high-cholesterol and high-fat foods. Coronary heart disease and other chronic diseases have shown impressive declines as a result. Although alcohol consumption patterns remain largely unchanged, exercise has increased. Despite these advances, obesity is currently endemic and will shortly supplant smoking as the major avoidable contributor to mortality. Poor sleep is an understudied path to poor health (Jarrin, McGrath, & Quon, 2014). Clearly, most people know that they need to practice good health behaviors, and many have tried to develop or change them. Not everyone is successful, however.

Increasingly, in health psychology, we will see efforts to identify the most potent and effective elements of behavior-change programs in order to incorporate them into cost-effective, efficient interventions that reach the largest number of people (Piper et al., 2018).

In particular, we can expect to see the design of interventions for mass consumption on the Internet and in the community, the workplace, the media, and the schools.

## A Focus on Those at Risk

As medical research identifies genetic and behavioral risk factors for chronic illness, the at-risk role will assume increasing importance. Individuals who are at risk for particular disorders need to learn how to cope with their risk status and how to change their modifiable risk-relevant behaviors. Health psychologists can aid in both these tasks.

Studies of people who are at risk for particular disorders are useful in identifying additional risk factors for various chronic disorders. Not everyone who is at risk for an illness will develop it, and by studying which people do and do not, researchers can identify the precipitating or promoting factors of these disorders.

## Prevention

Preventing poor health habits from developing is an essential goal of health care (National Academy of Medicine, 2012, April), to which health psychologists can and do make major contributions. Adolescence is a window of vulnerability for most bad health habits, and so closing this window is of paramount importance. **Behavioral immunization** programs are already in existence for smoking, drug abuse, and, in some cases, diet and eating disorders. Programs that expose fifth and sixth graders to antismoking or antidrug material before they begin these habits are somewhat successful in keeping some adolescents from undertaking such habits. Behavioral immunization for other health habits—including safe sex and diet—also holds promise.

For some health habits, we need to start earlier and teach parents how to reduce the risks of accidents in the home, how to practice good safety habits in automobiles, and how to help their children practice good health habits such as exercise, proper diet, regular immunizations and medical checkups, and regular dental care.

## A Focus on Older Adults

The aging of the population means that within the next 10 years, the United States and many other developed countries will have the largest cohort of older adults ever seen (see Table 15.1). Interventions should focus on enabling older adults to achieve the highest level of functioning possible through programs that emphasize diet, exercise, control of alcohol consumption, and other health habits.

## Refocusing Health Promotion Efforts

Some refocusing of health promotion efforts is in order. In the past, we have stressed mortality more than morbidity. Although the reduction of mortality, especially early mortality, is a priority, there will always be 10 major causes of death. Focusing our efforts on morbidity is important for a number of reasons.

One obvious reason is cost. Chronic diseases are expensive to treat, particularly when those diseases persist for years, even decades. For example, conditions such as rheumatoid arthritis and osteoarthritis have little impact on mortality rates but have a major impact on the functioning and well-being of the population, particularly the elderly. Maximizing the number of good years during which a person is free from the burdens of chronic illness produces a higher quality of life.

Priorities for the future include developing interventions that can address more than one behavioral risk factor at a time, addressing maintenance of behavior change, and integrating individual-level interventions into the broader environmental and health policies that support and sustain individual efforts.

In recent years, researchers and practitioners have focused on developing just-in-time interventions with the goal of providing the right type and amount of an intervention at just the right time, by responding to a person's changing internal (bodily) and external (context) environments (Nahum-Shani, Smith, Spring, Collins, & Witkiewitz, 2018). For example, the first step in a stop-smoking intervention might be delivered to a

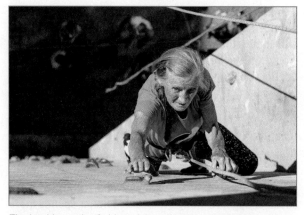

The health needs of older adults will take on increasing importance with the aging of the population. Helping the elderly achieve a high level of functioning through interventions that emphasize diet, exercise, and other health habits is a high priority for the future.
Alex Brylov/Shutterstock

smoker when she has developed bronchitis. The technological capacity offered by the Internet makes these just-in-time interventions increasingly likely and available.

## Promoting Resilience

Future health promotion efforts should place greater weight on the positive factors that reduce morbidity or delay mortality. For example, marriage would add several years to a man's life. Enhancing people's abilities to attract and maintain social support more generally is a priority for health psychology in the future. Internet interventions are one way of doing exactly this.

Studying how people spontaneously reduce stress and how they seek out opportunities for rest, renewal, and relaxation may provide knowledge for effective interventions. Personal resources, such as optimism or a sense of control, have proven to be protective against chronic illness. Can these resources be taught? Research suggests that they can (see, for example, Mann, 2001).

## Health Promotion and Medical Practice

A true philosophy of health promotion requires that this focus become an integral part of medical practice (McDaniel & deGruy, 2014). Although progress has been made, we are still far away from having a health care system that is oriented toward health promotion.

As noted in Chapter 3, there is as yet no formal diagnostic process for identifying and targeting preventive health behaviors on an individual basis. If the

**TABLE 15.1  |  Percent of Population Aged 65 and Over**

|  | 1970 (%) | 2010 (%) | 2050 (Projected) (%) |
|---|---|---|---|
| United States | 9.0 | 13.0 | 21.6 |
| India | 3.3 | 4.9 | 13.7 |
| China | 4.3 | 8.2 | 23.3 |
| Japan | 7.0 | 22.6 | 37.8 |
| United Kingdom | 13.0 | 16.6 | 22.9 |
| Western Europe | 13.1 | 18.4 | 28.9 |

*Source:* Authers, John. "Ways to Take Stock of it All." *Financial Times.* October 14, 2009.

annual physical that many people obtain were to include a simple review of the particular health issues and habits that the person should focus on, this step would, at the very least, alert each of us to attainable health goals and nudge us in the direction of taking necessary action.

## Health Disparities

Individual health behavior changes alone may not substantially improve the health of the general population. What is needed is individual change coupled with social change. Although the United States spends more on health care than any other country in the world (Figure 15.1), we have neither the longest life expectancy nor the lowest infant mortality rate (National Academy of Medicine, 2013). A ranking of nations by the Commonwealth Fund in terms of quality of health care in seven developed countries placed the United States last (Davis, Schoen, & Stremikis, 2010), and we are falling farther behind faster than any other country in the world (National Research Council, 2013).

Efforts to reduce and postpone morbidity and disability will be unsuccessful without attention to our country's and the world's large socioeconomic disparities in health and health care (House, 2015). Risk factors for some of the country's major disorders can show up as early as childhood and adolescence (Chen et al., 2006), and the accumulating effects of poor health habits related to SES on adult health outcomes are now well established (e.g., Kershaw, Mezuk, Abdou, Rafferty, & Jackson, 2010). The United States is only beginning to move toward universal health care coverage, the last of the industrialized nations to do so (Oberlander, 2010; Quadagno, 2004). Millions of people in the United States have difficulty paying their health care bills (Cohen & Bloom, 2010; U.S. Department of Commerce, 2009). Latinos and African Americans are especially affected (Bloom & Cohen, 2011). The United States is also the only country where health care for most people is financed by for-profit, minimally regulated private insurance companies (Quadagno, 2004).

The adverse effect of low socioeconomic status on health is true for both men and women at all age levels and across most countries of the world (House, 2015), and it is dramatically getting worse (Tavernise, 2016). Among the many risk factors tied to low SES are alcohol consumption, high levels of lipids, obesity, tobacco use, and fewer psychosocial resources, such as a sense of mastery, self-esteem, and social support. Each of

**FIGURE 15.1 | Public and Private Expenditure on Health**

*Source:* Organization for Economic Cooperation and Development. "Health Expenditure and Financing." Accessed July 9, 2019. https://stats.oecd.org/Index.aspx?DataSetCode=SHA.

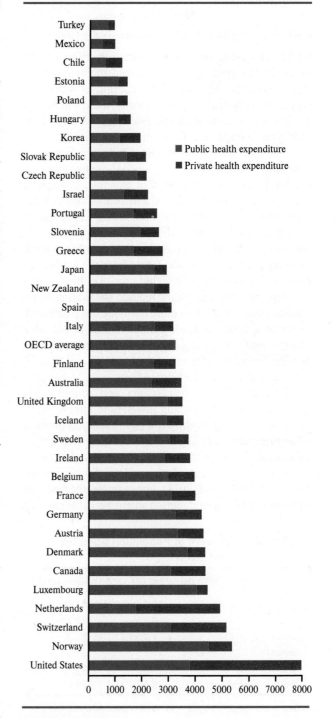

U.S. Dollars per Capita.

these has an effect on health (House, 2001; Kraus, Horberg, Goetz, & Keltner, 2011; Kubzansky, Berkman, Glass, & Seeman, 1998). Even the usually beneficial effects of social support may be muted in low SES populations (Fagundes et al., 2012). Low SES is linked to higher rates of chronic illness, low-birth-weight babies and infant mortality, risk of accidents, and many other causes of death and disability (Center for the Advancement of Health, 2002 December). The overwhelming majority of diseases and disorders show an SES gradient, with poor people experiencing greater risk (Minkler et al., 2006). And among diseases that lower- and upper-SES individuals are equally likely to develop, such as breast cancer, mortality is earlier among the more disadvantaged (Leclere, Rogers, & Peters, 1998).

Interventions targeted specifically to low-SES individuals to modify risk factors, such as smoking, drug use, alcohol consumption, and diet, as well as those targeted to more general risk factors such as poor education (Trumbetta, Seltzer, Gottesman, & McIntyre, 2010), need to assume high priority (Major, Mendes, & Dovidio, 2013).

There are substantial racial and ethnic differences in health as well (House, 2015). African Americans have poorer health at all ages (Klonoff, 2009), as well as higher levels of depression, hostility, anxiety, and other emotional risk factors for chronic disease. The life expectancy gap between African Americans and whites remains high, at a more than 4-year difference (National Center for Health Statistics, 2011). African Americans also have a higher infant mortality rate than whites and higher rates of most chronic diseases and disorders, with racial differences especially dramatic for hypertension, HIV, and diabetes (Wong, Shapiro, Boscardin, & Ettner, 2002). Some of this disadvantage is due to low SES, and some of the differences, as noted in Chapter 6, are due to the stress of discrimination (Fuller-Rowell, Evans, & Ong, 2012; Hao et al., 2011; Williams, Priest, & Anderson, 2016).

There are substantial SES and ethnic differences in the delivery of medical treatment as well (Garcia, Bernstein, & Bush, 2010; National Academy of Medicine, 2009). This problem is especially acute for the nation's unemployed workers (Driscoll & Bernstein, 2012). We currently have a two-tiered medical system: High-quality and high-technology care go to the well-to-do and not to the poor and unemployed.

The wars of the past few decades have meant that large numbers of veterans need special attention in the health care system. Veterans are more likely to have multiple chronic health conditions and serious psychological distress than the rest of the population (Kramarow & Pastor, 2012). As veterans age, their needs for services will increase correspondingly as well.

Another significant gap in health care and research concerns gender (Matthews, Gump, Block, & Allen, 1997). For many years, women were not included in medical trials of interventions and new drugs. For diseases that strike both men and women, such as coronary heart disease, evidence about treatments and dosage levels was available only for men. That picture has changed somewhat now, as Federal guidelines mandate that both genders be included in most clinical trials. But some discrimination remains. As one critical article put it, "Women are studied for what distinguishes them from men—their breasts and genitals" (Meyerowitz & Hart, 1993). Weak justification for such discrimination has sometimes been based on the fact that women live, on average, five years longer than men. But women are sick more than men, and their advantage in mortality has been decreasing in recent years. Women are less likely than men to have health insurance, and even if they do, their policies may fail to cover basic medical care, such as Pap smears for the detection of cervical cancer, a standard part of any gynecologic examination (National Academy of Medicine, 2011). More women are insured through their husbands' jobs than the reverse, but because of instability in marriage, coverage for women is irregular. These issues are especially problematic for African

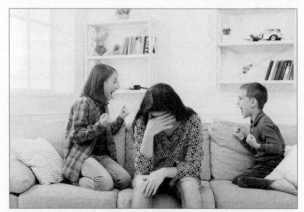

*Stressful living situations with noise, crowding, and crime take a particular toll on vulnerable populations, such as children, the elderly, and the poor. Increasingly, research must focus on interventions to alleviate the impact of these conditions.*
Prostock-studio/Shutterstock

American women (Meyer & Pavalko, 1996). Women's health care is fragmented. Whereas men may have all their needs met and tests done in a single visit, meeting women's health needs may require multiple visits to multiple specialists.

As noted, women have not been included as research subjects in studies of many major diseases, and they need to be. First, women may have different risk factors for major diseases, or existing risk factors may be more or less virulent (Grady, 2004, April 14). For example, smoking may be two to three times more hazardous for women than for men (Taubes, 1993). Consequently, women's symptoms, their age of onset for the same diseases, and their reactions to treatment and dosage levels of medications may all differ.

Stress takes a particular toll on women. The majority of American families find that both parents must work in order to make ends meet, yet, like all families, the two-career family must absorb an extra month a year of housework, home activities, and child care. Typically, this extra month a year is taken on by women (Hochschild, 1989). Moreover, increasing numbers of adult children have responsibility for their aging parents, and these responsibilities, too, more frequently fall to women than to men. These trends put the adult American female population under unprecedented stress, patterns that are increasing in other countries as well. Solutions to these dilemmas have yet to emerge.

In the future, we can expect to see that the health model fabricated around the white male heterosexual will give way to a multitude of models for women, minorities, and lesbian, gay, bisexual, and transgender (LGBT) people (National Academy of Medicine, 2011, March). Each group has its own health risk factors, its particular psychosocial concerns, and its vulnerabilities, including the stress of being marginalized. And as we articulate what the health goals may be for different groups in our population, we will develop a more comprehensive biopsychosocial model (National Academy of Medicine, 2011b).

## ■ STRESS AND ITS MANAGEMENT

The relation of stress to inflammatory processes and their effects on health represents a significant breakthrough of the past few decades (Gianaros & Manuck, 2010). Advances have been made in research on environmental and occupational stress. Stressors such as noise or crowding especially affect vulnerable populations. Thus, the health needs of children, the elderly,

and the poor have taken special priority in the study of stress and its reduction.

Occupational stress researchers have identified many of the job characteristics that are tied to stress, such as low control, high demands, and little opportunity for social support. As a consequence, promising workplace interventions have been developed to redesign jobs or reduce on-the-job stressors.

## Where Is Stress Research Headed?

Many important advances in stress research will come from research on the neurophysiology of stress, particularly the links between stress and corticosteroid functioning, dispositional differences in sympathetic nervous system activity, factors influencing the release of endogenous opioid peptides, and links to the immune system, including inflammatory processes. These studies will elucidate the pathways by which stress exerts adverse effects on health, which may lead to biologically sophisticated interventions. The pivotal role of depression and other negative affective states in development and course of chronic diseases, including cardiovascular disease, diabetes, and stroke, makes these states and the pathways linking them to illness outcomes of critical research importance (Valkanova & Ebmeier, 2013). Nearly one in five older adults, for example, has one or more mental health conditions that contribute to physical illness and complicate care (National Academy of Medicine, 2012, July).

One of the most significant advances in stress research is the discovery that social support can buffer stress. As the country is becoming increasingly single, marriage rates decline, and the population ages, this issue becomes more important. Fostering social support systems to offset social trends that isolate people, such as divorce, bereavement, and geographic mobility, should be a high priority for prevention. Reducing social isolation, promoting the benefits of social ties, alleviating factors that promote toxic social ties such as high-strain work environments, and ensuring that people who most need help are getting it can all help to promote a more healthful social fabric (Umberson & Montez, 2010). In addition, we should teach people how to provide support for others. Many people are aware that getting social support from others benefits their mental and physical health, but most people are not aware that providing social support to others also has health benefits, both for the people to whom they provide support and for themselves. Although this generalization does not extend to extreme cases of caregiving, at a moderate level, helping others through trying times with social support benefits both the provider and the recipient.

Self-help groups, both real and virtual via the Internet, can provide social support for those who otherwise lack it. Through these formats, people can discuss common problems and help each other work them out. Once oriented primarily around particular illnesses, such as cancer, or particular health problems, such as obesity, these groups are becoming increasingly available for those going through divorce, the loss of a child, and other specific stressful events.

## ■ HEALTH SERVICES

Health care reform remains one of the most urgent issues facing the United States (Obama, 2009). Our health care system is marked by at least three basic problems: Health care costs too much; the system is grossly inequitable, and health care consumers use health care services inappropriately (Center for the Advancement of Health, 2006 October).

### Building Better Consumers

Decades of research have indicated that people who are ill and those who are treated for illness are frequently not the same people. For financial or cultural reasons,

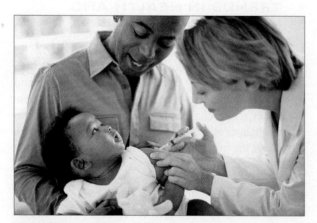

*Misinformation about supposed ill effects of vaccinations has proliferated on the Internet (Betsch & Sachse, 2013). An important part of being a good consumer of health care is being correctly informed about the science that underlies health care recommendation.*

Science Photo Library/Getty Images

many ill people do not find their way into the health care delivery system, and about half to two-thirds of people who seek and receive treatment have complaints that are related to psychological distress (Boyer & Lutfey, 2010). Health psychologists have important roles to play in creating responsible and informed health care consumers.

Increasingly, patients need to be co-managers in their own care, monitoring their symptoms and treatments in partnership with physicians and other health care practitioners. It does little good to diagnose a disorder correctly and prescribe appropriate treatment if the patient cannot or will not follow through on treatment recommendations. Moreover, as good health behaviors are critical to the achievement of good health and to secondary prevention among the chronically ill, the fact that 97 percent of patients fail to adhere to lifestyle recommendations is sobering.

Good consumers of health care need to watch out not only for themselves, but also for others. Health is a public good. This means getting vaccinations to avoid spreading disease, perhaps donating blood, or agreeing to be an organ donor (Sénémeaud, Georget, Guéguen, Callé, Plainfossé, Touati, & Mange, 2014).

Trends within medical care suggest that the problem of patient–provider communication may get worse, not better. Increasingly, patients are receiving their medical care through prepaid, colleague-centered services rather than through private, fee-for-service, client-centered practices. As noted in Chapters 8 and 9, these structural changes can improve the quality of medical care, but they may sacrifice the quality of communication.

Although the well-to-do can pay for emotionally satisfying care, the poor increasingly cannot. Health settings that rob patients of feelings of control can breed anger or depression, motivate people not to return for care, and contribute to a physiological state conducive to illness or its exacerbation. Thus, there is an expanding role for health psychologists in the design of health services.

## ■ MANAGEMENT OF SERIOUS ILLNESS

Chronic illness has become our major health problem and although programs are available to deal with problems posed by chronic illness, these efforts are as yet not systematically coordinated or widely available to the majority of chronically ill patients.

## Quality-of-Life Assessment

A chief goal for health psychologists in the coming years is to develop cost-effective interventions to improve quality of life, especially among the chronically ill. Initial assessment during the acute period is an important first step. Supplementing initial assessment with regular needs assessment over the long term can help identify potential problems, such as anxiety or depression, before they disrupt the patient's life and bring additional costs to the health care system. Adding social health indicators, such as the ability to perform social roles and participate in social activities, lends these assessments new and vital dimensions (Hahn et al., 2014). As these and related psychological states contribute to and aggravate several chronic diseases, as well as chronic pain, an intervention that fails to improve psychological functioning is unlikely to profoundly affect health or survival (Singer, 2000).

Health psychologists need to be involved in the ongoing controversies that surround complementary and alternative medicine. Increasingly, people are treating themselves in nontraditional ways, through herbal medicine, homeopathy, and other untested regimens. Some of these nontraditional methods have health or mental health benefits, but others may address primarily psychological needs, such as the feeling that something active is being done or that a caring provider is giving treatment. Health psychologists need not only to evaluate these complementary and alternative medical practices but also to help develop interventions that will address the psychological needs currently met by these treatments.

With the prevalence of chronic disease increasing and the aging of the population occurring rapidly, ethical issues surrounding death and dying—including assisted death, living wills, the patient's right to die, family decision making on death and dying, and euthanasia—will increasingly assume importance, and health psychologists have an important role to play in addressing these thorny issues.

## The Aging of the Population

The aging of the population poses multiple challenges for health psychologists. What kinds of living situations will older adults have, and what kinds of economic resources will they have available to them? How will these resources influence their health habits, their level of health, and their ability to seek treatment? How can we evaluate and monitor care in residential treatment settings, such as assisted living facilities and nursing homes, to guard against the risks of maltreatment (Olshansky, 2015)?

As our population ages, we can expect to see a higher incidence of chronic but not life-threatening conditions, such as chronic pain, hearing losses, incontinence, and blindness (Molton & Terrill, 2014). Some effort to control these disorders must necessarily focus on prevention. For example, the incidence of deafness is rising, attributable in part to the blasting rock music that teenagers in the 1950s and 1960s (who are now in their older years) listened to. Because rock music is not getting any quieter, and because adolescents now go to rock concerts and use headphones as well, prevention of deafness will take on increasing significance.

Sports-related concussions in youth and among professional athletes are problems whose dimensions are just beginning to be understood (Institute of Medicine, 2013). The damage to cognitive functioning may not be evident for years, but it can presage a debilitating older age. The risks are high: Estimates are that merely playing football for four months carries a risk of head injury as high as 20 percent (*The Economist*, March 5, 2016). Soccer (from headers), rugby, and ice hockey are among the sports with similar risks (*The Economist*, March 5, 2016). Problems with memory, attention, and impulsivity are early effects, with dementia a long-term prospect. These are just two examples of how aging affects health in ways that health psychologists can address (Figure 15.2).

## ■ TRENDS IN HEALTH AND HEALTH PSYCHOLOGY

### Research of the Future

The research of the future will be more integrative than ever. We can combine analyses at multiple levels and look, for example, at types of stressors, changes in stress hormones, brain changes in response to stress, and behavior changes all in the same people, which provides a glimpse at the full pathway from stress to coping through biology to behavior (e.g., Taylor et al., 2006). In the past, inferring these pathways involved cobbling together insights from multiple studies that differed from each other in many ways, and consequently, conclusions were speculative, rather than definitive. That has changed. Increasingly, we use meta-analysis to combine the results of many different studies, so results may be based on thousands of people, rather than dozens (Molloy, Noone, Caldwell, Welton, & Newell, 2018). Large longitudinal data sets give us opportunities to test whether psychosocial and

**FIGURE 15.2 | The World's Population Is Growing Rapidly, Especially in Less-Developed Countries, and Getting Older**    *Source:* United Nations, Department of Economic and Social Affairs, Population Division. "World Population Prospects The 2010 Revision." Last modified 2011. https://www.un.org/en/development/desa/population/publications/pdf/trends/WPP2010/WPP2010_Volume-I_Comprehensive-Tables.pdf.

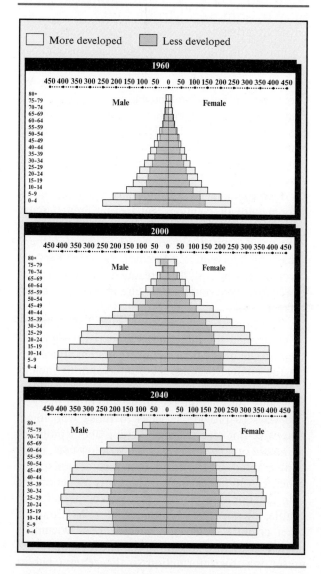

## The Changing Nature of Medical Practice

Health psychology needs to be continually responsive to changes in health trends and medical practice. The physical environment poses unprecedented challenges. For example, current levels of air pollution have chronic negative effects on lung development in children, leading to risks not only in childhood but in adulthood as well (Gauderman et al., 2004). Climate change affects patterns of illness. For example, tropical diseases such as malaria and diarrheal disorders are increasing in frequency and spreading north (Jack, 2007, April 25). Changes in society, technology, and microorganisms themselves are leading to the emergence of new diseases, the reemergence of diseases that were once controlled, and problems with drug-resistant strains of once-controlled disorders (Emerson & Purcell, 2004; Hien, de Jong, & Farrar, 2004).

Genetic testing availability means that an increasing number of people will know that they have a risk for illness before they develop that illness. How to disseminate that information both publicly through the media and individually to people at risk requires understanding social communication.

## The Impact of Technology    Technological advances in medicine have contributed greatly to the enormous costs of contemporary medicine. These complex aspects of medicine can themselves be daunting for

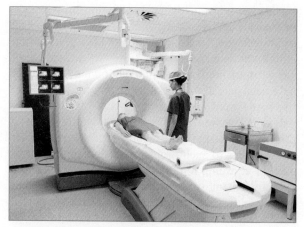

*The technologically complex aspects of medicine are often intimidating to patients, but when the purpose of the technology is fully explained and patients are committed to its use, it helps reduce this anxiety.*

Johnny Greig/E+/Getty Images

health-related predictors lead to the outcomes we expect. We have spent decades building this research base, and now it is available for producing the integrative research that allows us to go forward with confidence in our own conclusions. And technology enables us to get efficient online interventions to millions of people, rather than dozens.

many patients. Explaining the purposes of these technologies and using control-enhancing interventions so that people feel like active participants in their treatment can help reduce fear.

The increasing role of technology in health services presents great opportunities to reach more people with effective interventions. Changing diet, expanding social support opportunities, stop-smoking interventions, and online programs to reduce depression are just a few of the ways in which the Internet can be enlisted to improve health.

Advances in the decision sciences can be harnessed to improve health care decision making. For example, older adults choosing Medicare Part D coverage for prescriptions can be presented with as many as 35 options, and from this bewildering array, it may be difficult to pick the right plan. Together with economists, health psychologists can help make medical decision-making processes easier through the development of simple decision-making tools (Szrek & Bundorf, 2014; Thaler & Sunstein, 2009).

Comprehensive Intervention   A trend within medicine that affects health psychology is the movement toward **comprehensive intervention models**. An example is pain management programs, in which all available treatments for pain are brought together so that individual regimens can be developed for each patient. A second model is the hospice, in which palliative management technologies and psychotherapeutic technologies are available to the dying patient. Coordinated residential and outpatient rehabilitation programs for coronary heart disease patients, in which multiple health habits are dealt with simultaneously, constitute a third example.

Most comprehensive intervention models thus far have been geared to specific diseases or disorders, but this model may be employed for concerted attacks on risk factors as well. The mass media, youth prevention projects, educational interventions, and social engineering solutions to such problems as smoking, excessive alcohol consumption, and drug abuse, for example, can supplement programs that currently focus primarily on health risks that are already in place. The coordination of public health management at the institutional and community levels, with individual health and illness management for those already ill, is represented in Figure 15.3.

Although comprehensive interventions may provide the best quality of care, they are also expensive. Some hospitals have already dismantled their pain

management centers, for example, for lack of funds. For comprehensive intervention models to continue to define the highest quality of care, attention must be paid to **cost-effectiveness** as well as to **treatment effectiveness**.

## Systematic Documentation of Cost-Effectiveness and Treatment Effectiveness

An important professional goal of health psychology, therefore, is the continued documentation of the effectiveness of our interventions (Shadish, 2010). We know that our behavioral, cognitive, and psychotherapeutic technologies work, but we must communicate this success to others. This issue has taken on considerable significance as debate rages over to what degree behavioral and psychological interventions should be covered in managed health care systems.

**Cost containment** pressures have prompted the development of interventions that are time limited, symptom focused, and offered on an outpatient basis, a format that is not always conducive to change through behavioral intervention. Moreover, this trend has been accompanied by a shift in treatment decision-making power from behavioral health care providers to policy makers.

The pressures of cost containment push health psychology in the direction of research designed to keep people out of the health care system altogether. On the clinical practice side, interventions include self-help groups, peer counseling, self-management programs, Internet interventions, and other inexpensive ways to provide services to those who might otherwise not receive care. Writing about intensely traumatic or stressful events is also a low-cost, easily implemented intervention that has demonstrated benefits. Another example is the stress reduction and pain amelioration benefits that can be achieved by simple, inexpensive techniques of relaxation and other cognitive–behavioral interventions. Documenting effectiveness, developing convincing methods of presenting this information to the general public, and identifying the most critical components of behavioral interventions that produce the most behavior change at the lowest cost (Napolitano et al., 2008) will all contribute to establishing the effectiveness of health psychology interventions. Table 15.2 shows the reduction in health care visits that can occur as a result of health psychology interventions.

The potential for health psychology to make contributions to medicine and medical practice has never

**FIGURE 15.3 | Continuum of Care and Types and Levels of Intervention**   *Source:* Abrams, D. B., C. T. Orleans, R. S. Niaura, M. G. Goldstein, J. O. Prochaska, and W. Velicer. "Integrating Individual and Public Health Perspectives for Treatment of Tobacco Dependence Under Managed Health Care: A Combined Stepped-Care and Matching Model." *Annals of Behavioral Medicine,* 18, no. 4 (Spring 1996): 290–304.

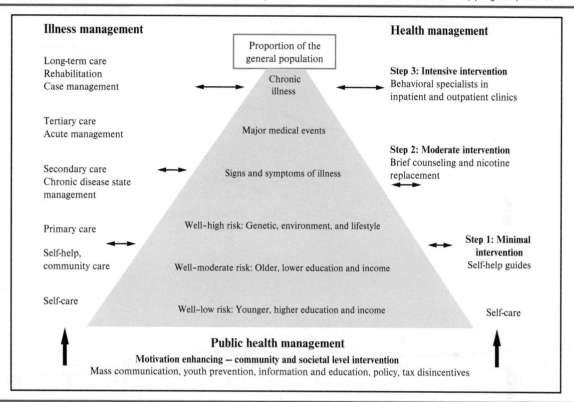

been greater. Evidence-based medicine is now the criterion for adopting medical standards. Evidence-based medicine refers to the conscientious, explicit, judicious

**TABLE 15.2 | The Bottom Line**

This chart shows the reduction in frequency of treatments that can result from clinical behavioral medicine interventions.

| Treatment | Frequency reduction (%) |
|---|---|
| Total ambulatory care visits | −17 |
| Visits for minor illnesses | −35 |
| Pediatric acute illness visits | −25 |
| Office visits for acute asthma | −49 |
| Office visits by arthritis patients | −40 |
| Cesarean sections | −56 |
| Epidural anesthesia during labor and delivery | −85 |
| Average hospital length of stay for surgical patients (in days) | −1.5 |

*Source:* American Psychological Society. "APS Observer: Special Issue HCI Report 4—Health Living." Last modified 1996.

use of the best scientific evidence for making decisions about the care of individual patients. This trend means that, with documentation of the success of health psychology interventions, the potential for empirical evidence to contribute to practice is enhanced.

## International Health

The world's population has increased from 2.5 billion in 1950 to over 7.5 billion at the present time (U.S. Census Bureau, May 2019). Increasingly, the population has shifted away from Europe, North America, and Latin America toward Africa and Asia. Life expectancy has increased almost everywhere in the world, with substantial improvements in developing countries. Significant challenges are created by these patterns, and increasingly, there is an important role for health psychologists in international health.

Disease prevalence varies greatly by country. Poverty, lack of education, and lack of health care resources contribute to a high incidence of acute infectious disease. Low rates of literacy and health literacy worsen these problems (Kiernan, Oppezzo, Resnicow, &

**FIGURE 15.4 | National Health Care Expenditures: Selected Calendar Years, 1990–2020\***

Sources: Centers for Medicare and Medicaid Services. "National Health Expenditures and Selected Economic Indicators, Levels and Average Annual Percent Change: Selected Calendar Years 1990–2013." Last modified 2014; Centers for Medicare and Medicaid Services. "National Health Expenditure Data." Last modified 2011. https://www.cms.gov/Research-Statistics-Data-and-Systems/Statistics-Trends-and-Reports/NationalHealthExpendData/index.html?redirect=/nationalhealthexpenddata/02_nationalhealthaccountshistorical.asp.

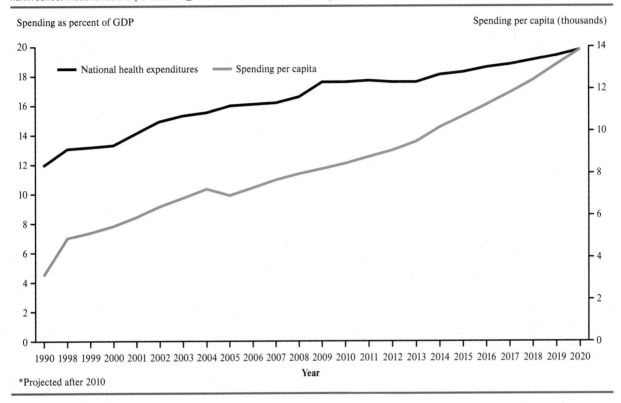

Spending as percent of GDP

Spending per capita (thousands)

National health expenditures — Spending per capita

*Projected after 2010

Alexander, 2018). Although smoking has declined in the United States, its incidence is rising in many developing countries. Whereas Americans are beginning to exercise more, countries that are becoming modernized are losing the exercise benefits that accompanied an active lifestyle. Many developing nations, such as China and India, are beginning to experience the burden of increases in chronic disease and poor health habits. Chronic disability is a major health cost in all countries. In developed countries with aging populations, lower back pain is the chief cause of disability, whereas in poorer and younger populations, depression is the primary cause of disability (*The Economist*, June 20, 2015).

Despite the ongoing importance of infectious disease, the health issues facing developing countries are looking increasingly like those of developed countries (*The Economist*, August 2017a). For example, the number of obese children in the world is predicted to surpass the number of malnourished children within the next 3 years (World Health Organization, 2017).

Chronic, noncommunicable conditions now account for about 70 percent of deaths in developing nations, as deaths from malaria and HIV have declined. Basic primary care, accordingly, becomes the essential focus of medicine in these countries, as it already is in developed countries (*The Economist*, April 2018). Telemedicine makes it easier to reach urban and isolated areas, so that, at the very least, an initial screening visit with a physician can begin to pinpoint what is wrong; chronic conditions, however, can necessitate ongoing care and contact that may not be available. Diabetes and mental illness, for example, are two conditions that often go undiagnosed and untreated (*The Economist*, August 2017b).

Health psychology can carry the hard-won intervention lessons from the United States to countries in which exactly the same problems are now beginning to emerge (National Academy of Medicine, 2011b). Moreover, health psychologists understand the significance of varying cultural norms and expectations, the ways social institutions function, and the roles that culturally specific attitudes and behaviors may play in health care practices and decisions (Cislaghi & Heise, 2018). Paying attention to these cultural factors is vital, because an intervention that works in one country may not have the right cultural focus for another country (Armistead et al., 2014). In the battle for a high level of international health, then, the health psychologist can make a substantial contribution.

## ■ BECOMING A HEALTH PSYCHOLOGIST

If you want to pursue a career in this field, what would you need to do?

### Undergraduate Experience

As an undergraduate interested in continuing health psychology, you would be wise to do several things. First, take all the health psychology courses that you can. Second, develop knowledge about the biological bases of behavior by taking courses in physiological psychology and neuroscience. Understanding the biological underpinnings of health psychology is important.

In addition, you should use your summers effectively. Find a psychologist who does research in health psychology, and see if you can get a research assistantship. Volunteer if you have to. You can look for summer employment opportunities in a medical school or hospital, which might give you patient contact or contact with medical care providers. Or you might try to find a managed care program that has internship opportunities. Even if you are involved only in paperwork, find out how the organization works. What kinds of patients does it see? How is the organization trying to reduce costs? How is the organization changing? Ask a lot of questions.

In addition, look for opportunities to get practical, hands-on field experience. If you're interested in exercise, for example, go to a fitness center. If you want to understand how people cope with HIV, volunteer at a local organization that assists people with HIV. If you're interested in aging, volunteer at senior citizen centers or other facilities for older adults.

### Graduate Experience

If you decide you want to go into the profession of health psychology, you will need to acquire a PhD. At this point, you should decide whether your interests lie chiefly in research, in clinical practice (i.e., direct contact with individual patients), or both (Novacek, 2016).

If your interest is in research, what kind of research excites you the most? Is it the study of how psychological and biological factors affect each other? Is it understanding how social support affects health? Is it research on increasing exercise or changing diet?

Many psychology departments now have graduate programs in health psychology, but others may require you to apply to a related program. Your choices are likely to be physiological psychology, which focuses heavily on the biology and neurological aspects of health psychology; social psychology, which examines social and psychological processes related to health; clinical psychology, in which interventions with patients will be one of your primary tasks; or developmental psychology, in which you may look especially at the health of children and the factors that affect it.

During your years in graduate school, if your interests are even partly in research, take courses in research methodology and statistics. You may take a course in epidemiology, as many health psychologists do, which would probably be taught in a school of public health. Most importantly, get practical experience. Work with a health psychologist on several research or clinical projects. Try to get into the field so that you gain experience not just in a university laboratory but also in a hospital, a clinic, or another health care delivery situation.

If you apply to a clinical psychology program, you will be expected to take the standard clinical curriculum, which includes courses and practical experience addressing major mental disorders and community intervention and therapy. Consequently, your patient contact not only will involve people with medical problems but also will be heavily geared toward people with depression, anxiety, psychoses, and other psychological disorders. You will need to complete a year's internship in a field setting, so if your interests are in health, you should try for a field setting in a hospital, clinic, or health maintenance organization that gives you direct patient contact.

At the time of your dissertation, you will be expected to mount a major research project on your own. By this time, you will have a clear idea of what your interests are and can pursue a health-related project in depth. This project will take you a year or more to complete.

If you are in clinical health psychology, your training, coupled with your internship, should help you get licensed in the state in which you choose to practice. You will have to take several hours of licensure exams, the exact form of which varies from state to state; on receipt of your license, you will be able to practice clinical psychology.

## Postgraduate Work

Following graduate school, you can look for a job, or you can get additional training in the form of postdoctoral research or clinical practice. Many health psychologists choose to acquire postdoctoral training, because training in health psychology at any one university depends heavily on the interests of the faculty who are there. You may, for example, specialize in stress and coping processes but be less well-informed about health behaviors. Or your program may provide you with lots of patient contact but very little in the way of training in neuroscience. You may decide that you want to concentrate on a particular disease, such as cancer or heart disease, but have insufficient knowledge about its risk factors, progression, and treatment. Identifying the gaps in your training reveals the type of postdoctoral training you should seek out.

Typically, postdoctoral training is undertaken at a laboratory different from the place at which you completed your PhD and takes place under the guidance of a senior scientist whose work you admire. You may spend up to 3 years in this person's lab, after which you should be ready for employment in health psychology.

## Employment

Many health psychologists go into academic settings or teach in medical schools. In academic positions, health psychologists are responsible for educating undergraduate and graduate students, physicians, nurses, and other health care workers. Most health psychologists in academic settings also conduct research to uncover the factors associated with the maintenance of health and the onset of and recovery from illness.

An increasing number of health psychologists work with medical patients in a hospital and in primary care (Fisher & Dickinson, 2014). Some are also involved in private practice, in which they provide therapy and other mental health services to people with medically related problems. The short-term cognitive–behavioral interventions that work well in modifying health behaviors, controlling pain, and managing issues in chronic illness are examples of activities that health psychologists in these settings undertake. Increasingly, health psychologists are employed in the workplace or as consultants to the workplace. They advise employers attempting to set up new health care systems about what kind of system will provide the best care for the least money. For example, they may establish work-site interventions to teach employees how to manage stress, stop smoking, and get more exercise. Health psychologists work with governmental agencies on how to reduce health care costs. They also advise health care services about how to improve patient satisfaction or reduce inappropriate use of health services.  •

## SUMMARY

1. Great progress in improving the health of the nation has been made, and health psychology has contributed meaningfully to the scientific and clinical bases of these improvements.

2. Health promotion priorities include modifying the most consequential risk factors and incorporating the most potent and effective elements of behavior change programs into low-cost and efficient interventions, including the use of technology such as mobile phones and the Internet.

3. Health psychology interventions focus on people at risk for particular disorders, on preventing poor health habits from developing, and on developing effective health promotion interventions with older adults. Health promotion efforts address not only mortality but also the reduction of morbidity and the importance of enhancing overall quality of life.

4. An effective health promotion program must involve not only health behavior change but also social change that makes high-quality health care available to all the population, especially those low in SES.

5. Research on stress will continue to focus on vulnerable populations and on trends in the economy and culture that increase stress on particular groups, such as children, women, older adults, racial and ethnic minorities, the unemployed, and the poor.

6. In the future, many important advances in stress research will come from research examining the biopsychosocial pathways by which stress adversely affects health.

7. A focus of health services research is to build better consumers and to reduce the improper use of services, and nonadherence to medication and lifestyle recommendations.

8. The management of chronic and terminal illness will increasingly focus on quality of life and appropriate ways to measure it. Ethical and psychosocial issues involving assisted suicide, living wills, the patient's right to die, family decision making in death and dying, and euthanasia will continue to be prominent.

9. A target for future work is identification of the health and lifestyle issues that will be created by the aging of the population. Anticipating medical disorders and developing interventions to offset their potential adverse effects should be targets for research now.

10. Health psychology needs to be responsive to changes in medical practice, including changes in disease demographics (such as age). The changing face of medicine creates challenges for health psychologists, who must anticipate the impact of technologically complex interventions and help prepare patients for them.

11. Important goals for health psychology include systematic documentation of treatment effectiveness using the criteria of evidence-based medicine, systematic documentation of the cost-effectiveness of interventions, and continued efforts to find ways to reduce health costs. In addition, there is an emerging and important role for health psychologists in the international health care arena.

12. Health psychology can be a rewarding career for anyone willing to gain the necessary education and experience in research and field settings.

## KEY TERMS

behavioral immunization
comprehensive intervention
  models
cost containment
cost-effectiveness
treatment effectiveness

# GLOSSARY

**abstinence violation effect**   A feeling of loss of control that results when one has violated self-imposed rules, such as not to smoke or drink.

**acquired immune deficiency syndrome (AIDS)**   Progressive impairment of the immune system by the human immunodeficiency virus (HIV); a diagnosis of AIDS is made on the basis of the presence of one or more specific opportunistic infections or a very low CD4 cell count.

**acupuncture**   A technique of healing and pain control, developed in China, in which long, thin needles are inserted into designated areas of the body to reduce discomfort in a target area.

**acute disorders**   Illnesses or other medical problems that occur over a short time, that are usually the result of an infectious process, and that are reversible.

**acute pain**   Short-term pain that usually results from a specific injury.

**acute stress paradigm**   A laboratory procedure whereby an individual goes through moderately stressful procedures (such as counting backward rapidly by 7s), so that stress-related changes in emotions and physiological and/or neuroendocrine processes may be assessed.

**addiction**   The state of physical or psychological dependence on a substance that develops when that substance is used over a period of time.

**adherence**   The degree to which an individual follows a recommended health-related or illness-related recommendation.

**adrenal glands**   Two small glands, located on top of the kidneys, that are part of the endocrine system and secrete several hormones, including cortisol, epinephrine, and norepinephrine, which are involved in responses to stress.

**aerobic exercise**   High-intensity, long-duration, and high-endurance exercise, believed to contribute to cardiovascular fitness and other positive health outcomes. Examples are jogging, bicycling, running, and swimming.

**aftereffects of stress**   Performance and attentional decrements that occur after a stressful event has subsided; believed to be produced by the residual physiological, emotional, and cognitive draining in response to stressful events.

**alcoholism**   The state of physical addiction to alcohol that manifests through such symptoms as stereotyped drinking, drinking to maintain blood alcohol at a particular level, increasing frequency and severity of withdrawal, drinking early in the day and in the middle of the night, a sense of loss of control over drinking, and a subjective craving for alcohol.

**allostatic load**   The accumulating adverse effects of stress, in conjunction with pre existing risks, on biological stress regulatory systems.

**angina pectoris**   Chest pain that occurs because the muscle tissue of the heart is deprived of adequate oxygen or because removal of carbon dioxide and other wastes interferes with the flow of blood and oxygen to the heart.

**anorexia nervosa**   A condition produced by excessive dieting and exercise that yields body weight grossly below optimal level, most common among adolescent girls.

**appraisal delay**   The time between recognizing that a symptom exists and deciding that it is serious.

**approach (confrontative, vigilant) coping style**   The tendency to cope with stressful events by tackling them directly and attempting to develop solutions; may ultimately be an especially effective method of coping, although it may produce accompanying distress.

**assertiveness training**   Techniques that train people how to be appropriately assertive in social situations; often included as part of health behavior modification programs, on the assumption that some poor health habits, such as excessive alcohol consumption or smoking, develop in part to control difficulties in being appropriately assertive.

**atherosclerosis**   A major cause of heart disease; caused by the narrowing of the arterial walls due to the formation of plaques that reduce the flow of blood through the arteries and interfere with the passage of nutrients from the capillaries into the cells.

**at risk**   A state of vulnerability to a particular health problem by virtue of heredity, health practices, or family environment.

**autoimmunity**   A condition in which the body produces an immune response against its own tissue constituents.

**avoidant (minimizing) coping style**   The tendency to cope with threatening events by withdrawing, minimizing, or avoiding them; believed to be an effective short-term, though not an effective long-term, response to stress.

**ayurvedic medicine**   An ancient approach to healing developed in India that focuses on balance among the mind, body, and spirit.

**behavioral assignments**   Home practice activities that clients perform on their own as part of an integrated therapeutic intervention for behavior modification.

**behavioral delay**   The time between deciding to seek treatment and actually doing so.

**behavioral immunization** Programs designed to inoculate people against adverse health habits by exposing them to mild versions of persuasive communications that try to engage them in a poor health practice and giving them techniques that they can use to respond effectively to these efforts.

**behavioral inoculation** Providing a person with a weak form of an argument, thus giving him or her the opportunity to develop counterarguments and successfully resist the message; similar to inoculation against disease.

**binge eating disorder** A serious eating disorder involving frequently consuming large amounts of food and feeling unable to stop eating.

**bingeing** A pattern of disordered eating that consists of episodes of uncontrollable eating. During such binges, a person rapidly consumes an excessive amount of food.

**biofeedback** A method whereby an individual is provided with ongoing, specific information or feedback about how a particular physiological process operates, so that he or she can learn how to modify that process.

**biomedical model** The viewpoint that illness can be explained on the basis of aberrant somatic processes and that psychological and social processes are largely independent of the disease process; the dominant model in medical practice until recently.

**biopsychosocial model** The view that biological, psychological, and social factors are all involved in any given state of health or illness.

**blood pressure** The force that blood exerts against vessel walls.

**body image** The perception and evaluation of one's body, one's physical functioning, and one's appearance.

**buffering hypothesis** The hypothesis that coping resources are useful primarily under conditions of high stress and not necessarily under conditions of low stress.

**bulimia** An eating syndrome characterized by alternating cycles of binge eating and purging through such techniques as vomiting and extreme dieting.

**cardiac invalidism** A psychological state that can result after a myocardial infarction or diagnosis of coronary heart disease, consisting of the perception that a patient's abilities and capacities are lower than they actually are; both patients and their spouses are vulnerable to these misperceptions.

**cardiac rehabilitation** An intervention program designed to help heart patients achieve their optimal physical, medical, psychological, social, emotional, vocational, and economic status after the diagnosis of heart disease or a heart attack.

**cardiopulmonary resuscitation (CPR)** A method of reviving the functioning of heart and lungs after a loss of consciousness in which the patient's pulse has ceased or lungs have failed to function appropriately.

**cardiovascular disease (CVD)** Chronically high blood pressure resulting from too much blood passing through too narrow vessels.

**cardiovascular system** The transport system of the body responsible for carrying oxygen and nutrients to the body and carrying away carbon dioxide and other wastes to the kidneys for excretion; composed of the heart, blood vessels, and blood.

**catecholamines** The neurotransmitters, epinephrine and norepinephrine, that promote sympathetic nervous system activity; released in substantial quantities during stressful times.

**cell-mediated immunity** A slow-acting immunologic reaction involving T lymphocytes from the thymus gland; effective in defending against viral infections that have invaded the cells, and against fungi, parasites, foreign tissues, and cancer.

**cerebellum** The part of the hindbrain responsible for the coordination of voluntary muscle movement, the maintenance of balance and equilibrium, and the maintenance of muscle tone and posture.

**cerebral cortex** The main portion of the brain, responsible for intelligence, memory, and the detection and interpretation of sensation.

**chiropractic medicine** A type of medicine that involves performing adjustments on the spine and joints to correct misalignments that are believed to both prevent and cure illness.

**chronic benign pain** Pain that typically persists for six months or longer and is relatively intractable to treatment. The pain varies in severity and may involve any of a number of muscle groups. Chronic low back pain and myofascial pain syndrome are examples.

**chronic illnesses** Illnesses that are long-lasting and usually irreversible.

**chronic pain** Pain that may begin after an injury but that does not respond to treatment and persists over time.

**chronic progressive pain** Pain that persists longer than six months and increases in severity over time. Typically, it is associated with malignancies or degenerative disorders, such as skeletal metastatic disease or rheumatoid arthritis.

**chronic strain** A stressful experience that is a usual but continually stressful aspect of life.

**classical conditioning** The pairing of a stimulus with an unconditioned reflex, such that over time the new stimulus acquires a conditioned response, evoking the same behavior; the process by which an automatic response is conditioned to a new stimulus.

**clinical thanatology** The clinical practice of counseling people who are dying on the basis of knowledge of reactions to dying.

**cognitive-behavioral therapy (CBT)** The use of principles from learning theory to modify the cognitions and behaviors associated with a behavior to be modified; cognitive–behavioral approaches are used to modify poor health habits, such as smoking, poor diet, and alcoholism.

**cognitive restructuring**  A method of modifying internal monologues in stress-producing situations; clients are trained to monitor what they say to themselves in stress-provoking situations and then to modify their cognitions in adaptive ways.

**colleague orientation**  A physician orientation toward gaining the esteem and regard of one's colleagues; fostered by any health care provider arrangement that does not involve direct reimbursement to physicians by patients.

**commonsense model of illness**  A model maintaining that people hold implicit commonsense beliefs about their symptoms and illnesses that result in organized illness representations or schemas and that influence their treatment decisions and adherence.

**complementary and alternative medicine (CAM)**  A diverse group of therapies, products, and medical treatments that are not generally considered part of conventional medicine, including prayer, potions, natural herb products, meditation, yoga, massage, homeopathic medicines, and acupuncture, among other treatments.

**comprehensive intervention models**  Models that pool and coordinate the medical and psychological expertise in a well-defined area of medical practice so as to make all available technology and expertise available to a patient; the pain management program is one example of a comprehensive intervention model.

**contingency contracting**  A procedure in which an individual forms a contract with another person, such as a therapist, detailing what rewards or punishments are contingent on the performance or nonperformance of a target behavior.

**control-enhancing interventions**  Interventions with patients who are awaiting treatment for the purpose of enhancing their perceptions of control over those treatments.

**controlled drinking**  Training in discriminating blood alcohol level so as to control the extent of drinking; may also include coping skills for dealing with situations that are high risk for high alcohol consumption; see also **placebo drinking.**

**conversion hysteria**  The viewpoint, originally advanced by Freud, that specific unconscious conflicts can produce physical disturbances symbolic of the repressed conflict; no longer a dominant viewpoint in health psychology.

**coping**  The process of trying to manage demands that are appraised as taxing or exceeding one's resources.

**coping outcomes**  The beneficial effects that are thought to result from successful coping; these include reducing stress, adjusting more successfully to it, maintaining emotional equilibrium, having satisfying relationships with others, and maintaining a positive self-image.

**coping style**  An individual's preferred method of dealing with stressful situations.

**coronary heart disease (CHD)**  A general term referring to illnesses caused by atherosclerosis, which is the narrowing of the coronary arteries, the vessels that supply the heart with blood.

**correlational research**  Measuring two variables and determining whether they are associated with each other. Studies relating smoking to lung cancer are correlational, for example.

**cost containment**  The effort to reduce or hold down health care costs.

**cost-effectiveness**  The formal evaluation of the effectiveness of an intervention relative to its cost and the cost of alternative interventions.

**counterirritation**  A pain control technique that involves inhibiting pain in one part of the body by stimulating or mildly irritating another area, sometimes adjacent to the area in which the pain is experienced.

**craving**  A strong desire to engage in a behavior or consume a substance, such as alcohol or tobacco, which appears, in part, to occur through the conditioning of physical dependence on environmental cues associated with the behavior.

**creative nonadherence**  The modification or supplementation of a prescribed treatment regimen on the basis of privately held theories about the disorder or its treatment.

**curative care**  Care designed to cure a patient's underlying disease.

**daily hassles**  Minor daily stressful events; believed to have a cumulative effect in increasing the likelihood of illness.

**death education**  Programs designed to inform people realistically about death and dying, the purpose of which is to reduce the terror connected with and avoidance of the topic.

**delay behavior**  The act of delaying seeking treatment for recognized symptoms.

**demand-control-support model**  Model of job stress developed by Karasek and associates that suggests that high demands, low control, and little support enhance risk for ill health, especially coronary artery disease.

**denial**  A defense mechanism involving the inability to recognize or deal with external threatening events; believed to be an early reaction to the diagnosis of a chronic or terminal illness.

**depression**  A mood disorder marked especially by sadness, a lack of interest or pleasure, inactivity, difficulty with thinking and concentration, a significant increase or decrease in appetite and time spent sleeping, feelings of dejection and hopelessness, and sometimes suicidal thoughts or an attempt to commit suicide.

**detoxification**  The process of withdrawing from alcohol, usually conducted in a supervised, medically monitored setting.

**diagnostic-related group (DRG)**    A patient classification scheme that specifies the nature and length of treatment for particular disorders; used by some third-party reimbursement systems to determine the amount of reimbursement.

**dietary supplements**    Preparations that contain nutrients, such as vitamins, minerals, or fiber, in amounts that are as high as or higher than the National Academy of Medicine daily recommendations.

**dietitians**    Trained and licensed individuals who apply principles of nutrition and food management to meal planning for institutions such as hospitals or for individuals who need help planning and managing special diets.

**direct effects hypothesis**    The theory that coping resources, such as social support, have beneficial psychological and health effects under conditions of both high stress and low stress.

**discriminative stimulus**    An environmental stimulus that is capable of eliciting a particular behavior; for example, the sight of food may act as a discriminative stimulus for eating.

**distraction**    A pain control method that may involve either focusing on a stimulus irrelevant to the pain experience or reinterpreting the pain experience; redirecting attention to reduce pain.

**double-blind experiment**    An experimental procedure in which neither the researcher nor the patient knows whether the patient received the real treatment or the placebo until precoded records indicating which patient received which are consulted; designed to reduce the possibility that expectations for success will increase evidence for success.

**emotion-focused coping**    Efforts to regulate emotions associated with a stressful encounter.

**emotional-approach coping**    The process of acknowledging, processing, and expressing the emotions experienced in conjunction with a stressor; generally has positive effects on psychological functioning and health.

**emotional support**    Indications from other people that one is loved, valued, and cared for; believed to be an important aspect of social support during times of stress.

**endocrine system**    A bodily system of ductless glands that secrete hormones into the blood to stimulate target organs; interacts with nervous system functioning.

**endogenous opioid peptides**    Opiate-like substances produced by the body.

**epidemiology**    The study of the frequency, distribution, and causes of infectious and noninfectious disease in a population, based on an investigation of the physical and social environment. Thus, for example, epidemiologists not only study who has what kind of cancer but also address questions such as why certain cancers are more prevalent in particular geographic areas than other cancers are.

**etiology**    The origins and causes of illness.

**euthanasia**    Ending the life of a person who has a painful terminal illness for the purpose of terminating the individual's suffering.

**evidence-based medicine**    Uses the scientific method to determine the best available treatments for disorders. Typically drawing on double-blind placebo-controlled clinical trials, evidence-based medicine is increasingly the standard for clinical decision making in health care.

**experiment**    A type of research in which a researcher randomly assigns people to two or more conditions, varies the treatments that people in each condition are given, and then measures the effect on some response.

**fear appeals**    Efforts to change attitudes by arousing fear to induce the motivation to change behavior; fear appeals are used to try to get people to change poor health habits.

**fight-or-flight response**    A response to a threat in which the body is rapidly aroused and motivated via the sympathetic nervous system and the endocrine system to attack or flee a threatening stimulus; the response was first described by Walter Cannon in 1932.

**functional somatic syndromes**    Syndromes marked by the symptoms, suffering, and disability they cause rather than by demonstrable tissue abnormality.

**gate-control theory of pain**    A theory detailing how the experience of pain is reflected in sensory, psychological, and behavioral responses.

**general adaptation syndrome**    Developed by Hans Selye, a profile of how organisms respond to stress; the general adaptation syndrome is characterized by three phases: a nonspecific mobilization phase, which promotes sympathetic nervous system activity; a resistance phase, during which the organism makes efforts to cope with the threat; and an exhaustion phase, which occurs if the organism fails to overcome the threat and depletes its physiological resources.

**gout**    A form of arthritis produced by a buildup of uric acid in the body, producing crystals that become lodged in the joints; the most commonly affected area is the big toe.

**grief**    A response to bereavement involving a feeling of hollowness and sometimes marked by preoccupation with the dead person, expressions of hostility toward others, and guilt over the death; may also involve restlessness, an inability to concentrate, and other adverse psychological and physical symptoms.

**guided imagery**    A technique of relaxation and pain control in which a person conjures up a picture that is held in mind during a painful or stressful experience.

**health**    The absence of disease or infirmity, coupled with a complete state of physical, mental, and social well-being; health psychologists recognize health to be a state that is actively achieved rather than the mere absence of illness.

**health behaviors**    Behaviors undertaken by people to enhance or maintain their health, such as exercise or the consumption of a healthy diet.

**health belief model**    A theory of health behaviors; the model predicts that whether a person practices a particular health habit can be understood by knowing the degree to which the person perceives a personal health threat and the perception that a particular health practice will be effective in reducing that threat.

**health habit**    A health-related behavior that is firmly established and often performed automatically, such as buckling a seat belt or brushing one's teeth.

**health locus of control**    The perception that one's health is under personal control; is controlled by powerful others, such as physicians; or is determined by external factors, including chance.

**health maintenance organization (HMO)**    An organizational arrangement for receiving health care services, by which an individual pays a standard monthly rate and then uses services as needed at no additional or at greatly reduced cost.

**health promotion**    A general philosophy maintaining that health is a personal and collective achievement; the process of enabling people to increase control over and improve their health. Health promotion may occur through individual efforts, through interaction with the medical system, and through a concerted health policy effort.

**health psychology**    The area within psychology devoted to understanding psychological influences on health, illness, and responses to those states, as well as the psychological origins and impacts of health policy and health interventions.

**holistic health**    A philosophy characterized by the belief that health is a positive state that is actively achieved; usually associated with certain nontraditional health practices.

**holistic medicine**    An approach to treatment that deals with the physical, psychological, and spiritual needs of the person.

**home care**    Care for dying patients in the home; the choice of care for the majority of terminally ill patients, though sometimes problematic for family members.

**homeopathy**    A system of alternative medicine that interprets disease and illness as caused by disturbances in a vital life force and treats patients using diluted preparations that cause symptoms similar to those from which the patient suffers.

**hospice**    An institution for dying patients that encourages personalized, warm, palliative care.

**hospice care**    An alternative to hospital and home care, designed to provide warm, personal comfort for terminally ill patients; may be residential or home-based.

**human immunodeficiency virus (HIV)**    The virus that is implicated in the development of AIDS.

**humoral immunity**    A fast-acting immunologic reaction mediated by B lymphocytes that secrete antibodies into the bloodstream; effective in defending against bacterial infections and viral infections that have not yet invaded the cells.

**hypertension**    Excessively high blood pressure that occurs when the supply of blood through the blood vessels is excessive, putting pressure on the vessel walls; a risk factor for a variety of medical problems, including coronary heart disease.

**hypnosis**    A pain management technique involving relaxation, suggestion, distraction, and the focusing of attention.

**hypothalamus**    The part of the forebrain responsible for regulating water balance and controlling hunger and sexual desire; assists in cardiac functioning, blood pressure regulation, and respiration regulation; plays a major role in regulation of the endocrine system, which controls the release of hormones, including those related to stress.

**illness delay**    The time between recognizing that a symptom implies an illness and the decision to seek treatment.

**illness representations**    An organized set of beliefs about an illness or a type of illness, including its nature, cause, duration, and consequences.

**immunity**    The body's resistance to injury from invading organisms, acquired from the mother at birth, through disease, or through vaccinations and inoculations.

**infant mortality rate**    The number of infant deaths per thousand infants.

**informational support**    The provision of information to a person experiencing stress by friends, family, and other people in the individual's social network; believed to help reduce the distressing and health-compromising effects of stress.

**integrative medicine**    The combination of practices of alternative medicine and conventional medicine.

**invisible support**    Support received from another person that is outside the recipient's awareness.

**ischemia**    A deficiency of blood to the heart due to obstruction or constriction of the coronary arteries; often associated with chest pain.

**John Henryism**    A personality predisposition to cope actively with psychosocial stressors; may become lethal when those active coping efforts are unsuccessful; the syndrome has been especially documented among lower-income Blacks at risk for or suffering from hypertension.

**kidney dialysis**    A procedure in which blood is filtered to remove toxic substances and excess fluid from the blood of patients whose kidneys do not function properly.

**lay referral network**    An informal network of family and friends who help an individual interpret and treat a disorder before the individual seeks formal medical treatment.

**life-skills-training approach**  A smoking prevention program characterized by the belief that training in self-esteem and coping skills will boost self-image to the point that smoking becomes unnecessary or inconsistent with lifestyle.

**lifestyle rebalancing**  Concerted lifestyle change in a healthy direction, usually including exercise, stress management, and a healthy diet; believed to contribute to relapse prevention after successful modification of a poor health habit, such as smoking or alcohol consumption.

**living will**  A will prepared by a person requesting that extraordinary life-sustaining procedures not be used in the event that the person's ability to make this decision is lost.

**longitudinal research**  The repeated observation and measurement of the same individuals over a period of time.

**lupus**  A chronic, inflammatory form of arthritis that may be managed by anti-inflammatory medications or immunosuppressive medications, depending on its severity.

**lymphatic system**  The drainage system of the body; the system is involved in immune functioning.

**managed care**  A health care arrangement in which an employer or employee pays a predetermined monthly fee to a health care or insurance agency that entitles the employee to use medical services at no additional (or a greatly reduced) cost.

**massage**  A relaxation technique that involves manipulating deep layers of muscles and soft tissue.

**matching hypothesis**  The hypothesis that social support is helpful to an individual to the extent that the kind of support offered satisfies the individual's specific needs.

**medical delay**  A delay in treating symptoms, which results from problems within the medical system, such as faulty diagnoses or lost test results.

**medical students' disease**  The relabeling of symptoms of fatigue and exhaustion as a particular illness resulting from learning about that illness; called medical students' disease because overworked medical students are vulnerable to this labeling effect.

**medulla**  The part of the hindbrain that controls autonomic functions such as regulation of heart rate, blood pressure, and respiration.

**meta-analysis**  Combines and contrasts results from multiple studies to identify consistencies in patterns of research findings.

**metabolic syndrome**  A pattern of risk factors for the chronic health problems of diabetes, heart disease, and hypertension, characterized by obesity, a high waist-to-hip ratio, and insulin resistance. Metabolic syndrome is exacerbated by inactivity, overeating, age, and hostility.

**mind–body relationship**  The philosophical position regarding whether the mind and body operate indistinguishably as a single system or whether they act as two separate systems; the view guiding health psychology is that the mind and the body are indistinguishable.

**mindfulness meditation**  A specific type of meditation that teaches people to strive for a state of mind marked by awareness and focus on the present moment, accepting and acknowledging it without becoming distracted or distressed by stress.

**modeling**  Learning gained from observing another person performing a target behavior.

**morbidity**  The number of cases of a disease that exist at a given point in time; it may be expressed as the number of new cases (incidence) or as the total number of existing cases (prevalence).

**mortality**  The number of deaths due to particular causes.

**myocardial infarction (MI)**  A heart attack produced when a clot has developed in a coronary vessel, blocking the flow of blood to the heart.

**negative affectivity**  A personality variable marked by a pervasive negative mood, including anxiety, depression, and hostility; believed to be implicated in the experience of symptoms, the seeking of medical treatment, and possibly illness.

**nervous system**  The system of the body responsible for the transmission of information from the brain to the rest of the body and from the rest of the body to the brain; it is composed of the central nervous system (the brain and the spinal cord) and the peripheral nervous system (which consists of the remainder of the nerves in the body).

**neurotransmitters**  Chemicals that regulate nervous system functioning.

**nociception**  The perception of pain.

**nonadherence**  The failure to comply fully with treatment recommendations for modification of a health habit or an illness state.

**nonspecific immune mechanisms**  A set of responses to infection or a disorder that is engaged by the presence of a biological invader.

**nurse-practitioners**  Nurses who, in addition to their training in traditional nursing, receive special training in primary care so they may provide routine medical care for patients.

**obesity**  An excessive accumulation of body fat, believed to contribute to a variety of health disorders, including cardiovascular disease.

**occupational therapists**  Trained and licensed individuals who work with emotionally and/or physically disabled people to determine skill levels and to develop a rehabilitation program to build on and expand these skills.

**operant conditioning**  The pairing of a voluntary, nonautomatic behavior with a new stimulus through reinforcement or punishment.

**opioid crisis**   The overprescription and overuse of opioid drugs, including prescription pain relievers, heroin, and synthetic opioids (such as fentanyl), resulting in high rates of addiction, disability, and death.

**osteoarthritis**   A form of arthritis that results when the articular cartilage begins to crack or wear away because of overuse of a particular joint; may also result from injury or other causes; usually affects the weight-bearing joints and is common among athletes and the elderly.

**pain behaviors**   Behaviors that result in response to pain, such as cutting back on work or taking drugs.

**pain control**   The ability to reduce the experience of pain, report of pain, emotional concern over pain, inability to tolerate pain, or presence of pain-related behaviors.

**pain management programs**   Coordinated, interdisciplinary efforts to modify chronic pain by bringing together neurological, cognitive, behavioral, and psychodynamic expertise concerning pain; such programs aim not only to make pain more manageable but also to modify the lifestyle that has evolved because of the pain.

**pain-prone personality**   A constellation of personality traits that predisposes a person to experience chronic pain.

**palliative care**   Care designed to make the patient comfortable, but not to cure or improve the patient's underlying disease; often part of terminal care.

**parasympathetic nervous system**   The part of the nervous system responsible for vegetative functions, the conservation of energy, and the damping down of the effects of the sympathetic nervous system.

**passive smoking**   See **secondhand smoke.**

**patient-centered care**   Care that involves providing patients with information, involving them in decisions regarding care, and consideration of psychosocial issues such as social support needs.

**patient education**   Programs designed to inform patients about their disorder and its treatment and to train them in methods for coping with a disorder and its corresponding limitations.

**perceived stress**   The perception that an event is stressful independent of its objective characteristics.

**person–environment fit**   The degree to which the needs and resources of a person and the needs and resources of an environment complement each other.

**phagocytosis**   The process by which phagocytes ingest and attempt to eliminate a foreign invader.

**physical dependence**   A state in which the body has adjusted to the use of a substance, incorporating it into the body's normal functioning.

**physical rehabilitation**   A program of activities for chronically ill or disabled persons geared toward helping them use their bodies as much as possible, sense changes in the environment and in themselves so as to make appropriate physical accommodations, learn new physical and management skills if necessary, pursue a treatment regimen, and learn how to control the expenditure of energy.

**physical therapists**   Trained and licensed individuals who help people with muscle, nerve, joint, or bone diseases to overcome their disabilities as much as possible.

**physicians' assistants**   Graduates of 2-year programs who perform routine health care functions, teach patients about their treatment regimens, and record medical information.

**pituitary gland**   A gland located at the base of and controlled by the brain that secretes the hormones responsible for growth and organ development.

**placebo**   A medical treatment that produces an effect in a patient because of its therapeutic intent and not its nature.

**placebo drinking**   The consumption of nonalcoholic beverages in social situations in which others are drinking alcohol.

**placebo effect**   The medically beneficial impact of an inert treatment.

**platelets**   Small disks found in vertebrate blood that contribute to blood coagulation.

**pons**   The part of the hindbrain that links the hindbrain to the midbrain and helps control respiration.

**post traumatic stress disorder (PTSD)**   A syndrome that results after exposure to a stressor of extreme magnitude, marked by emotional numbing, the reliving of aspects of the trauma, intense responses to other stressful events, and other symptoms, such as hyperalertness, sleep disturbance, guilt, or impaired memory or concentration.

**preferred-provider organization (PPO)**   A network of affiliated practitioners that has agreed to charge preestablished rates for particular medical services.

**premature death**   Death that occurs before the projected age of population.

**primary appraisal**   The perception of a new or changing environment as beneficial, neutral, or negative in its consequences; believed to be a first step in stress and coping.

**primary prevention**   Measures designed to combat risk factors for illness before an illness has a chance to develop.

**private, fee-for-service care**   The condition under which patients privately contract with physicians for services and pay them for services rendered.

**problem drinking**   Uncontrolled drinking that leads to social, psychological, and biomedical problems resulting from alcohol; the problem drinker may show some signs associated with alcoholism, but typically, problem drinking is considered to be a prealcoholic or a lesser alcoholic syndrome.

**problem-focused coping**   Attempts to do something constructive about the stressful situations that are harming or threatening an individual.

**prospective research**   A research strategy in which people are followed forward in time to examine the relationship between one set of variables and later occurrences. For example, prospective research can enable researchers to identify risk factors for diseases that develop at a later time.

**psychological control**   The perception that one has at one's disposal a response that will reduce, minimize, eliminate, or offset the adverse effects of an unpleasant event, such as a medical procedure.

**psychoneuroimmunology**   Study of the interactions among behavioral, neuroendocrine, and immunological processes of adaptation.

**psychosomatic medicine**   A field within psychiatry, related to health psychology, that developed in the early 1900s to study and treat particular diseases believed to be caused by emotional conflicts, such as ulcers, hypertension, and asthma. The term is now used more broadly to mean an approach to health-related problems and diseases that examine psychological as well as somatic origins.

**quality of life**   The degree to which a person is able to maximize his or her physical, psychological, vocational, and social functioning; an important indicator of recovery from or adjustment to chronic illness.

**randomized clinical trials**   An experimental study of the effects of a variable (such as a drug or treatment) administered to human participants who are randomly selected from a broad population and assigned on a random basis to either an experimental group or a control group. The goal is to determine the clinical efficacy and pharmacologic effects of the drug or procedure.

**reactivity**   The predisposition to react physiologically to stress; believed to be genetically based in part; high reactivity is believed to be a risk factor for a range of stress-related diseases.

**recurrent acute pain**   Pain that involves a series of intermittent episodes of pain that are acute in character but chronic inasmuch as the condition persists for more than 6 months; migraine headaches, temporomandibular disorder (involving the jaw), and trigeminal neuralgia (involving spasms of the facial muscles) are examples.

**relapse prevention**   A set of techniques designed to keep people from relapsing to prior poor health habits after initial successful behavior modification; includes training in coping skills for high-risk-for-relapse situations and lifestyle rebalancing.

**relaxation training**   Procedures that help people relax; include progressive muscle relaxation and deep breathing; may also include guided imagery and forms of meditation or hypnosis.

**renal system**   Part of the metabolic system; responsible for the regulation of bodily fluids and the elimination of wastes; regulates bodily fluids by removing surplus water, surplus electrolytes, and waste products generated by the metabolism of food.

**respiratory system**   The system of the body responsible for taking in oxygen, excreting carbon dioxide, and regulating the relative composition of the blood.

**retrospective designs**   A research strategy whereby people are studied for the relationship of past variables or conditions to current ones. Interviewing people with a particular disease and asking them about their childhood health behaviors or exposure to risks can identify conditions leading to an adult disease, for example.

**rheumatoid arthritis (RA)**   A crippling form of arthritis believed to result from an autoimmune process, usually attacking the small joints of the hands, feet, wrists, knees, ankles, and neck.

**role conflict**   Conflict that occurs when two or more social or occupational roles that an individual occupies produce conflicting standards for behavior.

**secondary appraisal**   The assessment of one's coping abilities and resources and the judgment as to whether they will be sufficient to meet the harm, threat, or challenge of a new or changing event.

**secondary gains**   Benefits of being treated for illness, including the ability to rest, to be freed from unpleasant tasks, and to be taken care of by others.

**secondhand smoke**   Smoke that is unintentionally inhaled by nonsmokers as a result of exposure to smokers; believed to cause health problems such as bronchitis, emphysema, and lung cancer.

**self-affirmation**   A process by which people focus on their personal values, which bolsters the self-concept.

**self-concept**   An integrated set of beliefs about one's personal qualities and attributes.

**self-control**   A state in which an individual desiring to change behavior learns how to modify the antecedents and the consequences of that target behavior.

**self-determination theory (SDT)**   The theory that autonomous motivation and perceived competence are fundamental to behavior change.

**self-efficacy**   The perception that one is able to perform a particular action.

**self-esteem**   A global evaluation of one's qualities and attributes.

**self-help aids**   Materials that can be used by an individual on his or her own without the aid of a therapist to assist in the modification of a personal habit; often used to combat smoking and other health-related risk factors.

**self-management**   Involvement of the patient in all aspects of a chronic illness including medication management, changes in social and vocational roles, and coping.

**self-monitoring**   Assessing the frequency, antecedents, and consequences of a target behavior to be modified; also known as self-observation.

**self-regulation**   The conscious and unconscious ways in which people control their own actions, emotions, and thoughts.

**self-reinforcement**   Systematically rewarding oneself to increase or strengthen a target behavior.

**self-talk**   Internal monologues; people tell themselves things that may undermine or help them implement appropriate health habits, such as "I can stop smoking" (positive self-talk) or "I'll never be able to do this" (negative self-talk).

**set point theory of weight**   The concept that each individual has an ideal biological weight that cannot be greatly modified.

**smoking prevention programs**   Programs designed to keep people from beginning to smoke, as opposed to programs that attempt to induce people to stop once they have already become smokers.

**social engineering**   Social or lifestyle change through legislation; for example, water purification is done through social engineering rather than by individual efforts.

**social influence intervention**   A preventive interventive that draws on the social learning principles of modeling and behavioral inoculation in inducing people not to smoke, for example; youngsters are exposed to older peer models who deliver antismoking messages after exposure to simulated peer pressure to smoke.

**social skills training**   Techniques that teach people how to relax and interact comfortably in social situations; often a part of health behavior modification programs, on the assumption that maladaptive health behaviors, such as alcohol consumption or smoking, may develop in part to control social anxiety.

**social support**   Information from other people that one is loved and cared for, esteemed and valued, and part of a network of communication and mutual obligation.

**social workers**   Trained and licensed individuals who help patients and their families deal with problems by providing therapy, making referrals, and engaging in social planning; medical social workers help patients and their families ease transitions between illness and recovery states.

**socialization**   The process by which people learn the norms, rules, and beliefs associated with their family and society; parents and social institutions are usually the major agents of socialization.

**somaticizers**   People who express distress and conflict through bodily symptoms.

**specific immune mechanisms**   Responses designed to respond to specific invaders; include cell-mediated and humoral immunity.

**stages of dying**   A theory, developed by Elisabeth Kübler-Ross, maintaining that people go through five temporal stages in adjusting to the prospect of death: denial, anger, bargaining, depression, and acceptance; believed to characterize some but not all dying people.

**stimulus-control interventions**   Interventions designed to modify behavior that involve the removal of discriminative stimuli that evoke a behavior targeted for change and the substitution of new discriminative stimuli that will evoke a desired behavior.

**stress**   Appraising events as harmful, threatening, or challenging, and assessing one's capacity to respond to those events; events that are perceived to tax or exceed one's resources are seen as stressful.

**stress carriers**   Individuals who create stress for others without necessarily increasing their own level of stress.

**stress eating**   Eating in response to stress; approximately half the population increases eating in response to stress.

**stress management**   A program for dealing with stress in which people learn how they appraise stressful events, develop skills for coping with stress, and practice putting these skills into effect.

**stress moderators**   Internal and external resources and vulnerabilities that modify how stress is experienced and its effects.

**stressful life events**   Events that confer threat or harm.

**stressors**   Events perceived to be stressful.

**stroke**   A condition that results from a disturbance in blood flow to the brain, often marked by resulting physical or cognitive impairments and, in the extreme, death.

**sudden infant death syndrome (SIDS)**   A common cause of death among infants, in which an infant simply stops breathing.

**support groups**   Groups of individuals who meet regularly and usually have a common problem or concern; support groups are believed to help people cope because they provide opportunities to share concerns and exchange information with similar others.

**symbolic immortality**   The sense that one is leaving a lasting impact on the world, as through one's children or one's work, or that one is joining the afterlife and becoming one with God.

**sympathetic nervous system**   The part of the nervous system that mobilizes the body for action.

**systems theory**    The view that all levels of an organization in any entity are linked to each other hierarchically and that change in any level will bring about change in other levels.

**tangible assistance**    The provision of material support by one person to another, such as services, financial assistance, or goods.

**teachable moment**    The idea that certain times are more effective for teaching particular health practices than others; pregnancy constitutes a teachable moment for getting women to stop smoking.

**tend-and-befriend**    A theory of responses to stress maintaining that in addition to fight-or-flight, humans respond to stress with social affiliation and nurturant behavior toward offspring; thought to depend on the stress hormone oxytocin; these responses may be especially true of women.

**terminal care**    Medical care of the terminally ill.

**thalamus**    The portion of the forebrain responsible for the recognition of sensory stimuli and the relay of sensory impulses to the cerebral cortex.

**thanatologists**    Those who study death and dying.

**theory**    A set of interrelated analytic statements that explain a set of phenomena, such as why people practice poor health behaviors.

**theory of planned behavior**    Derived from the theory of reasoned action, a theoretical viewpoint maintaining that a person's behavioral intentions and behaviors can be understood by knowing the person's attitudes toward the behavior, subjective norms regarding the behavior, and perceived behavioral control over that action.

**time management**    Skills for learning how to use one's time more effectively to accomplish one's goals.

**tolerance**    The process by which the body increasingly adapts to a substance, requiring larger and larger doses of it to obtain the same effects; a frequent characteristic of substance abuse, including alcohol and drug abuse.

**Traditional Chinese Medicine**    An ancient approach to healing developed in China that focuses on keeping life force (qi) in balance through techniques such as meditation, massage, and herbal medicine.

**transtheoretical model of behavior change**    An analysis of the health behavior change process that draws on the stages and processes people go through in order to bring about successful long-term behavior change. The stages include precontemplation, contemplation, preparation, action, and maintenance. Successful attitude or behavior change at each stage depends on the appropriateness of the intervention. For example, attitude-change materials help move people from precontemplation to contemplation, whereas relapse prevention techniques help move people from action to maintenance.

**treatment effectiveness**    Formal documentation of the success of an intervention.

**Type 1 diabetes**    An autoimmune disorder characterized by lack of insulin production by the beta cells of the pancreas.

**Type 2 diabetes**    A metabolic disorder characterized by high blood glucose in the context of insulin resistance; often co-occurs with risk for heart disease.

**wellness**    An optimum state of health achieved through balance among physical, mental, and social well-being.

**window of vulnerability**    The fact that, at certain times, people are more vulnerable to particular health problems. For example, early adolescence constitutes a window of vulnerability for beginning smoking, drug use, and alcohol abuse.

**withdrawal**    Unpleasant physical and psychological symptoms that people experience when they stop using a substance on which they have become physically dependent; symptoms include anxiety, craving, hallucinations, nausea, headaches, and shaking.

**worried well**    Individuals free from illness who are nonetheless concerned about their physical state and frequently and inappropriately use medical services.

**yoga**    A general term developed from Hindu philosophy for spiritual, mental, and physical discipline that includes breathing techniques, posture, strengthening exercises, and meditation.

**yo-yo dieting**    The process of chronically alternating between dieting and regular eating, leading to successive weight gains and losses; over time, yo-yo dieters increase their chances of becoming obese by altering their underlying metabolism.

# REFERENCES

ABC News. (2004). *Bitter medicine: Pills, profit, and the public health.* Retrieved from http://abcnews.go.com/onair/ABCNEWSSpecials/pharmaceuticals_020529_pjr_feature.html

Abdoli, S., Rahzani, K., Safaie, M., & Sattari, A. (2012). A randomized control trial: The effect of guided imagery with tape and perceived happy memory on chronic tension type headache. *Scandinavian Journal of Caring Sciences, 26,* 254–261.

Aboa-Éboulé, C., Brisson, C., Maunsell, E., Bourbonnais, R., Vézina, M., Milot, A. M., & Dagenais, G. R. (2011). Effort–reward imbalance at work and recurrent coronary heart disease events: A 4-year prospective study of post-myocardial infarction patients. *Psychosomatic Medicine, 73,* 436–447.

Abraham, C., & Graham-Rowe, E. (2009). Are worksite interventions effective in increasing physical activity? A systematic review and meta-analysis. *Health Psychology Review, 3,* 108–144.

Abrams, D. B., Orleans, C. T., Niaura, R. S., Goldstein, M. G., Prochaska, J. O., & Velicer, W. (1996). Integrating individual and public health perspectives for treatment of tobacco dependence under managed health care: A combined stepped-care and matching model. *Annals of Behavioral Medicine, 18,* 290–304.

Adams, K. F., Schatzkin, A., Harris, T. B., Kipnis, V., Mouw, T., Ballard-Barbash, R., & Leitzmann, M. F. (2006). Overweight, obesity, and mortality in a large prospective cohort of persons 50 to 71 years old. *The New England Journal of Medicine, 355,* 763–778.

Adams, M. A., Norman, G. J., Hovell, M. F., Sallis, J. F., & Patrick, K. (2009). Reconceptualizing decisional balance in an adolescent sun protection intervention: Mediating effects and theoretical interpretations. *Health Psychology, 28,* 217–225.

Adelman, R. C., & Verbrugge, L. M. (2000). Death makes news: The social impact of disease on newspaper coverage. *Journal of Health and Social Behavior, 41,* 347–367.

Ader, R. (1995). Historical perspectives on psychoneuroimmunology. In H. Friedman, T. W. Klein, & A. L. Friedman (Eds.), *Psychoneuroimmunology, stress, and infection* (pp. 1–24). Boca Raton, FL: CRC Press.

Adler, N., & Stewart, J. (Eds.). (2010). *The biology of disadvantage: Socioeconomic status and health* (Vol. 1186). Malden, MA: Wiley-Blackwell.

Adler, N. E., Boyce, T., Chesney, M. A., Cohen, C., Folkman, S., Kahn, R. L., & Syme, L. S. (1994). Socioeconomic status and health: The challenge of the gradient. *American Psychologist, 49,* 15–24.

Adler, S. (1991). Sudden unexpected nocturnal death syndrome among Hmong immigrants: Examining the role of the "nightmare." *The Journal of American Folklore, 104* (411), 54–71.

Afari, N., Ahumada, S. M., Wright, L. J., Mostoufi, S., Golnari, G., Reis, V., & Cuneo, J. G. (2014). Psychological trauma and functional somatic syndromes: A systematic review and meta-analysis. *Psychosomatic Medicine, 76,* 2–11.

Affleck, G., Tennen, H., Pfeiffer, C., & Fifield, C. (1987). Appraisals of control and predictability in adapting to a chronic disease. *Journal of Personality and Social Psychology, 53,* 273–279.

Aggio, D., Wallace, K., Boreham, N., Shankar, A., Steptoe, A., & Hamer, M. (2017). Objectively measured daily physical activity and postural changes as related to positive and negative affect using ambulatory monitoring assessments. *Psychosomatic Medicine, 79,* 792–797.

Agras, W. S., Berkowitz, R. I., Arnow, B. A., Telch, C. F., Marnell, M., Henderson, J., & Wilfley, D. E. (1996). Maintenance following a very-low-calorie diet. *Journal of Consulting and Clinical Psychology, 64,* 610–613.

Agras, W. S., Taylor, C. B., Kraemer, H. C., Southam, M. A., & Schneider, J. A. (1987). Relaxation training for essential hypertension at the work site: II. The poorly controlled hypertensive. *Psychosomatic Medicine, 49,* 264–273.

Ahlstrom, B., Dinh, T., Haselton, M. G., & Tomiyama, A. J. (2017). Understanding eating interventions through an evolutionary lens. *Health Psychology Review, 11,* 72–88.

Ahluwalia, J. S., Nollen, N., Kaur, H., James, A. S., Mayo, M. S., & Resnicow, K. (2007). Pathways to health: Cluster-randomized trial to increase fruit and vegetable consumption among smokers in public housing. *Health Psychology, 26,* 214–221.

Ahmedani, B. K., Peterson, E. L., Wells, K. E., & Williams, L. K. (2013). Examining the relationship between depression and asthma exacerbations in a prospective follow-up study. *Psychosomatic Medicine, 75,* 305–310.

Ahn, A. C., Colbert, A. P., Anderson, B. J., Martinsen, Ø. G., Hammerschlag, R., Cina, S., . . . Langevin, H. M. (2008). Electrical properties of acupuncture points and meridians: A systematic review. *Bioelectromagnetics, 29,* 245–256.

Ai, A. L., Wink, P., Tice, T. N., Bolling, S. F., & Shearer, M. (2009). Prayer and reverence in naturalistic, aesthetic, and socio-moral contexts predicted fewer complications following coronary artery bypass. *Journal of Behavioral Medicine, 32,* 570–581.

Aiken, L. H., & Marx, M. M. (1982). Hospices: Perspectives on the public policy debate. *American Psychologist, 37,* 1271–1279.

Ajzen, I., & Fishbein, M. (1980). *Understanding attitudes and predicting social behavior.* Englewood Cliffs, NJ: Prentice-Hall.

Ajzen, I., & Madden, T. J. (1986). Prediction of goal-directed behavior: Attitudes, intentions, and perceived behavioral control. *Journal of Experimental Social Psychology, 22,* 453–474.

Akil, H., Mayer, D. J., & Liebeskind, J. C. (1972). Comparison chez le Rat entre l'analgesie induite par stimulation de la substance grise periaqueducale et l'analgesie morphinique. *C. R. Academy of Science, 274,* 3603–3605.

Akil, H., Mayer, D. J., & Liebeskind, J. C. (1976). Antagonism of stimulation-produced analgesia by naloxone, a narcotic antagonist. *Science, 191,* 961–962.

Al'Absi, M. (2018). Stress and addiction: When a robust stress response indicates resiliency. *Psychosomatic Medicine, 80,* 2–16.

Alati, R., O'Callaghan, M., Najman, J. M., Williams, G. M., Bor, W., & Lawlor, D. A. (2005). Asthma and internalizing behavior problems in adolescence: A longitudinal study. *Psychosomatic Medicine, 67,* 462–470.

Albarracín, D., Durantini, M. R., Earl, A., Gunnoe, J. B., & Leeper, J. (2008). Beyond the most willing audience: A meta-intervention to increase exposure to HIV-prevention programs by vulnerable populations. *Health Psychology, 27,* 638–644.

Albarracín, D., McNatt, P. S., Klein, C. T. F., Ho, R. M., Mitchell, A. L., & Kumkale, G. C. (2003). Persuasive communications to change actions: An analysis of behavioral and cognitive impact in HIV prevention. *Health Psychology, 22,* 166–177.

Albarracin, D., Gillette, J. C., Earl, A. N., Glasman, L. R., Durantini, M. R., & Ho, M. H. (2005). A test of major assumptions about behavior change: A comprehensive look at the effects of passive and active HIV-prevention interventions since the beginning of the epidemic. *Psychological Bulletin, 131,* 856-897.

Albom, M. (1997). *Tuesdays with Morrie.* New York: Doubleday.

Alcoholics Anonymous. (2019, March). *Estimated worldwide A. A. individual and group membership.* Retrieved April 8, 2019, from http://www.aa.org/assets/en_US/smf-132_en.pdf

Alderman, M. H., & Lamport, B. (1988). Treatment of hypertension at the workplace: An opportunity to link service and research. *Health Psychology, 7* (Suppl.), 283-295.

Alexander, A. B., Stupiansky, N. W., Ott, M. A., Herbenick, D., Reece, M., & Zimet, G. D. (2014). What parents and their adolescent sons suggest for male HPV vaccine messaging. *Health Psychology, 33,* 448-456.

Alexander, F. (1950). *Psychosomatic medicine.* New York: Norton.

Alferi, S. M., Carver, C. S., Antoni, M. H., Weiss, S., & Duran, R. E. (2001). An exploratory study of social support, distress, and life disruption among low-income Hispanic women under treatment for early stage breast cancer. *Health Psychology, 20,* 41-46.

Ali, J., & Avison, W. (1997). Employment transitions and psychological distress: The contrasting experiences of single and married mothers. *Journal of Health and Social Behavior, 38,* 345-362.

Ainsworth, B., Steele, M., Stuart, B., Joseph, J., Miller, S., Morrison, L., . . . Yardley, L. (2016). Using an analysis of behavior change to inform effective digital intervention design: How did the PRIMIT website change hand hygiene behavior across 8993 users? *Annals of Behavioral Medicine, 51,* 423-431.

Allan, J. L., Johnston, M., & Campbell, N. (2015). Snack purchasing is healthier when the cognitive demands of choice are reduced: A randomized controlled trial. *Health Psychology, 34,* 750-755.

Allen, J., Markovitz, J., Jacobs, D. R., & Knox, S. S. (2001). Social support and health behavior in hostile black and white men and women. *Psychosomatic Medicine, 63,* 609-618.

Allen, J. E. (2003, April 7). Stroke therapy sets sights higher, farther. *Los Angeles Times,* pp. F1, F7.

Allen, M. S., Walter, E. E., & McDermott, M. S. (2017). Personality and sedentary behavior: A systematic review and meta-analysis. *Health Psychology, 36,* 255-263.

Almeida, N. D., Loucks, E. B., Kubzansky, L., Pruessner, J., Maselko, J., Meaney, M. J., & Buka, S. L. (2010). Quality of parental emotional care and calculated risk for coronary heart disease. *Psychosomatic Medicine, 72,* 148-155.

Alper, J. (2000). New insights into Type II diabetes. *Science, 289,* 37-39.

Alpert, J. J. (1964). Broken appointments. *Pediatrics, 34,* 127-132.

Alter, David. (2015). *Annals of Internal Medicine Tip Sheet.* Retrieved February 17, 2016, from http://annals.org

Altunç, U., Pittler, M. H., & Ernst, E. (2007). Homeopathy for childhood and adolescence ailments: Systematic review of randomized clinical trials. *Mayo Clinic Proceedings, 82,* 69-75.

Alzheimer's Association. (2016). *Alzheimer's & dementia: Global resources.* Retrieved February 6, 2016, from https://alz.org

Alzheimer's Association. (2016). *What is Alzheimer's?* Retrieved January 21, 2016, from https://alz.org

Alzheimer's Association. (2019). *Facts and figures.* Retrieved March 13, 2019, from https://www.alz.org/alzheimers-dementia/facts-figures

Ambrosone, C. B., Flevdenheim, J. L., Graham, S., Marshall, J. R., Vena, J. E., Glasure, J. R., . . . Shields, P. G. (1996). Cigarette smoking, N-acetyl-transferase 2, genetic polymorphisms, and breast cancer risk. *Journal of the American Medical Association, 276,* 1494-1501.

America, A., & Milling, L. S. (2008). The efficacy of vitamins for reducing or preventing depression symptoms in healthy individuals: Natural remedy or placebo? *Journal of Behavioral Medicine, 31,* 157-167.

American Association of Health Plans. (2001). *How to choose a health plan.* Retrieved from http://www.aahp.org

American Autoimmune Related Diseases Association. (2015). *Questions and answers.* Retrieved January 21, 2016, from http://www.aarda.org/q_and_a.php

American Cancer Society. (2014). *Tobacco use: Smoking cessation.* Atlanta, GA: Author.

American Cancer Society. (2006). *Common questions about diet and cancer.* Retrieved June 14, 2007, from http://www.cancer.org/docroot/PED/content/PED_3_2X_Common_Questions_About_diet_and_Cancer.asp

American Cancer Society. (2008). *Macrobiotic diet.* Retrieved October 22, 2012, from http://www.cancer.org/treatment/treatmentsandsideeffects/complementaryandalternativemedicine/dietandnutrition/macrobiotic-diet

American Cancer Society. (2009). *Cancer facts & figures, 2009.* Retrieved September 25, 2009, from http://www.cancer.org/downloads/STT/500809web.pdf

American Cancer Society. (2012). *Cancer facts & figures, 2012.* Retrieved March 26, 2012, from http://www.cancer.org/acs/groups/content/@epide-miologysurveilance/documents/document/acspc-031941.pdf

American Cancer Society. (2016, February). *American Cancer Society guidelines on nutrition and physical activity for cancer prevention.* Retrieved May 25, 2016, from http://www.cancer.org

American Cancer Society. (2017). *About cancer pain.* Retrieved April 29, 2019, from https://www.cancer.org/content/dam/CRC/PDF/Public/7161.pdf

American Cancer Society. (2018). *Cancer facts & figures 2018.* Retrieved April 1, 2019, from https://www.cancer.org/content/dam/cancer-org/research/cancer-facts-and-statistics/annual-cancer-facts-and-figures/2018/cancer-facts-and-figures-2018.pdf

American Cancer Society. (2019a). *Cancer facts & figures 2019.* Atlanta, GA: Author.

American Cancer Society. (2019b). *Key statistics for lung cancer.* Retrieved March 26, 2019, from https://www.cancer.org/cancer/non-small-cell-lung-cancer/about/key-statistics.html

American Diabetes Association. (2012). *Who is at greater risk for type 2 diabetes?* Retrieved June 12, 2012, from http://www.diabetes.org/diabetes-basics/prevention/risk-factors

American Diabetes Association. (2018). *Statistics about diabetes: Overall numbers, diabetes and prediabetes.* Retrieved from http://www.diabetes.org/diabetes-basics/statistics/

American Heart Association. (2000). *Heart and stroke a-z guide.* Dallas, TX: Author.

American Heart Association. (2004a). *Heart disease and stroke statistics— 2005 update.* Retrieved from http://www.americanheart.org/presenter.jhtml?identifier=1928

American Heart Association. (2004b). *Risk factors of cardiovascular disease.* Retrieved from http://www.americanheart.org/presenter.jhtml?identifier=3017033

American Heart Association. (2007). *Stroke statistics.* Retrieved April 5, 2007, from http://www.americanheart.org/presenter.jhtml? identifier=4725

American Heart Association. (2009). Heart disease and stroke statistics 2009 update: A report from the American Heart Association statistics committee and stroke statistics subcommittee. *Circulation, 119,* 21-181. Retrieved September 28, 2009, from http://circ.ahajournals.org/cgi/reprint/CIRCULATIONAHA.108.191261

American Heart Association. (2015, December). *Heart disease, stroke, and research statistics at-a-glance.* Retrieved April 30, 2016, from https://www.heart.org

American Heart Association. (2016). *Understand your risks to prevent a heart attack.* Retrieved March 25, 2019, from https://www.heart.org/en/health-topics/heart-attack/understand-your-risks-to-prevent-a-heart-attack

American Hospital Association. (2009). *Fast facts on US hospitals.* Retrieved October 13, 2009, from http://www.aha.org/aha/resource-center/Statistics-and-Studies/fast-facts.html

American Hospital Association. (2012). *TrendWatch chartbook: Trends affecting hospitals and health systems.* Retrieved March 21, 2012, from http://www.aha.org/research/reports/tw/chartbook/index.shtml

American Hospital Association. (2018). *TrendWatch chartbook 2018: Trends affecting hospitals and health systems.* Retrieved April 9, 2019, from https://www.aha.org/system/files/2018-07/2018-aha-chartbook.pdf

American Hospital Association. (2019, January). *Fast facts on U.S. hospitals, 2019.* Retrieved April 9, 2019, from https://www.aha.org/statistics/fast-facts-us-hospitals

American Institute of Stress. (n.d.). *Workplace stress.* Retrieved March 8, 2013, from http://www.stress.org/workplace-stress

American Kidney Fund. (2015). *Kidney disease statistics.* Retrieved March 26, 2019, from http://www.kidneyfund.org/assets/pdf/kidney-disease-statistics.pdf

American Lung Association. (2016). *Health effects of secondhand smoke.* Retrieved February 29, 2016, from http://www.lung.org

American Psychiatric Association. (2000). *Diagnostic and statistical manual of mental disorders* (4th ed., text revision). Washington, DC: Author.

American Psychological Association. (1996). *1993 APA directory survey, with new member updates for 1994 and 1995.* Washington, DC: American Psychological Association Research Office.

American Psychological Association. (2008). *Stress in America.* Washington, DC: American Psychological Association Research Office.

American Psychological Association Division 38. (2010). *About health psychology.* Retrieved March 23, 2010, from http://www.health-psych.org/AboutWhatWeDo.cfm

Ames, M. E., Leadbeater, B. J., & MacDonald, S. W. S. (2018). Health behavior changes in adolescence and young adulthood: Implications for cardiometabolic risk. *Health Psychology, 37,* 103–113.

Andersen, B. L., Cacioppo, J. T., & Roberts, D. C. (1995). Delay in seeking a cancer diagnosis: Delay stages and psychophysiological comparison processes. *British Journal of Social Psychology, 34,* 33–52.

Andersen, B. L., Woods, X. A., & Copeland, L. J. (1997). Sexual self-schema and sexual morbidity among gynecologic cancer survivors. *Journal of Consulting and Clinical Psychology, 65,* 1–9.

Anderson, K. O., Bradley, L. A., Young, L. D., McDaniel, L. K., & Wise, C. M. (1985). Rheumatoid arthritis: Review of psychological factors related to etiology, effects, and treatment. *Psychological Bulletin, 98,* 358–387.

Anderson, L. M., Symoniak, E. D., & Epstein, L. H. (2014). A randomized pilot trial of an integrated school-worksite weight control program. *Health Psychology, 33,* 1421–1425.

Anderson, R. A., Baron, R. S., & Logan, H. (1991). Distraction, control, and dental stress. *Journal of Applied Social Psychology, 21,* 156–171.

Andrews, J. A., & Duncan, S. C. (1997). Examining the reciprocal relation between academic motivation and substance use: Effects of family relationships, self-esteem, and general deviance. *Journal of Behavioral Medicine, 20,* 523–549.

Andrews, J. A., Tildesley, E., Hops, H., & Li, F. (2002). The influence of peers on young adult substance use. *Health Psychology, 21,* 349–357.

Aneshensel, C. S., Botticello, A. L., & Yamamoto-Mitani, N. (2004). When caregiving ends: The course of depressive symptoms after bereavement. *Journal of Health and Social Behavior, 45,* 422–440.

Angier, N. (2001, June 19). Researchers piecing together autoimmune disease puzzle. *New York Times,* pp. D1, D8.

Anschutz, D. J., Van Strien, T., & Engels, R. C. M. (2008). Exposure to slim images in mass media: Television commercials as reminders of restriction in restrained eaters. *Health Psychology, 27,* 401–408.

Anstey, K. J., Jorm, A. F., Réglade-Meslin, C., Maller, J., Kumar, R., Von Sanden, C., . . . Sachdev, P. (2006). Weekly alcohol consumption, brain atrophy, and white matter hyperintensities in a community-based sample aged 60 to 64 years. *Psychosomatic Medicine, 68,* 778–785.

Antoni, M. H., Carrico, A. W., Durán, R. E., Spitzer, S., Penedo, F., Ironson, G., . . . Schneiderman, N. (2006). Randomized clinical trial of cognitive behavioral stress management on human immunodeficiency virus viral load in gay men treated with highly active antiretroviral therapy. *Psychosomatic Medicine, 68,* 143–151.

Antoni, M. H., & Dhabhar, F. S. (2019). The impact of psychosocial stress and stress management on immune responses in patients with cancer. *Cancer, 125,* 1417–1431.

Antoni, M. H., Lechner, S. C., Kazi, A., Wimberly, S. R., Sifre, T., Urcuyo, K. R., . . . Carver, C. S. (2006). How stress management improves quality of life after treatment for breast cancer. *Journal of Consulting and Clinical Psychology, 74,* 1143–1152.

Antoni, M. H., Lehman, J. M., Kilbourne, K. M., Boyers, A. E., Culver, J. L., Alferi, S. M., . . . Carver, C. S. (2001). Cognitive–behavioral stress management intervention decreases the prevalence of depression and enhances benefit finding among women under treatment of early-stage breast cancer. *Health Psychology, 20,* 20–32.

Antoni, M. H., & Lutgendorf, S. (2007). Psychosocial factors and disease progression in cancer. *Current Directions in Psychological Science, 16,* 42–46.

Apanovitch, A. M., McCarthy, D., & Salovey, P. (2003). Using message framing to motivate HIV testing among low-income, ethnic minority women. *Health Psychology, 22,* 60–67.

Appleton, A. A., Buka, S. L., McCormick, M. C., Koenen, K. C., Loucks, E. B., & Kubzansky, L. D. (2012). The association between childhood emotional functioning and adulthood inflammation is modified by early-life socioeconomic status. *Health Psychology, 31,* 413–422.

Appleton, A. A., Buka, S. L., Loucks, E. B., Gilman, S. E., & Kubzansky, L. D. (2013). Divergent associations of adaptive and maladaptive emotion regulation strategies with inflammation. *Health Psychology, 32,* 748–756.

Armistead, L., Cook, S., Skinner, D., Toefy, Y., Anthony, E. R., Zimmerman, L., . . . Chow, L. (2014). Preliminary results from a family-based HIV prevention intervention for South African youth. *Health Psychology, 33,* 668–676.

Armitage, C. J. (2008). A volitional help sheet to encourage smoking cessation: A randomized exploratory trial. *Health Psychology, 27,* 557–566.

Armitage, C. J., Harris, P. R., & Arden, M. A. (2011). Evidence that self-affirmation reduces alcohol consumption: Randomized exploratory trial with a new, brief means of self-affirming. *Health Psychology, 30,* 633–641.

Arnst, C. (2004, February 23). Let them eat cake—if they want to. *Business Week,* pp. 110–111.

Arpawong, T. E., Richeimer, S. H., Weinstein, F., Elghamrawy, A., & Milam, J. E. (2013). Posttraumatic growth, quality of life, and treatment symptoms among cancer chemotherapy outpatients. *Health Psychology, 32,* 397–408.

Arthritis Foundation. (2012). *The heavy burden of arthritis in the U.S.* Retrieved April 2, 2013, from http://www.arthritis.org/files/images/AF_Connect/Departments/Public_Relations/Arthritis-Prevalence-Fact-Sheet-3-7-12.pdf

Ary, D. V., Biglan, A., Glasgow, R., Zoref, L., Black, C., Ochs, L., . . . James, L. (1990). The efficacy of social-influence prevention programs versus "standard care": Are new initiatives needed? *Journal of Behavioral Medicine, 13,* 281–296.

Asanuma, Y., Oeser, A., Shintani, A. K., Turner, E., Olsen, N., Fazio, S., . . . Stein, C. M. (2003). Premature coronary artery atherosclerosis in systematic lupus erythematosus. *The New England Journal of Medicine, 349,* 2407–2415.

Aschbacher, K., Patterson, T. L., von Känel, R., Dimsdale, J. E., Mills, P. J., Adler, K. A., . . . Grant, I. (2005). Coping processes and hemostatic reactivity to acute stress in dementia caregivers. *Psychosomatic Medicine, 67,* 964–971.

Ashkenazi, L., Toledano, R., Novack, V., Elluz, E., Abu-Salamae, I., & Ifergane, G. (2015). Emergency department companions of stroke patients: Implications on quality of care. *Medicine, 94,* 520.

Aslaksen, P. M., & Flaten, M. A. (2008). The roles of physiological and subjective stress in the effectiveness of a placebo on experimentally induced pain. *Psychosomatic Medicine, 70,* 811–818.

Aspinwall, L. G. (2011). Future-oriented thinking, proactive coping, and the management of potential threats to health and well-being. In S. Folkman (Ed.), *The Oxford handbook of stress, health, and coping.* New York: Oxford University Press.

Aspinwall, L. G., Leaf, S. L., Dola, E. R., Kohlmann, W., & Leachman, S. A. (2008). CDKN2A/p16 genetic test reporting improves early detection intention and practices in high-risk melanoma families. *Cancer Epidemiology, Biomarkers & Prevention, 17,* 1510–1519.

Aspinwall, L. G., Taber, J. M., Leaf, S. L., Kohlmann, W., & Leachman, S. A. (2013). Genetic testing for hereditary melanoma and pancreatic cancer: A longitudinal study of psychological outcome. *Psycho-Oncology, 22,* 276–289.

Aspinwall, L. G., & Taylor, S. E. (1997). A stitch in time: Self-regulation and proactive coping. *Psychological Bulletin, 121,* 417–436.

Association for Psychological Science. (1996). *APS observer: Special issue HCI report 4–Healthy living.* Washington, DC: Author.

Auerbach, S. M., Clore, J. N., Kiesler, D. J., Orr, T., Pegg, P. O., Quick, B. G., & Wagner, C. (2001). Relation of diabetic patients' health-related control appraisals and physician–patient interpersonal impacts to patients' metabolic control and satisfaction with treatment. *Journal of Behavioral Medicine, 25,* 17–32.

Awick, E. A., Ehlers, D., Fanning, J., Phillips, S. M., Wójcicki, T., Mackenzie, M. J., . . . McAuley, E. (2017). Effects of a home-based DVD-delivered physical activity program on self-esteem in older adults: Results from a randomized controlled trial. *Psychosomatic Medicine, 79,* 71–80.

Babyak, M., Blumenthal, J. A., Herman, S., Khatri, P., Doraiswamy, M., Moore, K., . . . Krishnan, K. R. (2000). Exercise treatment for major depression: Maintenance of therapeutic benefit at 10 months. *Psychosomatic Medicine, 62,* 633–638.

Bach, P. B., Schrag, D., Brawley, O. W., Galaznik, A., Yakrin, S., & Begg, C. B. (2002). Survival of blacks and whites after a cancer diagnosis. *The Journal of the American Medical Association, 287,* 2106–2113.

Bacon, C. G., Mittleman, M. A., Kawachi, I., Giovannucci, E., Glasser, D. B., & Rimm, E. B. (2006). A prospective study of risk factors for erectile dysfunction. *The Journal of Urology, 176,* 217–221.

Badr, H., Carmack, C. L., Kashy, D. A., Cristofanilli, M., & Revenson, T. A. (2010). Dyadic coping in metastatic breast cancer. *Health Psychology, 29,* 169–180.

Badr, H., & Krebs, P. (2013). A systematic review and meta-analysis of psychosocial interventions for couples coping with cancer. *Psycho-Oncology, 22,* 1688–1704.

Bages, N., Appels, A., & Falger, P. R. J. (1999). Vital exhaustion as a risk factor of myocardial infarction: A case–control study in Venezuela. *International Journal of Behavioral Medicine, 6,* 279–290.

Baig, E. (1997, February 17). The doctor is in cyberspace: Myriad sites offer feedback and support. *Business Week,* p. 102E8.

Bair, M. J., Robinson, R. L., Eckert, G. J., Stang, P. E., Croghan, T. W., & Kroenke, K. (2004). Impact of pain on depression treatment response in primary care. *Psychosomatic Medicine, 66,* 17–22.

Bair, M. J., Wu, J., Damush, T. M., Sutherland, J. M., & Kroenke, K. (2008). Association of depression and anxiety alone and in the combination with chronic musculoskeletal pain in primary care patients. *Psychosomatic Medicine, 70,* 890–897.

Baker, R. C., & Kirschenbaum, D. S. (1998). Weight control during the holidays: Highly consistent self-monitoring as a potentially useful coping mechanism. *Health Psychology, 17,* 367–370.

Bakker, A., Van der Heijden, P. G. M., Van Son, M. J. M., & Van Loey, N., E. E. (2013). Course of traumatic stress reactions in couples after a burn event to their young child. *Health Psychology, 32,* 1076–1083.

Baldwin, A. S., Rothman, A. J., Hertel, A. W., Linde, J. A., Jeffery, R. W., Finch, E. A., & Lando, H. A. (2006). Specifying the determinants of the initiation and maintenance of behavior change: An examination of self-efficacy, satisfaction, and smoking cessation. *Health Psychology, 25,* 626–634.

Baldwin, A. S., Rothman, A. J., Vander Weg, M. W., & Christensen, A. J. (2013). Examining causal components and a mediating process underlying self-generated health arguments for exercise and smoking cessation. *Health Psychology, 32,* 1209–1217.

Baldwin, J. R., Arseneault, L., Odgers, C., Belsky, D. W., Matthews, T., Ambler, A., . . . Danese, A. (2016). Childhood bullying victimization and subsequent overweight in young adulthood: A cohort study. *Psychosomatic Medicine, 78,* 1094–1103.

Balfour, L., White, D. R., Schiffrin, A., Dougherty, G., & Dufresne, J. (1993). Dietary disinhibition, perceived stress, and glucose control in young, Type I diabetic women. *Health Psychology, 12,* 33–38.

Balog, P., Falger, P. R. J., Szabó, G., Rafael, B., Székely, A., & Konkolÿ Thege, B. (2017). Are vital exhaustion and depression independent risk factors for cardiovascular disease morbidity? *Health Psychology, 36,* 740–748.

Bambauer, K. Z., Aupont, O., Stone, P. H., Locke, S. E., Mullan, M. G., Colagiovanni, J., & McLaughlin, T. J. (2005). The effect of a telephone counseling intervention on self-rated health of cardiac patients. *Psychosomatic Medicine, 67,* 539–545.

Band, R., Barrowclough, C., & Wearden, A. (2014). The impact of significant other expressed emotion on patient outcomes in chronic fatigue syndrome. *Health Psychology, 33,* 1092–1101.

Bandiera, F. C., Arheart, K. L., Caban-Martinez, A. J., Fleming, L. E., McCollister, K., Dietz, N. A., . . . Lee, D. J. (2010). Secondhand smoke exposure and depressive symptoms. *Psychosomatic Medicine, 72,* 68–72.

Bandura, A. (1969). *Principles of behavior modification.* New York: Holt, Rinehart & Winston.

Bandura, A. (1977). Self-efficacy: Toward a unifying theory of behavioral change. *Psychological Review, 84,* 191–215.

Bandura, A. (1991). Self-efficacy mechanism in physiological activation and health-promotion behavior. In J. Madden IV (Ed.), *Neurobiology of learning, emotion, and affect* (pp. 229–269). New York: Raven Press.

Bankier, B., Januzzi, J. L., & Littman, A. B. (2004). The high prevalence of multiple psychiatric disorders in stable outpatients with coronary heart disease. *Psychosomatic Medicine, 66,* 645–650.

Barefoot, J. C. (1992). Developments in the measurement of hostility. In H. S. Friedman (Ed.), *Hostility, coping, and health* (pp. 13–31). Washington, DC: American Psychological Association.

Barefoot, J. C., Maynard, K. E., Beckham, J. C., Brummett, B. H., Hooker, K., & Siegler, I. C. (1998). Trust, health, and longevity. *Journal of Behavioral Medicine, 21,* 517–526.

Barger, S. D. (2013). Social integration, social support and mortality in the U.S. National Health Interview Survey. *Psychosomatic Medicine, 75,* 510–517.

Bargh, J. A., & Morsella, E. (2008). The unconscious mind. *Perspectives on Psychological Science, 3,* 73–79.

Barlow, M. A., Liu, S. Y., & Wrosch, C. (2015). Chronic illness and loneliness in older adulthood: The role of self-protective control strategies. *Health Psychology, 34,* 870–879.

Barnes, P. M., Bloom, B., & Nahin, R. L. (2008). Complementary and alternative medicine use among adults and children: United States, 2007. *National Health Statistics Report, 10,* 1–23.

Barnes, P. M., Powell-Griner, E., McFann, K., & Nahin, R. L. (2004). Complementary and alternative medicine use among adults: United States, 2002. *Advance Data, 27,* 1–19.

Barnes, P. M., & Schoenborn, C. A. (2012). Trends in adults receiving a recommendation for exercise or other physical activity from a physician or other health professional. *NCHS Data Brief, 86,* 1–8.

Barnes, V. A., Davis, H. C., Murzynowski, J. B., & Treiber, F. A. (2004). Impact of meditation on resting and ambulatory blood pressure and heart rate in youth. *Psychosomatic Medicine, 66,* 909–914.

Barnett, R. C., Raudenbush, S. W., Brennan, R. T., Pleck, J. H., & Marshall, N. L. (1995). Change in job and marital experiences and change in psychological distress: A longitudinal study of dual-earner couples. *Journal of Personality and Social Psychology, 69,* 839–850.

Barrera, M., Jr., Toobert, D., Strycker, L., & Osuna, D. (2012). Effects of acculturation on a culturally adapted diabetes intervention for Latinas. *Health Psychology, 31,* 51–54.

Bar-Tal, Y., Stasiuk, K., & Maksymiuk, R. A. (2013). Patients' perceptions of physicians' epistemic authority when recommending flu inoculation. *Health Psychology, 32,* 706–709.

Barth, J., Schneider, S., & von Känel, R. (2010). Lack of social support in the etiology and the prognosis of coronary heart disease: A systematic review and meta-analysis. *Psychosomatic Medicine, 72,* 229–238.

Bartley, H., Faasse, K., Horne, R., & Petrie, K. J. (2016). You can't always get what you want: The influence of choice on nocebo and placebo responding. *Annals of Behavioral Medicine, 50,* 445–451.

Barton, B. K., & Schwebel, D. C. (2007). A contextual perspective on the etiology of children's unintentional injuries. *Health Psychology Review, 1,* 173–185.

Bartrop, R. W., Lockhurst, E., Lazarus, L., Kiloh, L. G., & Penny, R. (1977). Depressed lymphocyte function after bereavement. *Lancet, 1,* 834–836.

Basen-Enquist, K., Carmack, C. L., Li, Y., Brown, J., Jhingran, A., Hughes, D. C., & Waters, A. (2013). Social-cognitive theory predictors of exercise behavior in endometrial cancer survivors. *Health Psychology, 32,* 1137–1148.

Basu, N., Jones, G. T., Macfarlane, G. J., & Druce, K. L. (2017). Identification and validation of clinically relevant clusters of severe fatigue in rheumatoid arthritis. *Psychosomatic Medicine, 79,* 1051–1058.

Bates, D. W., Spell, N., Cullen, D. J., Burdick, E., Laird, N., Peterson, L. A., . . . Leape, L. L. (1997). The cost of adverse drug events in hospitalized patients. *Journal of the American Medical Association, 277,* 307–311.

Baucom, K. J. W., Queen, T. L., Wiebe, D. J., Turner, S. L., Wolfe, K. L., Godbey, E. I., & Berg, C. A. (2015). Depressive symptoms, daily stress, and adherence in late adolescents with type 1 diabetes. *Health Psychology, 34,* 522–530.

Baucom, K. J. W., Turner, S. L., Tracy, E. L., Berg, C. A., & Wiebe, D. J. (2018). Depressive symptoms and diabetes management from late adolescence to emerging adulthood. *Health Psychology, 37,* 716–724.

Bauman, K. E., Koch, G. G., & Fisher, L. A. (1989). Family cigarette smoking and test performance by adolescents. *Health Psychology, 8,* 97–105.

Beal, S. J., Dorn, L. D., Sucharew, H. J., Sontag-Padilla, L., Pabst, S., & Hillman, J. (2014). Characterizing the longitudinal relations between depressive and menstrual symptoms in adolescent girls. *Psychosomatic Medicine, 76,* 547–554.

Beatty, D. L., Hall, M. H., Kamarck, T. A., Buysse, D. J., Owens, J. F., Reis, S. E., . . . Matthews, K. A. (2011). Unfair treatment is associated with poor sleep in African American and Caucasian adults: Pittsburgh SleepSCORE Project. *Health Psychology, 30,* 351–359.

Beatty, D. M., Chang, Y., Brown, C., Bromberger, J. T., & Matthews, K. A. (2018). Everyday discrimination and metabolic syndrome incidence in a racially/ethnically diverse sample: Study of women's health across the nation. *Psychosomatic Medicine, 80,* 114–121.

Beatty Moody, D. L., Taylor, A. D., Leibel, D. K., Al-Najjar, E., Katzel, L. I., Davatzikos, C., . . . Waldstein, S. R. (2019). Lifetime discrimination burden, racial discrimination, and subclinical cerebrovascular disease among African Americans. *Health Psychology, 38,* 63–74.

Beatty Moody, D. L., Waldstein, S. R., Tobin, J. N., Cassells, A., Schwartz, J. C., & Brondolo, E. (2016). Lifetime racial/ethnic discrimination and ambulatory blood pressure: The moderating effect of age. *Health Psychology, 35,* 333–342.

Beauchamp, M. R., Harden, S. M., Wolf, S. A., Rhodes, R. E., Liu, Y., Dunlop, W. L., . . . Estabrooks, P. A. (2015). GrOup based physical Activity for oLder adults (GOAL) randomized controlled trial: Study protocol. *BMC Public Health, 15,* 592.

Becker, M. H., & Janz, N. K. (1987). On the effectiveness and utility of health hazard/health risk appraisal in clinical and nonclinical settings. *Health Services Research, 22,* 537–551.

Beckjord, E. B., Rutten, L. J. F., Arora, N. K., Moser, R. P., & Hesse, B. W. (2008). Information processing and negative affect: Evidence from the 2003 health information national trends survey. *Health Psychology, 27,* 249–257.

Beckner, V., Howard, I., Vella, L., & Mohr, D. C. (2010). Telephone-administered psychotherapy for depression in MS patients: Moderating role of social support. *Journal of Behavioral Medicine, 33,* 47–59.

Beecher, H. K. (1959). *Measurement of subjective responses.* New York: Oxford University Press.

Bejarano, C. M., & Cushing, C. C. (2018). Dietary motivation and hedonic hunger predict palatable food consumption: An intensive longitudinal study of adolescents. *Annals of Behavioral Medicine, 52,* 773–786.

Beltrán-Sánchez, H., Finch, C. E., & Crimmins, E. M. (2015). Twentieth century surge of excess adult male mortality. *Proceedings of the National Academy of Sciences, 112,* 8993–8998.

Bellavite, P., Marzotto, M., Chirumbolo, S., & Conforti, A. (2011). Advances in homeopathy and immunology: A review of clinical research. *Frontiers in Bioscience, 3,* 1363–1389.

Beller, J., & Wagner, A. (2018). Loneliness, social isolation, their synergistic interaction, and mortality. *Health Psychology, 37,* 808–813.

Belloc, N. D., & Breslow, L. (1972). Relationship of physical health status and family practices. *Preventive Medicine, 1,* 409–421.

Belluck, P. (2005, March 17). Children's life expectancy being cut short by obesity. *New York Times,* p. A15.

Benight, C. C., Antoni, M. H., Kilbourn, K., Ironson, G., Kumar, M. A., Fletcher, M. A., . . . Schneiderman, N. (1997). Coping self-efficacy buffers psychological and physiological disturbances in HIV-infected men following a natural disaster. *Health Psychology, 16,* 248–255.

Benjamin, E. J., Virani, S. S., Callaway, C. W., Chamberlain, A. M., Chang, A. R., Cheng, S., . . . Muntner, P. (2018). Heart disease and stroke statistics-2018 update: A report from the American Heart Association. *Circulation, 137,* e67–e492.

Benner, A. D., Wang, Y., Shen, Y., Boyle, A. E., Polk, R., & Cheng, Y. P. (2018). Racial/ethnic discrimination and well-being during adolescence: A meta-analytic review. *American Psychologist, 73,* 855–883.

Bennett, K. K., Compas, B. E., Beckjord, E., & Glinder, J. G. (2005). Selfblame among women with newly diagnosed breast cancer. *Journal of Behavioral Medicine, 28,* 313–323.

Bensley, L. S., & Wu, R. (1991). The role of psychological reactance in drinking following alcohol prevention messages. *Journal of Applied Social Psychology, 21,* 1111–1124.

Berg, C. A., Butner, J. E., Butler, J. M., King, P. S., Hughes, A. E., & Wiebe, D. J. (2013). Parental persuasive strategies in the face of daily problems in adolescent type 1 diabetes management. *Health Psychology, 32,* 719-728.

Bergeson, S. C., & Dean, J. D. (2006). A systems approach to patient-centered care. *Journal of the American Medical Association, 296,* 2848-2851.

Berkley-Patton, J. Y., Thompson, C. B., Moore, E., Hawes, S., Berman, M., Allsworth, J., . . . Catley, D. (2019). Feasibility and outcomes of an HIV testing intervention in African American churches. *AIDS and Behavior, 23,* 76-90.

Berkman, E. T., Dickenson, J., Falk, E. B., & Lieberman, M. D. (2011). Using SMS text messaging to assess moderators of smoking reduction: Validating a new tool for ecological measurement of health behaviors. *Health Psychology, 30,* 186-194.

Berli, C., Stadler, G., Shrout, P. E., Bolger, N., & Scholz, U. (2017). Mediators of physical activity adherence: Results from an action control intervention in couples. *Annals of Behavioral Medicine, 52,* 65-76.

Berlin, A. A., Kop, W. J., & Deuster, P. A. (2006). Depressive mood symptoms and fatigue after exercise withdrawal: The potential role of decreased fitness. *Psychosomatic Medicine, 68,* 224-230.

Berman, M. G., Askren, M. K., Jung, M., Therrien, B., Peltier, S., Noll, D., . . . Cimprich, B. (2014). Pretreatment worry and neurocognitive responses in women with breast cancer. *Health Psychology, 33,* 222-231.

Bernstein, E. E., & McNally, R. J. (2017). Acute aerobic exercise hastens emotional recovery from a subsequent stressor. *Health Psychology, 36,* 560-567.

Bernstein, L. (2018, November 29). U.S. life expectancy declines again, a dismal trend not seen since WWI. *The Washington Post.* Retrieved May 7, 2019, from https://www.washingtonpost.com/national/health-science/us-life-expectancy-declines-again-a-dismal-trend-not-seen-since-world-war-i/2018/11/28/ae58bc8c-f28c-11e8-bc7968604ed88993_story.html?utm_term=.34327d5e7bf1

Berntson, G. G., Norman, G. J., Hawkley, L. C., & Cacioppo, J. T. (2008). Spirituality and autonomic cardiac control. *Annals of Behavioral Medicine, 35,* 198-208.

Berry, L. L., Mirabito, A. M., & Baun, W. B. (2010). What's the hard return on employee wellness programs? *Harvard Business Review, 88,* 104-112, 142.

Betensky, J. D., & Contrada, R. J. (2010). Depressive symptoms, trait aggression, and cardiovascular reactivity to a laboratory stressor. *Annals of Behavioral Medicine, 39,* 184-191.

Betsch, C., & Sachse, K. (2013). Debunking vaccination myths: Strong risk negations can increase perceived vaccination risks. *Health Psychology, 32,* 146-155.

Beydoun, M. A., Poggi-Burke, A., Zonderman, A. B., Rostant, O. S., Evans, M. K., & Crews, D. C. (2017). Perceived discrimination and longitudinal change in kidney function among urban adults. *Psychosomatic Medicine, 79,* 824-834.

Biernat, M., Crosby, F. J., & Williams, J. C. (Eds.). (2004). The maternal wall: Research and policy perspective on discrimination against mothers. *Journal of Social Issues, 60.*

Biglan, A., McConnell, S., Severson, H. H., Bavry, J., & Ary, D. (1984). A situational analysis of adolescent smoking. *Journal of Behavioral Medicine, 7,* 109-114.

Billings, A. C., & Moos, R. H. (1984). Coping, stress, and social resources among adults with unipolar depression. *Journal of Personality and Social Psychology, 46,* 877-891.

Birch, S., Hesselink, J. K., Jonkman, F. A. M., Hekker, T. A. M., & Bos, A. A. T. (2004). Clinical research on acupuncture: Part 1. What have reviews of the efficacy and safety of acupuncture told us so far? *The Journal of Alternative and Complementary Medicine, 10,* 468-480.

Bishop, S. R. (2002). What do we really know about mindfulness-based stress reduction? *Psychosomatic Medicine, 64,* 71-84.

Bishop, S. R., & Warr, D. (2003). Coping, catastrophizing and chronic pain in breast cancer. *Journal of Behavioral Medicine, 26,* 265-281.

Bjorntorp, P. (1996). Behavior and metabolic disease. *International Journal of Behavioral Medicine, 3,* 285-302.

Blair, C., & Raver, C. C. (2012). Child development in the context of adversity: Experiential canalization of brain and behavior. *American Psychologist, 67,* 309-318.

Blakeslee, S. (1998, October 13). Placebos prove so powerful even experts are surprised. *New York Times,* p. F2.

Blanchard, C. M., Fortier, M., Sweet, S., O'Sullivan, T., Hogg, W., Reid, R. D., & Sigal, R. J. (2007). Explaining physical activity levels from a self-efficacy perspective: The physical activity counseling trial. *Annals of Behavioral Medicine, 34,* 323-328.

Blanchard, E. B., Andrasik, F., & Silver, B. V. (1980). Biofeedback and relaxation in the treatment of tension headaches: A reply to Belar. *Journal of Behavioral Medicine, 3,* 227-232.

Blanton, H., & Gerrard, M. (1997). Effect of sexual motivation on men's risk perception for sexually transmitted disease: There must be 50 ways to justify a lover. *Health Psychology, 16,* 374-379.

Blascovich, J. (1992). A biopsychosocial approach to arousal regulation. *Journal of Social and Clinical Psychology, 11,* 213-237.

Blascovich, J. (2008). Challenge and threat appraisal. In A. J. Eliot (Ed.), *Handbook of approach-avoidance motivation* (pp. 432-444). New York: Taylor & Francis Group.

Blashill, A. J., Goshe, B. M., Robbins, G. K., Mayer, K. H., & Safren, S. A. (2014). Body image disturbance and health behaviors among sexual minority men living with HIV. *Health Psychology, 33,* 667-680.

Blashill, A. J., Safren, S. A., Wilhelm, S., Jampel, J., Taylor, S. W., O'Cleirigh, C., & Mayer, K. H. (2017). Cognitive behavioral therapy for body image and self-care (CBT-BISC) in sexual minority men living with HIV: A randomized controlled trial. *Health Psychology, 36,* 937-946.

Blechert, J., Feige, B., Joos, A., Zeeck, A., & Tuschen-Caffier, B. (2011). Electrocortical processing of food and emotional pictures in anorexia nervosa and bulimia nervosa. *Psychosomatic Medicine, 73,* 415-421.

Bleil, M. E., Gianaros, P. J., Jennings, R., Flory, J. D., & Manuck, S. B. (2008). Trait negative affect: Toward an integrated model of understanding psychological risk for impairment in cardiac autonomic function. *Psychosomatic Medicine, 70,* 328-337.

Blissmer, B., & McAuley, E. (2002). Testing the requirements of stages of physical activity among adults: The comparative effectiveness of stage-matched, mismatched, standard care, and control interventions. *Annals of Behavioral Medicine, 24,* 181-189.

Blomhoff, S., Spetalen, S., Jacobsen, M. B., & Malt, U. F. (2001). Phobic anxiety changes the function of brain-gut axis in irritable bowel syndrome. *Psychosomatic Medicine, 63,* 959-965.

Bloom, B., & Cohen, R. A. (2011). Young adults seeking medical care: Do race and ethnicity matter? *NCHS Data Brief, 55,* 1-8.

Bluebond-Langner, M. (1977). Meanings of death to children. In H. Feifel (Ed.), *New meanings of death* (pp. 47-66). New York: McGraw-Hill.

Blumenthal, J. A., Emery, C. F., Smith, P. J., Keefe, F. J., Welty-Wolf, K., Mabe, S., & Palmer, S. M. (2014). The effects of a telehealth coping skills intervention on outcomes in chronic obstructive pulmonary disease: Primary results from the INSPIRE-II study. *Psychosomatic Medicine, 76,* 581-592.

Blumenthal, J. A., Smith, P. J., Mabe, S., Hinderliter, A., Welsh-Bohmer, K., Browndyke, J. N., . . . Sherwood, A. (2017). Lifestyle and neurocognition in older adults with cardiovascular risk factors and cognitive impairment. *Psychosomatic Medicine, 79,* 719-727.

Boehm, J. K., & Kubzansky, L. D. (2012). The heart's content: The association between positive psychological well-being and cardiovascular health. *Psychological Bulletin, 138,* 655-691.

Boehm, J. K., Soo, J., Zevon, E. S., Chen, Y., Kim, E. S., & Kubzansky, L. D. (2018). Longitudinal associations between psychological well-being and the consumption of fruits and vegetables. *Health Psychology, 37,* 959-967.

Boehm, J. K., Trudel-Fitzgerald, C., Kivimaki, M., & Kubzansky, L. D. (2015). The prospective association between positive psychological well-being and diabetes. *Health Psychology, 34,* 1013-1021.

Bogart, L. M. (2001). Relationship of stereotypic beliefs about physicians to health-care relevant behaviors and cognitions among African American women. *Journal of Behavioral Medicine, 245,* 573-586.

Bogart, L. M., Mutchler, M. G., McDavitt, B., Klein, D. J., Cunningham, W. E., Goggin, K. J., . . . Wagner, G. J. (2017). A randomized controlled trial of RISE, a community-based culturally congruent adherence intervention for black Americans living with HIV. *Annals of Behavioral Medicine, 51,* 868-878.

Bogart, L. M., Wagner, G. J., Galvan, F. H., & Klein, D. J. (2010). Longitudinal relationships between antiretroviral treatment adherence and discrimination due to HIV-serostatus, race, and sexual orientation among African-American men with HIV. *Annals of Behavioral Medicine, 40,* 184-190.

Bogg, T., & Slatcher, R. B. (2015). Activity mediates conscientiousness' relationship to diurnal cortisol slope in a national sample. *Health Psychology, 34,* 1195-1199.

Bold, K. W., Krishnan-Sarin, S., & Stoney, C. M. (2018). E-cigarette use as a potential cardiovascular disease risk behavior. *American Psychologist, 73,* 955-967.

Bolger, N., & Amarel, D. (2007). Effects of social support visibility on adjustment to stress: Experimental evidence. *Journal of Personality and Social Psychology, 92,* 458-475.

Bolger, N., Zuckerman, A., & Kessler, R. C. (2000). Invisible support and adjustment to stress. *Journal of Personality and Social Psychology, 79,* 953-961.

Bolles, R. C., & Fanselow, M. S. (1982). Endorphins and behavior. *Annual Review of Psychology, 33,* 87-101.

Bonanno, G. A., Keltner, D., Holen, A., & Horowitz, M. J. (1995). When avoiding unpleasant emotions might not be such a bad thing: Verbal-autonomic response dissociation and midlife conjugal bereavement. *Journal of Personality and Social Psychology, 69,* 975-989.

Bonanno, G. A., Wortman, C. B., Lehman, D. R., Tweed, R. G., Haring, M., Sonnega, J., . . . Neese, R. M. (2002). Resilience to loss and chronic grief: A prospective study from preloss to 18-months postloss. *Journal of Personality and Social Psychology, 83,* 1150-1164.

Bookwala, J., Marshall, K. I., & Manning, S. W. (2014). Who needs a friend? Marital status transitions and physical health outcomes in later life. *Health Psychology, 33,* 505-515.

Booth, T., Mõttus, R., Corley, J., Gow, A. J., Henderson, R. D., Maniega, S. M., & Deary, I. J. (2014). Personality, health, and brain integrity: The Lothian birth cohort study 1936. *Health Psychology, 33,* 1477-1486.

Borland, R. (2018). Misinterpreting theory and ignoring evidence: Fear appeals can actually work: A comment on Kok et al. (2018). *Health Psychology Review, 12,* 126-128.

Borrelli, B., Gaynor, S., Tooley, E., Armitage, C. J., Wearden, A., & Bartlett, Y. K. (2018). Identification of three different types of smokers who are not motivated to quit: Results from a latent class analysis. *Health Psychology, 37,* 179-187.

Bornschein, S., Hausteiner, C., Konrad, F., Förstl, H., & Zilker, T. (2006). Psychiatric morbidity and toxic burden in patients with environmental illness: A controlled study. *Psychosomatic Medicine, 68,* 104-109.

Boscarino, J., & Chang, J. (1999). Higher abnormal leukocyte and lymphocyte counts 20 years after exposure to severe stress: Research and clinical implications. *Psychosomatic Medicine, 61,* 378-386.

Bosch, J. A., Engeland, C. G., Cacioppo, J. T., & Marucha, P. T. (2007). Depressive symptoms predict mucosal wound healing. *Psychosomatic Medicine, 69,* 597-605.

Boskind-White, M., & White, W. C. (1983). *Bulimarexia: The binge/purge cycle.* New York: Norton.

Bosma, H., Marmot, M. G., Hemingway, H., Nicholson, A. C., Brunner, E., & Stanfeld, S. A. (1997). Low job control and risk of coronary heart disease in Whitehall II (prospective cohort) study. *British Medical Journal, 314,* 558-565.

Bosworth, H. B., Blalock, D. V., Hoyle, R. H., Czajkowski, S. M., & Voils, C. I. (2018). The role of psychological science in efforts to improve cardiovascular medication adherence. *American Psychologist, 73,* 968-980.

Bourassa, K. J., Sbarra, D. A., Ruiz, J. M., Karciroti, N., & Harburg, K. J. (2019). Mismatch in spouses' anger-coping response styles and risk of early mortality. *Psychosomatic Medicine, 81,* 26-33.

Boutelle, K. N., Kirschenbaum, D. S., Baker, R. C., & Mitchell, M. E. (1999). How can obese weight controllers minimize weight gain during the high risk holiday season? By self-monitoring very consistently. *Health Psychology, 18,* 364-368.

Bouton, M. E. (2000). A learning theory perspective on lapse, relapse, and the maintenance of behavior change. *Health Psychology, 19,* 57-63.

Bouwmans, M. E., Conradi, H. J., Bos, E. H., Oldenhinkel, A. J., & de Jonge, P. (2017). Bidirectionality between sleep symptoms and core depressive symptoms and their long-term course in major depression. *Psychosomatic Medicine, 79,* 336-344.

Bowen, A. M., Williams, M. L., Daniel, C. M., & Clayton, S. (2008). Internet based HIV prevention research targeting rural MSM: Feasibility, acceptability, and preliminary efficacy. *Journal of Behavioral Medicine, 31,* 463-477.

Bowen, D. J., Tomoyasu, N., Anderson, M., Carney, M., & Kristal, A. (1992). Effects of expectancies and personalized feedback on fat consumption, taste, and preference. *Journal of Applied Social Psychology, 22,* 1061-1079.

Bowen, K. S., Uchino, B. N., Birmingham, W., Carlisle, M., Smith, T. W., & Light, K. C. (2014). The stress-buffering effects of functional social support on ambulatory blood pressure. *Health Psychology, 33,* 1440-1443.

Bower, J. E. (2019). The role of neuro-immune interactions in cancer-related fatigue: Biobehavioral risk factors and mechanisms. *Cancer, 125,* 353-364.

Bower, J. E., Crosswell, A. D., & Slavich, G. M. (2013). Childhood adversity and cumulative life stress: Risk factors for cancer-related fatigue. *Clinical Psychological Science, 2,* 108-115.

Bower, J. E., Garet, D., Sternlieb, B., Ganz, P. A., Irwin, M. R., Olmstead, R., & Greendale, G. (2011). Yoga for persistent fatigue in breast cancer survivors: A randomized controlled trial. *Cancer, 118,* 3766-3775.

Bower, J. E., Kemeny, M. E., Taylor, S. E., & Fahey, J. L. (1997). Cognitive processing, discovery of meaning, CD 4 decline, and AIDS-related mortality among bereaved HIV-seropositive men. *Journal of Consulting and Clinical Psychology, 66,* 979-986.

Bower, J. E., Kemeny, M. E., Taylor, S. E., & Fahey, J. L. (2003). Finding positive meaning and its association with natural killer cell cytotoxicity among participants in bereavement-related disclosure intervention. *Annals of Behavioral Medicine, 25,* 146-155.

Boyce, W. T., Chesney, M., Alkon, A., Tschann, J. M., Adams, S., Chesterman, B., . . . Wara, D. (1995). Psychobiologic reactivity to stress and childhood respiratory illness: Results of two prospective studies. *Psychosomatic Medicine, 57,* 411-422.

Boyce, W. T., Chesterman, E. A., Martin, N., Folkman, S., Cohen, F., & Wara, D. (1993). Immunologic changes occurring at kindergarten entry predict respiratory illnesses after the Loma Prieta earthquake. *Journal of Developmental and Behavioral Pediatrics, 14,* 296-303.

Boyer, C. A., & Lutfey, K. E. (2010). Examining critical health policy issues within and beyond the clinical encounter: Patient–provider relationships and help-seeking behaviors. *Journal of Health and Social Behavior, 51,* S80–S93.

Boylan, J. M., Cundiff, J. M., & Matthews, K. A. (2018). Socioeconomic status and cardiovascular responses to standardized stressors: A systematic review and meta-analysis. *Psychosomatic Medicine, 80,* 278–293.

Boylan, J. M., & Ryff, C. D. (2013). Varieties of anger and the inverse link between education and inflammation: Toward an integrative framework. *Psychosomatic Medicine, 75,* 566–574.

Boyle, C. C., Stanton, A. L., Ganz, P. A., Crespi, C. M., & Bower, J. E. (2017). Improvements in emotion regulation following mindfulness meditation: Effects on depressive symptoms and perceived stress in younger breast cancer survivors. *Journal of Consulting and Clinical Psychology, 85,* 397–402.

Boyle, P. A., Barnes, L. L., Buchman, A. S., & Bennett, D. A. (2009). Purpose in life is associated with mortality among community-dwelling older persons. *Psychosomatic Medicine, 71,* 574–579.

Boyle, S. H., Michalek, J. E., & Suarez, E. C. (2006). Covariation of psychological attributes and incident coronary heart disease in U.S. Air Force veterans of the Vietnam War. *Psychosomatic Medicine, 68,* 844–850.

Boyle, S. H., Williams, R. B., Mark, D. B., Brummett, B. H., Siegler, I. C., Helms, M. J., & Barefoot, J. C. (2004). Hostility as a predictor of survival in patients with coronary artery disease. *Psychosomatic Medicine, 66,* 629–632.

Branegan, J. (1997, March 17). I want to draw the line myself. *Time,* pp. 30–31.

Bränström, R., Kvillemo, P., Brandberg, Y., & Moskowitz, J. T. (2010). Self-report mindfulness as a mediator of psychological well-being in a stress reduction intervention for cancer patients—A randomized study. *Annals of Behavioral Medicine, 39,* 151–161.

Brantley, P. J., Mosley, T. H., Jr., Bruce, B. K., McKnight, G. T., & Jones, G. N. (1990). Efficacy of behavioral management and patient education on vascular access cleansing compliance in hemodialysis patients. *Health Psychology, 9,* 103–113.

Brennan, P. L., & Moos, R. H. (1990). Life stressors, social resources, and late-life problem drinking. *Psychology and Aging, 5,* 491–501.

Brennan, P. L., & Moos, R. H. (1995). Life context, coping responses, and adaptive outcomes: A stress and coping perspective on late-life problem drinking. In T. Beresford & E. Gomberg (Eds.), *Alcohol and aging* (pp. 230–248). New York: Oxford University Press.

Breslau, N., & Davis, G. C. (1987). Posttraumatic stress disorder: The stressor criterion. *Journal of Nervous and Mental Disease, 175,* 255–264.

Breslow, L., & Enstrom, J. E. (1980). Persistence of health habits and their relationship to mortality. *Preventive Medicine, 9,* 469–483.

Brewer, N. T., Chapman, G. B., Gibbons, F. X., Gerrard, M., McCaul, K. D., & Weinstein, N. D. (2007). Meta-analysis of the relationship between risk perception and health behavior: The example of vaccination. *Health Psychology, 26,* 136–145.

Brindle, R. C., Cribbet, M. R., Samuelsson, L. B., Gao, C., Frank, E., Krafty, R. T., . . . Hall, M. H. (2018). The relationship between childhood trauma and poor sleep health in adulthood. *Psychosomatic Medicine, 80,* 200–207.

Brindle, R. C., Duggan, K. A., Cribbet, M. R., Kline, C. E., Krafty, R. T., Thayer, J. F., . . . Hall, M. H. (2018). Cardiovascular stress reactivity and carotid intima-media thickness: The buffering role of slow-wave sleep. *Psychosomatic Medicine, 80,* 301–306.

Brissette, I., & Cohen, S. (2002). The contribution of individual differences in hostility to the associations between daily interpersonal conflict, affect, and sleep. *Personality and Social Psychology Bulletin, 28,* 1265–1274.

Britton, A., & Marmot, M. (2004). Different measures of alcohol consumption and risk of coronary heart disease and all-cause mortality: 11-year follow-up of the Whitehall II Cohort Study. *Addiction, 99,* 109–116.

Britton, W. B., Haynes, P. L., Fridel, K. W., & Bootzin, R. R. (2010). Polysomnographic and subjective profiles of sleep continuity before and after mindfulness-based cognitive therapy in partially remitted depression. *Psychosomatic Medicine, 72,* 539–548.

Broadbent, E. (2017). Interactions with robots: The truths we reveal about ourselves. *Annual Review of Psychology, 68,* 627–652.

Broadbent, E., Ellis, C. J., Gamble, G., & Petrie, K. J. (2006). Changes in patient drawings of the heart identify slow recovery after myocardial infarction. *Psychosomatic Medicine, 68,* 910–913.

Broadbent, E., Niederhoffer, K., Hague, T., Corter, A., & Reynolds, L. (2009). Headache sufferers' drawings reflect distress, disability and illness perceptions. *Journal of Psychosomatic Research, 66,* 465–470.

Broadbent, E., Petrie, K. J., Alley, P. G., & Booth, R. J. (2003). Psychological stress impairs early wound repair following surgery. *Psychosomatic Medicine, 65,* 865–869.

Broadbent, E., Petrie, K. J., Ellis, C. J., Ying, J., & Gamble, G. (2004). A picture of health—myocardial infarction patients' drawings of their hearts and subsequent disability: A longitudinal study. *Journal of Psychosomatic Research, 57,* 583–587.

Broadwell, S. D., & Light, K. C. (1999). Family support and cardiovascular responses in married couples during conflict and other interactions. *International Journal of Behavioral Medicine, 6,* 40–63.

Brochu, P. M., Pearl, R. L., Puhl, R. M., & Brownell, K. D. (2014). Do media portrayals of obesity influence support for weight-related medical policy? *Health Psychology, 33,* 197–200.

Broderick, J. E., Junghaenel, D. U., & Schwartz, J. E. (2005). Written emotional expression produces health benefits in fibromyalgia patients. *Psychosomatic Medicine, 67,* 326–334.

Brody, G. H., Yu, T., Beach, S. R. H., Kogan, S. M., Windle, M., & Philbert, R. A. (2014). Harsh parenting and adolescent health: A longitudinal analysis with genetic moderation. *Health Psychology, 33,* 401–409.

Brody, G. H., Yu, T., Chen, E., & Miller, G. E. (2014). Prevention moderates associations between family risks and youth catecholamine levels. *Health Psychology, 33,* 1435–1439.

Brody, G. H., Yu, T., Chen, E., Ehrlich, K. B., & Miller, G. E. (2018). Racial discrimination, body mass index, and insulin resistance: A longitudinal analysis. *Health Psychology, 37,* 1107–1114.

Brody, J. E. (2002, January 22). Misunderstood opioids and needless pain. *New York Times,* p. D8.

Brondolo, E., Hausmann, L. R. M., Jhalani, J., Pencille, M., Atencio-Bacayon, J., Kumar, A., . . . Schwartz, J. (2011). Dimensions of perceived racism and self-reported health: Examination of racial/ethnic differences and potential mediators. *Annals of Behavioral Medicine, 42,* 14–28.

Brondolo, E., ver Halen, N. B., Pencille, M., Beatty, D., & Contrada, R. J. (2009). Coping with racism: A selective review of the literature and a theoretical and methodological critique. *Journal of Behavioral Medicine, 32,* 64–88.

Brooks, K. P., Gruenewald, T., Karlamangla, A., Hu, P., Koretz, B., & Seeman, T. E. (2014). Social relationships and allostatic load in the MIDUS study. *Health Psychology, 33,* 1373–1381.

Brooks, S., Rowley, S., Broadbent, E., & Petrie, K. J. (2012). Illness perception ratings of high-risk newborns by mothers and clinicians: Relationship to illness severity and maternal stress. *Health Psychology, 31,* 632–639.

Brosschot, J., Godaert, G., Benschop, R., Olff, M., Ballieux, R., & Heijnen, C. (1998). Experimental stress and immunological reactivity: A closer look at perceived uncontrollability. *Psychosomatic Medicine, 60,* 359–361.

Brown, J. L., & Vanable, P. A. (2008). Cognitive-behavioral stress management interventions for persons living with HIV: A review and critique of the literature. *Annals of Behavioral Medicine, 35,* 26–40.

Brown, K. W., Levy, A. R., Rosberger, Z., & Edgar, L. (2003). Psychological distress and cancer survival: A follow-up 10 years after diagnosis. *Psychosomatic Medicine, 65,* 636–643.

Brown, K. W., & Ryan, R. M. (2003). The benefits of being present: Mindfulness and its role in psychological well-being. *Journal of Personality and Social Psychology, 84,* 822–848.

Brown, S. L., Nesse, R. M., Vinokur, A. D., & Smith, D. M. (2003). Providing social support may be more beneficial than receiving it: Results from a prospective study of mortality. *Psychological Science, 14,* 320–327.

Brown, T. A., & Keel, P. K. (2012). Current and emerging directions in the treatment of eating disorders. *Journal of Substance Abuse, 6,* 33–61.

Brownell, K. D. (1982). Obesity: Understanding and treating a serious, prevalent and refractory disorder. *Journal of Consulting and Clinical Psychology, 50,* 820–840.

Brownell, K. D., & Frieden, T. R. (2009). Ounces of prevention—The public policy cases for taxes on sugared beverages. *The New England Journal of Medicine, 360,* 1805–1808.

Brownell, K. D., Marlatt, G. A., Lichtenstein, E., & Wilson, G. T. (1986). Understanding and preventing relapse. *American Psychologist, 41,* 765–782.

Brownell, K. D., & Napolitano, M. A. (1995). Distorting reality for children: Body size proportions of Barbie and Ken dolls. *International Journal of Eating Disorders, 18,* 295–298.

Brownell, K. D., & Wadden, T. A. (1992). Etiology and treatment of obesity: Understanding a serious, prevalent, and refractory disorder. *Journal of Consulting and Clinical Psychology, 60,* 505–517.

Browning, C. R., & Cagney, K. A. (2003). Moving beyond poverty: Neighborhood structure, social processes, and health. *Journal of Health and Social Behavior, 44,* 552–571.

Bruce, E. C., & Musselman, D. L. (2005). Depression, alterations in platelet function, and ischemic heart disease. *Psychosomatic Medicine, 67,* S34–S36.

Bruce, J. M., Bruce, A. S., Catley, D., Lynch, S., Goggin, K., Reed, D., . . . Jarmolowicz, D. P. (2015). Being kind to your future self: Probability discounting of health decision-making. *Annals of Behavioral Medicine, 50,* 297–309.

Bruce, J. M., Hancock, L. M., Arnett, P., & Lynch, S. (2010). Treatment adherence in multiple sclerosis: Associations with emotional status, personality, and cognition. *Journal of Behavioral Medicine, 33,* 219–227.

Bruehl, S., al'Absi, M., France, C. R., France, J., Harju, A., Burns, J. W., & Chung, O. Y. (2007). Anger management style and endogenous opioid function: Is gender a moderator? *Journal of Behavioral Medicine, 30,* 209–219.

Bruehl, S., Burns, J. W., Chung, O. Y., & Quartana, P. (2008). Anger management style and emotional reactivity to noxious stimuli among chronic pain patients and healthy controls: The role of endogenous opioids. *Health Psychology, 27,* 204–214.

Brumbach, B. H., Birmingham, W. C., Boonyasiriwat, W., Walters, S., & Kinney, A. Y. (2017). Intervention mediators in a randomized controlled trial to increase colonoscopy uptake among individuals at increased risk of familial colorectal cancer. *Annals of Behavioral Medicine, 51,* 694–706.

Brummett, B. H., Babyak, M. A., Barefoot, J. C., Bosworth, H. B., Clapp-Channing, N. E., Siegler, I. C., . . . Mark, D. B. (1998). Social support and hostility as predictors of depressive symptoms in cardiac patients one month after hospitalization: A prospective study. *Psychosomatic Medicine, 60,* 707–713.

Brummett, B. H., Babyak, M. A., Siegler, I. C., Vitaliano, P. P., Ballard, E. L., Gwyther, L. P., & Williams, R. B. (2006). Associations among perceptions of social support, negative affect, and quality of sleep in caregivers and noncaregivers. *Health Psychology, 25,* 220–225.

Brummett, B. H., Boyle, S. H., Ortel, T. L., Becker, R. C., Siegler, I. C., & Williams, R. B. (2010). Association of depressive symptoms, trait hostility, and gender with C-reactive and interleukin-6 responses after emotion recall. *Psychosomatic Medicine, 72,* 333–339.

Brummett, B. H., Siegler, I. C., Rohe, W. M., Barefoot, J. C., Vitaliano, P. P., Surwit, R. S., . . . Williams, R. B. (2005). Neighborhood characteristics moderate effects of caregiving on glucose functioning. *Psychosomatic Medicine, 67,* 752–758.

Bruzzese, J., Idalski Carcone, A., Lam, P., Ellis, D. A., & Naar-King, S. (2014). Adherence to asthma medication regimens in urban African American adolescents: Application of self-determination theory. *Health Psychology, 33,* 461–464.

Bryant, R. A., & Guthrie, R. M. (2005). Maladaptive appraisals as a risk factor for posttraumatic stress: A study of trainee firefighters. *Psychological Science, 16,* 749–752.

Bryck, R. L., & Fisher, P. A. (2012). Training the brain: Practical applications of neural plasticity from the intersection of cognitive neuroscience, developmental psychology, and prevention science. *American Psychologist, 62,* 87–100.

Buchman, A. S., Boyle, P. A., Wilson, R. S., Tang, Y., & Bennett, D. A. (2007). Frailty is associated with incident Alzheimer's disease and cognitive decline in the elderly. *Psychosomatic Medicine, 69,* 483–489.

Buchman, A. S., Kopf, D., Westphal, S., Lederbogen, F., Banaschewski, T., Esser, G., . . . Deuschle, M. (2010). Impact of early parental child-rearing behavior on young adults' cardiometabolic risk profile: A prospective study. *Psychosomatic Medicine, 72,* 156–162.

Buchwald, D., Herrell, R., Ashton, S., Belcourt, M., Schmaling, K., Sullivan, P., . . . Goldberg, J. (2001). A twin study of chronic fatigue. *Psychosomatic Medicine, 63,* 936–943.

Budman, S. H. (2000). Behavioral health care dot-com and beyond: Computer-mediated communications in mental health and substance abuse treatment. *American Psychologist, 55,* 1290–1300.

Buhle, J. T., Stevens, B. L., Friedman, J. J., & Wager, T. D. (2012). Distraction and placebo: Two separate routes to pain control. *Psychological Science, 23,* 246–253.

Bukberg, J., Penman, D., & Holland, J. C. (1984). Depression in hospitalized cancer patients. *Psychosomatic Medicine, 46,* 199–212.

Bulik, C. M., Thornton, L., Pinheiro, A. P., Plotnicov, K., Klump, K. L., Brandt, H., . . . Kaye, W. H. (2008). Suicide attempts in anorexia nervosa. *Psychosomatic Medicine, 70,* 378–383.

Bunde, J., & Martin, R. (2006). Depression and prehospital delay in the context of myocardial infarction. *Psychosomatic Medicine, 68,* 51–57.

Bureau of Labor Statistics. (2012a). *Labor force statistics from the current population survey.* Retrieved April 10, 2012, from http://data.bls.gov/timeseries/LNS12300000

Bureau of Labor Statistics. (2012b). *Social workers.* Retrieved March 15, 2013, from http://www.bls.gov/ooh/Community-and-Social-Service/Social-workers.htm#tab-1

Bureau of Labor Statistics. (2016, June 7). *The economics daily, employment-population ratio, 59.7 percent; unemployment rate, 4.7 percent in May.* Retrieved March 26, 2019, from https://www.bls.gov/opub/ted/2016/employment-population-ratio-59-point-7-percent-unemployment-rate-4-point-7-percent-in-may.htm

Bureau of Labor Statistics. (2019). *Physicians and surgeons: Occupational outlook handbook.* Retrieved April 9, 2019, from https://www.bls.gov/ooh/healthcare/physicians-and-surgeons.htm#tab-6

Burell, G., & Granlund, B. (2002). Women's hearts need special treatment. *International Journal of Behavioral Medicine, 9,* 228–242.

Burg, M. M., Barefoot, J., Berkman, L., Catellier, D. J., Czajkowski, S., Saab, P., . . . ENRICHD Investigators. (2005). Low perceived social support and post-myocardial infarction prognosis in the enhancing recovery in coronary heart disease clinical trial: The effects of treatment. *Psychosomatic Medicine, 67,* 879–888.

Burg, M. M., Benedetto, M. C., Rosenberg, R., & Soufer, R. (2003). Presurgical depression predicts medical mortality 6 months after coronary artery bypass graft surgery. *Psychosomatic Medicine, 65,* 111–118.

Burg, M. M., Brandt, C., Buta, E., Schwartz, J., Bathulapalli, H., Dziura, J., . . . Haskell, S. (2017). Risk for incident hypertension associated with PTSD in military veterans, and the effect of PTSD treatment. *Psychosomatic Medicine, 79,* 181–188.

Burg, M. M., Schwartz, J. E., Kronish, I. M., Diaz, K. M., Alcantara, C., Duer-Hefele, J., & Davidson, K. W. (2017). Does stress result in you exercising less? Or does exercising result in you being less stressed? Or is it both? Testing the bi-directional stress-exercise association at the group and person (N of 1) level. *Annals of Behavioral Medicine, 51,* 799–809.

Burgard, S. A., & Ailshire, J. A. (2009). Putting work to bed: Stressful experiences on the job and sleep quality. *Journal of Health and Social Behavior, 50,* 476–492.

Burgard, S. A., Brand, J. E., & House, J. S. (2007). Toward a better estimation of the effect of job loss on health. *Journal of Health and Social Behavior, 48,* 369–384.

Burgess, C., Morris, T., & Pettingale, K. W. (1988). Psychological response to cancer diagnosis: II. Evidence for coping styles. *Journal of Psychosomatic Research, 32,* 263–272.

Burish, T. G., & Lyles, J. N. (1979). Effectiveness of relaxation training in reducing the aversiveness of chemotherapy in the treatment of cancer. *Journal of Behavior Therapy and Experimental Psychiatry, 10,* 357–361.

Burns, J. W. (2000). Repression predicts outcome following multidisciplinary treatment of chronic pain. *Health Psychology, 19,* 75–84.

Burns, J. W., Elfant, E., & Quartana, P. J. (2010). Supression of pain-related thoughts and feelings during pain-induction: Sex differences in delayed pain responses. *Journal of Behavioral Medicine, 33,* 200–208.

Burns, J. W., Gerhart, J. I., Bruehl, S., Post, K. M., Smith, D. A., Porter, L. S., & Keefe, F. J. (2016). Anger arousal and behavioral anger regulation in everyday life among people with chronic low back pain: Relationships with spouse responses and negative affect. *Health Psychology, 35,* 29–40.

Burns, J. W., Holly, A., Quartana, P., Wolff, B., Gray, E., & Bruehl, S. (2008). Trait anger management style moderates effects of actual ("state") anger regulation on symptom-specific reactivity and recovery among chronic low back pain patients. *Psychosomatic Medicine, 70,* 898–905.

Burns, J. W., Quartana, P., & Bruehl, S. (2008). Anger inhibition and pain: Conceptualizations, evidence and new directions. *Journal of Behavioral Medicine, 31,* 259–279.

Burns, R. J., Deschênes, S. S., & Schmitz, N. (2015). Associations between depressive symptoms and social support in adults with diabetes: Comparing directionality hypotheses with a longitudinal cohort. *Annals of Behavioral Medicine, 50,* 348–357.

Burns, R. J., Deschenes, S. S., & Schmitz, N. (2016). Associations between coping strategies and mental health in individuals with type 2 diabetes: Prospective analyses. *Health Psychology, 35,* 78–86.

Burton, R. P. D. (1998). Global integrative meaning as a mediating factor in the relationship between social roles and psychological distress. *Journal of Health and Social Behavior, 39,* 201–215.

Bush, C., Ditto, B., & Feuerstein, M. (1985). A controlled evaluation of paraspinal EMG biofeedback in the treatment of chronic low back pain. *Health Psychology, 4,* 307–321.

Butler, L. D., Koopman, C., Classen, C., & Spiegel, D. (1999). Traumatic stress, life events, and emotional support in women with metastatic breast cancer: Cancer-related traumatic stress symptoms associated with past and current stressors. *Health Psychology, 18,* 555–560.

Buunk, B. P., Doosje, B. J., Jans, L. G. J. M., & Hopstaken, L. E. M. (1993). Perceived reciprocity, social support, and stress at work: The role of exchange and communal orientation. *Journal of Personality and Social Psychology, 65,* 801–811.

Cabizuca, M., Marques-Portella, C., Mendlowicz, M. V., Coutinho, E. S. F., & Figueira, I. (2009). Posttraumatic stress disorders in parents with children with chronic illness: A meta-analysis. *Health Psychology, 28,* 379–388.

Cacioppo, J. T., Cacioppo, S., & Capitanio, J. P. (2015). The neuroendocrinology of social isolation. *Annual Review of Psychology, 66,* 733–767.

Cacioppo, S., Grippo, A. J., London, S., Goossens, L., & Cacioppo, J. T. (2015). Loneliness: Clinical import and interventions. *Perspectives on Psychological Science, 10,* 238–249.

California Environmental Protection Agency. (2005). *Proposed identification of environmental tobacco smoke as a toxic air contaminant, part B: Health effects.* Retrieved October 20, 2009, from http://www.oehha.org/air/environmental_tobacco/pdf/app3partb2005.pdf

Callaghan, B. L. (2017). Generational patterns of stress: Help from our microbes? *Current Directions in Psychological Science, 26,* 323–329.

Calle, E. E., Rodriguez, C., Walker-Thurmond, K., & Thun, M. J. (2003). Overweight, obesity, and mortality from cancer in a prospectively studied cohort in U.S. adults. *The New England Journal of Medicine, 348,* 1625–1638.

Calvin, C. M., Batty, G. D., Lowe, G. D. O., & Deary, I. J. (2011). Childhood intelligence and midlife inflammatory and hemostatic biomarkers: The National Child Development Study (1958) cohort. *Health Psychology, 30,* 710–718.

Cameron, E. Z., Setsaas, T. H., & Linklater, W. L. (2009). Social bonds between unrelated females increase reproductive success in feral horses. *Proceedings of the National Academy of Sciences, 106,* 13850–13853.

Cameron, L., Leventhal, E. A., & Leventhal, H. (1995). Seeking medical care in response to symptoms and life stress. *Psychosomatic Medicine, 57,* 1–11.

Campos, B., & Kim, H. S. (2017). Incorporating the cultural diversity of family and close relationships into the study of health. *American Psychologist, 72,* 543–554.

Cankaya, B., Chapman, B. P., Talbot, N. L., Moynihan, J., & Duberstein, P. R. (2009). History of sudden unexpected loss is associated with elevated interleukin-6 and decreased insulin-like growth factor-1 in women in an urban primary care setting. *Psychosomatic Medicine, 71,* 914–919.

Cannon, W. B. (1932). *The wisdom of the body.* New York: Norton.

Carey, M. P., Coury-Doniger, P., Senn, T. E., Vanable, P. A., & Urban, M. A. (2008). Improving HIV rapid testing rates among STD clinic patients: A randomized controlled trial. *Health Psychology, 27,* 833–838.

Carlson, L. E., Speca, M., Patel, K. D., & Goodey, E. (2003). Mindfulness-based stress reduction in relation to quality of life, mood, symptoms of stress, and immune parameters in breast and prostate cancer outpatients. *Psychosomatic Medicine, 65,* 571–581.

Carmin, C. N., Weigartz, P. S., Hoff, J. A., & Kondos, G. T. (2003). Cardiac anxiety in patients self-referred for electron beam tomography. *Journal of Behavioral Medicine, 26,* 67–80.

Carmody, J., & Baer, R. A. (2008). Relationships between mindfulness practice and levels of mindfulness, medical and psychological symptoms and well-being in a mindfulness-based stress reduction program. *Journal of Behavioral Medicine, 31,* 23–33.

Carney, R. M., Freedland, K. E., Steinmeyer, B., Blumenthal, J. A., de Jonge, P., Davidson, K. W., . . . Jaffe, A. S. (2009). History of depression and survival after acute myocardial infarction. *Psychosomatic Medicine, 71,* 253–259.

Carpenter, K. M., Fowler, J. M., Maxwell, G. L., & Andersen, B. L. (2010). Direct and buffering effects of social support among gynecologic cancer survivors. *Annals of Behavioral Medicine, 39,* 79–90.

Carr, K. A., & Epstein, L. H. (2018). Influence of sedentary, social, and physical alternatives on food reinforcement. *Health Psychology, 37,* 125–131.

Carr, L. J., Dunsiger, S. I., Lewis, B., Ciccolo, J. T., Hartman, S., Bock, B., & Marcus, B. H. (2013). Randomized control trial testing an Internet physical activity intervention for sedentary adults. *Health Psychology, 32,* 328–336.

Carrico, A. W., Johnson, M. O., Moskowitz, J. T., Neilands, T. B., Morin, S. F., Charlebois, E. D., . . . NIMH Healthy Living Project Team. (2007). Affect regulation, stimulant use, and viral load among HIV-positive persons on anti-retroviral therapy. *Psychosomatic Medicine, 69,* 785–792.

Carrico, A. W., & Moskowitz, J. T. (2014). Positive affect promotes engagement in care after HIV diagnosis. *Health Psychology, 33,* 686–689.

Carroll, A. J., Carnethon, M. R., Liu, K., Jacobs, D. R., Jr., Colangelo, L. A., Stewart, J. C., . . . Hitsman, B. (2017). Interaction between smoking and depressive symptoms with subclinical heart disease in the Coronary Artery Risk Development in Young Adults (CARDIA) study. *Health Psychology, 36,* 101–111.

Carroll, D., Phillips, A. C., Der, G., Hunt, K., & Benzeval, M. (2011). Blood pressure reactions to acute mental stress and future blood pressure status: Data from the 12-year follow-up of the West of Scotland Study. *Psychosomatic Medicine, 73,* 737–742.

Carroll, J. E., Roux, A. V. D., Fitzpatrick, A. L., & Seeman, T. (2013). Low social support is associated with shorter leukocyte telomere length in late life: Multi-ethnic study of atherosclerosis. *Psychosomatic Medicine, 75,* 171–177.

Carroll, M. D., Kit, B. K., Lacher, D. A., & Yoon, S. S. (2013). Total and high-density lipoprotein cholesterol in adults: National health and nutrition examination survey, 2011–2012. *NCHS Data Brief, 132,* 1–8.

Carson, T. L., Wang, F., Cui, X., Jackson, B. E., Van Der Pol, W. J., Lefkowitz, E. J., . . . Baskin, M. L. (2018). Associations between race, perceived psychological stress, and the gut microbiota in a sample of generally healthy Black and White women: A pilot study on the role of race and perceived psychological stress. *Psychosomatic Medicine, 80,* 640–648.

Carter, J., Lacchetti, C., Andersen, B. L., Barton, D. L., Bolte, S., Damast, S., . . . Goldfarb, S. (2017). Interventions to address sexual problems in people with cancer: American Society of Clinical Oncology clinical practice guideline adaptation of Cancer Care Ontario guideline. *Journal of Clinical Oncology, 36,* 492–511.

Carver, C. S. (1997). You want to measure coping but your protocol's too long: Consider the Brief COPE. *International Journal of Behavioral Medicine, 4,* 92–100.

Carver, C. S., & Connor-Smith, J. (2010). Personality and coping. *Annual Review of Psychology, 61,* 679–704.

Case, A., & Deaton, A. (2015). Rising morbidity and mortality in midlife among white non-Hispanic Americans in the 21st century. *Proceedings of the National Academy of Sciences, 112,* 15078–15083.

Caska, C. M., Smith, T. W., Renshaw, K. D., Allen, S. N., Uchino, B. N., Birmingham, W., & Carlisle, M. (2014). Posttraumatic stress disorder and responses to couple conflict: Implications for cardiovascular risk. *Health Psychology, 33,* 1273–1280.

Cassileth, B. R., Lusk, E. J., Strouse, T. B., Miller, D. S., Brown, L. L., & Cross, P. A. (1985). A psychological analysis of cancer patients and their next-of-kin. *Cancer, 55,* 72–76.

Cassileth, B. R., Temoshok, L., Frederick, B. E., Walsh, W. P., Hurwitz, S., Guerry, D., . . . Sagebiel, R. W. (1988). Patient and physician delay in melanoma diagnosis. *Journal of the American Academy of Dermatology, 18,* 591–598.

Castro, C. M., Pruitt, L. A., Buman, M. P., & King, A. C. (2011). Physical activity program delivery by professionals versus volunteers: The TEAM randomized trial. *Health Psychology, 30,* 285–294.

Castro, F. G., Newcomb, M. D., McCreary, C., & Baezconde-Garbanati, L. (1989). Cigarette smokers do more than just smoke cigarettes. *Health Psychology, 8,* 107–129.

Catalano, R., Dooley, D., Wilson, C., & Hough, R. (1993). Job loss and alcohol abuse: A test using data from the epidemiologic catchment area. *Journal of Health and Social Behavior, 34,* 215–225.

Catalano, R., Hansen, H., & Hartig, T. (1999). The ecological effect of unemployment on the incidence of very low birthweight in Norway and Sweden. *Journal of Health and Social Behavior, 40,* 422–428.

Catania, J. A., Kegeles, S. M., & Coates, T. J. (1990). Towards an understanding of risk behavior: An AIDS risk reduction model (ARRM). *Health Education Quarterly, 17,* 53–72.

Celano, C. M., Albanese, A. M., Millstein, R. A., Mastromauro, C. A., Chung, W. J., Campbell, K. A., . . . Januzzi, J. L. (2018). Optimizing a positive psychology intervention to promote health behaviors after an acute coronary syndrome: The Positive Emotions after Acute Coronary Events III (PEACE-III) randomized factorial trial. *Psychosomatic Medicine, 80,* 526–534.

Celano, C. M., Beale, E. E., Beach, S. R., Belcher, A. M., Suarez, L., Motiwala, S. R., . . . Huffman, J. C. (2017). Associations between psychological constructs and cardiac biomarkers following acute coronary syndrome. *Psychosomatic Medicine, 79,* 318–326.

Center for the Advancement of Health. (2000a). *Selected evidence for behavioral approaches to chronic disease management in clinical settings. Cardiovascular disease.* Washington, DC: Author.

Center for the Advancement of Health. (2000b). *Selected evidence for behavioral approaches to chronic disease management in clinical settings: Chronic back pain.* Washington, DC: Author.

Center for the Advancement of Health. (2000c). *Selected evidence for behavioral approaches to chronic disease management in clinical settings: Depression.* Washington, DC: Author.

Center for the Advancement of Health. (2000d). *Selected evidence for behavioral risk reduction in clinical settings: Dietary practices.* Washington, DC: Author.

Center for the Advancement of Health. (2000e). *Smoking.* Washington, DC: Author.

Center for the Advancement of Health. (2002, December). Life lessons: Studying education's effect on health. *Facts of Life, 7,* 1.

Center for the Advancement of Health. (2004, May). *Is our people healthy?* Washington, DC: Author.

Center for the Advancement of Health. (2006, October). *November solutions. Good Behavior!* Washington, DC: Author.

Center for the Advancement of Health. (2008). Larger patients: In search of fewer lectures, better health care. *The Prepared Patient, 1,* 1–2.

Center for the Advancement of Health. (2009). Taking charge of your health records. *The Prepared Patient, 2,* 1–2.

Center to Advance Palliative Care. (2018). *Growth of palliative care in U.S. hospitals, 2018 snapshot (2000–2016).* Retrieved May 7, 2019, from https://media.capc.org/filer_public/27/2c/272c55c1-b69d-4eec-a932-562c2d2a4633/capc_2018_growth_snapshot_022118.pdf

Centers for Disease Control and Prevention. (2005, July). Annual smoking-attributable mortality, years of potential life lost, and productivity losses—United States, 1997–2001. *Morbidity and Mortality Weekly Report, 54*(25), 625–628. Retrieved October 26, 2006, from http://www.cdc.gov/mmwr/preview/mmwrhtml/mm5425a1.htm#tab

Centers for Disease Control and Prevention. (2008). Cigarette use among high school students—United States, 1991–2007. *Morbidity and Mortality Weekly Report, 57.* Retrieved October 19, 2009, from http://www.cdc.gov/mmwr/preview/mmwrhtml/mm5725a3.htm

Centers for Disease Control and Prevention. (2008, September). *Alcohol and public health.* Retrieved October 5, 2009, from http://www.cdc.gov/alcohol/index.htm

Centers for Disease Control and Prevention. (2009, April). *National vital statistics report, deaths: Final data for 2006.* Retrieved September 25, 2009, from http://www.cdc.gov/nchs/data/nvsr/nvsr57/nvsr57_14.pdf

Centers for Disease Control and Prevention. (2009a, June). *Estimates of healthcare-associated infections.* Retrieved February 2, 2011, from http://www.cdc.gov/hai

Centers for Disease Control and Prevention. (2009b, June). *Hepatitis B FAQs for the public.* Retrieved April 3, 2012, from http://www.cdc.gov/hepatitis/B/bFAQ.htm

Centers for Disease Control and Prevention. (2009a, August). *10 leading causes of injury death by age group highlighting unintentional injury deaths, United States–2006.* Retrieved September 30, 2009, from http://www.cdc.gov/injury/Images/LC-Charts/10lc%20-Unintentional%20Injury%202006-7_6_09-a.pdf

Centers for Disease Control and Prevention. (2009b, August). *HIV/AIDS in the United States.* Retrieved October 8, 2009, from http://www.cdc.gov/hiv/resources/factsheets/us.htm

Centers for Disease Control and Prevention. (2010). *Tobacco-related mortality.* Retrieved January 13, 2011, from http://www.cdc.gov/tobacco/data_statistics/fact_sheets/health_effects/tobacco_related_mortalmor/index.htm

Centers for Disease Control and Prevention. (2011a, September). *Rheumatoid arthritis.* Retrieved June 13, 2012, from http://www.cdc.gov/arthritis/basics/rheumatoid.htm#6

Centers for Disease Control and Prevention. (2011b, September). *National Health and Nutrition Examination Survey, 2009–2010.* Retrieved March 6, 2013, from http://www.cdc.gov/nchs/nhanes/nhanes2009-2010/nhanes09_10.htm

Centers for Disease Control and Prevention. (2011, November). *CDC responds to HIV/AIDS.* Retrieved June 12, 2012, from http://www.cdc.gov/hiv/aboutDHAP.htm

Centers for Disease Control and Prevention. (2012a, March). *Prevent unintentional poisoning.* Retrieved April 24, 2012, from http://www.cdc.gov/Features/PoisonPrevention

Centers for Disease Control and Prevention. (2012b, March). *HIV surveillance report, 2010.* Retrieved March 20, 2012, from http://www.cdc.gov/hiv/surveillance/resources/reports/2010report/pdf/2010_HIV_Surveillance_Report_vol_22.pdf#Page=21

Centers for Disease Control and Prevention. (2012, April). *Arthritis.* Retrieved May 29, 2012 from http://www.cdc.gov/chronicdisease/resources/publications/aag/arthritis.htm

Centers for Disease Control and Prevention. (2012, May). *Health, United States, 2011.* Retrieved August 8, 2012, from http://www.cdc.gov/nchs/data/hus/hus11.pdf#glance

Centers for Disease Control and Prevention. (2013). *Alcohol and public health: Alcohol-related disease impact (ARDI). Average for United States 2006–2010 alcohol-attributable deaths due to excessive alcohol use.* Retrieved April 3, 2019, from https://nccd.cdc.gov/DPH_ARDI/Default/Report.aspx?T=AAM&P=f6d7eda7-036e-4553-9968-9b17ffad620e&R=d7a9b303-48e9-4440-bf47-070a4827e1fd&M=8E1C5233-5640-4EE8-9247-1ECA7DA325B9&F=&D=.

Centers for Disease Control and Prevention. (2015, July). *Addressing the nation's most common cause of disability: At a glance 2015.* Retrieved May 25, 2016, from http://www.cdc.gov

Centers for Disease Control and Prevention. (2015, April). *Health expenditures, NCHS.* Retrieved January 26, 2016, from http://www.cdc.gov

Centers for Disease Control and Prevention. (2015, August). *Skin cancer statistics.* Retrieved February 17, 2016, from http://www.cdc.gov

Centers for Disease Control and Prevention. (2015, September). *Accidents or unintentional injuries.* Retrieved May 6, 2016, from http://www.cdc.gov

Centers for Disease Control and Prevention. (2015b, October). *Prescription drug overdose data.* Retrieved February 21, 2016, from http://www.cdc.gov

Centers for Disease Control and Prevention. (2015, October). *Rheumatoid arthritis (RA).* Retrieved May 25, 2016, from http://www.cdc.gov

Centers for Disease Control and Prevention. (2015, November). *Current cigarette smoking among adults: United States, 2005–2014.* Retrieved February 28, 2016, from http://www.cdc.gov

Centers for Disease Control and Prevention. (2016). *Percentage distribution of deaths, by place of death–United States, 2000–2014. Morbidity and Mortality Weekly Report, 65.* Retrieved from http://www.cdc.gov

Centers for Disease Control and Prevention. (2016, January). *Arthritis-related statistics.* Retrieved March 25, 2016, from http://www.cdc.gov

Centers for Disease Control and Prevention. (2016, January). *Excessive drinking is draining the U.S. economy.* Retrieved February 28, 2016, from http://www.cdc.gov

Centers for Disease Control and Prevention. (2016, February). *Asthma.* Retrieved April 30, 2016, from http://www.cdc.gov

Centers for Disease Control and Prevention. (2016, March). *HIV/AIDS: Statistics overview.* Retrieved May 25, 2016, from http://www.cdc.gov

Centers for Disease Control and Prevention. (2016, April). *Adolescent health.* Retrieved May 6, 2016, from http://www.cdc.gov

Centers for Disease Control and Prevention. (2016, April). *Cancer.* Retrieved April 30, 2016, from http://www.cdc.gov

Centers for Disease Control and Prevention. (2016, April). *Changes in life expectancy by race and Hispanic origin in the United States, 2013.* Retrieved May 6, 2016, from http://www.cdc.gov

Centers for Disease Control and Prevention. (2016, April). *Leading causes of death.* Retrieved May 25, 2016, from http://www.cdc.gov

Centers for Disease Control and Prevention. (2017a). *Current cigarette smoking among adults in the United States.* Retrieved April 8, 2019, from https://www.cdc.gov/tobacco/data_statistics/fact_sheets/adult_data/cig_smoking/index.htm

Centers for Disease Control and Prevention. (2017b). *High cholesterol facts.* Retrieved from https://www.cdc.gov/cholesterol/facts.htm

Centers for Disease Control and Prevention. (2017c). *National diabetes statistics report: Estimates of diabetes and its burden in the United States.* Retrieved May 5, 2019, from https://www.cdc.gov/diabetes/pdfs/data/statistics/national-diabetes-statistics-report.pdf

Centers for Disease Control and Prevention. (2017d). *National diabetes statistics report, 2017.* Retrieved May 25, 2019, from https://www.cdc.gov/diabetes/pdfs/data/statistics/national-diabetes-statistics-report.pdf

Centers for Disease Control and Prevention. (2017e). *Table 19. Leading causes of death and numbers of deaths, by sex, race, and Hispanic origin: United States 1980 and 2016.* Retrieved from https://www.cdc.gov/nchs/data/hus/2017/019.pdf

Centers for Disease Control and Prevention. (2017, June 5). *Sleep and sleep disorders: Data and statistics.* Retrieved April 1, 2019, from https://www.cdc.gov/sleep/about_us.html

Centers for Disease Control and Prevention. (2017, September 22). *CDC features: Take a stand on falls.* Retrieved April 1, 2019, from https://www.cdc.gov/features/older-adult-falls/index.html

Centers for Disease Control and Prevention. (2017, October). *Prevalence of obesity among adults and youth: United States, 2015–2016.* Retrieved April 8, 2019, from https://www.cdc.gov/nchs/data/databriefs/db288.pdf

Centers for Disease Control and Prevention. (2017, December). *Mortality in the United States, 2016.* Retrieved March 11, 2019, from https://www.cdc.gov/nchs/products/databriefs/db293.htm

Centers for Disease Control and Prevention. (2017, December 5). *Current HAI progress report.* Retrieved April 9, 2019, from https://www.cdc.gov/hai/data/portal/progress-report.html

Centers for Disease Control and Prevention (2018, May 15). *Most recent national asthma data.* Retrieved March 11, 2019, from https://www.cdc.gov/asthma/most_recent_national_asthma_data.htm

Centers for Disease Control and Prevention. (2018a, July). *Arthritis-related statistics.* Retrieved May 25, 2019, from https://www.cdc.gov/arthritis/data_statistics/arthritis-related-stats.htm

Centers for Disease Control and Prevention. (2018b, July). *Attempts to lose weight among adults in the United States, 2013-2016.* Retrieved April 8, 2019, from https://www.cdc.gov/nchs/data/databriefs/db313.pdf

Centers for Disease Control and Prevention. (2018, September). *Morbidity and Mortality Weekly Report: Prevalence of chronic pain and high-impact chronic pain among adults—United States, 2016.* Retrieved April 30, 2019, from https://www.cdc.gov/mmwr/volumes/67/wr/mm6736a2.htm

Center for Disease Control and Prevention. (2018a, November). *Mortality in the United States, 2017.* Retrieved May 30, 2019, from https://www.cdc.gov/nchs/products/databriefs/db328.htm

Centers for Disease Control and Prevention. (2018b, November). *HIV surveillance report, 2017;* vol. 29. Retrieved May 29, 2019, from http://www.cdc.gov/hiv/library/reports/hiv-surveillance.html.

Centers for Disease Control and Prevention. (2018, December). *Tuberculosis (TB) data and statistics.* Retrieved March 18, 2019, from https://www.cdc.gov/tb/statistics/default.htm

Centers for Disease Control and Prevention. (2019, January 30). *Arthritis: How CDC improves quality of life for people with arthritis.* Retrieved April 30, 2019, from https://www.cdc.gov/chronicdisease/resources/publications/factsheets/arthritis.htm

Centers for Disease Control and Prevention. (2019, January). *Osteoarthritis (OA).* Retrieved May 25, 2019, from https://www.cdc.gov/arthritis/basics/osteoarthritis.htm

Center for Drug Evaluation and Research. (2002). *Preventable adverse drug reactions: A focus on drug interactions.* Retrieved April 5, 2007, from http://www.fda.gov/cder/drug/drugReactions

Centers for Medicare and Medicaid Services. (2004). *National health expenditures and selected economic indicators, levels and average annual percent change: Selected calendar years 1990-2013.* Retrieved from http://www.cms.hhs.gov/statistics/nhe/projections-2003/t1.asp

Centers for Medicare and Medicaid Services. (2011). *National health expenditure data.* Retrieved March 21, 2012, from https://www.cms.gov/NationalHealthExpendData/downloads/proj2010.pdf

Centers for Medicare and Medicaid Services. (2015). *NHE fact sheet.* Retrieved February 20, 2016, from https://www.cms.gov

Centers for Medicare and Medicaid Services. (2018). *National health expenditures 2017 highlights.* Retrieved March 30, 2019, from https://www.cms.gov/Research-Statistics-Data-and-Systems/Statistics-Trends-and-Reports/NationalHealthExpendData/Downloads/highlights.pdf

Centers for Medicare and Medicaid Services. (2018, December). *National health accounts historical.* Retrieved March 26, 2019, from https://www.cms.gov/research-statistics-data-and-systems/statistics-trends-and-reports/nationalhealthexpenddata/nationalhealthaccountshistorical.html

Cepeda-Benito, A. (1993). Meta-analytical review of the efficacy of nicotine chewing gum in smoking treatment programs. *Journal of Consulting and Clinical Psychology, 61,* 822-830.

CerebralPalsy.Org. (n.d.). *Prevalence of cerebral palsy.* Retrieved March 26, 2019, from https://www.cerebralpalsy.org/about-cerebral-palsy/prevalence-and-incidence

CerebralPalsy.org. (2016). *My child.* Retrieved January 21, 2016, from https://www.cerebralpalsy.org

Cesana, G., Sega, R., Ferrario, M., Chiodini, P., Corrao, G., & Mancia, G. (2003). Job strain and blood pressure in employed men and women: A pooled analysis of four northern Italian population samples. *Psychosomatic Medicine, 65,* 558-563.

Chang, J., Yen, A. M., Lee, C., Chen, S. L., Chiu, S. Y., Fann, J. C., & Chen, H. (2013). Metabolic syndrome and the risk of suicide: A community-based integrated screening samples cohort study. *Psychosomatic Medicine, 75,* 807-814.

Chapman, C. R., & Gavrin, J. (1999). Suffering: The contributions of persisting pain. *Lancet, 353,* 2233-2237.

Charles, S. T., Gatz, M., Kato, K., & Pedersen, N. L. (2008). Physical health 25 years later: The predictive ability of neuroticism. *Health Psychology, 27,* 369-378.

Chattillion, E. A., Ceglowski, J., Roepke, S. K., von Känel, R., Losada, A., Mills, P., & Mausbach, B. T. (2013). Pleasant events, activity restriction, and blood pressure in dementia caregivers. *Health Psychology, 32,* 793-801.

Cheadle, A. C. D., Schetter, C. D., Lanzi, M. R. V., & Sahadeo, L. S. (2015). Spiritual and religious resources in African American women: Protection from depressive symptoms after childbirth. *Clinical Psychological Science,* 283-291.

Chen, E., Bloomberg, G. R., Fisher, E. B., Jr., & Strunk, R. C. L. (2003). Predictors of repeat hospitalizations in children with asthma: The role of psychosocial and socioenvironmental factors. *Health Psychology, 22,* 12-18.

Chen, E., Brody, G. H., & Miller, G. E. (2017). Childhood close family relationships and health. *American Psychologist, 72,* 555-566.

Chen, E., Fisher, E. B., Bacharier, L. B., & Strunk, R. C. (2003). Socioeconomic status, stress, and immune markers in adolescents with asthma. *Psychosomatic Medicine, 65,* 984-992.

Chen, E., Hanson, M. D., Paterson, L. Q., Griffin, M. J., Walker, H. A., & Miller, G. E. (2006). Socioeconomic status and inflammatory processes in childhood asthma: The role of psychological stress. *Journal of Allergy and Clinical Immunology, 117,* 1014-1020.

Chen, E., Hermann, C., Rodgers, D., Oliver-Welker, T., & Strunk, R. C. (2006). Symptom perception in childhood asthma: The role of anxiety and asthma severity. *Health Psychology, 25,* 389-395.

Chen, E., Matthews, K. A., Salomon, K., & Ewart, C. K. (2002). Cardiovascular reactivity during social and nonsocial stressors: Do children's personal goals and expressive skills matter? *Health Psychology, 21,* 16-24.

Chen, E., & Miller, G. E. (2012). "Shift-and-persist" strategies: Why low socioeconomic status isn't always bad for health. *Perspectives on Psychological Science, 7,* 135-158.

Chen, E., Miller, G. E., Lachman, M. E., Gruenewald, T. L., & Seeman, T. E. (2012). Protective factors for adults from low-childhood socioeconomic circumstances: The benefits of shift-and-persist for allostatic load. *Psychosomatic Medicine, 74,* 178-186.

Chen, L. H., Hedegaard, H., & Warner, M. (2014). Drug-poisoning deaths involving opioid analgesics: United States, 1999-2011. *NCHS Data Brief, 166,* 1-8.

Chen, Y., Wei, H., Bai, Y., Hsu, J., Huang, K., Su, T., . . . Chen, M. (2017). Risk of epilepsy in individuals with posttraumatic stress disorder. *Psychosomatic Medicine, 79,* 664-669.

Chen, Z., Sandercock, P., Pan, P., Counsell, C., Collins, R., Liu, L., . . . Peto, R. (2000). Indications of early aspirin use in acute ischemic stroke: A combined analysis of 40,000 randomized patients from the Chinese acute stroke trial and the international stroke trial. *Stroke, 31,* 1240-1249.

Cheng, C. (2003). Cognitive and motivational processes underlying coping flexibility: A dual-process model. *Journal of Personality and Social Psychology, 84,* 425-438.

Cheng, C., Hui, W., & Lam, S. (2004). Psychosocial factors and perceived severity of functional dyspeptic symptoms: A psychosocial interactionist model. *Psychosomatic Medicine, 66,* 85-91.

Cherkin, D. C., Sherman, K. J., Avins, A. L., Erro, J. H., Ichikawa, L., Barlow, W. E., . . . Deyo, R. A. (2009). A randomized trial comparing acupuncture, simulated acupuncture, and usual care for chronic low back pain. *Archives of Internal Medicine, 169,* 858–866.

Cherkin, D. C., Sherman, K. J., Deyo, R. A., & Shekelle, P. G. (2003). A review of the evidence for the effectiveness, safety, and cost of acupuncture, massage therapy, and spinal manipulation for back pain. *Annals of Internal Medicine, 138,* 898–906.

Cherrington, A., Wallston, K. A., & Rothman, R. L. (2010). Exploring the relationship between diabetes self-efficacy, depressive symptoms, and glycemic control among men and women with type 2 diabetes. *Journal of Behavioral Medicine, 33,* 81–89.

Cherry, D., Lucas, C., & Decker, S. L. (2010). Population aging and the use of office-based physician services. *NCHS Data Brief, 41,* 1–8.

Chesney, M. A., Chambers, D. B., Taylor, J. M., Johnson, L. M., & Folkman, S. (2003). Coping effectiveness training for men living with HIV: Results from a randomized clinical trial testing a group-based intervention. *Psychosomatic Medicine, 65,* 1038–1046.

Chetty, R., Stepner, M., Abraham, S., Lin, S., Scuderi, B., Turner, N., . . . Cutler, D. (2016). The association between income and life expectancy in the United States, 2001–2014. *JAMA, 315,* 1750–1766.

Cheung, N., Rogers, S., Mosley, T. H., Klein, R., Couper, D., & Wong, T. Y. (2009). Vital exhaustion and retinal microvascular changes in cardiovascular disease: Atherosclerosis risk in communities study. *Psychosomatic Medicine, 71,* 308–312.

Chevance, G., Stephan, Y., Héraud, N., & Boiché, J. (2018). Interaction between self-regulation, intentions and implicit attitudes in the prediction of physical activity among persons with obesity. *Health Psychology, 37,* 257–261.

Chiang, J. J., Eisenberger, N. I., Seeman, T. E., & Taylor, S. E. (2012). Negative and competitive social interactions are related to heightened proinflammatory cytokine activity. *Proceedings of the National Academy of Sciences, 109,* 1878–1882.

Chichlowska, K. L., Rose, K. M., Diez-Roux, A. V., Golden, S. H., McNeill, A.M., & Heiss, G. (2008). Individual and neighborhood socioeconomic status characteristics and prevalence of metabolic syndrome: The atherosclerosis risk in communities (ARIC) study. *Psychosomatic Medicine, 70,* 986–992.

Chiesa, A., & Serretti, A. (2009). Mindfulness-based stress reduction for stress management in healthy people: A review and meta-analysis. *The Journal of Alternative and Complementary Medicine, 15,* 593–600.

Chiou, W. B, Yang, C. C., & Wan, C. S, (2011). Ironic effects of dietary supplementation: Illusory invulnerability created by taking dietary supplements licenses health-risk behaviors. *Psychological Science, 8,* 1081–1086.

Chipperfield, J. G., & Perry, R. P. (2006). Primary and secondary-control strategies in later life: Predicting hospital outcomes in men and women. *Health Psychology, 25,* 226–236.

Chiros, C., & O'Brien, W. H. (2011). Acceptance, appraisals, and coping in relation to migraine headache: An evaluation of interrelationships using daily diary methods. *Journal of Behavioral Medicine, 34,* 307–320.

Chiu, C. J., Hu, S. C., Wray, L. A., & Wu, S. T. (2016). The short- and long-term effects of psychobehavioral correlates in buffering diabetes-related cognitive decline. *Annals of Behavioral Medicine, 50,* 436–444.

Chow, C. H. T., Wan, S., Pope, E., Meng, Z., Schmidt, L. A., Buckley, N., & Van Lieshout, R. J. (2018). Audiovisual interventions for parental preoperative anxiety: A systematic review and meta-analysis. *Health Psychology, 37,* 746–758.

Christakis, N. A., & Fowler, J. H. (2007). The spread of obesity in a large social network over 32 years. *The New England Journal of Medicine, 357,* 370–379.

Christakis, N. A., & Fowler, J. H. (2008). The collective dynamics of smoking in a large social network. *The New England Journal of Medicine, 358,* 2249–2258.

Christenfeld, N. (1997). Memory for pain and the delayed effects of distraction. *Health Psychology, 16,* 327–330.

Christensen, A. J., Ehlers, S. L., Raichle, K. A., Bertolatus, J. A., & Lawton, W. J. (2000). Predicting change in depression following renal transplantation: Effect of patient coping preferences. *Health Psychology, 19,* 348–353.

Christensen, A. J., Moran, P. J., Wiebe, J. S., Ehlers, S. L., & Lawton, W. J. (2002). Effect of a behavioral self-regulation intervention on patient adherence in hemodialysis. *Health Psychology, 21,* 393–397.

Christensen, A. J., Wiebe, J. S., & Lawton, W. J. (1997). Cynical hostility, powerful others, control expectancies and patient adherence in hemodialysis. *Psychosomatic Medicine, 59,* 307–312.

Christie-Mizell, C. A., & Perlata, R. L. (2009). The gender gap in alcohol consumption during late adolescence and young adulthood: Gendered attitudes and adult roles. *Journal of Health and Social Behavior, 50,* 410–426.

Chuang, Y. C., Ennett, S. T., Bauman, K. E., & Foshee, V. A. (2005). Neighborhood influences on adolescent cigarette and alcohol use: Mediating effects through parents and peer behaviors. *Journal of Health and Social Behavior, 46,* 187–204.

Chu, Q., Wong, C. C. Y., & Lu, Q. (2019). Acculturation moderates the effects of expressive writing on post-traumatic stress symptoms among Chinese American breast cancer survivors. *International Journal of Behavioral Medicine, 26,* 185–194.

Ciccone, D., Just, N., & Bandilla, E. (1999). A comparison of economic and social reward in patients with chronic nonmalignant back pain. *Psychosomatic Medicine, 61,* 552–563.

Ciere, Y., Snippe, E., Padberg, M., Jacobs, B., Visser, A., Sanderman, R., & Fleer, J. (2019). The role of state and trait positive affect and mindfulness in affective reactivity to pain in chronic migraine. *Health Psychology, 38,* 94–102.

Cislaghi, B., & Heise, L. (2018). Four avenues of normative influence: A research agenda for health promotion in low and mid-income countries. *Health Psychology, 37,* 562–573.

Clark, M. (1977). The new war on pain. *Newsweek,* pp. 48–58.

Clark, M. A., Rakowski, W., & Bonacore, L. B. (2003). Repeat mammography: Prevalence estimates and considerations for assessment. *Annals of Behavioral Medicine, 26,* 201–211.

Clark, R. (2006a). Perceived racism and vascular reactivity in black college women: Moderating effects of seeking social support. *Health Psychology, 25,* 20–25.

Clayton, K. M., Stewart, S. M., Wiebe, D. J., McConnel, C. E., Hughes, C. W., & White, P. C. (2013). Maternal depressive symptoms predict adolescent healthcare utilization and charges in youth with Type 1 diabetes (T1D). *Health Psychology, 32,* 1013–1022.

Cleary, E. H., & Stanton, A. L. (2015). Mediators of an Internet-based psychosocial intervention for women with breast cancer. *Health Psychology, 34,* 477–485.

Clemens, J. Q., Nadler, R. B., Schaeffer, A. J., Belani, J., Albaugh, J., & Bushman, W. (2000). Biofeedback, pelvic floor re-education, and bladder training for male chronic pelvic pain syndrome. *Urology, 56,* 951–955.

Clemmey, P. A., & Nicassio, P. M. (1997). Illness self-schemas in depressed and nondepressed rheumatoid arthritis patients. *Journal of Behavioral Medicine, 20,* 273–290.

Coan, J. A., Schaefer, H. S., & Davidson, R. J. (2006). Lending a hand: Social regulation of the neural response to threat. *Psychological Science, 17,* 1032–1039.

Cohen, F., & Lazarus, R. (1979). Coping with the stresses of illness. In G. C. Stone, F. Cohen, & N. E. Adler (Eds.), *Health psychology: A handbook* (pp. 217–254). San Francisco, CA: Jossey-Bass.

Cohen, G. L., & Sherman, D. K. (2014). The psychology of change: Self-affirmation and social psychological intervention. *Annual Review of Psychology, 65,* 333–371.

Cohen, J. (2018, July). Troublesome news: Numbers of uninsured on the rise. *Forbes.* Retrieved from https://www.forbes.com/sites/joshuacohen/2018/07/06/troublesome-news-numbers-of-uninsured-on-the-rise/#23e484f94309

Cohen, L., Baile, W. F., Henninger, E., Agarwal, S. K., Kudelka, A. P., Lenzi, R., . . . Marshall, G. D. (2003). Physiological and psychological effects of delivering medical news using a simulated physician–patient scenario. *Journal of Behavioral Medicine, 26,* 459–471.

Cohen, M. S., Chen, Y. Q., McCauley, M., Gamble, T., Hosseinipour, M. C., Kumarasamy, N., . . . Fleming, T. R. (2011). Prevention of HIV-1 infection with early antiretroviral therapy. *The New England Journal of Medicine, 365,* 493–505.

Cohen, R. A., & Adams, P. F. (2011). Use of the Internet for health information: United States, 2009. *NCHS Data Brief, 66,* 1–8.

Cohen, R. A., & Bloom, B. (2010). Access to and utilization of medical care for young adults aged 20–29 years: United States, 2008. *NCHS Data Brief, 29,* 1–8.

Cohen, R. A., Kirzinger, W. K., & Gindi, R. M. (2013). Strategies used by adults to reduce their prescription drug costs. *NCHS Data Brief, 119,* 1–8.

Cohen, R. Y., Brownell, K. D., & Felix, M. R. J. (1990). Age and sex differences in health habits and beliefs of schoolchildren. *Health Psychology, 9,* 208–224.

Cohen, S., Alper, C. M., Doyle, W. J., Adler, N., Treanor, J. J., & Turner, R. B. (2008). Objective and subjective socioeconomic status and susceptibility to the common cold. *Health Psychology, 27,* 268–274.

Cohen, S., Alper, C. M., Doyle, W. J., Treanor, J. J., & Turner, R. B. (2006). Positive emotional style predicts resistance to illness after experimental exposure to rhinovirus or influenza a virus. *Psychosomatic Medicine, 68,* 809–815.

Cohen, S., Doyle, W., & Skoner, D. (1999). Psychological stress, cytokine production, and severity of upper respiratory illness. *Psychosomatic Medicine, 61,* 175–180.

Cohen, S., Doyle, W. J., Skoner, D. P., Rabin, B. S., & Gwaltney, J. M., Jr. (1997). Social ties and susceptibility to the common cold. *Journal of the American Medical Association, 277,* 1940–1944.

Cohen, S., Glass, D. C., & Phillip, S. (1978). Environment and health. In H. E. Freeman, S. Levine, & L. G. Reeder (Eds.), *Handbook of medical sociology* (pp. 134–149). Englewood Cliffs, NJ: Prentice-Hall.

Cohen, S., Hamrick, N., Rodriguez, M. S., Feldman, P. J., Rabin, B. S., & Manuck, S. R. (2002). Reactivity and vulnerability to stress-associated risk for upper respiratory illness. *Psychosomatic Medicine, 64,* 302–310.

Cohen, S., & Herbert, T. B. (1996). Health psychology: Psychological factors and physical disease from the perspective of human psychoneuroimmunology. *Annual Review of Psychology, 47,* 113–142.

Cohen, S., & Hoberman, H. M. (1983). Positive events and social supports as buffers of life change stress. *Journal of Applied Social Psychology, 13,* 99–125.

Cohen, S., Janicki-Deverts, D., & Miller, G. E. (2007). Psychological stress and disease. *Journal of the American Medical Association, 298,* 1685–1687.

Cohen, S., Kamarck, T., & Mermelstein, R. (1983). A global measure of perceived stress. *Journal of Health and Social Behavior, 24,* 385–396.

Cohen, S., Kessler, R. C., & Gordon, L. U. (1995). Conceptualizing stress and its relation to disease. In S. Cohen, R. C. Kessler, & L. U. Gordon (Eds.), *Measuring stress: A guide for health and social scientists* (pp. 3–26). New York: Oxford University Press.

Cohen, S., & Lemay, E. P. (2007). Why would social networks be linked to affect and health practices? *Health Psychology, 26,* 410–417.

Cohen, S., & McKay, G. (1984). Social support, stress, and the buffering hypothesis. A theoretical analysis. In A. Baum, S. E. Taylor, & J. Singer (Eds.), *Handbook of psychology and health* (Vol. 4, pp. 253–268). Hillsdale, NJ: Erlbaum.

Cohen, S., & Pressman, S. D. (2006). Positive affect and health. *Current Directions in Psychological Science, 15,* 122–125.

Cohen, S., Sherrod, D. R., & Clark, M. S. (1986). Social skills and the stress-protective role of social support. *Journal of Personality and Social Psychology, 50,* 963–973.

Cohen, S., Tyrrell, D. A. J., & Smith, A. P. (1993). Negative life events, perceived stress, negative affect, and susceptibility to the common cold. *Journal of Personality and Social Psychology, 64,* 131–140.

Cohen, S., & Williamson, G. M. (1988). Perceived stress in a probability sample of the United States. In S. Spacapan & S. Oskamp (Eds.), *The social psychology of health* (pp. 31–67). Newbury Park, CA: Sage.

Cohen, S., & Williamson, G. M. (1991). Stress and infectious disease in humans. *Psychological Bulletin, 109,* 5–24.

Cohen, S., & Wills, T. A. (1985). Stress, social support, and the buffering hypothesis. *Psychological Bulletin, 98,* 310–357.

Coker, A. L., Bond, S., Madeleine, M. M., Luchok, K., & Pirisi, L. (2003). Psychological stress and cervical neoplasia risk. *Psychosomatic Medicine, 65,* 644–651.

Colagiuri, B., & Zachariae, R. (2010). Patient expectancy and post-chemotherapy nausea: A meta-analysis. *Annals of Behavioral Medicine, 40*(1), 3–14.

Cole, P. A., Pomerleau, C. S., & Harris, J. K. (1992). The effects of nonconcurrent and concurrent relaxation training on cardiovascular reactivity to a psychological stressor. *Journal of Behavioral Medicine, 15,* 407–427.

Cole, S. W. (2008). Psychosocial influences on HIV-1 disease progression: Neural, endocrine, and virologic mechanisms. *Psychosomatic Medicine, 70,* 562–568.

Cole, S. W., Kemeny, M. E., Fahey, J. L., Zack, J. A., & Naliboff, B. D. (2003). Psychological risk factors for HIV pathogenesis: Mediation by the autonomic nervous system. *Biological Psychiatry, 54,* 1444–1456.

Cole, S. W., Kemeny, M. E., Taylor, S. E., Visscher, B. R., & Fahey, J. L. (1996). Accelerated course of human immunodeficiency virus infection in gay men who conceal their homosexual identity. *Psychosomatic Medicine, 58,* 219–231.

Cole, S. W., Nagaraja, A. S., Lutgendorf, S. K., Green, P. A., & Sood, A. K. (2015). Sympathetic nervous system regulation of the tumour microenvironment. *Nature Reviews Cancer, 15,* 563–572.

Cole-Lewis, H. J., Kershaw, T. S., Earnshaw, V. A., Yonkers, K. A., Lin, H., & Ickovics, J. R. (2014). Pregnancy-specific stress, preterm birth, and gestational age among high risk-young women. *Health Psychology, 33,* 1033–1045.

Collins, G. (1997, May 30). Trial near in new legal tack in tobacco war. *New York Times,* p. A10.

Collins, R. L., Kanouse, D. E., Gifford, A. L., Senterfitt, J. W., Schuster, M. A., McCaffrey, D. F., . . . Wenger, N. S. (2001). Changes in health-promoting behavior following diagnosis with HIV: Prevalence and correlates in a national probability sample. *Health Psychology, 20,* 351–360.

Collins, R. L., Martino, S. C., Kovalchik, S. A., D'Amico, E. J., Shadel, W. G., Becker, K. M., & Tolpadi, A. (2017). Exposure to alcohol advertising and adolescents' drinking beliefs: Role of message interpretation. *Health Psychology, 36*(9), 890–897.

Collins, R. L., Taylor, S. E., & Skokan, L. A. (1990). A better world or a shattered vision? Changes in perspectives following victimization. *Social Cognition, 8,* 263–285.

Committee on the Use of Complementary and Alternative Medicine. (2005). *Complementary and alternative medicine in the United States.* Washington, DC: The National Academies Press. Retrieved March 27, 2013, from http://www.nap.edu/openbook.php?record_id=11182&page=R1

Compas, B. E., Worsham, N. L., Epping-Jordan, J. A. E., Grant, K. E., Mireault, G., Howell, D. C., & Malcarne, V. L. (1994). When mom or dad has cancer: Markers of psychological distress in cancer patients, spouses, and children. *Health Psychology, 13,* 507-515.

Compas, B. E., Worsham, N. L., Ey, S., & Howell, D. C. (1996). When mom or dad has cancer: II. Coping, cognitive appraisals, and psychological distress in children of cancer patients. *Health Psychology, 15,* 167-175.

Condit, C. M. (2011). When do people deploy genetic determinism? A review pointing to the need for multi-factorial theories of public utilization of scientific discourses. *Sociology Compass, 5,* 618-635.

Congressional Research Service. (2010). *U.S. military casualty statistics: Operation New Dawn, Operation Iraqi Freedom, and Operation Enduring Freedom.* Retrieved May 1, 2012, from www.fas.org/sgp/crs/natsec/RS22452.pdf

Conis, E. (2003, August). Chips for some, tofu for others. *Los Angeles Times,* p. F8.

Connell, L. E., & Francis, L. A. (2014). Positive parenting mitigates the effects of poor self-regulation on body mass index trajectories from ages 4-15 years. *Health Psychology, 33,* 757-764.

Conner, M., McEachan, R., Taylor, N., O'Hara, J., & Lawton, R. (2015). Role of affective attitudes and anticipated affective reactions in predicting health behaviors. *Health Psychology, 34,* 642-652.

Conner, M., Sandberg, T., & Norman, P. (2010). Using action planning to promote exercise behavior. *Annals of Behavioral Medicine, 40,* 65-76.

Conroy, D., & Hagger, M. S. (2018). Imagery interventions in health behavior: A meta-analysis. *Health Psychology, 37,* 668-679.

Conroy, D. E., Hedeker, D., McFadden, H. G., Pellegrini, C. A., Pfammatter, A. F., Phillips, S. M., . . . Spring, B. (2017). Lifestyle intervention effects on the frequency and duration of daily moderate-vigorous physical activity and leisure screen time. *Health Psychology, 36,* 299-308.

Conroy, D. E., Hyde, A. L., Doerksen, S. E., & Riebeiro, N. F. (2010). Implicit attitudes and explicit motivation prospectively predict physical activity. *Annals of Behavioral Medicine, 39,* 112-118.

Conroy, D. E., Maher, J. P., Elavsky, S., Hyde, A. L., & Doerksen, S. E. (2013). Sedentary behavior as a daily process regulated by habits and intentions. *Health Psychology, 32,* 1149-1157.

Contrada, R. J., Boulifard, D. A., Hekler, E. B., Idler, E. L., Spruill, T. M., Labouvie, E. W., & Krause, T. J. (2008). Psychosocial factors in heart surgery: Presurgical vulnerability and postsurgical recovery. *Health Psychology, 27,* 309-319.

Contrada, R. J., Goyal, T. M., Cather, C. C., Rafalson, L., Idler, E. L., & Krause, T. J. (2004). Psychosocial factors in outcomes of heart surgery: The impact of religious involvement and depressive symptoms. *Health Psychology, 23,* 227-238.

Cooper, J. K., Love, D. W., & Raffoul, P. R. (1982). Intentional prescription nonadherence (noncompliance) by the elderly. *Journal of the American Geriatric Society, 30,* 329-333.

Cooper, M. L., Wood, P. K., Orcutt, H. K., & Albino, A. (2003). Personality and the predisposition to engage in risky or problem behaviors during adolescence. *Journal of Personality and Social Psychology, 84,* 390-410.

Cooper, N., Tompson, S., O'Donnell, M. B., Vettel, J. M., Bassett, D. S., & Falk, E. B. (2018). Associations between coherent neural activity in the brain's value system during antismoking messages and reductions in smoking. *Health Psychology, 37,* 375-384.

Cooperman, N. A., & Simoni, J. M. (2005). Suicidal ideation and attempted suicide among women living with HIV/AIDS. *Journal of Behavioral Medicine, 28,* 149-156.

COPD International. (2015). *COPD.* Retrieved January 21, 2016, from http://www.copd-international.com.

Corathers, S. D., Kichler, J. C., Fino, N. F., Lang, W., Lawrence, J. M., Raymond, J. K., . . . Dolan, L. M. (2017). High health satisfaction among emerging adults with diabetes: Factors predicting resilience. *Health Psychology, 36,* 206-214.

Corbin, W. R., & Fromme, K. (2002). Alcohol use and serial monogamy as risks for sexually transmitted diseases in young adults. *Health Psychology, 21,* 229-236.

Cordova, M. J., Cunningham, L. L. C., Carlson, C. R., & Andrykowski, M. A. (2001). Posttraumatic growth following breast cancer: A controlled comparison study. *Health Psychology, 20,* 176-185.

Cornelius, T., Gettens, K., & Gorin, A. A. (2016). Dyadic dynamics in a randomized weight loss intervention. *Annals of Behavioral Medicine, 50,* 506-515.

Cornelius, T., Gettens, K., Lenz, E., Wojtanowski, A. C., Foster, G. D., & Gorin, A. A. (2018). How prescriptive support affects weight loss in weight-loss intervention participants and their untreated spouses. *Health Psychology, 37,* 775-781.

Cornelius, T., Voils, C. I., Birk, J. L., Romero, E. K., Edmondson, D. E., & Kronish, I. M. (2018). Identifying targets for cardiovascular medication adherence interventions through latent class analysis. *Health Psychology, 37,* 1006-1014.

Cosio, D., Jin, L., Siddique, J., & Mohr, D. C. (2011). The effect of telephone-administered cognitive-behavioral therapy on quality of life among patients with multiple sclerosis. *Annals of Behavioral Medicine, 41,* 227-234.

Cosser, S. (2008). *Google sets the standard for a happy work environment.* Retrieved March 8, 2013, from http://ezinearticles.com/?Google-Sets-The-Standard-For-A-Happy-Work-Environment&id=979201

Costa, P. T., Jr., Weiss, A., Duberstein, P. R., Friedman, B., & Siegler, I. C. (2014). Personality facets and all-cause mortality among medicare patients aged 66 to 102 years: A follow-up study of Weiss and Costa (2005). *Psychosomatic Medicine, 76,* 370-378.

Costanzo, E. S., Lutgendorf, S. K., Bradley, S. L., Rose, S. L., & Anderson, B. (2005). Cancer attributions, distress, and health practices among gynecologic cancer survivors. *Psychosomatic Medicine, 67,* 972-980.

Costanzo, E. S., Stawski, R. S., Ryff, C. D., Coe, C. L., & Almeida, D. M. (2012). Cancer survivors' responses to daily stressors: Implications for quality of life. *Health Psychology, 31,* 360-370.

Costello, D. M., Dierker, L. C., Jones, B. L., & Rose, J. S. (2008). Trajectories of smoking from adolescence to early adulthood and their psychosocial risk factors. *Health Psychology, 27,* 811-818.

Cotter, E. W., & Kelly, N. R. (2018). Stress-related eating, mindfulness, and obesity. *Health Psychology, 37,* 516-525.

Courneya, K. S., & Friedenreich, C. M. (2001). Framework PEACE: An organizational model for examining physical exercise across the cancer experience. *Annals of Behavioral Medicine, 23,* 263-272.

Courneya, K. S., McKenzie, D. C., Reid, R. D., Mackey, J. R., Gelmon, K., Freidenreich, C. M., . . . Segal, R. J. (2008). Barriers to supervised exercise training in a randomized trial of breast cancer patients receiving chemotherapy. *Annals of Behavioral Medicine, 35,* 116-122.

Courneya, K. S., Stevinson, C., McNeely, M. L., Sellar, C. M., Peddle, C. J. Friedenreich, C. M., . . . Reiman, T. (2010). Predictors of adherence to supervised exercise in lymphoma patients participating in a randomized controlled trial. *Annals of Behavioral Medicine, 40,* 30-39.

Cousins, N. (1979). *Anatomy of an illness.* New York: Norton.

Coutu, M. F., Dupuis, G., D'Antono, B., & Rochon-Goyer, L. (2003). Illness representation and change in dietary habits in hypercholesterolemic patients. *Journal of Behavioral Medicine, 26,* 133-152.

Cover, H., & Irwin, M. (1994). Immaturity and depression: Insomnia, retardation, and reduction of natural killer cell activity. *Journal of Behavioral Medicine, 17,* 217–223.

Covey, J. (2014). The role of dispositional factors in moderating message framing effects. *Health Psychology, 33,* 52–65.

Cox, M., Carmack, C., Hughes, D., Baum, G., Brown, J., Jhingran, A., Lu, K., & Basen-Engquist, K. (2015). Antecedents and mediators of physical activity in endometrial cancer survivors: Increasing physical activity through steps to health. *Health Psychology, 34,* 1022–1032.

Coyne, J. C., Jaarsma, T., Luttik, M. L., van Sonderen, E., van Veldhuisen, D. J., & Sanderman, R. (2011). Lack of prognostic value of Type D personality for mortality in a large sample of heart failure patients. *Psychosomatic Medicine, 73,* 557–562.

Crayton, E., Fahey, M., Ashworth, M., Besser, S. J., Weinman, J., & Wright, A. J. (2017). Psychological determinants of medication adherence in stroke survivors: A systematic review of observational studies. *Annals of Behavioral Medicine, 51,* 833–845.

Creed, F., Guthrie, E., Ratcliffe, J., Fernandes, L., Rigby, C., Tomenson, B.,…Thompson, D. G. (2005). Reported sexual abuse predicts impaired functioning but a good response to psychological treatments in patients with severe irritable bowel syndrome. *Psychosomatic Medicine, 67,* 490–499.

Crespo, N. C., Elder, J. P., Ayala, G. X., Slymen, D. J., Campbell, N. R., Sallis, J. F.,… Arredondo, E. M. (2012). Results of a multi-level intervention to prevent and control childhood obesity among Latino children: The Aventuras Para Niños study. *Annals of Behavioral Medicine, 43,* 84–100.

Creswell, J. D., Lam, S., Stanton, A. L., Taylor, S. E., Bower, J. E., & Sherman, D. K. (2007). Does self-affirmation, cognitive processing, or discovery of meaning explain cancer-related health benefits of expressive writing? *Personality and Social Psychology Bulletin, 33,* 238–250.

Creswell, J. D., Lindsay, E. K., Villalba, D. K., & Chin, B. (2019). Mindfulness training and physical health: Mechanisms and outcomes. *Psychosomatic Medicine, 81,* 224–232.

Creswell, J. D., Way, B. M., Eisenberger, N. I., & Lieberman, M. D. (2007). Neural correlates of dispositional mindfulness during affect labeling. *Psychosomatic Medicine, 69,* 560–565.

Crichton, F., Dodd, G., Schmid, G., Gamble, G., Cundy, T., & Petrie, K. J. (2014). The power of positive and negative expectations to influence reported symptoms of mood during exposure to wind farm sound. *Health Psychology, 33,* 1588–1592.

Crichton, F., Dodd, G., Schmid, G., Gamble, G., & Petrie, K. J. (2014). Can expectations produce symptoms from infrasound associated with wind turbines? *Health Psychology, 33,* 360–364.

Critser, G. (2003). *Fat land: How Americans became the fattest people in the world.* Boston, MA: Houghton Mifflin.

Crittenden, C. N., Murphy, M. L. M., & Cohen, S. (2018). Social integration and age-related decline in lung function. *Health Psychology, 37,* 472–480.

Croog, S. H., & Fitzgerald, E. F. (1978). Subjective stress and serious illness of a spouse: Wives of heart patients. *Journal of Health and Social Behavior, 9,* 166–178.

Crosby, R., & Noar, S. M. (2010). Theory development in health promotion: Are we there yet? *Journal of Behavioral Medicine, 33,* 259–263.

Crosnoe, R. (2002). Academic and health-related trajectories in adolescence: The intersection of gender and athletics. *Journal of Health and Social Behavior, 43,* 317–335.

Croyle, R. T., & Ditto, P. H. (1990). Illness cognition and behavior: An experimental approach. *Journal of Behavioral Medicine, 13,* 31–52.

Croyle, R. T., Loftus, E. F., Barger, S. D., Sun, Y. C., Hart, M., & Gettig, J. (2006). How well do people recall risk factor test results? Accuracy and bias among cholesterol screening participants. *Health Psychology, 25,* 425–432.

Croyle, R. T., Smith, K. R., Botkin, J. R., Baty, B., & Nash, J. (1997). Psychological responses to BRCA1 mutation testing: Preliminary findings. *Health Psychology, 16,* 63–72.

Cruess, D. G., Antoni, M., McGregor, B. A., Kilbourn, K. M., Boyers, A. E., Alferi, S. M.,… Kumar, M. (2000). Cognitive-behavioral stress management reduces serum cortisol by enhancing benefit finding among women being treated for early stage breast cancer. *Psychosomatic Medicine, 62,* 304–308.

Cruess, D. G., Burnham, K. E., Finitsis, D. J., Goshe, B. M., Strainge, L., Kalichman, M.,… Kalichman, S. C. (2017). A randomized clinical trial of a brief Internet-based group intervention to reduce sexual transmission risk behavior among HIV-positive gay and bisexual men. *Annals of Behavioral Medicine, 52,* 116–129.

Cruwys, T., Wakefield, J. R., Sani, F., Dingle, G. A., & Jetten, J. (2018). Social isolation predicts frequent attendance in primary care. *Annals of Behavioral Medicine, 52,* 817–829.

Cuijpers, P., van Straten, A., & Andersson, G. (2008). Internet-administered cognitive behavior therapy for health problems: A systematic review. *Journal of Behavioral Medicine, 31,* 169–177.

Cullen, K. W., & Zakeri, I. (2004). Fruit, vegetables, milk, and sweetened beverages consumption and access to à la carte/snack bar meals at school. *American Journal of Public Health, 94,* 463–467.

Cunningham, J. A., Lin, E., Ross, H. E., & Walsh, G. W. (2000). Factors associated with untreated remissions from alcohol abuse or dependence. *Addictive Behaviors, 25,* 317–321.

Curbow, B., Bowie, J., Garza, M. A., McDonnell, K., Scott, L. B., Coyne, C.A., & Chiappelli, T. (2004). Community-based cancer screening programs in older populations: Making progress but can we do better? *Preventive Medicine, 38,* 676–693.

Curran, S. L., Beacham, A. O., & Andrykowski, M. A. (2004). Ecological momentary assessment of fatigue following breast cancer treatment. *Journal of Behavioral Medicine, 27,* 425–444.

Currie, S. R., Wilson, K. G., & Curran, D. (2002). Clinical significance and predictors of treatment response to cognitive-behavior therapy for insomnia secondary to chronic pain. *Journal of Behavioral Medicine, 25,* 135–153.

Cuthbert, C. A., King-Shier, K. M., Ruether, J. D., Tapp, D. M., Wytsma-Fisher, K., Fung, T. S., & Culos-Reed, S. N. (2018). The effects of exercise on physical and psychological outcomes in cancer caregivers: Results from the RECHARGE randomized controlled trial. *Annals of Behavioral Medicine, 52,* 645–661.

Czaja, S. J., & Rubert, M. P. (2002). Telecommunications technology as an aid to family caregivers of persons with dementia. *Psychosomatic Medicine, 64,* 469–476.

Czekierda, K., Banik, A., Park, C. L., & Luszczynska, A. (2017). Meaning in life and physical health: Systematic review and meta-analysis. *Health Psychology Review, 11,* 387–418.

Dahlberg, C. C. (1977, June). Stroke. *Psychology Today,* pp. 121–128.

Dahlquist, L. M., McKenna, K. D., Jones, K. K., Dillinger, L., Weiss, K. E., & Ackerman, C. S. (2007). Active and passive distraction using a head-mounted display helmet: Effects on cold pressor pain in children. *Health Psychology, 26,* 794–801.

Dakof, G. A., & Taylor, S. E. (1990). Victims' perceptions of social support: What is helpful from whom? *Journal of Personality and Social Psychology, 58,* 80–89.

Daly, M., Delaney, L., Doran, P. P., Harmon, C., & MacLachlan, M. (2010). Naturalistic monitoring of the affect-heart rate relationship: A day reconstruction study. *Health Psychology, 29,* 186–195.

D'Amico, E. J., & Fromme, K. (1997). Health risk behaviors of adolescent and young adult siblings. *Health Psychology, 16,* 426–432.

Damush, T. M., Wu, J., Bair, M. J., Sutherland, J. M., & Kroenke, K. (2008). Self-management practices among primary care patients with musculoskeletal pain and depression. *Journal of Behavioral Medicine, 31,* 301–307.

D'Anna-Hernandez, K. L., Hoffman, M. C., Zerbe, G. O., Coussons-Read, M., Ross, R. G., & Laudenslager, M. L. (2012). Acculturation, maternal cortisol, and birth outcomes in women of Mexican descent. *Psychosomatic Medicine, 74,* 296–304.

Dantzer, R., Cohen, S., Russo, S., & Dinan, T. (2018). Resilience and immunity. *Brain, Behavior, and Immunity, 74,* 28–42.

Dar, R., Leventhal, E. A., & Leventhal, H. (1993). Schematic processes in pain perception. *Cognitive Therapy and Research, 17,* 341–357.

Darbes, L. A., & Lewis, M. A. (2005). HIV-specific social support predicts less sexual risk behavior in gay male couples. *Health Psychology, 24,* 617–622.

Dar-Nimrod, I., & Heine, S. J. (2011). Genetic essentialism: On the deceptive determinism of DNA. *Psychological Bulletin, 137,* 800–818.

Darrow, S. M., Verhoeven, J. E., Révész, D., Lindqvist, D., Penninx, B. W., Delucchi, K. L., . . . Mathews, C. A. (2016). The association between psychiatric disorders and telomere length: A meta-analysis involving 14,827 persons. *Psychosomatic Medicine, 78,* 776–787.

Davidson, K. W., Goldstein, M., Kaplan, R. M., Kaufmann, P. G., Knatterud, G. L., Orleans, C. T., . . . Whitlock, E. P. (2003). Evidence-based behavioral medicine: What is it and how do we achieve it? *Annals of Behavioral Medicine, 26,* 161–171.

Davidson, K. W., Hall, P., & MacGregor, M. (1996). Gender differences in the relation between interview-derived hostility scores and resting blood pressure. *Journal of Behavioral* Medicine, *19,* 185–202.

Davidson, K. W., MacGregor, M. W., Stuhr, J., & Gidron, Y. (1999). Increasing constructive anger verbal behavior decreases resting blood pressure: A secondary analysis of a randomized controlled hostility intervention. *International Journal of Behavioral Medicine, 6,* 268–278.

Davidson, R. J., & Kaszniak, A. W. (2015). Conceptual and methodological issues in research on mindfulness and meditation. *American Psychologist, 7,* 581–592.

Davis, K., Schoen, C., & Stremikis, K. (2010). *Mirror, mirror on the wall: How the performance of the U.S health care system compares internationally, 2010 update.* The Commonwealth Fund.

Davis, K. C., Jacques-Tiura, A. J., Stappenbeck, C. A., Danube, C. L., Morrison, D. M., Norris, J., & George, W. H. (2016). Men's condom use resistance: Alcohol effects on theory of planned behavior constructs. *Health Psychology, 35,* 178–186.

Davis, M., Matthews, K., & McGrath, C. (2000). Hostile attitudes predict elevated vascular resistance during interpersonal stress in men and women. *Psychosomatic Medicine, 62,* 17–25.

Davis, M. C., Matthews, K. A., Meilahn, E. N., & Kiss, J. E. (1995). Are job characteristics related to fibrinogen levels in middle-aged women? *Health Psychology, 14,* 310–318.

Davison, G. C., Williams, M. E., Nezami, E., Bice, T. L., & DeQuattro, V. L. (1991). Relaxation, reduction in angry articulated thoughts, and improvements in borderline hypertension and heart rate. *Journal of Behavioral Medicine, 14,* 453–468.

Davison, K. K., Schmalz, D. L., & Downs, D. S. (2010). Hop, skip . . . no! Explaining adolescent girls' disinclination for physical activity. *Annals of Behavioral Medicine, 39,* 290–302.

Deatrick, J. A., Hobbie, W., Ogle, S., Fisher, M. J., Barakat, L., Hardie, T., & Ginsberg, J. P. (2014). Competence in caregivers of adolescent and young adult childhood brain tumor survivors. *Health Psychology, 33,* 1103–1112.

De Bloom, J., Geurts, S. A. E., & Kompier, M. A. J. (2012). Effects of short vacations, vacation activities and experiences on employee health and well-being. *Stress and Health, 28,* 305–318.

De Graaf, R., & Bijl, R. V. (2002). Determinants of mental distress in adults with a severe auditory impairment: Difference between prelingual and postlingual deafness. *Psychosomatic Medicine, 64,* 61–70.

De Jonge, P., Latour, C., & Huyse, F. J. (2003). Implementing psychiatric interventions on a medical ward: Effects on patients' quality of life and length of hospital stay. *Psychosomatic Medicine, 65,* 997–1002.

De Koning, L., Malik, V. S., Kellogg, M. D., Rimm, E. B., Willett, W. C., & Hu, F. B. (2012). Sweetened beverage consumption, incident coronary heart disease and biomarkers of risk in men. *Circulation, 125,* 1735–1741.

De Moor, C., Sterner, J., Hall, M., Warneke, C., Gilani, Z., Amato, R., & Cohen, L. (2002). A pilot study of the effects of expressive writing on psychological and behavioral adjustment in patients in a phase II trial of vaccine therapy for metastatic renal cell carcinoma. *Health Psychology, 21,* 615–619.

De Peuter, S., Lemaigre, V., Van Diest, I., & Van den Bergh, O. (2008). Illness-specific catastrophic thinking and overperception in asthma. *Health Psychology, 27,* 93–99.

De Visser, R. O., Graber, R., Hart, A., Abraham, C., Scanlon, T., Watten, P., & Memon, A. (2015). Using qualitative methods within a mixed-methods approach to developing and evaluating interventions to address harmful alcohol use among young people. *Health Psychology,* 34(4), 349–360.

Deary, I. J., Batty, G. D., Pattie, A., & Gale, C. R. (2008). More intelligent, more dependable children live longer: A 55-year longitudinal study of a representative sample of the Scottish nation. *Psychological Science, 19,* 874–880.

Deci, E. L., & Ryan, R. M. (1985). *Intrinsic motivation and self-determination in human behavior.* New York: Plenum.

Dedert, E. A., Calhoun, P. S., Watkins, L. L., Sherwood, A., & Beckham, J. C. (2010). Posttraumatic stress disorder, cardiovascular, and metabolic disease: A review of the evidence. *Annals of Behavioral Medicine, 39,* 61–78.

De la Monte, S. M. (2012). Contributions of brain insulin resistance and deficiency in amyloid-related neurodegeneration in Alzheimer's disease. *Drugs, 72,* 49–66.

Demakakos, P., Zaninotto, P., & Nouwen, A. (2014). Is the association between depressive symptoms and glucose metabolism bidirectional? Evidence from the English longitudinal study of ageing. *Psychosomatic Medicine, 76,* 555–561.

Denford, S., Taylor, R. S., Campbell, J. L., & Greaves, C. J. (2014). Effective behavior change techniques in asthma self-care interventions: Systematic review and meta-regression. *Health Psychology, 33,* 577–587.

Dennis, P. A., Watkins, L. L., Calhoun, P. S., Oddone, A., Sherwood, A., Dennis, M. F., Rissling, M. B., & Beckham, J. C. (2014). Posttraumatic stress, heart rate variability, and the mediating role of behavioral risks. *Psychosomatic Medicine, 76,* 629–637.

Denollet, J. (2000). Type D personality: A potential risk factor refined. *Journal of Psychosomatic Research, 49,* 255–266.

Denollet, J., Pedersen, S. S., Vrints, C. J., & Conraads, V. M. (2006). Usefulness of type D personality in predicting five-year cardiac events above and beyond concurrent symptoms of stress in patients with coronary heart disease. *American Journal of Cardiology, 97,* 970–973.

Denollet, J., Pedersen, S. S., Vrints, C. J., & Conraads, V. M. (2013). Predictive value of social inhibition and negative affectivity for cardiovascular events and mortality in patients with coronary artery disease: The type D personality construct. *Psychosomatic Medicine, 75,* 873–881.

Department for Professional Employees. (April, 2006). *Fact sheet 2006, professional women: Vital statistics.* Retrieved April 13, 2007, from http://www.dpeaflcio.org/programs/factsheets/fs_2006_Professional_ Women.htm#_edn14

Derbyshire, S. W. G. (2014). The use of neuroimaging to advance the understanding of chronic pain: From description to mechanism. *Psychosomatic Medicine, 76,* 402-403.

DeRosa, C. J., & Marks, G. (1998). Preventative counseling of HIV-positive men and self-disclosure of serostatus to sex partners: New opportunities for prevention. *Health Psychology, 17,* 224-231.

Dersh, J., Polatin, P. B., & Gatchel, R. J. (2002). Chronic pain and psychopathology: Research findings and theoretical considerations. *Psychosomatic Medicine, 64,* 773-786.

Des Jarlais, D. C., & Semaan, S. (2008). HIV prevention for injecting drug users: The first 25 years and counting. *Psychosomatic Medicine, 70,* 606-611.

Deschênes, S. S., Burns, R. J., Pouwer, F., & Schmitz, N. (2017). Diabetes complications and depressive symptoms. *Psychosomatic Medicine, 79,* 603-612.

Detweiler, J. B., Bedell, B. T., Salovey, P., Pronin, E., & Rothman, A. J. (1999). Message framing and sunscreen use: Gain-framed messages motivate beach-goers. *Health Psychology, 18,* 189-196.

Deverts, D. J., Cohen, S., DiLillo, V. G., Lewis, C. E., Kiefe, C., Whooley, M., & Matthews, K. A. (2010). Depressive symptoms, race, and circulating C-reactive protein: The coronary artery risk development in young adults (CARDIA) study. *Psychosomatic Medicine, 72,* 734-741.

Devine, C. M., Connors, M. M., Sobal, J., & Bisogni, C. A. (2003). Sandwiching it in: Spillover of work onto food choices and family roles in low- and moderate-income urban households. *Social Science and Medicine, 56,* 617-630.

Dew, M. A., Hoch, C. C., Buysse, D. J., Monk, T. H., Begley, A. E., Houck, P. R., . . . Reynolds, C. F. (2003). Healthy older adults' sleep predicts all-cause mortality at 4 to 19 years of follow-up. *Psychosomatic Medicine, 65,* 63-73.

Di Giorgio, A., Hudson, M., Jerjes, W., & Cleare, A. J. (2005). 24-hour pituitary and adrenal hormone profiles in chronic fatigue syndrome. *Psychosomatic Medicine, 67,* 433-440.

Diabetes Prevention Program Research Group. (2002). Reduction in the incidence of type 2 diabetes with lifestyle intervention or metformin. *The New England Journal of Medicine, 346,* 393-403.

Diamond, J., Massey, K. L., & Covey, D. (1989). Symptom awareness and blood glucose estimation in diabetic adults. *Health Psychology, 8,* 15-26.

Dias, J. A., Griffith, R. A., Ng, J. J., Reinert, S. E., Friedmann, P. D., & Moulton, A. W. (2002). Patients' use of the Internet for medical information. *Journal of General Internal Medicine, 17,* 180-185.

Dickens, C., McGowan, L., Clark-Carter, D., & Creed, F. (2002). Depression and rheumatoid arthritis: A systematic review of the literature with meta-analysis. *Psychosomatic Medicine, 64,* 52-60.

Dickens, C., McGowan, L., & Dale, S. (2003). Impact of depression on experimental pain perception: A systematic review of the literature with meta-analysis. *Psychosomatic Medicine, 65,* 369-375.

Dickens, C., McGowan, L., Percival, C., Tomenson, B., Cotter, L., Heagerty, A., & Creed, F. (2008). New onset depression following myocardial infarction predicts cardiac mortality. *Psychosomatic Medicine, 70,* 450-455.

Dickerson, S. S., Kemeny, M. E., Aziz, N., Kim, K. H., & Fahey, J. L. (2004). Immunological effects of induced shame and guilt. *Psychosomatic Medicine, 66,* 124-131.

DiClemente, R. J., Crittenden, C. P., Rose, E., Sales, J. M., Wingood, G. M., Crosby, R. A., & Salazar, L. F. (2008). Psychosocial predictors of HIV-associated sexual behavior and the efficacy of prevention interventions in adolescents at-risk for HIV infection: What works and what doesn't work? *Psychosomatic Medicine, 70,* 598-605.

Diefenbach, M. A., Leventhal, E. A., Leventhal, H., & Patrick-Miller, L. (1996). Negative affect relates to cross-sectional but not longitudinal symptom reporting: Data from elderly adults. *Health Psychology, 15,* 282-288.

Dientsbier, R. A. (1989). Arousal and physiological toughness: Implications for mental and physical health. *Psychological Review, 96,* 84-100.

Dietz, W. H., & Gortmaker, S. L. (2001). Preventing obesity in children and adolescents. *Annual Review of Public Health, 22,* 337-353.

DiFulvio, G. T., Linowski, S. A., Mazziotti, J. S., & Puleo, E. (2012). Effectiveness of the Brief Alcohol and Screening Intervention for College Students (BASICS) program with a mandated population. *Journal of American College Health, 60,* 269-280.

Dillard, A. J., Ferrer, R. A., Ubel, P. A., & Fagerlin, A. (2012). Risk perception measures' associations with behavior intentions, affect, and cognition following colon cancer screening messages. *Health Psychology, 31,* 106-113.

Dillon, P., Phillips, L. A., Gallagher, P., Smith, S. M., Stewart, D., & Cousins, G. (2018). Assessing the multidimensional relationship between medication beliefs and adherence in older adults with hypertension using polynomial regression. *Annals of Behavioral Medicine, 52,* 146-156.

DiLorenzo, T. A., Schnur, J., Montgomery, G. H., Erblich, J., Winkel, G., & Bovbjerg, D. H. (2006). A model of disease-specific worry in heritable disease: The influence of family history, perceived risk and worry about other illnesses. *Journal of Behavioral Medicine, 29,* 37-49.

DiMatteo, M. R. (2004). Social support and patient adherence to medical treatment: A meta-analysis. *Health Psychology, 23,* 207-218.

DiMatteo, M. R., & DiNicola, D. D. (1982). *Achieving patient compliance: The psychology of the medical practitioner's role.* New York: Pergamon Press.

DiMatteo, M. R., Friedman, H. S., & Taranta, A. (1979). Sensitivity to bodily nonverbal communication as a factor in practitioner-patient rapport. *Journal of Nonverbal Behavior, 4,* 18-26.

DiMatteo, M. R., Giordani, P. J., Lepper, H. S., & Croghan, T. W. (2002). Patient adherence and medical treatment outcomes: A meta-analysis. *Medical Care, 40,* 794-811.

DiMatteo, M. R., Haskard-Zolnierek, K. B., & Martin, L. R. (2012). Improving patient adherence: A three-factor model to health practice. *Health Psychology Review, 6,* 74-91.

DiMatteo, M. R., Hays, R. D., & Prince, L. M. (1986). Relationship of physicians' nonverbal communication skill to patient satisfaction, appointment noncompliance, and physical workload. *Health Psychology, 5,* 581-594.

DiMatteo, M. R., Lepper, H. S., & Croghan, T. W. (2000). Depression is a risk factor for noncompliance with medical treatment. *Archives of Internal Medicine, 160,* 2101-2107.

Dimidjian, S., & Segal, Z. V. (2015). Prospects for a clinical science of mindfulness-based intervention. *American Psychologist, 70,* 593-620.

Dinan, T. G., & Cryan, J. F. (2017). Brain-gut-microbiota axis and mental health. *Psychosomatic Medicine, 79,* 920-926.

Dinescu, D., Horn, E. E., Duncan, G., & Turkheimer, E. (2016). Socioeconomic modifiers of genetic and environmental influences on body mass index in adult twins. *Health Psychology, 35,* 157-166.

Dishman, R. K. (1982). Compliance/adherence in health-related exercise. *Health Psychology, 1,* 237-267.

Dishman, R. K., Vandenberg, R. J., Motl, R. W., & Nigg, C. R. (2010). Using constructs of the transtheoretical model to predict classes of change in regular physical activity: A multi-ethnic longitudinal cohort study. *Annals of Behavioral Medicine, 40,* 150-163.

Ditto, P. H., Druley, J. A., Moore, K. A., Danks, H. J., & Smucker, W. D. (1996). Fates worse than death: The role of valued life activities in health-state evaluations. *Health Psychology, 15,* 332-343.

Ditto, P. H., & Hawkins, N. A. (2005). Advance directives and cancer decision making near the end of life. *Health Psychology, 24* (Suppl.), S63-S70.

Ditto, P. H., Munro, G. D., Apanovich, A. M., Scepansky, J. A., & Lockhart.

L. K. (2003). Spontaneous skepticism: The interplay of motivation and expectation in response to favorable and unfavorable medical diagnoses. *Personality and Social Psychology Bulletin, 29,* 1120-1132.

Ditto, P. H., Smucker, W. D., Danks, J. H., Jacobson, J. A., Houts, R. M., Fagerlin, A., . . . Gready, R. M. (2003). Stability of older adults' preferences for life-sustaining medical treatment. *Health Psychology, 22,* 605-615.

Ditzen, B., Hoppmann, C., & Klumb, P. (2008). Positive couple interactions and daily cortisol: On the stress-protecting role of intimacy. *Psychosomatic Medicine, 70,* 883-889.

Ditzen, B., Neumann, I. D., Bodenmann, G., von Dawans, B., Turner, R. A., Ehlert, U., & Heinrichs, M. (2007). Effects of different kinds of couple interaction on cortisol and heart rate responses to stress in women. *Psychoneuroendocrinology, 32,* 565-574.

Dixon, K. E., Keefe, F. J., Scipio, C. D., Perri, L. M., & Abernethy, A. P. (2007). Psychological interventions for arthritis pain management in adults: A meta-analysis. *Health Psychology, 26,* 241-250.

Doan, S. N., Dich, N., & Evans, G. W. (2014). Childhood cumulative risk and later allostatic load: Mediating role of substance use. *Health Psychology, 33,* 1402-1409.

Dobson, K. S. (Ed.). (2010). *Handbook of cognitive behavioral therapies.* New York: Guilford.

Dohrenwend, B. P., Yager, T. J., Wall, M. M., & Adams, B. G. (2013). The roles of combat exposure, personal vulnerability, and involvement in harm to civilians or prisoners in Vietnam-war-related posttraumatic stress disorder. *Clinical Psychological Science,* 223-238.

Dolezsar, C. M., McGrath, J. J., Herzig, A. J. M., & Miller, S. B. (2014). Perceived racial discrimination and hypertension: A comprehensive systematic review. *Health Psychology, 33,* 20-34.

Donahue, R. G., Lampert, R., Dornelas, E., Clemow, L., & Burg, M. M. (2010). Rationale and design of a randomized clinical trial comparing stress reduction treatment to usual cardiac care: The reducing variability to implantable cardioverter defibrillator shock-treated ventricular arrhythmias (RISTA) trial. *Psychosomatic Medicine, 72,* 172-177.

Donaldson, S. I., Graham, J. W., & Hansen, W. B. (1994). Testing the generalizability of intervening mechanism theories: Understanding the effects of adolescent drug use prevention interventions. *Journal of Behavioral Medicine, 17,* 195-216.

Donaldson, S. I., Graham, J. W., Piccinin, A. M., & Hansen, W. B. (1995). Resistance-skills training and onset of alcohol use: Evidence for beneficial and potentially harmful effects in public schools and in private Catholic schools. *Health Psychology, 14,* 291-300.

Donovan, J. E., & Jessor, R. (1985). Structure of problem behavior in adolescence and young adulthood. *Journal of Consulting and Clinical Psychology, 53,* 890-904.

Dore, G. A., Elias, M. F., Robbins, M. A., Budge, M. M., & Elias, P. K. (2008). Relation between central adiposity and cognitive function in the Maine-Syracuse study: Attenuation by physical activity. *Annals of Behavioral Medicine, 35,* 341-350.

Dorgan, C., & Editue, A. (1995). *Statistical record of health and medicine: 1995.* Detroit, MI: Orale Research.

Dornelas, E. A., & Sears, S. F. (2018). Living with heart despite recurrent challenges: Psychological care for adults with advanced cardiac disease. *American Psychologist, 73,* 1007-1018.

Dorough, A. E., Winett, R. A., Anderson, E. S., Davy, B. M., Martin, E. C., & Hedrick, V. (2014). Dash to wellness: Emphasizing self-regulation through e-health in adults with prehypertension. *Health Psychology, 33,* 249-254.

Dracup, K., & Moser, D. (1991). Treatment-seeking behavior among those with signs and symptoms of acute myocardial infarction. *Heart and Lung, 20,* 570-575.

Driscoll, A. K., & Bernstein, A. B. (2012). Health and access to care among employed and unemployed adults: United States, 2009-2010. *NCHS Data Brief, 83,* 1-8.

Droomers, M., Schrijvers, C. T. M., & Mackenbach, J. P. (2002). Why do lower educated people continue smoking? Explanations from the longitudinal GLOBE study. *Health Psychology, 21,* 263-272.

Drossman, D. A., Leserman, J., Li, Z., Keefe, F., Hu, Y. J. B., & Toomey, T. C. (2000). Effects of coping on health outcome among women with gastrointestinal disorders. *Psychosomatic Medicine, 62,* 309-317.

D'Souza, P. J., Lumley, M. A., Kraft, C. A., & Dooley, J. A. (2008). Relaxation training and written emotional disclosure for tension or migraine headaches: A randomized, controlled trial. *Annals of Behavioral Medicine, 36,* 21-32.

DuBenske, L. L., Gustafson, D. H., Namkoong, K., Hawkins, R. P., Atwood, K., Brown, R. L., & Cleary, J. F. (2014). CHESS improves cancer caregivers' burden and mood: Results of an eHealth RCT. *Health Psychology, 33,* 1261-1272.

Duffy, K. A., McLaughlin, K. A., & Green, P. A. (2018). Early life adversity and health-risk behaviors: Proposed psychological and neural mechanisms. *Annals of the New York Academy of Sciences, 1428,* 151-169.

Duggan, K. A., Reynolds, C. A., Kern, M. L., & Friedman, H. S. (2014). Childhood sleep duration and lifelong mortality risk. *Health Psychology, 33,* 1195-1203.

DuHamel, K. N., Manne, S., Nereo, N., Ostroff, J., Martini, R., Parsons, S., . . . Redd, W. H. (2004). Cognitive processing among mothers of children undergoing bone marrow/stem cell transplantation. *Psychosomatic Medicine, 66,* 92-103.

Duits, A. A., Boeke, S., Taams, M. A., Passchier, J., & Erdman, R. A. M. (1997). Prediction of quality of life after coronary artery bypass graft surgery: A review and evaluation of multiple, recent studies. *Psychosomatic Medicine, 59,* 257-268.

Duivis, H. E., Kupper, N., Vermunt, J. K., Penninx, B. W., Bosch, N. M., Riese, H., & de Jonge, P. (2015). Depression trajectories, inflammation, and lifestyle factors in adolescence: The tracking adolescents' individual lives survey. *Health Psychology, 34,* 1047-1057.

Dunbar, F. (1943). *Psychosomatic diagnosis.* New York: Hoeber.

Duncan, S. C., Duncan, T. E., Strycker, L. A., & Chaumeton, N. R. (2002). Relations between youth antisocial and prosocial activities. *Journal of Behavioral Medicine, 25,* 425-438.

Dunkel Schetter, C., & Dolbier, C. (2011). Resilience in the context of chronic stress and health in adults. *Social and Personality Psychology Compass, 5,* 634-652.

Dunkel Schetter, C., Feinstein, L. G., Taylor, S. E., & Falke, R. L. (1992). Patterns of coping with cancer. *Health Psychology, 11,* 79-87.

Dunn, M. J., Rodriguez, E. M., Barnwell, A. S., Grossenbacher, J. C., Vannatta, K., Gerhardt, C. A., & Compas, B. E. (2012). Posttraumatic stress symptoms in parents of children with cancer within six months of diagnosis. *Health Psychology, 31,* 176-185.

Dunton, G. F., Liao, Y., Intille, S., Huh, J., & Leventhal, A. (2015). Momentary assessment of contextual influences on affective response during physical activity. *Health Psychology, 34,* 1145-1153.

Dupont, A., Bower, J. E., Stanton, A. L., & Ganz, P. A. (2014). Cancer-related intrusive thoughts predict behavioral symptoms following breast cancer treatment. *Health Psychology, 33,* 155-163.

DuPont, R. L. (1988). The counselor's dilemma: Treating chemical dependence at college. In T. M. Rivinus (Ed.), *Alcoholism/chemical dependency and the college student* (pp. 41-61). New York: Haworth Press.

Duschek, S., Schuepbach, D., Doll, A., Werner, N. S., & Reyes del Paso, G. A. (2011). Self-regulation of cerebral blood flow by means of transcranial doppler sonography biofeedback. *Annals of Behavioral Medicine, 41,* 235-242.

Dutton, G. (2012). Pain management market ripe with immediate opportunities, *Genetic Engineering and Biotechnology News*. Retrieved April 2, 2013, from http://www.genengnews.com/gen articles/pain-management-market-ripe-with-immediate-opportunities/4123

Duxbury, M. L., Armstrong, G. D., Dren, D. J., & Henley, S. J. (1984). Head nurse leadership style with staff nurse burnout and job satisfaction in neonatal intensive care units. *Nursing Research, 33,* 97-101.

Dwyer, L. L., Harris-Kojetin, L. D., & Valverde, R. H. (2014). Differences in adult day services center participant characteristics by center ownership: United States, 2012. *NCHS Data Brief, 164,* 1-8.

Eaker, E. D., Sullivan, L. M., Kelly-Hayes, M., D'Agostino, R. B., & Benjamin, E. J. (2007). Marital status, marital strain, and risk of coronary heart disease or total mortality: The Framingham offspring study. *Psychosomatic Medicine, 69,* 509-513.

Eakin, E. G., Bull, S. S., Riley, K. M., Reeves, M. M., McLaughlin, P., & Gutierrez, S. (2007). Resources for health: A primary-care-based diet and physical activity intervention targeting urban Latinos with multiple chronic conditions. *Health Psychology, 26,* 392-400.

Eakin, E., Reeves, M., Winkler, E., Lawler, S., & Owen, N. (2010). Maintenance of physical activity and dietary change following a telephone-delivered intervention. *Health Psychology, 29,* 566-573.

Earnshaw, V. A., Bogart, L. M., Dovidio, J. F., & Williams, D. R. (2013). Stigma and racial/ethnic HIV disparities: Moving toward resilience. *American Psychologist, 68,* 225-236.

*The Economist.* (2012, April 14). Medicine and its rivals: The believers, pp. 68-69.

*The Economist.* (2012, May 19). African child mortality: The best story in development, p. 56.

*The Economist.* (2012, October 20). Assisted suicide: Over my dead body, pp. 55-56.

*The Economist.* (2013, March 23). Open skies, bottomless pits, p. 72.

*The Economist.* (2013, July 13). Altered states, p. 70.

*The Economist.* (2015, June 27). Campaigns to let doctors help the suffering and terminally ill to die are gathering momentum across the West, p. 16.

*The Economist.* (2015, July 11). Quitting is so hard, p. 18.

Edwards, K. M., Burns, V. E., Adkins, A. E., Carroll, D., Drayson, M., & Ring, C. (2008). Meningococcal A vaccination response is enhanced by acute stress in men. *Psychosomatic Medicine, 70,* 147-151.

Edwards, R. R. (2008). The association of perceived discrimination with low back pain. *Journal of Behavioral Medicine, 31,* 379-389.

Edwards, S., Hucklebridge, F., Clow, A., & Evans, P. (2003). Components of the diurnal cortisol cycle in relation to upper respiratory symptoms and perceived stress. *Psychosomatic Medicine, 65,* 320-327.

Egede, L. E. (2005). Effect of comorbid chronic diseases on prevalence and odds of depression in adults with diabetes. *Psychosomatic Medicine, 67,* 46-51.

Ehrlich, K. B., Hoyt, L. T., Sumner, J. A., McDade, T. W., & Adam, E. K. (2015). Quality of relationships with parents and friends in adolescence predicts metabolic risk in young adulthood. *Health Psychology, 345,* 896-904.

Eichstaedt, J. C., Schwartz, H. A., Kern, M. L., Park, G., Labarthe, D. R., Merchant, R. M., & Seligman, M. E. P. (2015). Psychological language on twitter predicts county-level heart disease mortality. *Psychological Science,* 1-11.

Eifert, G. H., Hodson, S. E., Tracey, D. R., Seville, J. L., & Gunawardane, K. (1996). Heart-focused anxiety, illness beliefs, and behavioral impairment: Comparing healthy heart-anxious patients with cardiac and surgical inpatients. *Journal of Behavioral Medicine, 19,* 385-400.

Eisenberg, D., & Sieger, M. (2003, June 9). The doctor won't see you now. *Time,* pp. 46-60.

Eisenlohr-Moul, T. A., Burris, J. L., & Evans, D. R. (2013). Pain acceptance, psychological functioning, and self-regulatory fatigue in temporomandibular disorder. *Health Psychology, 32,* 1236-1239.

Ekkekakis, P., Hall, E. F, VanLanduyt, L. M., & Petruzzello, S. J. (2000). Walking in (affective) circles: Can short walks enhance affect? *Journal of Behavioral Medicine, 23,* 245-275.

Ekmann, A., Osler, M., & Avlund, K. (2012). The predictive value of fatigue for nonfatal ischemic heart disease and all-cause mortality. *Psychosomatic Medicine, 74,* 464-470.

Ekstedt, M., Åkerstedt, T., & Söderström, M. (2004). Microarousals during sleep are associated with increased levels of lipids, cortisol, and blood pressure. *Psychosomatic Medicine, 66,* 925-931.

El-Serag, H. B., Sweet, S., Winchester, C. C., & Dent, J. (2013). Update on the epidemiology of gastro-oesophageal reflux disease: A systematic review. *Gut, 63,* 871-880.

Elbejjani, M., Fuhrer, R., Abrahamowicz, M., Mazoyer, B., Crivello, F., Tzourio, C., & Dufouil, C. (2017). Life-course socioeconomic position and hippocampal atrophy in a prospective cohort of older adults. *Psychosomatic Medicine, 79,* 14-23.

Elder, J. P., Ayala, G. X., Campbell, N. R., Slymen, D., Lopez-Madurga, E. T., Engelberg, M., & Baquero, B. (2005). Interpersonal and print nutrition communication for Spanish-dominant Latino population: Secretos de la buena vida. *Health Psychology, 24,* 49-57.

Ellington, L., & Wiebe, D. (1999). Neuroticism, symptom presentation, and medical decision making. *Health Psychology, 18,* 634-643.

Elliot, A. J., Turiano, N. A., Infurna, F. J., Lachman, M. E., & Chapman, B. P. (2018). Lifetime trauma, perceived control, and all-cause mortality: Results from the Midlife in the United States Study. *Health Psychology, 37*(3), 262-270.

Ellis, E. M., Elwyn, G., Nelson, W. L., Scalia, P., Kobrin, S. C., & Ferrer, R. A. (2018). Interventions to engage affective forecasting in health-related decision making: A meta-analysis. *Annals of Behavioral Medicine, 52*(2), 157-174.

Ellis, E. M., Homish, G. G., Parks, K. A., Collins, R. L., & Kiviniemi, M. T. (2015). Increasing condom use by changing people's feelings about them: An experimental study. *Health Psychology, 34,* 941-950.

El-Sheikh, M., Bagley, E. J., Keiley, M., Elmore-Staton, L., Chen, E., & Buckhalt, J. A. (2013). Economic adversity and children's sleep problems: Multiple indicators and moderation effects. *Health Psychology, 32,* 849-859.

Emerson, S. U., & Purcell, R. H. (2004). Running like water—the omnipresence of hepatitis E. *The New England Journal of Medicine, 351,* 2367-2368.

Emeny, R. T., Zierer, A., Lacruz, M. E., Baumert, J., Herder, C., Gornitzka, G., Koenig, W., Thorand, B., & Ladwig, K., for the KORA Investigators (2013). Job strain-associated inflammatory burden and long-term risk of coronary events: Findings from the MONICA/KORA Ausburg case-cohort study. *Psychosomatic Medicine, 75,* 317-325.

Emery, C. F., Kiecolt-Glaser, J. K., Glaser, R., Malarkey, W. B., & Frid, D. J. (2005). Exercise accelerates wound healing among healthy older adults: A preliminary investigation. *Journal of Gerontology: Medical Sciences,* 60A, 1432-1436.

Emmons, C., Biernat, M., Teidje, L. B., Lang, E. L., & Wortman, C. B. (1990). Stress, support, and coping among women professionals with preschool children. In J. Eckenrode & S. Gore (Eds.), *Stress between work and family* (pp. 61-93). New York: Plenum Press.

Emmons, K. (2012). Behavioral medicine and the health of our nation: Accelerating our impact. *Annals of Behavioral Medicine, 43,* 153-161.

Emslie, C., Hunt, K., & Lyons, A. (2013). The role of alcohol in forging and maintaining friendships amongst Scottish men in midlife. *Health Psychology, 32,* 33-41.

Endrighi, R., Hamer, M., & Steptoe, A. (2011). Associations of trait optimism with diurnal neuroendocrine activity, cortisol responses to mental stress, and subjective stress measures in healthy men and women. *Psychosomatic Medicine, 73,* 672–678.

Endrighi, R., Hamer, M., & Steptoe, A. (2016). Post-menopausal women exhibit greater interleukin-6 responses to mental stress than older men, *Annals of Behavioral Medicine, 50,* 564–571.

Eng, P. M., Fitzmaurice, G., Kubzansky, L. D., Rimm, E. B., & Kawachi, I. (2003). Anger in expression and risk of stroke and coronary heart disease among male health professionals. *Psychosomatic Medicine, 65,* 100–110.

Engebretson, T. O., & Matthews, K. A. (1992). Dimensions of hostility in men, women, and boys: Relationships to personality and cardiovascular responses to stress. *Psychosomatic Medicine, 54,* 311–323.

Ennett, S. T., & Bauman, K. E. (1993). Peer group structure and adolescent cigarette smoking: A social network analysis. *Journal of Health and Social Behavior, 34,* 226–236.

Enright, M. F., Resnick, R., DeLeon, P. H., Sciara, A. D., & Tanney, F. (1990). The practice of psychology in hospital settings. *American Psychologist, 45,* 1059–1065.

Environmental Health Perspectives. (2004). *Study finds that combined exposure to second-hand smoke and urban air pollutants during pregnancy adversely affects birth outcomes.* Retrieved from http://ehp. niehs.nih. gov/press/012304.html

Epel, E. S., McEwen, B., Seeman, T., Matthews, K., Catellazzo, G., Brownell, K., ... Ickovics, J. R. (2000). Stress and body shape: Stress-induced cortisol secretion is consistently greater among women with central fat. *Psychosomatic Medicine, 62,* 623–632.

Epilepsy Foundation. (2018, April 24). *The latest stats about epilepsy from the CDC: Who has epilepsy and seizure control?* Retrieved March 13, 2019, from https://www.epilepsy.com/article/2018/4/latest-stats-about-epilepsy-cdc-who-has-epilepsy-and-seizure-control

Epker, J., & Gatchel, R. J. (2000). Coping profile differences in the biopsychosocial functioning of patients with temporomandibular disorder. *Psychosomatic Medicine, 62,* 69–75.

Epping-Jordan, J. A., Compas, B. E., & Howell, D. C. (1994). Predictors of cancer progression in young adult men and women: Avoidance, intrusive thoughts, and psychological symptoms. *Health Psychology, 13,* 539–547.

Epstein, E. M., Sloan, D. M., & Marx, B. P. (2005). Getting to the heart of the matter: Written disclosure, gender, and heart rate. *Psychosomatic Medicine, 67,* 413–419.

Epstein, R. M., Shields, C. G., Meldrum, S. C., Fiscella, K., Carroll, J., Carney, P. A., & Duberstein, P. R. (2006). Physicians' responses to patients' medically unexplained symptoms. *Psychosomatic Medicine, 68,* 269–276.

Epton, T., & Harris, P. R. (2008). Self-affirmation promotes health behavior change. *Health Psychology, 27,* 746–752.

Epton, T., Harris, P. R., Kane, R., van Koningsbruggen, G. M., & Sheeran, P. (2015). The impact of self-affirmation on health-behavior change: A meta-analysis. *Health Psychology, 34,* 187–196.

Erickson, K. I., Voss, M. W., Prakash, R. S., Basak, C., Szabo, A., Chaddock, L., ... Kramer, A. F. (2011). Exercise training increases size of hippocampus and improves memory. *Proceedings of the National Academy of Sciences, 108,* 3017–3022.

Erlich, K. B., Hoyt, L. T., Sumner, J. A., McDade, T. W., & Adam, E. K. (2015). Quality of relationships with parents and friends in adolescence predicts metabolic risk in young adulthood. *Health Psychology, 34,* 896–904.

Ernst, E. (2009). Acupuncture: What does the most reliable evidence tell us? *Journal of Pain and Symptom Management, 37,* 709–714.

Ernst, E., Lee, M. S., & Choi, T. Y. (2011). Acupuncture: Does it alleviate pain and are there serious risks? A review of reviews. *Pain, 152,* 755–764.

Ernst, E., Pittler, M. H., Wider, B., & Boddy, K. (2007). Acupuncture: Its evidence-base is changing. *American Journal of Chinese Medicine, 35,* 21–25.

Ervin, R. B., Kit, B. K., Carroll, M. D., & Ogden, C. L. (2012). Consumption of added sugar among U.S. children and adolescents, 2005–2008. *NCHS Data Brief, 87,* 1–8.

Ervin, R. B., & Ogden, C. L. (2013). Consumption of added sugars among U.S. adults 2005–2010. *NCHS Data Brief, 122,* 1–7.

Esposito-Del Puente, A., Lillioja, S., Bogardus, C., McCubbin, J. A., Feinglos, M. N., Kuhn, C. M., & Surwit, R. S. (1994). Glycemic response to stress is altered in euglycemic Pima Indians. *International Journal of Obesity, 18,* 766–770.

Estabrooks, P. A., Lee, R. E., & Gyurcsik, N. C. (2003). Resources for physical activity participation: Does availability and accessibility differ by neighborhood socioeconomic status? *Annals of Behavioral Medicine, 25,* 100–104.

Esterl, M. (2015, April 15). More teens use e-cigarettes than traditional smokes. *The Wall Street Journal,* p. 83.

Esterling, B. A., Kiecolt-Glaser, J. K., Bodnar, J. C., & Glaser, R. (1994). Chronic stress, social support, and persistent alterations in the natural killer cell response to cytokines in older adults. *Health Psychology, 13,* 291–298.

Esterling, B. A., Kiecolt-Glaser, J. K., & Glaser, R. (1996). Psychosocial modulation of cytokine-induced natural killer cell activity in older adults. *Psychosomatic Medicine, 58,* 264–272.

Eunice Kennedy Shriver National Institute of Child Health and Human Development. (2017). *Sudden infant death syndrome (SIDS).* Retrieved May 8, 2019, from https://www.nichd.nih.gov/health/topics/sids

Euesden, J., Matcham, F., Hotopf, M., Steer, S., Cope, A. P., Lewis, C. M., & Scott, I. C. (2017). The relationship between mental health, disease severity, and genetic risk for depression in early rheumatoid arthritis. *Psychosomatic Medicine, 79,* 638–645.

Euteneuer, F., Mills, P. J., Pung, M. A., Rief, W., & Dimsdale, J. E. (2014). Neighborhood problems and nocturnal blood pressure dipping. *Health Psychology, 33,* 1366–1372.

Evans, G. W., Exner-Cortens, D., Kim, P., & Bartholomew, D. (2013). Childhood poverty and blood pressure reactivity to and recovery from an acute stressor in late adolescence: The mediating role of family conflict. *Psychosomatic Medicine, 75,* 691–700.

Evans, G. W., & Wener, R. E. (2006). Rail commuting duration and passenger stress. *Health Psychology, 25,* 408–412.

Everson, S. A., Lovallo, W. R., Sausen, K. P., & Wilson, M. F. (1992). Hemodynamic characteristics of young men at risk for hypertension at rest and during laboratory stressors. *Health Psychology, 11,* 24–31.

Ewart, C. K. (1991). Familial transmission of essential hypertension: Genes, environments, and chronic anger. *Annals of Behavioral Medicine, 13,* 40–47.

Ewart, C. K., Elder, G. J., Jorgensen, R. S., & Fitzgerald, S. T. (2017). The role of agonistic striving in the association between cortisol and high blood pressure. *Psychosomatic Medicine, 79,* 416–425.

Ewart, C. K., Elder, G. J., Laird, K. T., Shelby, G. D., & Walker, L. S. (2014). Can agonistic striving lead to unexplained illness? Implicit goals, pain tolerance, and somatic symptoms in adolescents and adults. *Health Psychology, 33,* 977–985.

Ewart, C. K., & Jorgensen, R. S. (2004). Agonistic interpersonal striving: Social–cognitive mechanism of cardiovascular risk in youth? *Health Psychology, 23,* 75–85.

Faasse, K., Cundy, T., Gamble, G., & Petrie, K. J. (2013). The effect of an apparent change to a branded or generic medication on drug effectiveness and side effects. *Psychosomatic Medicine, 75,* 90–96.

Faasse, K., Parkes, B., Kearney, J., & Petrie, K. J. (2018). The influence of social modeling, gender, and empathy on treatment side effects. *Annals of Behavioral Medicine, 52,* 560–570.

Facebook. (2012). *Key facts.* Retrieved March 13, 2013, from http://newsroom.fb.com/Key-Facts

Facts of Life. (2002, July). *Cover your hide: Too much sun can lead to skin cancer.* Center for the Advancement of Health, 7(7).

Facts of Life. (2002, November). *Food for thought: Prevention of eating disorders in children.* Center for the Advancement of Health, 7(11).

Facts of Life. (2003, March). *Talking the talk: Improving patient-provider communication.* Center for the Advancement of Health, 8(3).

Facts of Life. (2003, November). *Health education: Schools learn the hard way.* Center for the Advancement of Health, 8(11).

Facts of Life. (2003, December). *Potential health benefits of moderate drinking.* Center for the Advancement of Health, 8(12).

Facts of Life. (2004, May). *On the road to improving traffic safety.* Center for the Advancement of Health, 9(5).

Facts of Life. (2004, December). *Weighing the data: Obesity affects elderly, too.* Center for the Advancement of Health, 9(12).

Facts of Life. (2005, July). *Smoking cessation: Beyond the patch.* Center for the Advancement of Health, 10(7).

Facts of Life. (2006, November). *An aging marketplace.* Center for the Advancement of Health, 11(11).

Facts of Life. (2007, February). *Statins: Still going strong.* Center for the Advancement of Health, 12(2).

Fagan, J., Galea, S., Ahern, J., Bonner, S., & Vlahov, D. (2003). Relationship of self-reported asthma severity and urgent health care utilization to psychological sequelae of the September 11, 2001 terrorist attacks on the World Trade Center among New York City area residents. *Psychosomatic Medicine, 65,* 993–996.

Fagerlin, A., Ditto, P. H., Danks, J. H., Houts, R. M., & Smucker, W. D. (2001). Projection in surrogate decisions about life-sustaining medical treatments. *Health Psychology, 20,* 166–175.

Fagundes, C. P., Bennett, J. M., Alfano, C. M., Glaser, R., Povoski, S. P., Lipari, A. M., . . . Kiecolt-Glaser, J. K. (2012). Social support and socioeconomic status interact to predict Epstein-Barr virus latency in women awaiting diagnosis or newly diagnosed with breast cancer. *Health Psychology, 31,* 11–19.

Fagundes, C. P., Murdock, K. W., Chirinos, D. A., & Green, P. A. (2017). Biobehavioral pathways to cancer incidence, progression, and quality of life. *Current Directions in Psychological Science, 26,* 548–553.

Fakhouri, T. H. I., Ogden, C. L., Carroll, M. D., Kit, B. K., & Flegal, K. M. (2012). Prevalence of obesity among older adults in the United States, 2007–2010. *NCHS Data Brief, 106,* 1–8.

Falba, T. (2005). Health events and the smoking cessation of middle aged Americans. *Journal of Behavioral Medicine, 28,* 21–33.

Fales, J. L., Rice, S., Aaron, R. V., & Palermo, T. M. (2018). Traditional and cyber-victimization among adolescents with and without chronic pain. *Health Psychology, 37,* 291–300.

Falk, E. B., Berkman, E. T., Mann, T., Harrison, B., & Lieberman, M. D. (2010). Predicting persuasion-induced behavior change from the brain. *The Journal of Neuroscience, 30,* 8421–8424.

Falk, E. B., Berkman, E. T., Whalen, D., & Lieberman, M. D. (2011). Neural activity during health messaging predicts reductions in smoking above and beyond self-report. *Health Psychology, 30,* 177–185.

Falkenstein, A., Tran, B., Ludi, D., Molkara, A., Nguyen, H., Tabuenca, A., & Sweeny, K. (2016). Characteristics and correlates of word use in physician–patient communication. *Annals of Behavioral Medicine, 50,* 664–677.

Fang, C. Y., Ross, E. A., Pathak, H. B., Godwin, A. K., & Tseng, M. (2014). Acculturative stress and inflammation among Chinese immigrant women. *Psychosomatic Medicine, 76,* 320–326.

Faria, N. R., Rambaut, A., Suchard, M. A., Baele, G., Bedford, T., Ward, M. J., . . . Lemey, P. (2014). The early spread and epidemic ignition of HIV-1 in human populations. *Science, 346,* 56–61.

Favreau, H,, Bacon, S. L., Labrecque, M., & Lavoie, K. L. (2014). Prospective impact of panic disorder and panic-anxiety on asthma control, health service use, and quality of life in adult patients with asthma over a 4-year follow-up. *Psychosomatic Medicine, 76,* 147–155.

Federal Tax Increase. (2009). *Higher cost of tobacco products, cigarettes increases quit attempts.* Retrieved August 9, 2012, from http://www.cdc.gov/tobacco/basic_information/tobacco_industry/tax_increase/index.htm

Federspiel, J. F. (1983). *The ballad of Typhoid Mary.* New York: Dutton.

Feeney, B. C., & Collins, N. L. (2015). A new look at social support: A theoretical perspective on thriving through relationships. *Personality and Social Psychology Review, 19,* 113–147.

Feeney, B. C., Dooley, C., Finucane, C., & Kenny, R. A. (2015). Stressful life events and orthostatic blood pressure recovery in older adults. *Health Psychology, 34,* 765–774.

Feinglos, M. N., & Surwit, R. S. (1988). *Behavior and diabetes mellitus.* Kalamazoo, MI: Upjohn.

Feldman, P., Cohen, S., Doyle, W., Skoner, D., & Gwaltney, J. (1999). The impact of personality on the reporting of unfounded symptoms and illness. *Journal of Personality and Social Psychology, 77,* 370–378.

Feldman, P. J., Dunkel-Schetter, C., Sandman, C. A., & Wadhwa, P. D. (2000). Maternal social support predicts birth weight and fetal growth in human pregnancy. *Psychosomatic Medicine, 62,* 715–725.

Feldman, P. J., & Steptoe, A. (2004). How neighborhoods and physical functioning are related: The roles of neighborhood socioeconomic status, perceived neighborhood strain, and individual health risk factors. *Annals of Behavioral Medicine, 27,* 91–99.

Felitti, V. J., Anda, R. F., Nordenberg, D., Williamson, D. F., Apitz, A. M., Edwards, V., . . . Marks, J. S. (1998). Relationship of childhood abuse and household dysfunction to many of the leading causes of death in adults. *American Journal of Preventive Medicine, 14,* 245–258.

Fernandes, H. A., Richard, N. M., & Edelstein, K. (2019). Cognitive rehabilitation for cancer-related cognitive dysfunction: A systematic review. *Supportive Care in Cancer, 27,* 3253–3279.

Fernandez, A. B., Soufer, R., Collins, D., Soufer, A., Ranjbaran, H., & Burg, M. M. (2010). Tendency to angry rumination predicts stress-provoked endothelin-1 increase in patients with coronary artery disease. *Psychosomatic Medicine, 72,* 348–353.

Fernandez, E., & Turk, D. C. (1992). Sensory and affective components of pain: Separation and synthesis. *Psychological Bulletin, 112,* 205–217.

Fernández-Mendoza, J., Vela-Bueno, A., Vgontzas, A. N., Ramos-Platón, M. J., Olavarrieta-Bernardino, S., Bixler, E. O., & De la Cruz-Troca, J. J. (2010). Cognitive–emotional hyperarousal as a premorbid characteristic of individuals vulnerable to insomnia. *Psychosomatic Medicine, 72,* 397–403.

Ferrer, R. A., Huedo-Medina, T. B., Johnson, B. T., Ryan, S., & Pescatello, L. S. (2011). Exercise interventions for cancer survivors: A metaanalysis of quality of life outcomes. *Annals of Behavioral Medicine, 41,* 32–47.

Ferris, P. A., Kline, T. J. B., & Bourdage, J. S. (2012). He said, she said: Work, biopsychosocial, and lifestyle contributions to coronary heart disease risk. *Health Psychology, 31,* 503–511.

Ferro, M. A., & Boyle, M. H. (2013). Self-concept among youth with a chronic illness: A meta-analytic review. *Health Psychology, 32,* 839–848.

Fife, B. L., & Wright, E. R. (2000). The dimensionality of stigma: A comparison of its impact on the self of persons with HIV/AIDS and cancer. *Journal of Health and Social Behavior, 41,* 50–67.

Fifield, J., McQuinlan, J., Tennen, H., Sheehan, T. J., Reisine, S., Hesselbrock, V., & Rothfield, N. (2001). History of affective disorder and the temporal trajectory of fatigue in rheumatoid arthritis. *Annals of Behavioral Medicine, 23,* 34–41.

Fillingham, R. B., & Maixner, W. (1996). The influence of resting blood pressure and gender on pain responses. *Psychosomatic Medicine, 58,* 326–332.

Finan, P. H., Zautra, A. J., & Davis, M. C. (2009). Daily affect relations in fibromyalgia patients reveal positive affective disturbance. *Psychosomatic Medicine, 71,* 474–482.

*Financial Times.* (2009, October 14). Ways to take stock of it all. p. 9.

Findley, T. (1953). The placebo and the physician. *Medical Clinics of North America, 37,* 1821–1826.

Fink, P., Toft, T., Hansen, M. S., Ornbol, E., & Olesen, F. (2007). Symptoms and syndromes of bodily distress: An exploratory study of 978 internal medical, neurological, and primary care patients. *Psychosomatic Medicine, 69,* 30–39.

Finney, J. W., & Moos, R. H. (1995). Entering treatment for alcohol abuse: A stress and coping method. *Addiction, 90,* 1223–1240.

Firestein, G. S. (2003). Evolving concepts of rheumatoid arthritis. *Nature, 423,* 356–361.

Fishbain, D., Cutler, R., Rosomoff, H., & Rosomoff, R. (1998). Do antidepressants have an analgesic effect in psychogenic pain and somatoform pain disorder? A meta-analysis. *Psychosomatic Medicine, 60,* 503–509.

Fishbein, M., & Ajzen, I. (1975). *Belief, attitude, intention, and behavior: An introduction to theory and research.* Reading, MA: Addison-Wesley.

Fisher, J. D., & Fisher, W. A. (1992). Changing AIDS-risk behavior. *Psychological Bulletin, 111,* 455–474.

Fisher, J. D., Fisher, W. A., Amico, K. R., & Harman, J. J. (2006). An information-motivation-behavioral skills model of adherence to antiretroviral therapy. *Health Psychology, 25,* 462–473.

Fisher, J. D., Fisher, W. A., Bryan, A. D., & Misovich, S. J. (2002). Information-motivation-behavioral skills model-based HIV risk behavior change intervention for inner-city high school youth. *Health Psychology, 21,* 177–186.

Fisher, L., & Dickinson, W. P. (2014). Psychology and primary care: New collaborations for providing effective care for adults with chronic health conditions. *American Psychologist, 69,* 355–363.

Fisher, L., Soubhi, H., Mansi, O., Paradis, G., Gauvin, L., & Potvin, L. (1998). Family process in health research: Extending a family typology to a new cultural context. *Health Psychology, 17,* 358–366.

Fisher, W. A., Fisher, J. D., & Harman, J. J. (2003). The information-motivation-behavioral skills model: A general social psychological approach to understanding and promoting health behavior. In J. Suls & K. Wallston (Eds.), *Social psychological foundations of health and illness* (pp. 82–105). Oxford, UK: Blackwell.

Fiske, S. T., & Taylor, S. E. (2013). *Social cognition: From brain to culture* (2nd ed.). London: Sage Publication.

Fitzgerald, S. T., Haythornthwaite, J. A., Suchday, S., & Ewart, C. K. (2003). Anger in young black and white workers: Effects of job control, dissatisfaction, and support. *Journal of Behavioral Medicine, 26,* 283–296.

Fjeldsoe, B. S., Miller, Y. D., & Marshall, A. L. (2013). Social cognitive mediators of the effect of the MobileMums intervention on physical activity. *Health Psychology, 32,* 729–738.

Flay, B. R., Koepke, D., Thomson, S. J., Santi, S., Best, J. A., & Brown, K. S. (1992). Six year follow-up of the first Waterloo school smoking prevention trial. *American Journal of Public Health, 68,* 458–478.

Flegal, K. M., Graubard, B. I., Williamson, D. F., & Gail, M. H. (2007). Cause-specific excess deaths associated with underweight, overweight, and obesity. *Journal of the American Medical Association, 298,* 2028–2037.

Fleming, R., Baum, A., Davidson, L. M., Rectanus, E., & McArdle, S. (1987). Chronic stress as a factor in physiologic reactivity to challenge. *Health Psychology, 6,* 221–237.

Fleming, R., Leventhal, H., Glynn, K., & Ershler, J. (1989). The role of cigarettes in the initiation and progression of early substance use. *Addictive Behaviors, 14,* 261–272.

Fletcher, J. B., & Reback, C. J. (2015). Depression mediates and moderates effects of methamphetamine use on sexual risk taking among treatment-seeking gay and bisexual men. *Health Psychology, 34,* 865–869.

Flor, H. (2014). Psychological pain interventions and neurophysiology: Implications for a mechanism-based approach. *American Psychologist, 69,* 188–198.

Flor, H., Birbaumer, N., & Turk, D. C. (1990). The psychology of chronic pain. *Advances in Behavior Research and Therapy, 12,* 47–84.

Flores, G. (2006). Language barriers to health care in the United States. *The New England Journal of Medicine, 355,* 229–231.

Flory, J. D., & Manuck, S. B. (2009). Impulsiveness and cigarette smoking. *Psychosomatic Medicine, 71,* 431–437.

Floyd, A., & Moyer, A. (2010). Group versus individual exercise interventions for women with breast cancer: A meta-anlysis. *Health Psychology Review, 4,* 22–41.

Fluharty, M., Taylor, A. E., Grabski, M., & Munafò, M. R. (2016). The association of cigarette smoking with depression and anxiety: A systematic review. *Nicotine & Tobacco Research, 19,* 3–13.

Fogel, J., Albert, S. M., Schnabel, F., Ditkoff, B. A., & Neuget, A. I. (2002). Internet use and support in women with breast cancer. *Health Psychology, 21,* 398–404.

Foldes-Busque, G., Denis, I., Poitras, J., Fleet, R. P., Archambault, P. M., & Dionne, C. E. (2018). The revised-panic screening score for emergency department patients with noncardiac chest pain. *Health Psychology, 37,* 828–838.

Folkman, S., Chesney, M., McKusick, L., Ironson, G., Johnson, D. S., & Coates, T. J. (1991). Translating coping theory into intervention. In J. Eckenrode (Ed.), *The social context of coping* (pp. 239–259). New York: Plenum.

Folkman, S., & Lazarus, R. S. (1980). An analysis of coping in a middle-aged community sample. *Journal of Health and Social Behavior, 21,* 219–239.

Folkman, S., & Moskowitz, J. T. (2004). Coping: Pitfalls and promise. *Annual Review of Psychology, 55,* 745–774.

Folkman, S., Schaefer, C., & Lazarus, R. S. (1979). Cognitive processes as mediators of stress and coping. In V. Hamilton & D. M. Warburton (Eds.), *Human stress and cognition: An information processing approach* (pp. 265–298). London: Wiley.

Forest, A. L., & Wood, J. V. (2012). When social networking is not working: Individuals with low self-esteem recognize but do not reap the benefits of self-disclosure on Facebook. *Psychological Science, 23,* 295–302.

Forsyth, J., Schoenthaler, A., Chaplin, W. F., Ogedegbe, G., & Ravenell, J. (2014). Percieved discrimination and medication adherence in black hypertensive patients: The role of stress and depression. *Psychosomatic Medicine, 76,* 229–236.

Fournier, M., d'Arripe-Longueville, F., Rovere, C., Easthope, C. S., Schwabe, L., El Methni, J., & Radel, R. (2017). Effects of circadian cortisol on the development of a health habit. *Health Psychology, 36,* 1059–1064.

Fradkin, C., Wallander, J. L., Elliott, M. N., Tortolero, S., Cuccaro, P., & Schuster, M. A. (2015). Associations between socioeconomic status and obesity in diverse, young adolescents: Variation across race/ethnicity and gender. *Health Psychology, 34,* 1–9.

Frances, R. J., Franklin, J., & Flavin, D. (1986). Suicide and alcoholism. *Annals of the New York Academy of Sciences, 487,* 316–326.

Francis, L. A., & Birch, L. L. (2005). Maternal influences on daughters' restrained eating behavior. *Health Psychology, 24,* 548–554.

Frankenhaeuser, M., Lundberg, U., Fredrikson, M., Melin, B., Tuomisto, M., Myrsten, A., . . . Wallin, L. (1989). Stress on and off the job as related to sex and occupational status in white-collar workers. *Journal of Organizational Behavior, 10,* 321–346.

Franzen, P. L., Gianaros, P. J., Marsland, A. L., Hall, M. H., Siegle, G. J., Dahl, R. E., & Buysse, D. J. (2011). Cardiovascular reactivity to acute psychological stress following sleep deprivation. *Psychosomatic Medicine, 73,* 679-682.

Fraser, S. N., & Rodgers, W. M. (2010). An examination of psychosocial correlates of exercise tolerance in cardiac rehabilitation participants. *Journal of Behavioral Medicine, 33,* 159-167.

Frass, M., Strassl, R. P., Friehs, H., Müllner, M., Kundi, M., & Kaye, A. D. (2012). Use and acceptance of complementary and alternative medicine among the general population and medical personnel: A systematic review. *The Ochsner Journal, 12,* 45-56.

Fredrickson, B. L., Maynard, K. E., Helms, M. J., Haney, T. L., Siegler, I. C., & Barefoot, J. C. (2000). Hostility predicts magnitude and duration of blood pressure response to anger. *Journal of Behavioral Medicine, 23,* 229-243.

Fredrickson, B. L., Tugade, M. M., Waugh, C. E., & Larkin, G. R. (2003). What good are positive emotions in crises? A prospective study of resilience and emotions following the terrorist attacks on the United States on September 11th, 2001. *Journal of Personality and Social Psychology, 84,* 365-376.

Freedland, K. E. (2017). A new era of health psychology. *Health Psychology, 36,* 1-4.

Freedman, V. A. (1993). Kin and nursing home lengths of stay: A backward recurrence time approach. *Journal of Health and Social Behavior, 34,* 138-152.

Freidson, E. (1961). *Patients' views of medical practice.* New York: Russell Sage Foundation.

French, A. P., & Tupin, J. P. (1974). Therapeutic application of a simple relaxation method. *American Journal of Psychotherapy, 28,* 282-287.

French, D. P., Cameron, E., Benton, J. S., Deaton, C., & Harvie, M. (2017). Can communicating personalised disease risk promote healthy behaviour change? A systematic review of systematic reviews. *Annals of Behavioral Medicine, 51,* 718-729.

French, J. R. P., Jr., & Caplan, R. D. (1973). Organizational stress and the individual strain. In A. J. Marrow (Ed.), *The failure of success.* New York: Amacon.

Frenzel, M. P., McCaul, K. D., Glasgow, R. E., & Schafer, L. C. (1988). The relationship of stress and coping to regimen adherence and glycemic control of diabetes. *Journal of Social and Clinical Psychology, 6,* 77-87.

Frestad, D., & Prescott, E. (2017). Vital exhaustion and coronary heart disease risk. *Psychosomatic Medicine, 79,* 260-272.

Fried, A. B., & Dunn, M. E. (2012). The expectancy challenge alcohol literacy curriculum (ECALC): A single session group intervention to reduce alcohol use. *Psychology of Addictive Behaviors, 26,* 615-620.

Friedberg, F., Napoli, A., Coronel, J., Adamowicz, J., Seva, V., Caikauskaite, I., & Meng, H. (2013). Chronic fatigue self-management in primary care: A randomized trial. *Psychosomatic Medicine, 75,* 650-657.

Friedman, E. M., & Herd, P. (2010). Income, education and inflammation: Differential associations in a national probability sample (the MIDUS study). *Psychosomatic Medicine, 72,* 290-300.

Friedman, E. M., Love, G. D., Rosenkranz, M. A., Urry, H. L., Davidson, R. J., Singer, B. H., & Ryff, C. D. (2007). Socioeconomic status predicts objective and subjective sleep quality in aging women. *Psychosomatic Medicine, 69,* 682-691.

Friedman, H. S., & Booth-Kewley, S. (1987). The "disease-prone" personality: A meta-analytic view of the construct. *American Psychologist, 42,* 539-555.

Friedman, H. S., & Silver, R. C. (Eds.). (2007). *Foundations of health psychology.* Oxford: Oxford University Press.

Friedman, H. S., Tucker, J. S., Schwartz, J. E., Martin, L. R., Tomlinson-Keasey, C., Wingard, D. L., & Criqui, M. H. (1995). Childhood conscientiousness and longevity: Health behaviors and cause of death. *Journal of Personality and Social Psychology, 68,* 696-703.

Friedman, H. S., Tucker, J. S., Tomlinson-Keasey, C., Schwartz, J. E., Wingard, D. L., & Criqui, M. H. (1993). Does childhood personality predict longevity? *Journal of Personality and Social Psychology, 65,* 176-185.

Frieser, M. J., Wilson, S., & Vrieze, S. (2018). Behavioral impact of return of genetic test results for complex disease: Systematic review and meta-analysis. *Health Psychology, 37,* 1134-1144.

Fritz, H. L. (2000). Gender-linked personality traits predict mental health and functional status following a first coronary event. *Health Psychology, 19,* 420-428.

Fromm, K., Andrykowski, M. A., & Hunt, J. (1996). Positive and negative psychosocial sequelae of bone marrow transplantation: Implications for quality of life assessment. *Journal of Behavioral Medicine, 19,* 221-240.

Frosch, D. L., Kimmel, S., & Volpp, K. (2008). What role do lay beliefs about hypertension etiology play in perceptions of medication effectiveness? *Health Psychology, 27,* 320-326.

Fryar, C. D., Chen, T., & Li, X. (2012). Prevalence of uncontrolled risk factors for cardiovascular disease: United States, 1999-2010. *NCHS Data Brief, 103,* 1-8.

Fuglestad, P. T., Rothman, A. J., & Jeffery, R. W. (2008). Getting there and hanging on: The effect of regulatory focus on performance in smoking and weight loss interventions. *Health Psychology, 27,* S260-S270.

Fukudo, S., Lane, J. D., Anderson, N. B., Kuhn, C. M., Schanberg, S. M., McCown, N., . . . Williams, R. B., Jr. (1992). Accentuated vagal antagonism of beta-adrenergic effects on ventricular repolarization: Evidence of weaker antagonism in hostile Type A men. *Circulation, 85,* 2045-2053.

Fuller-Rowell, T. E., Evans, G. W., & Ong, A. D. (2012). Poverty and health: The mediating role of perceived discrimination. *Psychological Science, 23,* 734-739.

Fung, T. T., Willett, W. C., Stampfer, M. J., Manson, J. E., & Hu, F. B. (2001). Dietary patterns and the risk of coronary heart disease in women. *Archives of Internal Medicine, 161,* 1857-1862.

Fyrand, L., Moum, T., Finset, A., & Glennas, A. (2002). The impact of disability and disease duration on social support of women with rheumatoid arthritis. *Journal of Behavioral Medicine, 25,* 251-268.

Gable, S. L., Gosnell, C. L., Maisel, N. C., & Strachman, A. (2012). Safely testing the alarm: Close others' responses to personal positive events. *Journal of Personality and Social Psychology, 103,* 963-981.

Gabriele, J. M., Carpenter, B. D., Tate, D. F., & Fisher, E. B. (2011). Directive and non-directive e-coach support for weight loss in overweight adults. *Annals of Behavioral Medicine, 41,* 252-263.

Gagné, C., & Harnois, I. (2013). The contribution of psychosocial variables in explaining preschoolers' physical activity. *Health Psychology, 32,* 657-665.

Gahche, J., Bailey, R., Burt, V., Hughes, J., Yetley, E., Dwyer, J., . . . Sempos, C. (2011). Dietary supplement use among U.S. adults has increased since NHANES III (1988-1994). *NCHS Data Brief, 61,* 1-8.

Gahche, J., Fakhouri, T., Carroll, D. D., Burt, V. L., Wang, C., & Fulton, J. E. (2014). Cardiorespiratory fitness levels among U.S. youth aged 12-15 years: United States, 1999-2004 and 2012. *NCHS Data Brief, 153,* 1-7.

Gale, C. R., Batty, G. D., & Deary, I. J. (2008). Locus of control at age 10 years and health outcomes and behaviors at age 30 years: The 1970 British cohort study. *Psychosomatic Medicine, 70,* 397-403.

Galesic, M., Garcia-Retamero, R., & Gigerenzer, G. (2009). Using icon arrays to communicate medical risks: Overcoming low numeracy. *Health Psychology, 29,* 210-216.

Gallacher, J. E. J., Yarnell, J. W. G., Sweetnam, P. M., Elwood, P. C., & Stansfeld, S. A. (1999). Anger and incident heart disease in the Caerphilly study. *Psychosomatic Medicine, 61,* 446-453.

Gallagher, K. M., & Updegraff, J. A. (2012). Health message framing effects on attitudes, intentions, and behavior: A meta-analytic review. *Annals of Behavioral Medicine, 43,* 101-116.

Gallagher, K. M., Updegraff, J. A., Rothman, A. J., & Sims, L. (2011). Perceived susceptibility to breast cancer moderates the effect of gain- and loss-framed messages on use of screening mammography. *Health Psychology, 30,* 145-152.

Gallagher, S., Phillips, A. C., Drayson, M. T., & Carroll, D. (2009). Caregiving for children with developmental disabilities is associated with a poor antibody response to influenza vaccination. *Psychosomatic Medicine, 71,* 341-344.

Gallo, L. C., Fortmann, A. L., de los Monteros, K. E., Mills, P. J., Barrett-Connor, E., Roesch, S. C., & Matthews, K. A. (2012). Individual and neighborhood socioeconomic status and inflammation in Mexican American women: What is the role of obesity? *Psychosomatic Medicine, 74,* 535-542.

Gallo, L. C., Fortmann, A. L., & Mattei, J. (2014). Allostatic load and the assessment of cumulative biological risk in behavioral medicine: Challenges and opportunities. *Psychosomatic Medicine, 76,* 478-480.

Gallo, L. C., & Matthews, K. A. (2006). Adolescents' attachment orientation influences ambulatory blood pressure responses to everyday social interactions. *Psychosomatic Medicine, 68,* 253-261.

Gallo, L. C., Matthews, K. A., Kuller, L. H., Sutton-Tyrell, K., & Edmundowicz, D. (2001). Educational attainment and coronary and aortic calcification in postmenopausal women. *Psychosomatic Medicine, 63,* 925-935.

Gallo, L. C., Roesch, S. C., Fortmann, A. L., Carnethon, M. R., Penedo, F. J., Perreira, K., & Isasi, C. R. (2014). Associations of chronic stress burden, perceived stress, and traumatic stress with cardiovascular disease prevalence and risk factors in the Hispanic community health study/study of Latinos sociocultural ancillary study. *Psychosomatic Medicine, 76,* 468-475.

Gallo, L. C., Troxel, W. M., Kuller, L. H., Sutton-Tyrell, K., Edmundowicz, D., & Matthews, K. A. (2003). Marital status, marital quality and atherosclerotic burden in postmenopausal women. *Psychosomatic Medicine, 65,* 952-962.

Gallo, L. C., Troxel, W. M., Matthews, K. A., Jansen-McWilliams, L., Kuller, L. H., & Sutton-Tyrell, K. (2003). Occupation and subclinical carotid artery disease in women: Are clerical workers at greater risk? *Health Psychology, 22,* 19-29.

Gallup Poll. (2009). *Religion.* Retrieved October 15, 2009, from http://www.gallup.com/poll/1690/Religion.aspx

Gana, K., Bailly, N., Saada, Y., Joulain, M., Trouillet, R., Hervè, C., & Alaphilippe, D. (2013). Relationship between life satisfaction and physical health in older adults: A longitudinal test of cross-lagged and simultaneous effects. *Health Psychology, 32,* 896-904.

Garcia, T. C., Bernstein, A. B., & Bush, M. A. (2010). Emergency department visitors and visits: Who used the emergency room in 2007? *NCHS Data Brief, 38,* 1-8.

Garcia-Linares, M. I., Sanchez-Lorente, S., Coe, C. L., & Martinez, M. (2004). Intimate male partner violence impairs immune control over herpes simplex virus type 1 in physically and psychologically abused women. *Psychosomatic Medicine, 66,* 965-972.

Garcia-Retamero, R., Wicki, B., Cokely, E. T., & Hanson, B. (2014). Factors predicting surgeons' preferred and actual roles in interactions with their patients. *Health Psychology, 33,* 920-928.

Garfield, L. D., Scherrer, J. F., Hauptman, P. J., Freedland, K. E., Owen, R., Bucholz, K. K., & Lustman, P. J. (2014). Association of anxiety disorders and depression with incident heart failure. *Psychosomatic Medicine, 76,* 122-127.

Garfinkel, P. E., & Garner, D. M. (1983). The multidetermined nature of anorexia nervosa. In P. L. Darby, P. E. Garfinkel, D. M. Garner, & D. V. Coscina (Eds.), *Anorexia nervosa: Recent developments in research.* New York: Liss.

Garner, D. M., & Wooley, S. C. (1991). Confronting the failure of behavioral and dietary treatments for obesity. *Clinical Psychology Review, 11,* 729-780.

Gasperi, M., Herbert, M., Schur, E., Buchwald, D., & Afari, N. (2017). Genetic and environment influences on sleep, pain, and depression symptoms in a community sample of twins. *Psychosomatic Medicine, 79,* 646-654.

Gathright, E. C., Dolansky, M. A., Gunstad, J., Redle, J. D., Josephson, R. A., Moore, S. M., & Hughes, J. W. (2017). The impact of medication nonadherence on the relationship between mortality risk and depression in heart failure. *Health Psychology, 36,* 839-847.

Gauderman, W. J., Avol, E., Gilliland, F., Vora, H., Thomas, D., Berhane, K., . . . Peters, J. (2004). The effect of air pollution on lung development from 10 to 18 years of age. *The New England Journal of Medicine, 351,* 1057-1067.

Gaynes, B. N., Pence, B. W., Eron, J. J., & Miller, W. C. (2008). Prevalence and comorbidity of psychiatric diagnoses based on reference standard in an HIV+ patient population. *Psychosomatic Medicine, 70,* 505-511.

Gaziano, J. M., Sesso, H. D., Christen, W. G., Bubes, V., Smith. J. P., MacFadyen, J., . . . Buring, J. E. (2012). Multivitamins in the prevention of cancer in men: The Physicians' Health Study II randomized controlled trial. *The Journal of the American Medical Association, 308,* 1871-1880.

Gebauer, J. E., Sedikides, C., & Neberich, W. (2012). Religiosity, social self-esteem, and psychological adjustment: On the cross-cultural specificity of the psychological benefits of religiosity. *Psychological Science, 23,* 158-160.

Geers, A. L., Rose, J. P., Fowler, S. L., Rasinski, H. M., Brown, J. A., & Helfer, S. G. (2013). Why does choice enhance treatment effectiveness? Using placebo treatments to demonstrate the role of personal control. *Journal of Personality and Social Psychology, 105,* 549-566.

Geers, A. L., Van Wasshenova, E., Murray, A. B., Mahas, R., Fahlman, M., & Boardley, D. (2017). Affective associations as predictors of health behavior in urban minority youth. *Health Psychology, 36,* 996-1005.

Geers, A. L., Wellman, J. A., Fowler, S. L., Rasinski, H. M., & Helfer, S. G. (2011). Placebo expectations and the detection of somatic information. *Journal of Behavioral Medicine, 34,* 208-217.

Gemming, M. G., Runyan, C. W., Hunter, W. W., & Campbell, B. J. (1984). A community health education approach to occupant protection. *Health Education Quarterly, 11,* 147-158.

George, L. K., Ellison, C. G., & Larson, D. B. (2002). Explaining the relationships between religious involvement and health. *Psychology Inquiry, 13,* 190-200.

Gerend, M. A., & Maner, J. K. (2011). Fear, anger, fruits, and veggies: Interactive effects of emotion and message framing on health behavior. *Health Psychology, 30,* 420-423.

Gerend, M. A., Shepherd, J. E., & Monday, K. A. (2008). Behavioral frequency moderates the effects of message framing on HPV vaccine acceptability. *Annals of Behavioral Medicine, 35,* 221-229.

Gerend, M. A., & Shepherd, M. A. (2015). When different message frames motivate different routes to the same health outcome. *Annals of Behavioral Medicine, 50,* 319-329.

Gerend, M. A., Shepherd, M. A., & Shepherd, J. E. (2013). The multidimensional nature of perceived barriers: Global versus practical barriers to HPV vaccination. *Health Psychology, 32,* 361-369.

Gerrard, M., Gibbons, F. X., Lane, D. J., & Stock, M. L. (2005). Smoking cessation: Social comparison level predicts success for adult smokers. *Health Psychology, 24,* 623-629.

Gerhart, J. I., Burns, J. W., Post, K. M., Smith, D. A., Porter, L. S., Burgess, H. J., . . . Keefe, F. J. (2016). Relationships between sleep quality and pain-related factors for people with chronic low back pain: Tests of reciprocal and time of day effects. *Annals of Behavioral Medicine, 51,* 365–375.

Gerhart, J. I., Sanchez Varela, V., Burns, J., Hobfoll, S. E., & Fung, H. C. (2015). Anger, provider responses, and pain: Prospective analysis of stem cell transplant patients. *Health Psychology, 34,* 197–206.

Gianaros, P. J., & Hackman, D. (2013). Contributions of neuroscience to the study of socioeconomic health disparities. *Psychosomatic Medicine, 75,* 610–615.

Gianaros, P. J., & Manuck, S. B. (2010). Neurobiological pathways linking socioeconomic position and health. *Psychosomatic Medicine, 72,* 450–461.

Gibbons, F. X., & Eggleston, T. J. (1996). Smoker networks and the "typical smoker": A prospective analysis of smoking cessation. *Health Psychology, 15,* 469–477.

Gibbons, F. X., & Gerrard, M. (1995). Predicting young adults' health risk behavior. *Journal of Personality and Social Psychology, 69,* 505–517.

Gibbons, F. X., Gerrard, M., Lane, D. J., Mahler, H. I. M., & Kulik, J. A. (2005). Using UV photography to reduce use of tanning booths: A test of cognitive mediation. *Health Psychology, 24,* 358–363.

Gibbons, F. X., Kingsbury, J. H., Weng, C., Gerrard, M., Cutrona, C., Willis, T. A., & Stock, M. (2014). Effects of perceived racial discrimination on health status and health behavior: A differential mediation hypothesis. *Health Psychology, 33,* 11–19.

Gidron, Y., & Davidson, K. (1996). Development and preliminary testing of a brief intervention for modifying CHD-predictive hostility components. *Journal of Behavioral Medicine, 19,* 203–220.

Gidron, Y., Davidson, K., & Bata, I. (1999). The short-term effects of a hostility-reduction intervention on male coronary heart disease patients. *Health Psychology, 18,* 416–420.

Giese-Davis, J., Sephton, S. E., Abercrombie, H. C., Durán, R. E. F., & Spiegel, D. (2004). Repression and high anxiety are associated with aberrant diurnal cortisol rhythms in women with metastatic breast cancer. *Health Psychology, 23,* 645–650.

Giese-Davis, J., Wilhelm, F. H., Conrad, A., Abercrombie, H. C., Sephton, S., Yutsis, M., . . . Spiegel, D. (2006). Depression and stress reactivity in metastatic breast cancer. *Psychosomatic Medicine, 68,* 675–683.

Gil, K. M., Carson, J. W., Porter, L. S., Scipio, C., Bediako, S. M., & Orringer, E. (2004). Daily mood and stress predict pain, health care use, and work activity in African American adults with sickle-cell disease. *Health Psychology, 23,* 267–274.

Gil, K. M., Wilson, J. J., Edens, J. L., Webster, D. A., Abrams, M. A., Orringer, E., . . . Janal, M. N. (1996). Effects of cognitive coping skills training on coping strategies and experimental pain sensitivity in African American adults with sickle cell disease. *Health Psychology, 15,* 3–10.

Gil, S., & Caspi, Y. (2006). Personality traits, coping style, and perceived threat as predictors of posttraumatic stress disorder after exposure to a terrorist attack: A prospective study. *Psychosomatic Medicine, 68,* 904–909.

Gilbertson, M. W., Paulus, L. A., Williston, S. K., Gurvits, T. V., Lasko, N. B., Pitman, R. K., & Orr, S. P. (2006). Neurocognitive function in monozygotic twins discordant for combat exposure: Relationship to posttraumatic stress disorders. *Journal of Abnormal Psychology, 115,* 484–495.

Gill, T. M., Baker, D. I., Gottschalk, M., Peduzzi, P. N., Allore, H., & Byers, A.(2002). A randomized trial of a prehabilitation program to prevent functional decline among frail community-living older persons. *The New England Journal of Medicine, 347,* 1068–1074.

Gilliam, W., Burns, J. W., Quartana, P., Matsuura, J., Nappi, C., & Wolff, B. (2010). Interactive effects of catastrophizing and suppression on responses to acute pain: A test of an appraisal × emotion regulation model. *Journal of Behavioral Medicine, 33,* 191–199.

Gilliam, W. P., Burns, J. W., Gagnon, C., Stanos, S., Matsuura, J., & Beckman, N. (2013). Strategic self-presentation may enhance effects of interdisciplinary chronic pain treatment. *Health Psychology, 32,* 156–163.

Gillum, R. F., & Ingram, D. D. (2006). Frequency of attendance at religious services, hypertension, and blood pressure: The third national health and nutrition examination survey. *Psychosomatic Medicine, 68,* 382–385.

Gindi, R. M., & Jones, L. I. (2014). Reasons for emergency room use among U.S. children: National health interview survey, 2012. *NCHS Data Brief,* 160.

Gindi, R. M., Whitney, K. K., & Cohen, R. A. (2013). Health insurance coverage and adverse experiences with physician ability: United States, 2012. *NCHS Data Brief,* 138.

Girdler, S. S., Jamner, L. D., Jarvik, M., Soles, J. R., & Shapiro, D. (1997). Smoking status and nicotine administration differentially modify hemodynamic stress reactivity in men and women. *Psychosomatic Medicine, 59,* 294–306.

Glantz, S. A. (2004). Effect of public smoking ban in Helena, Montana: Author's reply. *British Medical Journal, 328,* 1380.

Glanz, K., Croyle, R. T., Chollette, V. Y., & Pinn, V. W. (2003). Cancer-related health disparities in women. *American Journal of Public Health, 93,* 292–298.

Glaros, A. G., & Burton, E. (2004). Parafunctional clenching, pain, and effort in temporomandibular disorders. *Journal of Behavioral Medicine, 27,* 91–100.

Glaser, R., Kiecolt-Glaser, J. K., Speicher, C. E., & Holliday, J. E. (1985). Stress, loneliness, and changes in herpesvirus latency. *Journal of Behavioral Medicine, 8,* 249–260.

Glasgow, R. E. (2008). What types of evidence are most needed to advance behavioral medicine? *Annals of Behavioral Medicine, 35,* 19–25.

Glasgow, R. E., Strycker, L. A., Kurz, D., Faber, A., Bell, H., Dickman, J. M., . . . Osuna, D. (2010). Recruitment for an Internet-based diabetes self-management program: Scientific and ethical implications. *Annals of Behavioral Medicine, 40,* 40–48.

Glasgow, R. E., Toobert, D. J., Hampson, S. E., & Wilson, W. (1995). Behavioral research on diabetes at the Oregon Research Institute. *Annals of Behavioral Medicine, 17,* 32–40.

Glass, T. A., deLeon, C. M., Marottoli, R. A., & Berkman, L. F. (1999). Population based study of social and productive activities as predictors of survival among elderly Americans. *British Medical Journal, 319,* 478–483.

Glenn, B. A., Herrmann, A. K., Crespi, C. M., Mojica, C. M., Chang, L. C., Maxwell, A. E., & Bastani, R. (2011). Changes in risk perceptions in relation to self-reported colorectal cancer screening among first-degree relatives of colorectal cancer cases enrolled in a randomized trial. *Health Psychology, 30,* 481–491.

Global Information Incorporated. (2007*). Pain management: World prescription drug markets.* Retrieved from http://www.theinfoshop.com/study/tv12667_pain_management.html

Glombiewski, J. A., Tersek, J., & Rief, W. (2008). Muscular reactivity and specificity in chronic back pain patients. *Psychosomatic Medicine, 70,* 125–131.

Gluck, M. E., Geliebter, A., Hung, J., & Yahav, E. (2004). Cortisol, hunger, and desire to binge eat following a cold stress test in obese women with binge eating disorder. *Psychosomatic Medicine, 66,* 876–881.

Gluck, M. E., Yahav, E., Hashim, S. A., & Geliebter, A. (2014). Ghrelin levels after a cold pressor stress test in obese women with binge eating disorder. *Psychosomatic Medicine, 76,* 74–79.

Glynn, L. M., Dunkel-Schetter, C., Hobel, C. J., & Sandman, C. A. (2008). Pattern of perceived stress and anxiety in pregnancy predicts preterm birth. *Health Psychology, 27,* 43–51.

Goldbacher, E. M., Bromberger, J., & Matthews, K. A. (2009). Lifetime history of major depression predicts the development of the metabolic syndrome in middle-aged women. *Psychosomatic Medicine, 71,* 266–272.

Goldbacher, E. M., Matthews, K. A., & Salomon, K. (2005). Central adiposity is associated with cardiovascular reactivity to stress in adolescents. *Health Psychology, 24,* 375–384.

Goldberg, J. H., Halpern-Felsher, B. L., & Millstein, S. G. (2002). Beyond invulnerability: The importance of benefits in adolescents' decision to drink alcohol. *Health Psychology, 21,* 477–484.

Goldberg, R. J. (1981). Management of depression in the patient with advanced cancer. *Journal of the American Medical Association, 246,* 373–376.

Golden, J. S., & Johnston, G. D. (1970). Problems of distortion in doctor-patient communications. *Psychiatry in Medicine, 1,* 127–149.

Golden-Kreutz, D. M., Thornton, L. M., Gregorio, S. W., Frierson, G. M., Jim, H. S., Carpenter, K. M., . . . Andersen, B. L. (2005). Traumatic stress, perceived global stress, and life events: Prospectively predicting quality of life in breast cancer patients. *Health Psychology, 24,* 288–296.

Goldschmidt, A. B., Wall, M. M., Loth, K. A., Bucchianeri, M. M., & Neumark-Sztainer, D. (2014). The course of binge eating from adolescence to young adulthood. *Health Psychology, 33,* 457–460.

Gollwitzer, P. M. (1999). Implementation intentions: Strong effects of simple plans. *American Psychologist, 54,* 493–503.

Gonder-Frederick, L. A., Carter, W. R., Cox, D. J., & Clarke, W. L. (1990). Environmental stress and blood glucose change in insulin-dependent diabetes mellitus. *Health Psychology, 9,* 503–515.

Gonder-Frederick, L. A., Cox, D. J., Bobbitt, S. A., & Pennebaker, J. W. (1986). Blood glucose symptom beliefs of diabetic patients: Accuracy and implications. *Health Psychology, 5,* 327–341.

Gonzalez, J. S., Shreck, E., Psaros, C., & Safren, S. A. (2015). Distress and type 2 diabetes-treatment adherence: A mediating role for perceived control. *Health Psychology, 34,* 505–513.

Gonzalez, J. S., Psaros, C., Batchelder, A., Applebaum, A., Newville, H., & Safren, S. A. (2011). Clinician-assessed depression and HAART adherence in HIV-infected individuals in methadone maintenance treatment. *Annals of Behavioral Medicine, 42,* 120–126.

Gonzalez, P., Núñez, A., Wang-Letzkus, M., Lim, J., Flores, K. F., & Napoles, A. M. (2016). Coping with breast cancer: Reflections from Chinese American, Korean American, and Mexican American women. *Health Psychology, 35,* 19–28.

Goode, E. (2015, October 13). Anorexia may be habit, not resolve, study finds: Evidence that brain circuits have a role in self-destructive choices. *The New York Times,* p. A17.

Goodman, E., & Capitman, J. (2000). Depressive symptoms and cigarette smoking among teens. *Pediatrics, 106,* 748–755.

Goodman, E., Daniels, S. R., & Dolan, L. M. (2007). Socioeconomic disparities in insulin resistance: Results from the Princeton school district study. *Psychosomatic Medicine, 69,* 61–67.

Goodman, E., McEwen, B. S., Huang, B., Dolan, L. M., & Adler, N. E. (2005). Social inequalities in biomarkers of cardiovascular risk in adolescence. *Psychosomatic Medicine, 67,* 9–15.

Goodnough, A. (2009, December 17). A state's lower smoking rate draws attention. *The New York Times,* p. A29.

Goodwin, R. D., Cox, B. J., & Clara, I. (2006). Neuroticism and physical disorders among adults in the community: Results from the national comorbidity survey. *Journal of Behavioral Medicine, 29,* 229–238.

Gordon, C. M., Carey, M. P., & Carey, K. B. (1997). Effects of a drinking event on behavioral skills and condom attitudes in men: Implications for HIV risk from a controlled experiment. *Health Psychology, 16,* 490–495.

Gordon, W. A., & Diller, L. (1983). Stroke: Coping with a cognitive deficit. In T. G. Burish & L. A. Bradley (Eds.), *Coping with chronic disease: Research and applications* (pp. 113–135). New York: Academic Press.

Gordon, W. A., & Hibbard, M. R. (1991). The theory and practice of cognitive remediation. In J. S. Kreutzer & P. H. Wehman (Eds.), *Cognitive rehabilitation for persons with traumatic brain injury: A functional approach* (pp. 13–22). Baltimore, MD: Paul H. Brookes Publishing Co.

Gore-Felton, C., & Koopman, C. (2008). Behavioral mediation of the relationship between psychosocial factors and HIV disease progression. *Psychosomatic Medicine, 70,* 569–574.

Gorin, A. A., Powers, T. A., Koestner, R., Wing, R. R., & Raynor, H. A. (2014). Autonomy support, self-regulation, and weight loss. *Health Psychology, 33,* 332–339.

Gorin, A. A., Raynor, H. A., Fava, J., Maguire, K., Robichaud, E., Trautvetter, J., . . . Wing, R. R. (2013). Randomized controlled trial of a comprehensive home environment-focused weight-loss program for adults. *Health Psychology, 32,* 128–137.

Gorin, S. S. (2005). Correlates of colorectal cancer screening compliance among urban Hispanics. *Journal of Behavioral Medicine, 28,* 125–137.

Gorin, S. S., Haggstrom, D., Han, P. K., Fairfield, K. M., Krebs, P., & Clauser, S. B. (2017). Cancer care coordination: A systematic review and meta-analysis of over 30 years of empirical studies. *Annals of Behavioral Medicine, 51,* 532–546.

Gorin, S. S., Krebs, P., Badr, H., Janke, E. A., Jim, H. S., Spring, B., . . . Jacobsen, P. B. (2012). Meta-analysis of psychosocial interventions to reduce pain in patients with cancer. *Journal of Clinical Oncology, 30,* 539–547

Gorman, C. (1996, September 19). Damage control. *Time.*

Gorman, C. (1999, March 29). Get some sleep. *Time,* p. 225.

Gorst, S. L., Coates, E., & Armitage, C. J. (2016). "It's a sort of lifeline": Chronic obstructive pulmonary disease patients' experiences of home telehealth. *Health Psychology, 35,* 60–68.

Gottlieb, B. H. (Ed.). (1988). *Marshalling social support: Formats, processes, and effects.* Newbury Park, CA: Sage.

Gouin, J. P., Glaser, R., Malarkey, W. B., Beversdorf, D., & Kiecolt-Glaser, J. (2012). Chronic stress, daily stressors, and circulating inflammatory markers. *Health Psychology, 31,* 264–268.

Gould, R. (1972). The phases of adult life: A study in developmental psychology. *American Journal of Psychiatry, 129,* 521–531.

Grady, D. (2002, May 23). Hormones may explain difficulty dieters have keeping weight off. *New York Times,* pp. A1, A24.

Grady, D. (2004, April 14). Lung cancer affects sexes differently. *New York Times,* p. A18.

Grady, D. (2012, April 30). Diabetes is harder to treat in children. *New York Times,* p. A10.

Grady, D. (2018, November 19). How can we unleash the immune system? *New York Times.* Retrieved May 8, 2019, from https://www.nytimes.com/2018/11/19/health/cancer-immunotherapy-drugs.html

Graham, J. E., Lobel, M., Glass, P., & Lokshina, I. (2008). Effects of written anger expression in chronic pain patients: Making meaning from pain. *Journal of Behavioral Medicine, 31,* 201–212.

Grande, G., Romppel, M., Vesper, J. M., Schubmann, R., Glaesmer, H., & Herrmann-Lingen, C. (2011). Type D personality and all-cause mortality in cardiac patients—Data from a German cohort study. *Psychosomatic Medicine, 73,* 548–556.

Grandner, M. A., & Kripke, D. F. (2004). Self-reported sleep complaints with long and short sleep: A nationally representative sample. *Psychosomatic Medicine, 66,* 239–241.

Granö, N., Vahtera, J., Virtanen, M., Keltikangas-Järvinen, L., & Kivimäki, M. (2008). Association of hostility with sleep duration and sleep disturbances in an employee population. *International Journal of Behavioral Medicine, 15*, 73-80.

Grant, J. A., & Rainville, P. (2009). Pain sensitivity and analgesic effects of mindful states in Zen mediators: A cross-sectional study. *Psychosomatic Medicine, 71*, 106-114.

Grassi, L., & Molinari, S. (1986). Intrafamilial dynamics and neoplasia: Prospects for a multidisciplinary analysis. *Rivista di Psichiatria, 21*, 329-341.

Graugaard, P., & Finset, A. (2000). Trait anxiety and reactions to patient-centered and doctor-centered styles of communication: An experimental study. *Psychosomatic Medicine, 62*, 33-39.

Green, J. H. (1978). *Basic clinical physiology* (3rd ed.). New York: Oxford University Press.

Greenberg, E. S., & Grunberg, L. (1995). Work alienation and problem alcohol behavior. *Journal of Health and Social Behavior, 36*, 83-102.

Greene, K. (2011, June 14). Toll of caring for elderly increases. *The Wall Street Journal*, p. D3.

Greene, R. E., Houston, B. K., & Holleran, S. A. (1995). Aggressiveness, dominance, developmental factors, and serum cholesterol level in college males. *Journal of Behavioral Medicine, 18*, 569-580.

Greer, J., & Halgin, R. (2006). Predictors of physician–patient agreement on symptom etiology in primary care. *Psychosomatic Medicine, 68*, 277-282.

Greer, J. A., Jacobs, J. M., El-Jawahri, A., Nipp, R. D., Gallagher, E. R., Pirl, W. F., & Temel, J. S. (2018). Role of patient coping strategies in understanding the effects of early palliative care on quality of life and mood. *Journal of Clinical Oncology, 36*, 53-60.

Greer, T. M., Brondolo, E., & Brown, P. (2014). Systemic racism moderates effects of provider racial biases on adherence to hypertension treatment for African Americans. *Health Psychology, 33*, 35-42.

Griffiths, S. E., Parsons, J., Naughton, F., Fulton, E. A., Tombor, I., & Brown, K. E. (2018). Are digital interventions for smoking cessation in pregnancy effective? A systematic review and meta-analysis. *Health Psychology Review, 12*, 333-356.

Grogan, S., Flett, K., Clark-Carter, D., Conner, M., Davey, R., Richardson, D., & Rajaratnam, G. (2011). A randomized controlled trial of an appearance-related smoking intervention. *Health Psychology, 30*, 805-809.

Gross, A. M., Eudy, C., & Drabman, R. S. (1982). Training parents to be physical therapists with their physically handicapped child. *Journal of Behavioral Medicine, 5*, 321-328.

Grossardt, B. R., Bower, J. H., Geda, Y. E., Colligan, R. C., & Rocca, W. A. (2009). Pessimistic, anxious, and depressive personality traits predict all-cause mortality: The Mayo Clinic cohort study of personality and aging. *Psychosomatic Medicine, 71*, 491-500.

Grossman, H. Y., Brink, S., & Hauser, S. T. (1987). Self-efficacy in adolescent girls and boys with insulin-dependent diabetes mellitus. *Diabetes Care, 10*, 324-329.

Grossman, P., Niemann, L., Schmidt, S., & Walach, H. (2004). Mindfulness-based stress reduction and health benefits: A meta-analysis. *Journal of Psychosomatic Research, 57*, 35-43.

Grossman, P., Tiefenthaler-Gilmer, U., Raysz, A., & Kesper, U. (2007). Mindfulness training as an intervention for fibromyalgia: Evidence of postintervention and 3-year follow-up benefits in well-being. *Psychotherapy and Psychosomatics, 76*, 226-233.

Groth-Marnat, G., & Fletcher, A. (2000). Influence of neuroticism, catastrophizing, pain, duration, and receipt of compensation on short-term response to nerve block treatment for chronic back pain. *Journal of Behavioral Medicine, 23*, 339-350.

Gruenewald, T. L., Kemeny, M. E., Aziz, N., & Fahey, J. L. (2004). Acute threat to the social self: Shame, social self-esteem, and cortisol activity. *Psychosomatic Medicine, 66*, 915-924.

Grunberg, N. E., & Acri, J. B. (1991). Conceptual and methodological considerations for tobacco addiction research. *British Journal of Addiction, 86*, 637-641.

Grunberg, N. E., & Straub, R. O. (1992). The role of gender and taste class in the effects of stress on eating. *Health Psychology, 11* 97-100.

Grunfeld, E. A., Drudge-Coates, L., Rixon, L., Eaton, E., & Cooper, A. F. (2013). "*The only way I know how to live is to work*": A qualitative study of work following treatment for prostate cancer. *Health Psychology, 32*, 75-82.

Grzywacz, J. G., Almeida, D. M., Neupert, S. D., & Ettner, S. L. (2004). Socioeconomic status and health: A micro-level analysis of exposure and vulnerability to daily stressors. *Journal of Health and Social Behavior, 45*, 1-16.

Gu, Q., Dillon, C. F., & Burt, V. L. (2010). Prescription drug use continues to increase: U.S. prescription drug data for 2007-2008. *NCHS Data Brief, 42*, 1-8.

Guéguen, N., Meineri, S., & Charles-Sire, V. (2010). Improving medication adherence by using practitioner nonverbal techniques: A field experiment on the effect of touch. *Journal of Behavioral Medicine, 33*, 466-473.

Guilamo-Ramos, V., Jaccard, J., Pena, J., & Goldberg, V. (2005). Acculturation-related variables, sexual initiation, and subsequent sexual behavior among Puerto Rican, Mexican, and Cuban youth. *Health Psychology, 24*, 88-95.

Gujral, S., McAuley, E., Oberlin, L. E., Kramer, A. F., & Erickson, K. I. (2018). Role of brain structure in predicting adherence to a physical activity regimen. *Psychosomatic Medicine, 80*, 69-77.

Gump, B. B., & Matthews, K. A. (1998). Vigilance and cardiovascular reactivity to subsequent stressors in men: A preliminary study. *Health Psychology, 17*, 93-96.

Gunthert, K. C., Cohen, L. H., & Armeli, S. (1999). The role of neuroticism in daily stress and coping. *Journal of Personality and Social Psychology, 77*, 1087-1100.

Gupta, S. (2002, August 26). Don't ignore heart-attack blues. *Time*, p. 71.

Gupta, S. (2004, October 24). Click to get sick? *Time*, p. 102.

Gurevich, M., Devins, G. M., Wilson, C., McCready, D., Marmar, C. R., & Rodin, G. M. (2004). Stress responses syndromes in women undergoing mammography: A comparison of women with and without a history of breast cancer. *Psychosomatic Medicine, 66*, 104-112.

Guyll, M., & Contrada, R. J. (1998). Trait hostility and ambulatory cardiovascular activity: Responses to social interaction. *Health Psychology, 17*, 30-39.

Gwyther, H., Bobrowicz-Campos, E., Luis Alves Apóstolo, J., Marcucci, M., Cano, A., & Holland, C. (2018). A realist review to understand the efficacy and outcomes of interventions designed to minimise, reverse or prevent the progression of frailty. *Health Psychology Review, 12*, 382-404.

Haase, C. M., Poulin, M. J., & Heckhausen, J. (2012). Happiness as a motivator: Positive affect predicts primary control striving for career and educational goals. *Personality and Social Psychology Bulletin, 38*, 1093-1104.

Habibović, M., Denollet, J., Cuijpers, P., van der Voort, P. H., Herrman, J.-P., Bouwels, L., . . . Pedersen, S. S. (2017). Web-based distress management for implantable cardioverter defibrillator patients: A randomized controlled trial. *Health Psychology, 36*, 392-401.

Hackett, T. P., & Cassem, N. H. (1973). Psychological adaptation to convalescence in myocardial infarction patients. In J. P. Naughton, H. K. Hellerstein, & I. C. Mohler (Eds.), *Exercise testing and exercise training in coronary heart disease.* New York: Academic Press.

Hadjistavropoulos, T., Craig, K. D., Duck, S., Cano, A., Goubert, L., Jackson, P. L., . . . Fitzgerald, T. D. (2011). A biopsychosocial formulation of pain communication. *Psychological Bulletin, 137*, 910-939.

Haemmerli, K., Znoj, H., & Berger, T. (2010). Internet-based support for infertile patients: A randomized controlled study. *Journal of Behavioral Medicine, 33,* 135–146.

Haerens, L., Deforche, B., Maes, L., Brug, J., Vandelanotte, C., & De Bourdeaudhuij, I. (2007). A computer-tailored dietary fat intake intervention for adolescents: Results of a randomized controlled trial. *Annals of Behavioral Medicine, 34,* 253–262.

Hafez, D., Heisler, M., Choi, H., Ankuda, C. K., Winkelman, T., & Kullgren, J. T. (2018). Association between purpose in life and glucose control among older adults. *Annals of Behavioral Medicine, 52,* 309–318.

Hagedoorn, M., Dagan, M., Puterman, E., Hoff, C., Meijerink, W. J. H. J., Delongis, A., & Sanderman, R. (2011). Relationship satisfaction in couples confronted with colorectal cancer: The interplay of past and current spousal support. *Journal of Behavioral Medicine, 34,* 288–297.

Hagger-Johnson, G., Mõttus, R., Craig, L. C., A., Starr, J. M., & Deary, I. J. (2012). Pathways from childhood intelligence and socioeconomic status to late-life cardiovascular disease risk. *Health Psychology, 31,* 403–412.

Hahn, E. A., DeWalt, D. A., Bode, R. K., Garcia, S. F., DeVillis, R. F., Correia, H., & PROMIS Cooperative Group. (2014). New English and Spanish social health measures will facilitate evaluating health determinants. *Health Psychology, 33,* 490–499.

Hajjari, P., Mattsson, S., McIntyre, K. M., McKinley, P. S., Shapiro, P. A., Gorenstein, E. E., . . . Sloan, R. P. (2016). The effect of hostility reduction on autonomic control of the heart and vasculature: A randomized controlled trial. *Psychosomatic Medicine, 78,* 481–491.

Halkitis, P. N., Cook, S. H., Ristuccia, A., Despotoulis, J., Levy, M. D., Bates, F. C., & Kapadia, F. (2018). Psychometric analysis of the Life Worries Scale for a new generation of sexual minority men: The P18 Cohort Study. *Health Psychology, 37,* 89–101.

Halford, W. K., Cuddihy, S., & Mortimer, R. H. (1990). Psychological stress and blood glucose regulation in Type I diabetic patients. *Health Psychology, 9,* 516–528.

Halim, M. L., Yoshikawa, H., & Amodio, D. M. (2013). Cross-generational effects of discrimination among immigrant mothers: Perceived discrimination predicts child's healthcare visits for illness. *Health Psychology, 32,* 203–211.

Hall, J. A., Epstein, A. M., DeCiantis, M. L., & McNeil, B. J. (1993). Physicians' liking for their patients: More evidence for the role of affect in medical care. *Health Psychology, 12,* 140–146.

Hall, J. A., Irish, J. T., Roter, D. L., Ehrlich, C. M., & Miller, L. H. (1994). Gender in medical encounters: An analysis of physician and patient communication in a primary care setting. *Health Psychology, 13,* 384–392.

Hall, K. S., Crowley, G. M., McConnell, E. S., Bosworth, H. B., Sloane, R., Ekelund, C. C., & Morey, M. C. (2010). Change in goal ratings as a mediating variable between self-efficacy and physical activity in older men. *Annals of Behavioral Medicine, 39,* 267–273.

Hall, M., Vasko, R., Buysse, D., Ombao, H., Chen, Q., Cashmere, J. D., . . . Thayer, J. F. (2004). Acute stress affects heart rate variability during sleep. *Psychosomatic Medicine, 66,* 56–62.

Hall, M. H., Brindle, R. C., & Buysse, D. J. (2018). Sleep and cardiovascular disease: Emerging opportunities for psychology. *American Psychologist, 73,* 994–1006.

Hall, M. J., Levant, S., & DeFrances, C. J. (2013). Trends in inpatient hospital deaths: National hospital discharge survey, 2000-2010. *NCHS Data Brief, 118,* 1–8.

Hall, P. A., Dubin, J. A., Crossley, M., Holmqvist, M. E., & D'Arcy, C. (2009). Does executive function explain the IQ-mortality association? Evidence from the Canadian study on health and aging. *Psychosomatic Medicine, 71,* 196–204.

Hall, P. A., Erickson, K. I., & Gianaros, P. J. (2017). The neurobiology of health communication. *Psychosomatic Medicine, 79,* 376–378.

Halpern-Felsher, B. L., Millstein, S. G., Ellen, J. M., Adler, N. E., Tschann, J. M., & Biehl, M. (2001). The role of behavioral experience in judging risks. *Health Psychology, 20,* 120–126.

Ham, B. (Ed.). (2003). Health behavior information transfer. *Habit, 6.* Retrieved from http://www.cfah.org/habit

Hamburg, D. A., & Adams, J. E. (1967). A perspective on coping behavior: Seeking and utilizing information in major transitions. *Archives of General Psychiatry, 19,* 277–284.

Hamer, M., Stamatakis, E., Kivimäki, M., Kengne, A. P., & Batty, G. D. (2010). Psychological distress, glycated hemoglobin, and mortality in adults with and without diabetes. *Psychosomatic Medicine, 72,* 882–886.

Hamer, M., & Steptoe, A. (2007). Association between physical fitness, parasympathetic control, and proinflammatory responses to mental stress. *Psychosomatic Medicine, 69,* 660–666.

Hamilton, K., Kirkpatrick, A., Rebar, A., & Hagger, M. S. (2017). Child sun safety: Application of an integrated behavior change model. *Health Psychology, 36,* 916–926.

Hamilton, N. A., Catley, D., & Karlson, C. (2007). Sleep and the affective response to stress and pain. *Health Psychology, 26,* 288–295.

Hamilton, V. L., Broman, C. L., Hoffman, W. S., & Renner, D. S. (1990). Hard times and vulnerable people: Initial effects of plant closing on autoworkers' mental health. *Journal of Health and Social Behavior, 31,* 123–140.

Hampson, S. E., Edmonds, G. W., Goldberg, L. R., Dubanoski, J. P., & Hillier, T. A. (2015). A life-span behavioral mechanism relating childhood conscientiousness to adult clinical health. *Health Psychology, 34,* 887–895.

Hampson, S. E., Edmons, G. W., Goldberg, L. R., Dubanoski, J. P., & Hillier, T. A. (2015). A life-span behavioral mechanism relating childhood conscientiousness to adult clinical health. *Health Psychology, 34,* 887–895.

Hampson, S. E., Glasgow, R. E., & Toobert, D. J. (1990). Personal models of diabetes and their relations to self-care activities. *Health Psychology, 9,* 632–646.

Hampson, S. E., Glasgow, R. E., & Zeiss, A. M. (1994). Personal models of osteoarthritis and their relation to self-management activities and quality of life. *Journal of Behavioral Medicine, 17,* 143–158.

Hamrick, N., Cohen, S., & Rodriguez, M. S. (2002). Being popular can be healthy or unhealthy: Stress, social network diversity, and incidence of upper respiratory infection. *Health Psychology, 21,* 294–298.

Han, S., & Shavitt, S. (1994). Persuasion and culture: Advertising appeals in individualistic and collectivistic societies. *Journal of Experimental Social Psychology, 30,* 326–350.

Hanoch, Y., Wood, S., Barnes, A., Liu, P. J., & Rice, T. (2011). Choosing the right medicare prescription drug plan: The effect of age, strategy selection, and choice set size. *Health Psychology, 30,* 719–727.

Hansen, R. N., Oster, G., Edelsberg, J., Woody, G. E., & Sullivan, S. D. (2011). *Economic costs of nonmedical use of prescription opioids.* Retrieved on February 21, 2016, from http://www.ncbi.nlm.nih.gov

Hanson, C. L., Henggeler, S. W., & Burghen, G. A. (1987). Models of associations between psychosocial variables and health-outcome measures of adolescents with IDDM. *Diabetes Care, 10,* 752–758.

Hanson, C. L., & Pichert, J. W. (1986). Perceived stress and diabetes control in adolescents. *Health Psychology, 5,* 439–452.

Hanson, M. D., & Chen, E. (2007). Socioeconomic status and health behaviors in adolescence: A review of the literature. *Journal of Behavioral Medicine, 30,* 263–285.

Hanson, M. D., & Chen, E. (2010). Daily stress, cortisol, and sleep: The moderating role of childhood psychosocial environments. *Health Psychology, 29,* 394–402.

Hao, Y., Landrine, H., Smith, T., Kaw, C., Corral, I., & Stein, K. (2011). Residential segregation and disparities in health-related quality of life among Black and White cancer survivors. *Health Psychology, 30,* 137–144.

Harburg, E., Julius, M., Kacirotti, N., Gleiberman, L., & Schork, M. A. (2003). Expressive/suppressive anger-coping responses, gender, and types of mortality: A 17-year follow-up (Tecumseh, Michigan, 1971–1988). *Psychosomatic Medicine, 65,* 588–597.

Hardcastle, S. J., Fortier, M., Blake, N., & Hagger, M. S. (2017). Identifying content-based and relational techniques to change behaviour in motivational interviewing. *Health Psychology Review, 11*(1), 1–16.

Harris-Kojetin, L., Sengupta, M., Lendon, J. P., Rome, V., Valverde, R., & Caffrey, C. (2019). Long-term care providers and services users in the United States, 2015–2016. *National Center for Health Statistics. Vital Health Statistics, 3*(43), 1–78.

Harris, P. R., Brearley, I., Sheeran, P., Barker, M., Klein, W. M. P., Creswell, J. D., . . . Bond, R. (2014). Combining self-affirmation with implementation intentions to promote fruit and vegetable consumption. *Health Psychology, 33,* 729–736.

Harris, P. R., Mayle, K., Mabbott, L., & Napper, L. (2007). Self-affirmation reduces smokers' defensiveness to graphic on-pack cigarette warning labels. *Health Psychology, 26,* 437–446.

Hartman, M., Martin, A. B., Espinosa, N., Catlin, A., & The National Health Care Spending Team (2017). National health care spending in 2016: Spending and enrollment growth slow after initial coverage expansions. *Health Affairs, 37,* 150–160.

Harvey, A. G., Bryant, R. A., & Tarrier, N. (2003). Cognitive behaviour therapy for posttraumatic stress disorder. *Clinical Psychology Review, 23,* 501–522.

Hatzenbuehler, M. L., Nolen-Hoeksema, S., & Erickson, S. J. (2008). Minority stress predictors of HIV risk behavior, substance use, and depressive symptoms: Results from a prospective study of bereaved gay men. *Health Psychology, 27,* 455–462.

Harvey, C. J., Gehrman, P., & Espie, C. A. (2014). Who is predisposed to insomnia: A review of familial aggregation, stress-reactivity, personality and coping style. *Sleep Medicine Reviews, 18,* 237–247.

Hatzenbuehler, M. L., O'Cleirigh, C., Mayer, K. H., Mimiaga, M. J., & Safren, S. A. (2011). Prospective associations between HIV-related stigma, transmission risk behaviors, and adverse mental health outcomes in men who have sex with men. *Annals of Behavioral Medicine, 42,* 227–234.

Haug, M. R., & Folmar, S. J. (1986). Longevity, gender, and life quality. *Journal of Health and Social Behavior, 27,* 332–345.

Haug, M. R., & Ory, M. G. (1987). Issues in elderly patient–provider interactions. *Research on Aging, 9,* 3–44.

Haukkala, A., Konttinen, H., Lehto, E., Uutela, A., Kawachi, I., & Laatikainen, T. (2013). Sense of coherence, depressive symptoms, cardiovascular diseases, and all-cause mortality. *Psychosomatic Medicine, 75,* 429–435.

Hausteiner, C., Klupsch, D., Emeny, R., Baumert, J., Ladwig, K. H., & for the KORA Investigators. (2010). Clustering of negative affectivity and social inhibition in the community; prevalance of Type D personality as a cardiovascular risk marker. *Psychosomatic Medicine, 72,* 163–171.

Hawkins, M. A. W., Gunstad, J., Calvo, D., & Spitznagel, M. B. (2016). Higher fasting glucose is associated with poorer cognition among healthy young adults. *Health Psychology, 35,* 199–202.

Hawkley, L. C., Thisted, R. A., & Cacioppo, J. T. (2009). Loneliness predicts reduced physical activity: Cross-sectional & longitudinal analyses. *Health Psychology, 28,* 354–363.

Hayes-Bautista, D. E. (1976). Modifying the treatment: Patient compliance, patient control, and medical care. *Social Science and Medicine, 10,* 233–238.

Hayes, S. C. (2016). Acceptance and commitment therapy, relational frame theory, and the third wave of behavioral and cognitive therapies-republished article. *Behavior Therapy, 47,* 869–885.

Haynes, R. B., McKibbon, K. A., & Kanani, R. (1996). Systematic review of randomized controlled trials of the effects on patient adherence and outcomes of interventions to assist patients to follow prescriptions for medications. *The Cochrane Library, 2,* 1–26.

Haythornthwaite, J., Lawrence, J., & Fauerbach, J. (2001). Brief cognitive interventions for burn pain. *Annals of Behavioral Medicine, 23,* 42–49.

Hazuda, H. P., Gerety, M. B., Lee, S., Mulrow, C. D., & Lichtenstein, M. J. (2002). Measuring subclinical disability in older Mexican Americans. *Psychosomatic Medicine, 64,* 520–30.

Healy, M. (2014, November 17). Working while others sleep? Obesity may be a higher risk; here's why. *Los Angeles Times.*

Healy, M. (2015, January 15). Sedentary behavior trumps fat as a killer. *Los Angeles Times.*

Healy, M. (2015, February 13). Diet and exercise alone are no cure for obesity, experts say. *Los Angeles Times.*

Healy, M. (2015, July 15). Study ties sugary drinks to 25,000 U.S. deaths. *Los Angeles Times,* p. A13.

Healy, M. (2016, January 31). Number of overweight children grows globally. *Los Angeles Times,* p. A5.

Heaney, C. A., Israel, B. A., & House, J. A. (1994). Chronic job insecurity among automobile workers: Effects on job satisfaction and health. *Social Science and Medicine, 38,* 1431–1437.

Heatherton, T. F., & Sargent, J. D. (2009). Does watching smoking in movies promote teenage smoking? *Current Directions in Psychological Science, 18,* 63–67.

Heckman, C. J., Handorf, E. A., Darlow, S. D., Ritterband, L. M., & Manne, S. L. (2017). An online skin cancer risk-reduction intervention for young adults: Mechanisms of effects. *Health Psychology, 36,* 215–225.

Heckman, T. G. (2003). The chronic illness quality of life (CIQOL) model: Explaining life satisfaction in people living with HIV disease. *Health Psychology, 22,* 140–147.

Heckman, T. G., Anderson, E. S., Sikkema, K. J., Kochman, A., Kalichman, S. C., & Anderson, T. (2004). Emotional distress in nonmetropolitan persons living with HIV disease enrolled in a telephone-delivered, coping improvement group intervention. *Health Psychology, 23,* 94–100.

Heckman, T. G., Markowitz, J. C., Heckman, B. D., Woldu, H., Anderson, T., Lovejoy, T. I., . . . Yarber, W. (2018). A randomized clinical trial showing persisting reductions in depressive symptoms in HIV-infected rural adults following brief telephone-administered interpersonal psychotherapy. *Annals of Behavioral Medicine, 52,* 299–308.

Heckman, T. G., Miller, J., Kochman, A., Kalichman, S. C., Carlson, B., & Silverthorn, M. (2002). Thoughts of suicide among HIV-infected rural persons enrolled in telephone-delivered mental health intervention. *Annals of Behavioral Medicine, 24,* 141–148.

Heim, C., Nater, U. M., Maloney, E., Boneva, R., Jones, J. F., & Reeves, W. C. (2009). Childhood trauma and risk for chronic fatigue syndrome: Association with neuroendocrine dysfunction. *Archives of General Psychiatry, 66,* 72–80.

Heim, E., Valach, L., & Schaffner, L. (1997). Coping and psychosocial adaptation: Longitudinal effects over time and stages in breast cancer. *Psychosomatic Medicine, 59,* 408–418.

Heisler, M., Wagner, T. H., & Piette, J. D. (2005). Patient strategies to cope with high prescription medication costs: Who is cutting back on necessities, increasing debt, or underusing medications? *Journal of Behavioral Medicine, 28,* 43–51.

Heisz, J. J., Vandermorris, S., Wu, J., McIntosh, A. R., & Ryan, J. D. (2015). Age differences in the association of physical activity, sociocognitive engagement, and TV viewing on face memory. *Health Psychology, 34,* 83–88.

Hekler, E. B., Lambert, J., Leventhal, E., Leventhal, H., Jahn, E., & Contrada, R. J. (2008). Commonsense illness beliefs, adherence behaviors, and hypertension control among African Americans. *Journal of Behavioral Medicine, 31,* 391–400.

Helgeson, V. S. (1993). Implications of agency and communion for patient and spouse adjustment to a first coronary event. *Journal of Personality and Social Psychology, 64,* 807–816.

Helgeson, V. S. (2003). Cognitive adaptation, psychological adjustment and disease progression among angioplasty patients: 4 years later. *Health Psychology, 22,* 30–38.

Helgeson, V. S., & Cohen, S. (1996). Social support and adjustment to cancer: Reconciling descriptive, correlational, and intervention research. *Health Psychology, 15,* 135–148.

Helgeson, V. S., Cohen, S., Schulz, R., & Yasko, J. (2000). Group support interventions for women with breast cancer: Who benefits from what? *Health Psychology, 19,* 107–117.

Helgeson, V. S., Cohen, S., Schulz, R., & Yasko, J. (2001). Long-term effects of educational and peer discussion group interventions on adjustment to breast cancer. *Health Psychology, 20,* 387–392.

Helgeson, V. S., Escobar, O., Siminerio, L., & Becker, D. (2010). Relation of stressful life events to metabolic control among adolescents with diabetes: 5-year longitudinal study. *Health Psychology, 29,* 153–159.

Helgeson, V. S., & Fritz, H. L. (1999). Cognitive adaptation as a predictor of new coronary events after percutaneous transluminal coronary angioplasty. *Psychosomatic Medicine, 61,* 488–495.

Helgeson, V. S., & Lepore, S. J. (1997). Men's adjustment to prostate cancer: The role of agency and unmitigated agency. *Sex Roles, 37,* 251–267.

Helgeson, V. S., Palladino, D. K., Reynolds, K. A., Becker, D. J., Escobar, O., & Siminerio, L. (2014). Relationships and health among emerging adults with and without Type 1 diabetes. *Health Psychology, 33,* 1125–1133.

Hellsten, L., Nigg, C., Norman, G., Burbank, P., Braun, L., Breger, R., . . . Wang, T. (2008). Accumulation of behavioral validation evidence for physical activity state of change. *Health Psychology, 27,* S43–S53.

Helmers, K. F., & Krantz, D. S. (1996). Defensive hostility, gender and cardiovascular levels and responses to stress. *Annals of Behavioral Medicine, 18,* 246–254.

Hemmingsson, T., Kriebel, D., Melin, B., Allebeck, P., & Lundberg, I. (2008). How does IQ affect onset of smoking and cessation of smoking—Linking the Swedish 1969 conscription cohort to the Swedish survey of living conditions. *Psychosomatic Medicine, 70,* 805–810.

Henry J Kaiser Family Foundation. (2017, February 27). *Total HMO enrollment.* Retrieved April 9, 2019, from https://www.kff.org/other/state-indicator/total-hmo-enrollment/?currentTimeframe=0&sortModel=%7B%22colId%22%3A%22Location%22%2C%22sort%22%3A%22asc%22%7D

Henry, J. P., & Cassel, J. C. (1969). Psychosocial factors in essential hypertension: Recent epidemiologic and animal experimental evidence. *American Journal of Epidemiology, 90,* 171–200.

Hendrickson, C. M., Neylan, T. C., Na, B., Regan, M., Zhang, Q., & Cohen, B. E. (2013). Lifetime trauma exposure and prospective cardiovascular events and all-cause mortality: Findings from the heart and soul study. *Psychosomatic Medicine, 75,* 849–855.

Hepatitis B Foundation. (2018). *Hepatitis B fast facts.* Retrieved March 26, 2019, from http://www.hepb.org/assets/Uploads/Hepatitis-B-Fast-Facts-8-28-18-FINAL.pdf

Heppner, W. L., Ji, L., Reitzel, L. R., Castro, Y., Correa-Fernandez, V., Vidrine, J. I., . . . Wetter, D. W. (2011). The role of prepartum motivation in the maintenance of postpartum smoking abstinence. *Health Psychology, 30,* 736–745.

Herbert, T. B., & Cohen, S. (1993). Stress and immunity in humans: A meta-analytic review. *Psychosomatic Medicine, 5,* 364–379.

Herman, S., Blumenthal, J. A., Babyak, M., Khatri, P., Craighead, W. E., Krishnan, K. R., & Doraiswamy, P. M. (2002). Exercise therapy for depression in middle-aged and older adults: Predictors of early dropout and treatment failure. *Health Psychology, 21,* 553–563.

Hermand, D., Mullet, E., & Lavieville, S. (1997). Perception of the combined effects of smoking and alcohol on health. *Journal of Health Psychology, 2,* 481–491.

Hermann, C., & Blanchard, E. B. (2002). Biofeedback in the treatment of headache and other childhood pain. *Applied Psychophysiology and Biofeedback, 27,* 143–162.

Hernandez, A., & Sachs-Ericsson, N. (2006). Ethnic differences in pain reports and the moderating role of depression in a community sample of Hispanic and Caucasian participants with serious health problems. *Psychosomatic Medicine, 68,* 121–128.

Herrmann-Lingen, C. (2017). Past, present, and future of psychosomatic movements in an ever-changing world: Presidential address. *Psychosomatic Medicine, 79,* 960–970.

Herschbach, P., Duran, G., Waadt, S., Zettler, A., Amm, C., & Marten-Mittag, B. (1997). Psychometric properties of the questionnaire on stress in patients with diabetes-revised (QSD-F). *Health Psychology, 16,* 171–174.

Hersey, J. C., Niederdeppe, J., Evans, W. D., Nonnemaker, J., Blahut, S., Holden, D., . . . Haviland, M. L. (2005). The theory of "truth": How counterindustry media campaigns affect smoking behavior among teens. *Health Psychology, 24,* 22–31.

Hertel, A. W., Finch, E. A., Kelly, K. M., King, C., Lando, H., Linde, J. A., . . . Rothman, A. J. (2008). The impact of expectations and satisfaction on the initiation and maintenance of smoking cessation: An experimental test. *Health Psychology, 27,* S197–S206.

Hewig, J., Cooper, S., Trippe, R. H., Hecht, H., Straube, T., & Miltner, W. H. R. (2008). Drive for thinness and attention toward specific body parts in a nonclinical sample. *Psychosomatic Medicine, 70,* 729–736.

Hien, T. T., de Jong, M., & Farrar, J. (2004). Avian influenza—A challenge to global health care structures. *The New England Journal of Medicine, 351,* 2363–2365.

Higgins, T. J., Middleton, K. R., Winner, L., & Janelle, C. M. (2014). Physical activity interventions differentially affect exercise task and barrier self-efficacy: A meta-analysis. *Health Psychology, 33,* 891–903.

Hill, L. K., Sherwood, A., McNeilly, M., Anderson, N. B., Blumenthal, J. A., & Hinderliter, A. L. (2018). Impact of racial discrimination and hostility on adrenergic receptor responsiveness in African American adults. *Psychosomatic Medicine, 80,* 208–215.

Hill, P. L., & Roberts, B. W. (2011). The role of adherence in the relationship between conscientiousness and perceived health. *Health Psychology, 30,* 797–804.

Hill, P. L., Sin, N. L., Turiano, N. A., Burrow, A. L., & Almeida, D. M. (2018). Sense of purpose moderates the associations between daily stressors and daily well-being. *Annals of Behavioral Medicine, 52,* 724–729.

Hill, P. L., Turiano, N. A., Hurd, M. D., Mroczek, D. K., & Roberts, B. W. (2011). Conscientiousness and longevity: An examination of possible mediators. *Health Psychology, 30,* 536–541.

Hill, T. D., Ellison, C. G., Burdette, A. M., & Musick, M. A. (2007). Religious involvement and healthy lifestyles: Evidence from the survey of Texas adults. *Annals of Behavioral Medicine, 34,* 217–222.

Hill-Briggs, F. (2003). Problem solving in diabetes self-management: A model of chronic illness self-management behavior. *Annals of Behavior Medicine, 25,* 182–193.

Hill-Briggs, F., Gary, T. L., Bone, L. R., Hill, M. N., Levine, D. M., & Brancati, F. L. (2005). Medication adherence and diabetes control in urban African Americans with type 2 diabetes. *Health Psychology, 24,* 349-357.

Hilliard, M. E., Eakin, M. N., Borrelli, B., Green, A., & Riekert, K. A. (2015) Medication beliefs mediate between depressive symptoms and medication adherence in cystic fibrosis. *Health Psychology, 34,* 496-504.

Hilliard, M. E., Holmes, C. S., Chen, R., Maher, K., Robinson, E., & Streisand, R. (2013). Disentangling the roles of parental monitoring and family conflict in adolescents' management of type 1 diabetes. *Health Psychology, 32,* 388-396.

Hilmert, C. J., Dunkel Schetter, C., Dominguez, T. P., Abdou, C., Hobel, C. J., Glynn, L., & Sandman, C. (2008). Stress and blood pressure during pregnancy: Racial differences and associations with birthweight. *Psychosomatic Medicine, 70,* 57-64.

Hilton, L., Hempel, S., Ewing, B. A., Apaydin, E., Xenakis, L., Newberry, S., . . . Maglione, M. A. (2016). Mindfulness meditation for chronic pain: Systematic review and meta-analysis. *Annals of Behavioral Medicine, 51,* 199-213.

Hing, E., & Uddin, S. (2011). Physician assistant and advance practice nurse care in hospital outpatient departments: United States, 2008-2009. *NCHS Data Brief, 77,* 1-8.

Hinton, J. M. (1967). *Dying.* Baltimore, MD: Penguin.

Hintsanen, M., Elovainio, M., Puttonen, S., Kivimäki, M., Koskinen, T., Raitakari, O. T., & Keltikangas-Jarvinen, L. (2007). Effort-reward imbalance, heart rate, and heart-rate variability: The cardiovascular risk in young Finns study. *International Journal of Behavioral Medicine, 14,* 202-212.

Hintsanen, M., Kivimäki, M., Elovainio, M., Pulkki-Råback, L., Keskivaara, P., Juonala, M., . . . Keltikangas-Järvinen, L. (2005). Job strain and early atherosclerosis: The cardiovascular risk in young Finns study. *Psychosomatic Medicine, 67,* 740-747.

Hirokawa, K., Nagayoshi, M., Ohira, T., Kajiura, M., Kitamura, A., Kiyama, M., & Iso, H. (2014). Menopausal status in relation to cardiovascular stress reactivity in healthy Japanese patients. *Psychosomatic Medicine, 76,* 701-708.

Hobfoll, S. E., Jackson, A. P., Lavin, J., Britton, P. J., & Shepherd, J. B. (1993). Safer sex knowledge, behavior, and attitudes of inner-city women. *Health Psychology, 12,* 481-488.

Hochbaum, G. (1958). *Public participation in medical screening programs* (DHEW Publication No. 572, Public Health Service). Washington, DC: U.S. Government Printing Office.

Hochschild, A. (1989). *The second shift: Working parents and the revolution at home.* New York: Viking Penguin.

Hoelscher, T. J., Lichstein, K. L., & Rosenthal, T. L. (1986). Home relaxation practice in hypertension treatment: Objective assessment and compliance induction. *Journal of Consulting and Clinical Psychology, 54,* 217-221.

Holahan, C. J., & Moos, R. H. (1990). Life stressors, resistance factors, and improved psychological functioning: An extension of the stress resistance paradigm. *Journal of Personality and Social Psychology, 58,* 909-917.

Holahan, C. J., & Moos, R. H. (1991). Life stressors, personal and social resources, and depression: A four-year structural model. *Journal of Abnormal Psychology, 100,* 31-38.

Holland, J. C. (2002). History of psycho-oncology: Overcoming attitudinal and conceptual barriers. *Psychosomatic Medicine, 64,* 206-221.

Holmes, J., Powell-Griner, E., Lethbridge-Cejku, M., & Heyman, K. (2009). Aging differently: Physical limitations among adults aged 50 years and over: United States, 2001-2007. *NCHS Data Brief, 20,* 1-7.

Holmes, J. A., & Stevenson, C. A. Z. (1990). Differential effects of avoidant and attentional coping strategies on adaptation to chronic and recent-onset pain. *Health Psychology, 9,* 577-584.

Holmes, T. H., & Rahe, R. H. (1967). The social readjustment rating scale. *Journal of Psychosomatic Research, 11,* 213-218.

Holt, C. L., Clark, E. M., Kreuter, M. W., & Rubio, D. M. (2003). Spiritual health locus of control and breast cancer beliefs among urban African American women. *Health Psychology, 22,* 294-299.

Holt-Lunstad, J., Robles, T. F., & Sbarra, D. A. (2017). Advancing social connection as a public health priority in the United States. *American Psychologist, 72,* 517-530.

Holt-Lunstad, J., Smith, T. W., & Uchino, B. N. (2008). Can hostility interfere with the health benefits of giving and receiving social support? The impact of cynical hostility on cardiovascular reactivity during social support interactions among friends. *Annals of Behavioral Medicine, 35,* 319-330.

Hölzel, B. K., Lazar, S. W., Gard, T., Schuman-Olivier, Z., Vago, D. R., & Ott, U. (2011). How does mindfulness meditation work? Proposing mechanisms of action from a conceptual and neural perspective. *Perspectives on Psychological Science, 6,* 537-559.

Hong, S., Nelesen, R. A., Krohn, P. L., Mills, P. J., & Dimsdale, J. E. (2006). The association of social status and blood pressure with markers of vascular inflammation. *Psychosomatic Medicine, 68,* 517-523.

Hopko, D. R., Clark, C. G., Cannity, K., & Bell, J. L. (2016). Pretreatment depression severity in breast cancer patients and its relation to treatment response to behavior therapy. *Health Psychology, 35,* 10-18.

Horan, M. J., & Roccella, E. J. (1988). Non-pharmacologic treatment of hypertension in the United States. *Health Psychology, 7* (Suppl.), 267-282.

Horrell, B., Stephens, C., & Breheny, M. (2015). Capability to care: Supporting the health of informational caregivers for older people. *Health Psychology, 34,* 339-348.

Horvath, K. J., Bowen, A. M., & Williams, M. L. (2006). Virtual and physical venues as contexts for HIV risk among rural men who have sex with men. *Health Psychology, 25,* 237-242.

Hostinar, C. E., Ross, K. M., Chen, E., & Miller, G. E. (2017). Early-life socioeconomic disadvantage and metabolic health disparities. *Psychosomatic Medicine, 79,* 514-523.

Hoth, K. F., Wamboldt, F. S., Strand, M., Ford, D. W., Sandhaus, R. A., Strange, C., Bekelman, D. B., & Holm, K. E. (2013). Prospective impact of illness uncertainty on outcomes in chronic lung disease. *Health Psychology, 32,* 1170-1174.

Hou, W. K., & Wan, J. H. Y. (2012). Perceived control mediates the prospective impact of relationship quality in the year after colorectal cancer diagnosis. *Annals of Behavioral Medicine, 43,* 129-138.

Houle, J. N. (2013). Depressive symptoms and all-cause mortality in a nationally representative longitudinal study with time-varying covariates. *Psychosomatic Medicine, 75,* 297-304.

House, J. A. (1981). *Work stress and social support.* Reading, MA: Addison-Wesley.

House, J. S. (2001). Understanding social factors and inequalities in health: 20th century progress and 21st century prospects. *Journal of Health and Social Behavior, 43,* 125-142.

House, J. S. (2015). *Beyond Obamacare: Life, death, and social policy.* New York: Russell Sage Foundation.

House, J. S., Landis, K. R., & Umberson, D. (1988). Social relationships and health. *Science, 241,* 540-545.

Houston, B. K., & Vavak, C. R. (1991). Cynical hostility: Developmental factors, psychosocial correlates, and health behaviors. *Health Psychology, 10,* 9-17.

Howe, L. C., Goyer, J. P., & Crum, A. J. (2017). Harnessing the placebo effect: Exploring the influence of physician characteristics on placebo response. *Health Psychology, 36,* 1074-1082.

Howren, B. M., & Suls, J. (2011). The symptom perception hypothesis revised: Depression and anxiety play different roles in concurrent and retrospective physical symptom reporting. *Journal of Personality and Social Psychology, 100,* 182-195.

Howren, B., Suls, J., & Martin, R. (2009). Depressive symptomatology, rather than neuroticism, predicts inflated physical symptom reports in community-residing women. *Psychosomatic Medicine, 71,* 951–957.

Hoyert, D. L. (2012). 75 years of mortality in the United States, 1935–2010. *NCHS Data Brief, 88,* 1–8.

Hoyt, M. A., & Stanton, A. L. (2012). Adjustment to chronic illness. In A. Baum, T. A. Revenson, & J. Singer (Eds.), *Handbook of health psychology* (2nd ed., pp. 219–246). New York: Taylor & Francis.

Hoyt, M. A., Thomas, K. S., Epstein, D. R., & Dirksen, S. R. (2009). Coping style and sleep quality in men with cancer. *Annals of Behavioral Medicine, 37,* 88–93.

Hu, F. B., Stampfer, M. J., Manson, J. E., Grodstein, F., Colditz, G. A., Speizer, F. E., & Willett, W. C. (2000). Trends in the incidence of coronary heart disease and changes in diet and lifestyle in women. *The New England Journal of Medicine, 343,* 530–537.

Hu, F. B., Willett, W. C., Li, T., Stampfer, M. J., Colditz, G. A., & Manson, J. E. (2004). Adiposity as compared with physical activity in predicting mortality among women. *The New England Journal of Medicine, 351,* 2694–2703.

Huebner, D. M., Kegeles, S. M., Rebchook, G. M., Peterson, J. L., Neilands, T. B., Johnson, W. D., & Eke, A. N. (2014). Social oppression, psychological vulnerability, and unprotected intercourse among Black men who have sex with men. *Health Psychology, 33,* 1568–1578.

Hughes, J. R. (1993). Pharmacotherapy for smoking cessation: Unvalidated assumptions, anomalies, and suggestions for future research. *Journal of Consulting and Clinical Psychology, 61,* 751–760.

Hughes, J. W., Fresco, D. M., Myerscough, R., van Dulmen, M. H. M., Carlson, L. E., & Josephson, R. (2013). Randomized controlled trial of mindfulness-based stress reduction for prehypertension. *Psychosomatic Medicine, 75,* 721–728.

Hughes, M. E., & Waite, L. J. (2002). Health in household context: Living arrangements and health in late middle age. *Journal of Health and Social Behavior, 43,* 1–21.

Huizink, A. C., Robles de Medina, P. G., Mulder, E. J. H., Visser, G. H. A., & Buitelaar, J. K. (2002). Coping in normal pregnancy. *Annals of Behavioral Medicine, 24,* 132–140.

Hundt, N. E., Renn, B. N., Sansgiry, S., Petersen, N. J., Stanley, M. A., Kauth, M. R., . . . Cully, J. A. (2018). Predictors of response to brief CBT in patients with cardiopulmonary conditions. *Health Psychology, 37,* 866–873.

Hunnicutt, J. N., Ulbricht, C. M., Tjia, J., & Lapane, K. L. (2017). Pain and pharmacologic pain management in long-stay nursing home residents. *Pain, 158,* 1091–1099.

Hunt, K., McCann, C., Gray, C. M., Mutrie, N., & Wyke, S. (2013). "You've got to walk before you run": Positive evaluations of a walking program as part of a gender-sensitized, weight-management program delivered to men through professional football clubs. *Health Psychology, 32,* 57–65.

Huntington, R., & Metcalf, P. (1979). *Celebrations of death: The anthropology of mortuary ritual.* New York: Cambridge University Press.

Huntington's Disease Society of America. (2019). *What is Huntington's disease? Overview of Huntington's disease.* Retrieved March 26, 2019, from https://hdsa.org/what-is-hd/overview-of-huntingtons-disease/

Hutchison, K. E., McGeary, J., Smolen, A., Bryan, A., & Swift, R. M. (2002). The DRD4 VNTR polymorphism moderates craving after alcohol consumption. *Health Psychology, 21,* 139–146.

Huth, C., Thorand, B., Baumert, J., Kruse, J., Emeny, R. T., Schneider, A., & Ladwig, K. (2014). Job strain as a risk factor for the onset of type 2 diabetes mellitus: Findings from the MONICA/KORA Augsburg cohort study. *Psychosomatic Medicine, 76,* 562–568.

Hwang, B., Moser, D. K., & Dracup, K. (2014). Knowledge is insufficient for self-care among heart failure patients with psychological distress. *Health Psychology, 33,* 588–596.

Iacovino, J. M., Bogdan, R., & Oltmanns, T. F. (2016). Personality predicts health declines through stressful life events during late mid-life. *Journal of Personality, 84,* 536–546.

Ickovics, J. R., Viscoli, C. M., & Horwitz, R. I. (1997). Functional recovery after myocardial infarction in men: The independent effects of social class. *Annals of Behavioral Medicine, 127,* 518–525.

Idler, E. L., Boulifard, D. A., & Contrada, R. J. (2012). Mending broken hearts: Marriage and survival following cardiac surgery. *Journal of Health and Social Behavior, 53,* 33–49.

Ikeda, H., Stark, J., Fischer, H., Wagner, M., Drdla, R., Jäger, T., & Sandkühler, J. (2006). Synaptic amplifier of inflammatory pain in the spinal dorsal horn. *Science, 312,* 1659–1662.

Ikram, U. Z., Snijder, M. B., Agyemang, C., Schene, A. H., Peters, R. J., Stronks, K., & Kunst, A. E. (2017). Perceived ethnic discrimination and the metabolic syndrome in ethnic minority groups: The healthy life in an urban setting study. *Psychosomatic Medicine, 79,* 101–111.

Inagaki, T. K., & Orehek, E. (2017). On the benefits of giving social support: When, why, and how support providers gain by caring for others. *Current Directions in Psychological Science, 26,* 109–113.

Inauen, J., Shrout, P. E., Bolger, N., Stadler, G., & Scholz, U. (2016). Mind the gap? An intensive longitudinal study of between-person and within-person intention-behavior relations. *Annals of Behavioral Medicine, 50,* 516–522.

Infurna, F. J., & Gerstorf, D. (2014). Perceived control relates to better functional health and lower cardio-metabolic risk: The mediating role of physical activity. *Health Psychology, 33,* 85–94.

Infurna, F. J., Gerstorf, D., Ram, N., Schupp, J., & Wagner, G. G. (2011). Long-term antecedents and outcomes of perceived control. *Psychology and Aging, 26,* 559–575.

Ingelfinger, J. R. (2004). Pediatric antecedents of adult cardiovascular disease-awareness and intervention. *The New England Journal of Medicine, 350,* 2123–2126.

Ingersoll, K. S., & Cohen, J. (2008). The impact of medication regiment factors on adherence to chronic treatment: A review of literature. *Journal of Behavioral Medicine, 31,* 213–224.

Ingram, R. E., Atkinson, J. H., Slater, M. A., Saccuzzo, D. P., & Garfin, S. R. (1990). Negative and positive cognition in depressed and nondepressed chronic-pain patients. *Health Psychology, 9,* 300–314.

Institute of Highway Safety. (2017). *Decline in fatal car accidents.* Retrieved from https://www.hg.org/legal-articles/decline-in-fatal-car-accidents-34822

International Foundation for Gastrointestinal Disorders. (2014). *Gastroesophageal reflux disease.* Retrieved March 18, 2019, from https://www.aboutgerd.org/images/pdfs/GERD-Infograph.jpg

Irish, L. A., Dougall, A. L., Delahanty, D. L., & Hall, M. H. (2013). The impact of sleep complaints on physical health and immune outcomes in rescue workers: A 1-year prospective study. *Psychosomatic Medicine, 75,* 196–201.

Ironson, G., & Hayward, H. (2008). Do positive psychosocial factors predict disease progression in HIV-1? A review of the evidence. *Psychosomatic Medicine, 70,* 546–554.

Ironson, G., Fitch, C., & Stuetzle, R. (2017). Depression and survival in a 17-year longitudinal study of people with HIV: Moderating effects of race and education. *Psychosomatic Medicine, 79,* 749–756.

Ironson, G., O'Cleirigh, C., Fletcher, M., Laurenceau, J. P., Balbin, E., Klimas, N., . . . Solomon, G. (2005). Psychosocial factors predict CD4 and viral load change in men and women with human immunodeficiency virus in the era of highly active antiretroviral treatment. *Psychosomatic Medicine, 67,* 1013–1021.

Ironson, G., O'Cleirigh, C., Weiss, A., Schneiderman, N., & Costa, P. T. (2008). Personality and HIV disease progression: Role of NEO-PI-R openness, extraversion, and profiles of engagement. *Psychosomatic Medicine, 70,* 245–253.

Ironson, G., Stuetzle, R., Ironson, D., Balbin, E., Kremer, H., George, A., . . . Fletcher, M. A. (2011). View of God as benevolent and forgiving or punishing and judgmental predicts HIV disease progression. *Journal of Behavioral Medicine, 34,* 414–425.

Ironson, G., Wynings, C., Schneiderman, N., Baum, A., Rodriguez, M., Greenwood, D., . . . Fletcher, M. A. (1997). Posttraumatic stress symptoms, intrusive thoughts, loss, and immune function after Hurricane Andrew. *Psychosomatic Medicine, 59,* 128–141.

Irvin, J. E., Bowers, C. A., Dunn, M. E., & Wang, M. C. (1999). Efficacy of relapse prevention: A meta-analytic review. *Journal of Consulting and Clinical Psychology, 67,* 563–570.

Irwin, M. R. (2015). Why sleep is important for health: A psychoneuroimmunology perspective. In S. T. Fiske, D. L. Schacter, & S. E. Taylor. *Annual Review of Psychology, 66,* 115–142.

Irwin, M. R., Cole, J. C., & Nicassio, P. M. (2006). Comparative meta-analysis of behavioral interventions for insomnia and their efficacy in middle-aged adults and in older adults 55+ years of age. *Health Psychology, 25,* 3–14.

Irwin, M. R., Pike, J. L., Cole, J. C., & Oxman, M. N. (2003). Effects of a behavioral intervention, tai chi chih, on Varicella-Zoster virus specific immunity and health functioning in older adults. *Psychosomatic Medicine, 65,* 824–830.

Itkowitz, N. I., Kerns, R. D., & Otis, J. D. (2003). Support and coronary heart disease: The importance of significant other responses. *Journal of Behavioral Medicine, 26,* 19–30.

Ivanovski, B., & Malhi, G. S. (2007). The psychological and neurophysiological concomitants of mindfulness forms of meditation. *Acta Neuropsychiatrica, 19,* 76–91.

Jachuck, S. J., Brierley, H., Jachuck, S., & Willcox, P. M. (1982). The effect of hypotensive drugs on the quality of life. *Journal of the Royal College of General Practitioners, 32,* 103–105.

Jakubowski, K. P., Cundiff, J. M., & Matthews, K. A. (2018). Cumulative childhood adversity and adult cardiometabolic disease: A meta-analysis. *Health Psychology, 37,* 701–715.

Jack, A. (2007, April 25). Climate change bites. *Financial Times,* p. 9.

Jackson, K. M., & Aiken, L. S. (2006). Evaluation of a multicomponent appearance-based sun-protective intervention for young women: Uncovering the mechanisms of program efficacy. *Health Psychology, 25,* 34–46.

Jacobs, N., Rijsdijk, F., Derom, C., Vlietinck, R., Delespaul, P., Van Os, J., & Myin-Germeys, I. (2006). Genes making one feel blue in the flow of daily life: A momentary assessment study of gene–stress interaction. *Psychosomatic Medicine, 68,* 201–206.

Jacobs, T. L., Shaver, P. R., Epel, E. S., Zanesco, A. P., Aichele, S. R., Bird well, D. A., & Saron, C. D. (2013). Self-reported mindfulness and cortisol during a Shamatha meditation retreat. *Health Psychology, 33,* 1104–1109.

Jacobsen, P. B., & Andrykowski, M. A. (2015). Tertiary prevention in cancer care: Understanding and addressing the psychological dimensions of cancer during the active treatment period. *American Psychologist, 70,* 134–145.

James, S. A., Hartnett, S. A., & Kalsbeek, W. D. (1983). John Henryism and blood pressure differences among Black men. *Journal of Behavioral Medicine, 6,* 259–278.

James, S. A., Keenan, N. L., Strogatz, D. S., Browning, S. R., & Garrett, J. M. (1992). Socioeconomic status, John Henryism, and blood pressure in Black adults: The Pitt County study. *American Journal of Epidemiology, 135,* 59–67.

Jameson, M. (2004, January 19). No standing pat. *Los Angeles Times,* p. F7.

Jamieson, J. P., Mendes, W. B., & Nock, M. K. (2013). Improving acute stress responses: The power of reappraisal. *Current Directions in Psychological Science, 22,* 51–56.

Janicki-Deverts, D., Cohen, S., Matthews, K. A., & Cullen, M. R. (2008). History of unemployment predicts future elevations in C-reactive protein among male participants in the coronary artery risk development in young adults (CARDIA) study. *Annals of Behavioral Medicine, 36,* 176–185.

Janicki-Deverts, D., Cohen, S., Matthews, K. A., & Jacobs, D. R., Jr. (2012). Sex differences in the association of childhood socioeconomic status with adult blood pressure change: The CARDIA Study. *Psychosomatic Medicine, 74,* 728–735.

Janis, I. L. (1958). *Psychological stress.* New York: Wiley.

Janssen, I., Powell, L. H., Jasielec, M. S., Matthews, K. A., Hollenberg, S. M., Sutton-Tyrrell, K., & Everson-Rose, S. A. (2012). Progression of coronary artery calcification in Black and White women: Do the stresses and rewards of multiple roles matter? *Annals of Behavioral Medicine, 43,* 39–49.

Jaremka, L. M., Andridge, R. R., Fagundes, C. P., Alfano, C. M., Povoski, S. P., Lipari, A. M., & Kiecolt-Glaser, J. K. (2014). Pain, depression, and fatigue: Loneliness as a longitudinal risk factor. *Health Psychology, 33,* 948–957.

Jaremka, L. M., Derry, H. M., Bornstein, R., Prakash, R. S., Peng, J., Belury, M. A., & Kiecolt-Glaser, J. K. (2014). Omega-3 supplementation and loneliness-related memory problems: Secondary analyses of a randomized controlled trial. *Psychosomatic Medicine, 76,* 650–658.

Jarrin, D. C., McGrath, J. J., & Quon, E. C. (2014). Objective and subjective socioeconomic gradients exist for sleep in children and adolescents. *Health Psychology, 33,* 301–305.

Jay, S. M., Elliott, C. H., Woody, P. D., & Siegel, S. (1991). An investigation of cognitive-behavior therapy combined with oral Valium for children undergoing painful medical procedures. *Health Psychology, 10,* 317–322.

Jeffery, R. W., Hennrikus, D. J., Lando, H. A., Murray, D. M., & Liu, J. W. (2000). Reconciling conflicting findings regarding postcessation weight concerns and success in smoking cessation. *Health Psychology, 19,* 242–246.

Jeffery, R. W., Pirie, P. L., Rosenthal, B. S., Gerber, W. M., & Murray, D. M. (1982). Nutritional education in supermarkets: An unsuccessful attempt to influence knowledge and produce sales. *Journal of Behavioral Medicine, 5,* 189–200.

Jemmott, J. B., III, Croyle, R. T., & Ditto, P. H. (1988). Commonsense epidemiology: Self-based judgments from laypersons and physicians. *Health Psychology, 7,* 55–73.

Jemmott, J. B., III, Jemmott, L. S., & Fong, G. (1992). Reductions in HIV risk–associated sexual behaviors among Black male adolescents: Effects of an AIDS prevention intervention. *American Journal of Public Health, 82,* 372–377.

Jemmott, J. B., III, Jemmott, L. S., O'Leary, A., Ngwane, Z., Lewis, D. A., Bellamy, S. L., & Teitelman, A. (2015). HIV/STI risk-reduction intervention efficacy with South African adolescents over 54 months. *Health Psychology, 34,* 610–621.

Jensen-Johansen, M. B., O'Toole, M. S., Christensen, S., Valdimarsdottir, H., Zakowski, S., Bovbjerg, D. H., . . . Zachariae, R. (2018). Expressive writing intervention and self-reported physical health outcomes—Results from a nationwide randomized controlled trial with breast cancer patients. *PLoS One, 13*(2), e0192729.

Jensen, M., & Patterson, D. R. (2006). Hypnotic treatment of chronic pain. *Journal of Behavioral Medicine, 29,* 95–124.

Jensen, M. P., & Patterson, D. R. (2014). Hypnotic approaches for chronic pain management: Clinical implications of recent research findings. *American Psychologist, 69,* 167–177.

Jim, H. S. L., Jacobsen, P. B., Phillips, K. M., Wenham, R. M., Roberts, W., & Small, B. J. (2013). Lagged relationships among sleep disturbance, fatigue, and depressed mood during chemotherapy. *Health Psychology, 32,* 768–774.

Jimerson, D. C., Mantzoros, C., Wolfe, B. E., & Metzger, E. D. (2000). Decreased serum leptin in bulimia nervosa. *The Journal of Clinical Endocrinology & Metabolism, 85,* 4511–4514.

Joben, J., Wrosch, C., & Scheier, M. F. (2014). Associations between dispositional optimism and diurnal cortisol in a community sample: When stress is perceived as higher than normal. *Health Psychology, 33,* 382–391.

Johansson, E., & Lindberg, P. (2000). Low back pain patients in primary care: Subgroups based on the multidimensional pain inventory. *International Journal of Behavioral Medicine, 7,* 340–352.

John-Henderson, N. A., Kamarck, T. W., Muldoon, M. F., & Manuck, S. B. (2016). Early life family conflict, social interactions and carotid artery intima-media thickness in adulthood. *Psychosomatic Medicine, 78,* 319–326.

Johnsen, L., Spring, B., Pingitore, R., Sommerfeld, B. K., & MacKirnan, D. (2002). Smoking as subculture? Influence on Hispanic and non-Hispanic white women's attitudes toward smoking and obesity. *Health Psychology, 21,* 279–287.

Johnson, J. (1982). The effects of a patient education course on persons with a chronic illness. *Cancer Nursing, 5,* 117–123.

Johnson, J. E. (1984). Psychological interventions and coping with surgery. In A. Baum, S. E. Taylor, & J. E. Singer (Eds.), *Handbook of psychology and health* (Vol. 4, pp. 167–188). Hillsdale, NJ: Erlbaum.

Johnson, J. E., Cohen, P., Pine, D. S., Klein, D. F., Kasen, S., & Brook, J. S. (2000). Association between cigarette smoking and anxiety disorders during adolescence and early adulthood. *Journal of the American Medical Association, 284,* 2348–2351.

Johnson, J. E., & Leventhal, H. (1974). Effects of accurate expectations and behavioral instructions on reactions during a noxious medical examination. *Journal of Personality and Social Psychology, 29,* 710–718.

Johnson, M. K. (2004). Further evidence on adolescent employment and substance use: Differences by race and ethnicity. *Journal of Health and Social Behavior, 45,* 187–197.

Johnson, M. O., Neilands, T. B., Dilworth, S. E., Morin, S. F., Remien, R. H., & Chesney, M. A. (2007). The role of self-efficacy in HIV treatment adherence: Validation of the HIV treatment adherence self-efficacy scale (HIV-ASES). *Journal of Behavioral Medicine, 30,* 359–370.

Johnson, R. J., McCaul, K. D., & Klein, W. M. P. (2002). Risk involvement and risk perception among adolescents and young adults. *Journal of Behavioral Medicine, 25,* 67–82.

Johnson, S. B. (2012). Increasing psychology's role in integrated care. *Monitor on Psychology,* p. 5.

Johnson, S. B., Freund, A., Silverstein, J., Hansen, C. A., & Malone, J. (1990). Adherence-health status relationships in childhood diabetes. *Health Psychology, 9,* 606–631.

Johnson, S. B., Park, H. S., Gross, C. P., & Yu, J. B. (2017). Use of alternative medicine for cancer and its impact on survival. *Journal of the National Cancer Institute, 110,* 121–124.

Johnson, S. S., Paiva, A. L., Mauriello, L., Prochaska, J. O., Redding, C., & Velicer, W. F. (2014). Coaction in multiple behavior change interventions: Consistency across multiple studies on weight management and obesity prevention. *Health Psychology, 33,* 475–480.

Jokela, M., Elovainio, M., Nyberg, S. T., Tabak, A. G., Hintsa, T., Batty, G. D., & Kivimaki, M. (2014). Personality and risk of diabetes in adults: Pooled analysis of 5 cohort studies. *Health Psychology, 33,* 1618–1621.

Jokela, M., Elovainio, M., Singh-Manoux, A., & Kivimäki, M. (2009). IQ, socioeconomic status, and early death: The US national longitudinal survey of youth. *Psychosomatic Medicine, 71,* 322–328.

Jonas, B. S., & Mussolino, M. E. (2000). Symptoms of depression as a prospective risk factor of stroke. *Psychosomatic Medicine, 62,* 463–471.

Jones, A. L., Moss, A. J., & Harris-Kojetin, L. D. (2011). Use of advance directives in long-term care populations. *NCHS Data Brief, 54,* 1–8.

Jones, D. J., Beach, S. R. H., Forehand, R., & Foster, S. E. (2003). Self-reported health in HIV-positive African American women: The role of family stress and depressive symptoms. *Journal of Behavioral Medicine, 26,* 577–599.

Jorgensen, R. S., Frankowski, J. J., & Carey, M. P. (1999). Sense of coherence, negative life events and appraisal of physical health among university students. *Personality and Individual Differences, 27,* 1079–1089.

Joseph, N. T., Matthews, K. A., & Myers, H. F. (2014). Conceptualizing health consequences of Hurricane Katrina from the perspective of socioeconomic status decline. *Health Psychology, 33,* 139–146.

Jun, H. J., Subramanian, S. V., Gortmaker, S., & Kawachi, I. (2004). A multilevel analysis of women's status and self-rated health in the United States. *Journal of the American Medical Women's Association, 59,* 172–180.

Jung, M. E., Latimer-Cheung, A. E., Bourne, J. E., & Martin Ginis, K. A. (2016). Targeted messages increase dairy consumption in adults: A randomized controlled trial. *Annals of Behavioral Medicine, 51,* 57–66.

Kabat-Zinn, J., & Chapman-Waldrop, A. (1988). Compliance with an outpatient stress reduction program: Rates and predictors of program completion. *Journal of Behavioral Medicine, 11,* 333–352.

Kahana, E., Lawrence, R. H., Kahana, B., Kercher, K., Wisniewski, A., Stoller, E., . . . Stange, K. (2002). Long-term impact of preventive proactivity on quality of life of the old-old. *Psychosomatic Medicine, 64,* 382–394.

Kahn, R. L. (1981). *Work and health.* New York: Wiley.

Kahn, R. L., & Juster, F. T. (2002). Well-being: Concepts and measures. *Journal of Social Issues, 58,* 627–644.

Kaiser Family Foundation. (2017, April). *Views and experiences with end-of-life medical care in the U.S.* Retrieved May 8, 2019, from https://www.kff.org/report-section/views-and-experiences-with-end-of-life-medical-care-in-the-us-findings/

Kaiser Family Foundation and Health Research and Education Trust. (2011). *Employer health benefits: Annual survey 2011.* Retrieved March 13, 2013, from http://ehbs.kff.org/pdf/2011/8225.pdf

Kaiser State Health Facts. (2011). *Total HMO enrollment, July 2011.* Retrieved August 6, 2012, from http://www.statehealthfacts.org/comparemaptable.jsp?cat=7&ind=348

Kalaydjian, A., & Merikangas, K. (2008). Physical and mental comorbidity of headache in a national representative sample of U.S. adults. *Psychosomatic Medicine, 70,* 773–780.

Kalichman, S. C. (2008). Co-occurrence of treatment nonadherence and continued HIV transmission risk behavior: Implications for positive prevention interventions. *Psychosomatic Medicine, 70,* 593–597.

Kalichman, S. C., Benotsch, E. G., Weinhardt, L., Austin, J., Luke, W., & Cherry, C. (2003). Health related Internet use, coping, social support, and health indicators in people living with HIV/AIDS: Preliminary results from community survey. *Health Psychology, 22,* 111–116.

Kalichman, S. C., Cain, D., Weinhardt, L., Benotsch, E., Presser, K., Zweben, A., . . . Swain, G. R. (2005). Experimental components analysis of brief theory-based HIV/AIDS risk-reduction counseling for sexually transmitted infection patients. *Health Psychology, 24,* 198–208.

Kalichman, S. C., Carey, M. P., & Johnson, B. T. (1996). Prevention of sexually transmitted HIV infection: A meta-analytic review of the behavioral outcome literature. *Annals of Behavioral Medicine, 18,* 6–15.

Kalichman, S. C., Cherry, C., Cain, D., Weinhardt, L. S., Benotsch, E., Pope, H., & Kalichman, M. (2006). Health information on the Internet and people living with HIV/AIDS: Information evaluation and coping styles. *Health Psychology, 25,* 205–210.

Kalichman, S. C., DiMarco, M., Austin, J., Luke, W., & DiFonzo, K. (2003). Stress, social support, and HIV-status disclosure to family and friends among HIV-positive men and women. *Journal of Behavioral Medicine, 26,* 315–332.

Kalichman, S. C., Eaton, L., Cain, D., Cherry, C., Fuhrel, A., Kaufman, & Pope, H. (2007). Changes in HIV treatment beliefs and sexual risk behaviors among gay and bisexual men, 1997–2005. *Health Psychology, 26,* 650–656.

Kalichman, S. C., & Grebler, T. (2010). Stress and poverty predictors of treatment adherence among people with low-literacy living with HIV/AIDS. *Psychosomatic Medicine, 72,* 810–816.

Kamarck, T. W., Muldoon, M. F., Shiffman, S. S., & Sutton-Tyrrell, K. (2007). Experiences of demand and control during daily life are predictors of carotid atherosclerotic progression among healthy men. *Health Psychology, 26,* 324–332.

Kamarck, T. W., Muldoon, M. F., Shiffman, S., Sutton-Tyrell, K., Gwaltney, C., & Janieki, D. L. (2004). Experiences of demand and control in daily life as correlates of subclinical carotid atherosclerosis in a healthy older sample. *Health Psychology, 23,* 24–32.

Kanaan, R. A. A., Lepine, J. P., & Wessely, S. C. (2007). The association or otherwise of the functional somatic syndromes. *Psychosomatic Medicine, 69,* 855–859.

Kang, Y., O'Donnell, M. B., Strecher, V. J., Taylor, S. E., Lieberman, M. D., & Falk, E. B. (2017). Self-transcendent values and neural responses to threatening health messages. *Psychosomatic Medicine, 79,* 379–387.

Kaplan, G. A., & Reynolds, P. (1988). Depression and cancer mortality and morbidity: Prospective evidence from the Alameda County Study. *Journal of Behavioral Medicine, 11,* 1–13.

Kaplan, K. (2014, September 5). U.S. obesity rates finally hold steady. *The New York Times,* p. A6.

Kaplan, K. (2015, October 22). Analysis links stroke risk to stressful jobs. *The New York Times,* p. A9.

Kaplan, R. M. (1990). Behavior as the central outcome in health care. *American Psychologist, 45,* 1211–1220.

Kaplan, R. M. (2000). Two pathways to prevention. *American Psychologist, 55,* 382–396.

Kaplan, R. M. (2003). The significance of quality of life in health care. *Quality of Life Research,* 12 (Suppl. 1), 3–16.

Kaplan, R. M., Ries, A. L., Prewitt, L. M., & Eakin, E. (1994). Self-efficacy expectations predict survival for patients with chronic obstructive pulmonary disease. *Health Psychology, 13,* 366–368.

Kaplan, R. M., & Simon, H. J. (1990). Compliance in medical care: Reconsideration of self-predictions. *Annals of Behavioral Medicine, 12,* 66–71.

Kaptein, A. A., Bijsterbosch, J., Scharloo, M., Hampson, S. E., Kroon, H. M., & Kloppenburg, M., (2010). Using the common sense model of illness perceptions to examine osteoarthritis change: A 6-year longitudinal study. *Health Psychology, 29,* 56–64.

Kapuku, G. K., Davis, H., Murdison, K., Robinson, V., & Harshfield, G. (2012). Stress reduces diastolic function in youth. *Psychosomatic Medicine, 74,* 588–595.

Karasek, R., Baker, D., Marxer, F., Ahlbom, A., & Theorell, T. (1981). Job decision latitude, job demands, and cardiovascular disease: A prospective study of Swedish men. *American Journal of Public Health, 71,* 694–705.

Karatsoreos, I. N., & McEwen, B. S. (2011). Psychobiological allostasis: Resistance, resilience, and vulnerability. *Trends in Cognitive Sciences, 15,* 576–584.

Karlamangla, A. S., Singer, B. H., & Seeman, T. E. (2006). Reduction in allostatic load in older adults is associated with lower all-cause mortality risk: MacArthur studies of successful aging. *Psychosomatic Medicine, 68,* 500–507.

Karlan, W. A., Brondolo, E., & Schwartz, J. (2003). Workplace social support and ambulatory cardiovascular activity in New York City traffic agents. *Psychosomatic Medicine, 65,* 167–176.

Karlson, C. W., Gallagher, M. W., Olson, C. A., & Hamilton, N. A. (2013). Insomnia symptoms and well being: Longitudinal follow-up. *Health Psychology, 32,* 311–319.

Kärmeniemi, M., Lankila, T., Ikäheimo, T., Koivumaa-Honkanen, H., & Korpelainen, R. (2018). The built environment as a determinant of physical activity: A systematic review of longitudinal studies and natural experiments. *Annals of Behavioral Medicine, 52,* 239–251.

Karoly, P., Okun, M. A., Enders, C., & Tennen, H. (2014). Effects of pain intensity on goal schemas and goal pursuit: A daily diary study. *Health Psychology, 33,* 968–976.

Karoly, P., & Ruehlman, L. S. (1996). Motivational implications of pain: Chronicity, psychological distress, and work goal construal in a national sample of adults. *Health Psychology, 15,* 383–390.

Kashdan, T. B., & Nezlek, J. B. (2012). Whether, when, and how is spirituality related to well-being? Moving beyond single occasion questionnaires to understanding daily process. *Personality and Social Psychology Bulletin, 38,* 1523–1535.

Kasl, S. V., & Berkman, L. (1983). Health consequences of the experience of migration. *Annual Review of Public Health, 4,* 69–90.

Kassem, N. O., & Lee, J. W. (2004). Understanding soft drink consumption among male adolescents using the theory of planned behavior. *Journal of Behavioral Medicine, 27,* 273–296.

Kastenbaum, R. (1977). Death and development through the lifespan. In H. Feifel (Ed.), *New meanings of death* (pp. 17–46). New York: McGraw-Hill.

Katon, W. J., Richardson, L., Lozano, P., & McCauley, E. (2004). The relationship of asthma and anxiety disorder. *Psychosomatic Medicine, 66,* 349–355.

Katon, W., Russo, J., Lin, E. H. B., Heckbert, S. R., Karter, A. J., Williams, L. H., . . . Von Korff, M. (2009). Diabetes and poor disease control: Is comorbid depression associated with poor medication adherence or lack of treatment intensification? *Psychosomatic Medicine, 71,* 965–972.

Katon, W., Von Korff, W., Lin, E., Lipscomb, P., Russo, J., Wagner, E., & Polk, E. (1990). Distressed high utilizers of medical care: *DSM-III-R* diagnosis and treatment needs. *General Hospital Psychiatry, 12,* 355–362.

Katz, J. (2017, June 6). U.S. drug deaths climbing faster than ever. *The New York Times,* pp. A1, A12.

Katz, R. C., Flasher, L., Cacciapaglia, H., & Nelson, S. (2001). The psychological impact of cancer and lupus: A cross validation study that extends the generality of "benefit finding" in patients with chronic disease. *Journal of Behavioral Medicine, 24,* 561–571.

Katzman, M. A., Bara-Carril, N., Rabe-Hesketh, S., Schmidt, U., Troop, N., & Treasure, J. (2010). A randomized controlled two-stage trial in the treatment of bulimia nervosa, comparing CBT versus motivational enhancement in phase 1 followed by group versus individual CBT in phase 2. *Psychosomatic Medicine, 72,* 656–663.

Kaufman, M. R. (1970). Practicing good manners and compassion. *Medical Insight, 2,* 56–61.

Kavalieratos, D., Corbelli, J., Zhang, D., Dionne-Odom, J. N., Ernecoff, N. C., . . . Schenker, Y. (2016). Association between palliative care and patient and caregiver outcomes: A systematic review and meta-analysis. *Journal of the American Medical Association, 316,* 2104–2114.

Kaysen, D., Pantalone, D. W., Chawla, N., Lindgren, K. P., Clum, G. A., Lee, C., & Resick, P. A. (2008). Posttraumatic stress disorder, alcohol use, and physical concerns. *Journal of Behavioral Medicine, 31,* 115–125.

Keane, T. M., & Wolfe, J. (1990). Comorbidity in post-traumatic stress disorder: An analysis of community and clinical studies. *Journal of Applied Social Psychology, 20,* 1776–1788.

Keefe, F. J., Caldwell, D. S., Queen, K. T., Gil, K. M., Martinez, S., Crisson, J. E., . . . Nunley, J. (1987). Pain coping strategies in osteoarthritis patients. *Journal of Consulting and Clinical Psychology, 55,* 208-212.

Keefe, F. J., Dunsmore, J., & Burnett, R. (1992). Behavioral and cognitive-behavioral approaches to chronic pain: Recent advances and future directions. *Journal of Consulting and Clinical Psychology, 60,* 528-536.

Kehler, M. D., & Hadjistavropoulos, H. D. (2009). Is health anxiety a significant problem for individuals with multiple sclerosis? *Journal of Behavioral Medicine, 32,* 150-161.

Kellerman, J., Rigler, D., & Siegel, S. E. (1979). Psychological responses of children to isolation in a protected environment. *Journal of Behavioral Medicine, 2,* 263-274.

Kelley, J. M., Lembo, A. J., Ablon, S., Villanueva, J. J., Conboy, L. A., Levy, R., . . . Kaptchuk, T. J. (2009). Patient and practitioner influences on the placebo effect in irritable bowel syndrome. *Psychosomatic Medicine, 71,* 789-797.

Kelly, J. A., Lawrence, J. S., Hood, H. V., & Brasfield, T. L. (1989). Behavioral intention to reduce AIDS risk activities. *Journal of Consulting and Clinical Psychology, 57,* 60-67.

Kemeny, M. E. (2003). The psychobiology of stress. *Current Directions, 12,* 124-129.

Kemps, E., Tiggemann, M., & Hollitt, S. (2014). Biased attentional processing of food cues and modification in obese individuals. *Health Psychology, 33,* 1391-1401.

Keng, S. L., Smoski, M. J., & Robins, C. J. (2011). Effects of mindfulness on psychological health: A review of empirical studies. *Clinical Psychology Review, 31,* 1041-56.

Kent, D. G., Uchino, B. N., Trettevik, R., Cronan, S., & Hogan, J. N. (2018). Social support and sleep: A meta-analysis. *Health Psychology, 37,* 787-798.

Kerameas, K., Vartanian, L. R., Herman, C. P., & Polivy, J. (2015). The effect of portion size and unit size on food intake: Unit bias or segmentation effect? *Health Psychology, 34,* 670-676.

Kerckhoff, A. C., & Back, K. W. (1968). *The June bug: A study of hysterical contagion.* New York: Appleton-Century-Crofts.

Kern, M. L., Friedman, H. S., Martin, L. R., Reynolds, C. A., & Luong, G. (2009). Conscientiousness, career success, and longevity: A lifespan analysis. *Annals of Behavioral Medicine, 37,* 154-163.

Kern, M. L., Reynolds, C. A., & Friedman, H. S. (2010). Predictors of physical activity patterns across adulthood: A growth curve analysis. *Personality and Social Psychology Bulletin, 36,* 1058-1072.

Kerns, R. D., Rosenberg, R., & Otis, J. D. (2002). Self-appraised problem solving and pain-relevant social support as predictors of the experience of chronic pain. *Annals of Behavioral Medicine, 24,* 100-105.

Kershaw, K. N., Mezuk, B., Abdou, C. M., Rafferty, J. A., & Jackson, J. S. (2010). Socioeconomic position, health behaviors, and C-reactive protein: A moderated-mediation analysis. *Health Psychology, 29,* 307-316.

Kershaw, T. S., Ethier, K. A., Niccolai, L. M., Lewis J. B., & Ickovics, J. R. (2003). Misperceived risk among female adolescents: Social and psychological factors associated with sexual risk accuracy. *Health Psychology, 22,* 523-532.

Kershaw, T. S., Ethier, K. A., Niccolai, L. M., Lewis, J. B., Milan, S., Meade, C., & Ickovics, J. R. (2010). Let's stay together: Relationship dissolution and sexually transmitted diseases among parenting and non-parenting adolescents. *Journal of Behavioral Medicine, 33,* 454-465.

Kershaw, T. S., Mood, D. W., Newth, G., Ronis, D. L., Sandra, M. G., Vaishampayan, U., & Northouse, L. L. (2008). Longitudinal analysis of a model to predict quality of life in prostate cancer patients and their spouses. *Annals of Behavioral Medicine, 36,* 117-128.

Kerst, W. F., & Waters, A. J. (2014). Attentional retaining administered in the field reduces smokers' attentional bias and craving. *Health Psychology, 33,* 1232-1240.

Kessler, R. C., Berglund, P. A., Chiu, W. T., Deitz, A. C., Hudson, J. I., Shahly, V., & Aguilar-Gaxiola, S. (2013). The prevalence and correlates of binge eating disorder in the World Health Organization world mental health surveys. *Biological Psychiatry, 73,* 904-914.

Kessler, R. C., Kendler, K. S., Heath, A. C., Neale, M. C., & Eaves, L. J. (1992). Social support, depressed mood, and adjustment to stress: A genetic epidemiological investigation. *Journal of Personality and Social Psychology, 62,* 257-272.

Kessler, R. C., Turner, J. B., & House, J. S. (1987). Intervening processes in the relationship between unemployment and health. *Psychological Medicine, 17,* 949-961.

Kessler, R. C., Turner, J. B., & House, J. S. (1988). Effects of unemployment on health in a community survey: Main, modifying, and mediating effects. *Journal of Social Issues, 44,* 69-85.

Key, B. L., Campbell, T. S., Bacon, S. L., & Gerin, W. (2008). The influence of trait and state rumination on cardiovascular recovery from a negative emotional stressor. *Journal of Behavioral Medicine, 31,* 237-248.

Khaddouma, A., Gordon, K. C., Fish, L. J., Bilheimer, A., Gonzalez, A., & Pollak, K. I. (2015). Relationships among spousal communication, self-efficacy, and motivation among expectant Latino fathers who smoke. *Health Psychology, 34,* 1038-1042.

Khan, C. M., Stephens, M. A. P., Franks, M. M., Rook, K. S., & Salem, J. K. (2013). Influences of spousal support and control on diabetes management through physical activity. *Health Psychology, 32,* 739-747.

Kiecolt-Glaser, J. K. (2018). Marriage, divorce, and the immune system. *American Psychologist, 73,* 1098-1108.

Kiecolt-Glaser, J. K., Christian, L., Preston, H., Houts, C. R., Malarkey, W. B., Emery, C. F., & Glaser, R. (2010). Stress, inflammation, and yoga practice. *Psychosomatic Medicine, 72,* 113-121.

Kiecolt-Glaser, J. K., Derry, H. M., & Fagundes, C. P. (2015). Inflammation: Depression fans the flames and feasts on the heat. *American Journal of Psychiatry, 172,* 1075-1091.

Kiecolt-Glaser, J. K., Fisher, L., Ogrocki, P., Stout, J. C., Speicher, C. E., & Glaser, R. (1987). Marital quality, marital disruption, and immune function. *Psychosomatic Medicine, 49,* 13-34.

Kiecolt-Glaser, J. K., & Glaser, R. (1987). Psychosocial influences on herpes virus latency. In E. Kurstak, Z. J. Lipowski, & P. V. Morozov (Eds.), *Viruses, immunity, and mental disorders* (pp. 403-412). New York: Plenum.

Kiecolt-Glaser, J. K., Glaser, R., Cacioppo, J. T., MacCallum, R. C., Snydersmith, M., Kim, C., & Malarkey, W. B. (1997). Marital conflict in older adults: Endocrinological and immunological correlates. *Psychosomatic Medicine, 59,* 339-349.

Kiecolt-Glaser, J. K., Glaser, R., Gravenstein, S., Malarkey, W. B., & Sheridan, J. (1996). Chronic stress alters the immune response to influenza virus vaccine in older adults. *Proceedings of the National Academy of Science, 93,* 3043-3047.

Kiecolt-Glaser, J. K., Glaser, R., Williger, D., Stout, J., Messick, G., Sheppard, S., . . . Donnerberg, R. (1985). Psychosocial enhancement of immuno-competence in a geriatric population. *Health Psychology, 4,* 25-41.

Kiecolt-Glaser, J. K., Loving, T. J., Stowell, J. R., Malarkey, W. B., Lemeshow, S., Dickinson, S. L., & Glaser, R. (2005). Hostile marital interactions, proinflammatory cytokine production, and wound healing. *Archives of General Psychiatry, 62,* 1377-1384.

Kiecolt-Glaser, J. K., Malarkey, W. B., Chee, M. A., Newton, T., Cacioppo, J. T., Mao, H. Y., & Glaser, R. (1993). Negative behavior during marital conflict is associated with immunological down-regulation. *Psychosomatic Medicine, 55,* 395-409.

Kiecolt-Glaser, J. K., Marucha, P. T., Malarkey, W. B., Mercado, A. M., & Glaser, R. (1995). Slowing of wound healing by psychological stress. *Lancet, 346,* 1194-1196.

Kiecolt-Glaser, J. K., McGuire, L., Robles, T. F., & Glaser, R. (2002). Psychoneuroimmunology and psychosomatic medicine: Back to the future. *Psychosomatic Medicine, 64,* 15–28.

Kiecolt-Glaser, J. K., & Newton, T. L. (2001). Marriage and health: His and hers. *Psychological Bulletin, 127,* 472–503.

Kiecolt-Glaser, J. K., & Wilson, S. J. (2016). Psychiatric disorders, morbidity, and mortality: Tracing mechanistic pathways to accelerated aging. *Psychosomatic Medicine, 78,* 772–775.

Kiene, S. M., Fisher, W. A., Shuper, P. A., Cornman, D. H., Christie, S., MacDonald, S., & Fisher, J. D. (2013). Understanding HIV transmission risk behavior among HIV-infected South Africans receiving antiretroviral therapy. *Health Psychology, 32,* 860–868.

Kiene, S. M., Tennen, H., & Armeli, S. (2008). Today I'll use a condom, but who knows about tomorrow: A daily process study of variability in predictions of condom use. *Health Psychology, 27,* 463–472.

Kiernan, M., Oppezzo, M. A., Resnicow, K., & Alexander, G. L. (2018). Effects of a methodological infographic on research participants' knowledge, transparency, and trust. *Health Psychology, 37,* 782–786.

Kim, E. S., Kubzansky, L. D., & Smith, J. (2015). Life satisfaction and use of preventive health care services. *Health Psychology, 34,* 779–782.

Kim, J., Knight, B. G., & Longmire, C. V. (2007). The role of familism in stress and coping processes among African American and White dementia caregivers: Effects on mental and physical health. *Health Psychology, 26,* 564–576.

Kim, Y., Valdimarsdottir, H. B., & Bovbjerg, D. H. (2003). Family histories of breast cancer, coping styles, and psychological adjustment. *Journal of Behavioral Medicine, 26,* 225–243.

Kincaid, E. (2017, September 13). How to fix the ER. *The Wall Street Journal,* pp. R1, R2.

King, A. C., Hekler, E. B., Castro, C. M., Buman, M. P., Marcus, B. H., Friedman, R. H., & Napolitano, M. A. (2014). Exercise advice by humans versus computers: Maintenance effects at 18 months. *Health Psychology, 33,* 192–196.

King, K. B., & Reis, H. T. (2012). Marriage and long-term survival after coronary artery bypass grafting. *Health Psychology, 31,* 55–62.

Kiplinger's Retirement Report. (2019, January). Your questions answered. *Kiplinger's Retirement Report,* p. 11.

Kirby, J. B. (2002). The influence of parental separation on smoking initiation in adolescents. *Journal of Health and Social Behavior, 43,* 56–71.

Kirby, J. B., & Kaneda, T. (2005). Neighborhood socioeconomic disadvantage and access to health care. *Journal of Health and Social Behavior, 46,* 15–31.

Kirkham, J. A., Smith, J. A., & Havsteen-Franklin, D. (2015). Painting pain: An interpretative phenomenological analysis of representations of living with chronic pain. *Health Psychology, 34,* 398–406.

Kirschbaum, C., Klauer, T., Filipp, S., & Hellhammer, D. H. (1995). Sex-specific effects of social support on cortisol and subjective responses to acute psychological stress. *Psychosomatic Medicine, 57,* 23–31.

Kitayama, S., Park, J., Boylan, J. M., Miyamoto, Y., Levine, C. S., Markus, H. R., & Ryff, C. D. (2015). Expression of anger and ill health in two cultures: An examination of inflammation and cardiovascular risk. *Psychological Science, 26,* 1–10.

Kitzmann, K. M., Dalton, W. T., Stanley, C. M., Beech, B. M., Reeves, T. P., Buscemi, J., . . . Midgett, E. L. (2010). Lifestyle interventions for youth who are overweight: A meta-analytic review. *Health Psychology, 29,* 91–101.

Kivimäki, M., Head, J., Ferrie, J. E., Brunner, E., Marmot, M. G., Vahtera, J., & Shipley, M. J. (2006). Why is evidence on job strain and coronary heart disease mixed? An illustration of measurement challenges in the Whitehall II study. *Psychosomatic Medicine, 68,* 398–401.

Kiviniemi, M. T., Klasko-Foster, L., Erwin, D. O., & Jandorf, L. (2018). Decision-making and socioeconomic disparities in colonoscopy screening in African Americans. *Health Psychology, 37,* 481–490.

Kivimäki, M., Vahtera, J., Elovainio, M., Lillrank, B., & Kevin, M. V. (2002). Death or illness of a family member, violence, interpersonal conflict, and financial difficulties as predictors of sickness absence. Longitudinal cohort study on psychological and behavioral links. *Psychosomatic Medicine, 64,* 817–825.

Kiviniemi, M. T., Voss-Humke, A. M., & Seifert, A. L. (2007). How do I feel about the behavior? The interplay of affective associations with behaviors and cognitive beliefs as influences on physical activity behavior. *Health Psychology, 26,* 152–158.

Kivlahan, D. R., Marlatt, G. A., Fromme, K., Coppel, D. B., & Williams, E. (1990). Secondary prevention with college drinkers: Evaluation of an alcohol skills training program. *Journal of Consulting and Clinical Psychology, 58,* 805–810.

Klonoff, E. A. (2009). Disparities in the provision of medical care: An outcome in search of an explanation. *Journal of Behavioral Medicine, 32,* 48–63.

Klonoff, E. A. (2014). Introduction to the special section on discrimination. *Health Psychology, 33,* 1–2.

Klonoff, E. A., & Landrine, H. (1992). Sex roles, occupational roles, and symptom-reporting: A test of competing hypotheses on sex differences. *Journal of Behavioral Medicine, 15,* 355–364.

Klonoff, E. A., & Landrine, H. (1999). Acculturation and cigarette smoking among African Americans: Replication and implications for prevention and cessation programs. *Journal of Behavioral Medicine, 22,* 195–204.

Klopfer, B. (1959). Psychological variables in human cancer. *Journal of Projective Techniques, 21,* 331–340.

Klumb, P., Hoppmann, C., & Staats, M. (2006). Work hours affect spouse's cortisol secretion—For better and for worse. *Psychosomatic Medicine, 68,* 742–746.

Knowles, L. M., Ruiz, J. M., & O'Connor, M. F. (2019). A systematic review of the association between bereavement and biomarkers of immune function. *Psychosomatic Medicine, 81,* 415–433.

Kobayashi, L. C., & Steptoe, A. (2018). Social isolation, loneliness, and health behaviors at older ages: Longitudinal cohort study. *Annals of Behavioral Medicine, 52,* 582–593.

Koenig, L. B., & Vaillant, G. E. (2009). A prospective study of church attendance and health over the lifespan. *Health Psychology, 28,* 117–124.

Koenig, L. J., Pals, S. L., Bush, T., Pratt-Palmore, M., Stratford, D., & Ellerbrock, T. V. (2008). Randomized controlled trial of an intervention to prevent adherence failure among HIV-infected patients initiating antiretroviral therapy. *Health Psychology, 27,* 159–169.

Kogan, S. M., Cho, J., & Oshri, A. (2016). The influence of childhood adversity on rural black men's sexual risk behavior. *Annals of Behavioral Medicine, 50,* 813–822.

Kojima, M., Wakai, K., Tokudome, S., Tamakoshi, K., Toyoshima, H., Watanabe, Y., . . . JACC Study Group. (2005). Perceived psychologic stress and colorectal cancer mortality: Findings from the Japan collaborative cohort study. *Psychosomatic Medicine, 67,* 72–77.

Kok, G., Peters, G. J. Y., Kessels, L. T., Ten Hoor, G. A., & Ruiter, R. A. (2018). Ignoring theory and misinterpreting evidence: The false belief in fear appeals. *Health Psychology Review, 12,* 111–125.

Kolata, G. (2018, July, 3). The limits of online genetic tests. *The New York Times,* pp. D1, D3.

Kontis, V., Bennett, J. E., Mathers, C. D., Li, G., Foreman, K., & Ezzati, M. (2017). Future life expectancy in 35 industrialised countries: Projections with a Bayesian model ensemble. *Lancet, 389,* 1323–1335.

Kopelman, P. G. (2000). Obesity as a medical problem. *Nature, 404,* 635–643.

Korn, L., Betsch, C., Böhm, R., & Meier, N. W. (2018). Social nudging: The effect of social feedback interventions on vaccine uptake. *Health Psychology, 37,* 1045-1054.

Korotana, L. M., Dobson, K. S., Pusch, D., & Josephson, T. (2016). A review of primary care interventions to improve health outcomes in adult survivors of adverse childhood experiences. *Clinical Psychology Review, 46,* 59-90.

Koschwanez, H. E., Kerse, N., Darragh, M., Jarrett, P., Booth, R. J., & Broadbent, E. (2013). Expressive writing and wound healing in older adults: A randomized controlled trial. *Psychosomatic Medicine, 75,* 581-590.

Koton, S., Tanne, D., Bornstein, N. M., & Green, M. S. (2004). Triggering risk factors for ischemic stroke: A case-crossover study. *Neurology, 63,* 2006-2010.

Kouyanou, K., Pither, C., & Wessely, S. (1997). Iatrogenic factors and chronic pain. *Psychosomatic Medicine, 59,* 597-604.

Kowal, J., & Fortier, M. S. (2007). Physical activity behavior change in middle-aged and older women: The role of barriers and of environmental characteristics. *Journal of Behavioral Medicine, 30,* 232-242.

Kozo, J., Sallis, J. F., Conway, T. L., Kerr, J., Cain, K., Saelens, B. E., . . . Owen, N. (2012). Sedentary behaviors of adults in relation to neighborhood walkability and income. *Health Psychology, 31,* 704-713.

Kramarow, E. A., & Pastor, P. N. (2012). The health of male veterans and nonveterans aged 25-64: United States, 2007-2010. *NCHS Data Brief, 101,* 1-8.

Krantz, D. S., & Deckel, A. W. (1983). Coping with coronary heart disease and stroke. In T. G. Burish & L. A. Bradley (Eds.), *Coping with chronic disease: Research and applications* (pp. 85-112). New York: Academic Press.

Kraus, M. W., Horberg, E. J., Goetz, J. L., & Keltner, D. (2011). Social class rank, threat vigilance, and hostile reactivity. *Personality and Social Psychology Bulletin, 37,* 1376-1388.

Krause, N., Ingersoll-Dayton, B., Liang, J., & Sugisawa, H. (1999). Religion, social support, and health among the Japanese elderly. *Journal of Health and Social Behavior, 40,* 405-421.

Krause, N., & Markides, K. S. (1985). Employment and psychological well-being in Mexican American women. *Journal of Health and Social Behavior, 26,* 15-26.

Kreibig, S. D., Whooley, M. A., & Gross, J. J. (2014). Social integration and mortality in patients with coronary heart disease: Findings from the heart and soul study. *Psychosomatic Medicine, 76,* 659-668.

Kristal-Boneh, E., Melamed, S., Bernheim, J., Peled, I., & Green, M. S. (1995). Reduced ambulatory heart rate response to physical work and complaints of fatigue among hypertensive males treated with beta-blockers. *Journal of Behavioral Medicine, 18,* 113-126.

Kristof, N. D. (2012, April 25). Veterans and brain disease. *The New York Times,* A23.

Kroeber, A. L. (1948). *Anthropology.* New York: Harcourt.

Kroenke, C. H., Kubzansky, L. D., Schernhammer, E. S., Holmes, M. D., & Kawachi, I. (2006). Social networks, social support, and survival after breast cancer diagnosis. *Journal of Clinical Oncology, 24,* 1105-1111.

Krohne, H. W., & Slangen, K. E. (2005). Influence of social support on adaptation to surgery. *Health Psychology, 24,* 101-105.

Kronish, I. M., Rieckmann, N., Schwartz, J. E., Schwartz, D. R., & Davidson, K. W. (2009). Is depression after an acute coronary syndrome simply a marker of known prognostic factors for mortality? *Psychosomatic Medicine, 71,* 697-703.

Kross, E., & Ayduk, O. (2011). Making meaning out of negative experiences by self-distancing. *Current Directions in Psychological Science, 20,* 187-191.

Krousel-Wood, M., Islam, T., Muntner, P. Holt, E., Joyce, C., Morisky, D. E., . . . Frohlich, E. D. (2010). Association of depression with antihypertensive medication adherence in older adults: Cross-sectional and longitudinal findings from CoSMO. *Annals of Behavioral Medicine, 40,* 248-257.

Krukowski, R. A., Harvey-Berino, J., Bursac, Z., Ashikaga, T., & West, D. S. (2013). Patterns of success: Online self-monitoring in a web-based behavioral weight control program. *Health Psychology, 32,* 164-170.

Kübler-Ross, E. (1969). *On death and dying.* New York: Macmillan.

Kübler-Ross, E. (1975). *Death: The final stage of growth.* Englewood Cliffs, NJ: Prentice-Hall.

Ku, P. W., Fox, K. R., Gardiner, P. A., & Chen, L. J. (2015). Late-life exercise and difficulty with activities of daily living: An 8-year nationwide follow-up study in Taiwan. *Annals of Behavioral Medicine, 50,* 237-246.

Kuba, K., Esser, P., Mehnert, A., Hinz, A., Johansen, C., Lordick, F., & Götze, H. (2019). Risk for depression and anxiety in long-term survivors of hematologic cancer. *Health Psychology, 38,* 187-195.

Kubzansky, L. D., Berkman, L. F., Glass, T. A., & Seeman, T. E. (1998). Is educational attainment associated with shared determinants of health in the elderly? Findings from the MacArthur studies of successful aging. *Psychosomatic Medicine, 60,* 578-585.

Kubzansky, L. D., Gilthorpe, M. S., & Goodman, E. (2012). A prospective study of psychological distress and weight status in adolescents/young adults. *Annals of Behavioral Medicine, 43,* 219-228.

Kubzansky, L. D., Koenen, K. C., Jones, C., & Eaton, W. W. (2009). A prospective study of posttraumatic stress disorder symptoms and coronary heart disease in women. *Health Psychology, 28,* 125-130.

Kubzansky, L. D., Sparrow, D., Vokonas, P., & Kawachi, I. (2001). Is the glass half empty or half full? A prospective study of optimism and coronary heart disease in the normative aging study. *Psychosomatic Medicine, 63,* 910-916.

Kuhl, E. S., Clifford, L. M., Bandstra, N. F., Filigno, S. S., Yeomans-Maldonado, G., Rausch, J. R., & Stark, L. J. (2014). Examination of the association between lifestyle behavior changes and weight outcomes in preschoolers receiving treatment for obesity. *Health Psychology, 33,* 95-98.

Kulik, J. A., & Mahler, H. I. M. (1987). Effects of preoperative roommate assignment on preoperative anxiety and recovery from coronary-bypass surgery. *Health Psychology, 6,* 525-543.

Kulik, J. A., & Mahler, H. I. M. (1989). Social support and recovery from surgery. *Health Psychology, 8,* 221-238.

Kulik, J. A., & Mahler, H. I. M. (1993). Emotional support as a moderator of adjustment and compliance after coronary artery bypass surgery: A longitudinal study. *Journal of Behavioral Medicine, 16,* 45-64.

Kulik, J. A., Moore, P. J., & Mahler, H. I. M. (1993). Stress and affiliation: Hospital roommate effects on preoperative anxiety and social interaction. *Health Psychology, 12,* 118-124.

Kulkarni, S. C., Levin-Rector, A., Ezzati, M., & Murray, C. J. (2011). Falling behind: Life expectancy in US counties from 2000 to 2007 in an international context. *Population Health Metrics, 9,* 1-12.

Kumanyika, S. K., Van Horn, L., Bowen, D., Perri, M. G., Rolls, B. J., Czajkowski, S. M., & Schron, E. (2000). Maintenance of dietary behavior change. *Health Psychology, 19,* 42-56.

Kumari, M., Badrick, E., Chandola, T., Adler, N., Epel, E., Seeman, T., . . . Marmot, M. G. (2010). Measures of social position and cortisol secretion in an aging population: Findings from the Whitehall II study. *Psychosomatic Medicine, 72,* 27-34.

Kupper, N., & Denollet, J. (2018). Type D personality as a risk factor in coronary heart disease: A review of current evidence. *Current Cardiology Reports, 20,* 104.

Kutner, N. G. (1987). Issues in the application of high cost medical technology: The case of organ transplantation. *Journal of Health and Social Behavior, 28,* 23-36.

Kwan, B. M., Stevens, C. J., & Bryan, A. D. (2017). What to expect when you're exercising: An experimental test of the anticipated affect-exercise relationship. *Health Psychology, 36,* 309–319.

Lacroix, J. M., Martin, B., Avendano, M., & Goldstein, R. (1991). Symptom schemata in chronic respiratory patients. *Health Psychology, 10,* 268–273.

Lacourt, T. E., Houtveen, J. H., Smeets, H. M., Lipovsky, M. M., & van Doornen, L. J. (2015). Infection load as a predisposing factor for somatoform disorders: Evidence from a Dutch General Practice Registry. *Psychosomatic Medicine, 75,* 759–764.

Lai, H., Lai, S., Krongrad, A., Trapido, E., Page, J. B., & McCoy, C. B. (1999). The effect of marital status on survival in late-stage cancer patients: An analysis based on surveillance, epidemiology, and end results (SEER) data, in the United States. *International Journal of Behavioral Medicine, 6,* 150–176.

Lallukka, T., Martikainen, P., Reunanen, A., Roos, E., Sarlo-Lahteenkorva, S., & Lahelma, E. (2006). Associations between working conditions and angina pectoris symptoms among employed women. *Psychosomatic Medicine, 68,* 348–354.

Lam, T. H., Stewart, M., & Ho, L. M. (2001). Smoking and high-risk sexual behavior among young adults in Hong Kong. *Journal of Behavioral Medicine, 24,* 503–518.

Lambiase, M. J., Kubzansky, L. D., & Thurston, R. C. (2015). Positive psychological health and stroke risk: The benefits of emotional vitality. *Health Psychology, 34,* 1043–1046.

Lamprecht, F., & Sack, M. (2002). Posttraumatic stress disorder revisited. *Psychosomatic Medicine, 64,* 222–237.

Landro, L. (2012, April 16). The simple idea that is transforming health care. *The Wall Street Journal,* pp. R1, R2.

Landro, L. (2019, February 7). Health-care technology. *The Wall Street Journal,* pp. R1, R2.

Lane, R. D., Laukes, C., Marcus, F. I., Chesney, M. A., Sechrest, L., Gear, K., . . . Steptoe, A. (2006). Psychological stress preceding idiopathic ventricular fibrillation. *Psychosomatic Medicine, 67,* 359–365.

Lane, R. D., Waldstein, S. R., Chesney, M. A., Jennings, J. R., Lovallo, W. R., Kozel, P. J., . . . Cameron, O. G. (2009). The rebirth of neuroscience in psychosomatic medicine, part I: Historical context, methods, and relevant basic science. *Psychosomatic Medicine, 71,* 117–134.

Langens, T. A., & Schüler, J. (2007). Effects of written emotional expression: The role of positive expectancies. *Health Psychology, 26,* 174–182.

Langford, A. T., Solid, C. A., Gann, L. C., Rabinowitz, E. P., Williams, S. K., & Seixas, A. A. (2018). Beliefs about the causes of hypertension and associations with pro-health behaviors. *Health Psychology, 37,* 1092–1101.

Langford, D. J., Cooper, B., Paul, S., Humphreys, J., Keagy, C., Conley, Y. P., . . . Dunn, L. B. (2017). Evaluation of coping as a mediator of the relationship between stressful life events and cancer-related distress. *Health Psychology, 36,* 1147–1160.

Langston, C. A. (1994). Capitalizing on and coping with daily-life events: Expressive responses to positive events. *Journal of Personality and Social Psychology, 67,* 1112–1125.

Lankford, T. R. (1979). *Integrated science for health students* (2nd ed.). Reston, VA: Reston.

Lantz, P. M., Weigers, M. E., & House, J. S. (1997). Education and income differentials in breast and cervical cancer screening: Policy implications for rural women. *Medical Care, 35,* 219–236.

Larimer, M. E., Palmer, R. S., & Marlatt, G. A. (1999). Relapse prevention: An overview of Marlatt's cognitive–behavioral model. *Alcohol Research and Health, 23,* 151–160.

Larkin, K. T., & Zayfert, C. (1996). Anger management training with mild essential hypertensive patients. *Journal of Behavioral Medicine, 19,* 415–434.

Larsen, D. (1990, March 18). Future of fear. *Los Angeles Times,* pp. E1, E8.

Latimer, A. E., Williams-Piehota, P., Katulak, N. A., Cox, A., Mowad, L., Higgins, E. T., & Salovey, P. (2008). Promoting fruit and vegetable intake through messages tailored to individual differences in regulatory focus. *Annals of Behavioral Medicine, 35,* 363–369.

Lau, R. R., Kane, R., Berry, S., Ware, J. E., Jr., & Roy, D. (1980). Channeling health: A review of televised health campaigns. *Health Education Quarterly, 7,* 56–89.

Laubmeier, K. K., Zakowski, S. G., & Blair, J. P. (2004). The role of spirituality in the psychological adjustment to cancer: A test of the transactional model of stress and coping. *International Journal of Behavioral Medicine, 11,* 48–55.

Lauver, D. R., Henriques, J. B., Settersten, L., & Bumann, M. C. (2003). Psychosocial variables, external barriers, and stage of mammography adoption. *Health Psychology, 22,* 649–653.

Laveist, T. A., & Nuru-Jeter, A. (2002). Is doctor–patient race concordance associated with greater satisfaction with care? *Journal of Health and Social Behavior, 43,* 296–306.

Laviano, A., Seelaender, M., Sanchez-Lara, K., Gioulbasanis, I., Molfino, A., & Fanelli, F. R. (2011). Beyond anorexia-cachexia. Nutrition and modulation of cancer patients' metabolism: Supplementary, complementary or alternative anti-neoplastic therapy? *European Journal of Pharmacology, 668,* 587–590.

Lavoie, K. L., Bouchard, A., Joseph, M., Campbell, T. S., Favereau, H., & Bacon, S. L. (2008). Association of asthma self-efficacy to asthma control and quality of life. *Annals of Behavioral Medicine, 36,* 100–106.

Lavoie, K. L., Paine, N. J., Pelletier, R., Arsenault, A., Diodati, J. G., Campbell, T. S., . . . Bacon, S. L. (2018). Relationship between antidepressant therapy and risk for cardiovascular events in patients with and without cardiovascular disease. *Health Psychology, 37,* 989–999.

Lavretsky, H., Epel, E. S., Siddarth, P., Nazarian, N., St. Cyr, N., Khalsa, D. S., . . . Irwin, M. R. (2013). A pilot study of yogic meditation for family dementia caregivers with depressive symptoms: Effects on mental health, cognition, and telomerase activity. *International Journal of Geriatric Psychiatry, 28,* 57–65.

Lawler, S. P., Winkler, E., Reeves, M. M., Owen, N., Graves, N., & Eakin, E. G. (2010). Multiple health behavior changes and co-variation in a telephone counseling trial. *Annals of Behavioral Medicine, 39,* 250–257.

Lawlor, D. A., O'Callaghan, M. J., Mamun, A. A., Williams, G. M., Bor, W., & Najman, J. M. (2005). Socioeconomic position, cognitive function, and clustering of cardiovascular risk factors in adolescence: Findings from the Mater University study of pregnancy and its outcomes. *Psychosomatic Medicine, 67,* 862–868.

Laws, H. B., Sayer, A. G., Pietromonaco, P. R., & Powers, S. I. (2015). Longitudinal changes in spouses' HPA responses: Convergence in cortisol patterns during the early years of marriage. *Health Psychology, 34,* 1076–1089.

Lazarus, R. S. (1983). The costs and benefits of denial. In S. Bresnitz (Ed.), *Denial of stress* (pp. 1–30). New York: International Universities Press.

Lazarus, R. S., & Folkman, S. (1984b). *Stress, appraisal, and coping.* New York: Springer.

Lazarus, R. S., & Launier, R. (1978). Stress-related transactions between person and environment. In L. A. Pervin & M. Lewis (Eds.), *Internal and external determinants of behavior* (pp. 287–327). New York: Plenum.

Lebel, S., Beattie, S., Ares, I., & Bielajew, C. (2013). Young and worried: Age and fear of recurrence in breast cancer survivors. *Health Psychology, 32,* 695–705.

Leclere, F. B., Rogers, R. G., & Peters, K. (1998). Neighborhood social context and racial differences in women's heart disease mortality. *Journal of Health and Social Behavior, 39,* 91–107.

Lee, A. A., Piette, J. D., Heisler, M., Janevic, M. R., & Rosland, A. M. (2019). Diabetes self-management and glycemic control: The role of autonomy support from informal health supporters. *Health Psychology, 38,* 122-132.

Lee, J. H., Park, S. K., Ryoo, J. H., Oh, C. M., Kang, J. G., Mansur, R. B., . . . Jung, J. Y. (2018). Sleep duration and quality as related to left ventricular structure and function. *Psychosomatic Medicine, 80,* 78-86.

Lee, J. L., Eaton, C. K., Loiselle Rich, K., Reed-Knight, B., Liverman, R. S., Mee, L. L., . . . Blount, R. L. (2017). The interactive effect of parent personality and medication knowledge on adherence in children awaiting solid organ transplantation. *Health Psychology, 36,* 445-448.

Lee, M. B., Wu, Z., Rotheram-Borus, M., Detels, R., Guan, J., & Li, L. (2004). HIV-related stigma among market workers in China. *Health Psychology, 24,* 435-438.

Lee, R., Yu, H., Gao, X., Cao, J., Tao, H., Yu, B., . . . Lin, P. (2019). The negative affectivity dimension of Type D personality is associated with in-stent neoatherosclerosis in coronary patients with percutaneous coronary intervention: An optical coherence tomography study. *Journal of Psychosomatic Research, 120,* 20-28.

Lee, W. K., Milloy, M. J. S., Walsh, J., Nguyen, P., Wood, E., & Kerr, T. (2016). Psychosocial factors in adherence to antiretroviral therapy among HIV-positive people who use drugs. *Health Psychology, 35,* 290-297.

Lehman, A. J., Pratt, D. D., DeLongis, A., Collins, J. B., Shojania, K., Koehler, B., . . . Esdaile, J. M. (2011). Do spouses know how much fatigue, pain, and physical limitation their partners with rheumatoid arthritis experience? Implications for social support. *Arthritis Care & Research, 63,* 120-127.

Lehman, C. D., Rodin, J., McEwen, B., & Brinton, R. (1991). Impact of environmental stress on the expression of insulin-dependent diabetes mellitus. *Behavioral Neuroscience, 105,* 241-245.

Leigh, H., & Reiser, M. F. (1986). Comparison of theoretically oriented and patient-oriented behavioral science courses. *Journal of Medical Education, 61,* 169-174.

Lelutiu-Weinberger, C., Gamarel, K. E., Golub, S. A., & Parsons, J. T. (2015). Race-based differentials in the impact of mental health and stigma on HIV risk among young men who have sex with men. *Health Psychology, 34,* 847-856.

Lemogne, C., Consoli, S. M., Geoffroy-Perez, B., Coeuret-Pellicer, M., Nabi, H., & Cordier, S. (2013). Personality and the risk of cancer: A 16-year follow-up study of the GAZEL cohort. *Psychosomatic Medicine, 75,* 262-271.

Lemoine, J., & Mougne, C. (1983). Why has death stalked the refugees? *Natural History, 92,* 6-19.

Lenert, L., & Skoczen, S. (2002). The Internet as a research tool: Worth the price of admission? *Annals of Behavioral Medicine, 24,* 251-256.

Lennon, M. C., & Rosenfield, S. (1992). Women and mental health: The interaction of job and family conditions. *Journal of Health and Social Behavior, 33,* 316-327.

Lepore, S. J., Ragan, J. D., & Jones, S. (2000). Talking facilitates cognitive-emotional processes of adaptation to an acute stressor. *Journal of Personality and Social Psychology, 78,* 499-508.

Lepore, S. J., & Smyth, J. (Eds.). (2002). *The writing cure: How expressive writing influences health and well-being.* Washington, DC: American Psychological Association.

Lerman, C., Caporaso, N. E., Audrain, J., Main, D., Bowman, E. D., Lockshin, B., . . . Shields, P. G. (1999). Evidence suggesting the role of specific genetic factors in cigarette smoking. *Health Psychology, 18,* 14-20.

Leserman, J. (2008). Role of depression, stress, and trauma in HIV disease progression. *Psychosomatic Medicine, 70,* 539-545.

Leung, Y. W., Ceccato, N., Stewart, D. E., & Grace, S. L. (2007). A prospective examination of patterns and correlates of exercise maintenance in coronary artery disease patients. *Journal of Behavioral Medicine, 30,* 411-421.

Levenson, J. L., McClish, D. K., Dahman, B. A., Bovbjerg, V. E., Citero, V. D. A., Penberthy, L. T., . . . Smith, W. R. (2008). Depression and anxiety in adults with sickle cell disease: The PiSCES project. *Psychosomatic Medicine, 70,* 192-196.

Leventhal, E. A., Easterling, D., Leventhal, H., & Cameron, L. (1995). Conservation of energy, uncertainty reduction, and swift utilization of medical care among the elderly: Study II. *Medical Care, 33,* 988-1000.

Leventhal, E. A., Hansell, S., Diefenbach, M., Leventhal, H., & Glass, D. C. (1996). Negative affect and self-report of physical symptoms: Two longitudinal studies of older adults. *Health Psychology, 15,* 193-199.

Leventhal, E. A., Leventhal, H., Schacham, S., & Easterling, D. V. (1989). Active coping reduces reports of pain from childbirth. *Journal of Consulting and Clinical Psychology, 57,* 365-371.

Leventhal, H. (1970). Findings and theory in the study of fear communications. In L. Berkowitz (Ed.), *Advances in experimental social psychology* (Vol. 5, pp. 120-186). New York: Academic Press.

Leventhal, H., Diefenbach, M., & Leventhal, E. A. (1992). Illness cognition: Using common sense to understand treatment adherence and affect cognition interactions. *Cognitive Therapy and Research, 16,* 143-163.

Leventhal, H., Leventhal, E. A., & Breland, J. Y. (2011). Cognitive science speaks to the "common-sense" of chronic illness management. *Annals of Behavioral Medicine, 41,* 152-163.

Leventhal, H., Meyer, D., & Nerenz, D. (1980). The common sense representation of illness danger. In S. Rachman (Ed.), *Contributions to medical psychology* (Vol. II, pp. 7-30). New York: Pergamon Press.

Leventhal, H., & Nerenz, D. R. (1982). A model for stress research and some implications for the control of stress disorders. In D. Meichenbaum & M. Jaremko (Eds.), *Stress prevention and management: A cognitive behavioral approach.* New York: Plenum.

Leventhal, H., Nerenz, D., & Strauss, A. (1982). Self-regulation and the mechanisms for symptom appraisal. In D. Mechanic (Ed.), *Monograph series in psychosocial epidemiology, 3: Symptoms, illness behavior, and help-seeking* (pp. 55-86). New York: Neale Watson.

Leventhal, H., Weinman, J., Leventhal, E. A., & Phillips, L. A. (2008). Health psychology: The search for pathways between behavior and health. *Annual Review of Psychology, 59,* 477-505.

Levey, N. N. (2015, March 23). Diabetes study touts benefits of Obamacare. *New York Times,* p. A6.

Levine, J. D., Gordon, N. C., & Fields, H. L. (1978). The mechanism of placebo analgesia. *Lancet, 2,* 654-657.

Levinson, R. M., McCollum, K. T., & Kutner, N. G. (1984). Gender homophily in preferences for physicians. *Sex Roles, 10,* 315-325.

Levitsky, L. L. (2004). Childhood immunizations and chronic illness. *The New England Journal of Medicine, 350,* 1380-1382.

Levy, B. R., Hausdorff, J. M., Hencke, R., & Wei, J. Y. (2000). Reducing cardiovascular stress with positive self-stereotypes of aging. *The Journals of Gerontology:* Series B, *55,* 205-213.

Levy, S. M., Herberman, R. B., Whiteside, T., Sanzo, K., Lee, J., & Kirkwood, J. (1990). Perceived social support and tumor estrogen/progesterone receptor status as predictors of natural killer cell activity in breast cancer patients. *Psychosomatic Medicine, 52,* 73-85.

Levy, S. M., Lee, J. K., Bagley, C., & Lippman, M. (1988). Survival hazards analysis in first recurrent breast cancer patients: Seven-year follow-up. *Psychosomatic Medicine, 50,* 520-528.

Lewin, K. (1946). Action research and minority problems. *Journal of Social Issues, 2,* 34-36.

Lewis, J. A., Manne, S. L., DuHamel, K. N., Vickburgh, S. M. J., Bovbjerg, D. H., Currie, V., . . . Redd, W. H. (2001). Social support, intrusive thoughts, and quality of life in breast cancer survivors. *Journal of Behavioral Medicine, 24,* 231-245.

Lewis, J. W., Terman, S. W., Shavit, Y., Nelson, L. R., & Liebeskind, J. C. (1984). Neural, neurochemical, and hormonal bases of stress-induced analgesia. In L. Kruger & J. C. Liebeskind (Eds.), *Advances in pain research and therapy* (Vol. 6, pp. 277–288). New York: Raven Press.

Lewis, M. A., & Rook, K. S. (1999). Social control in personal relationships: Impact on health behaviors and psychological distress. *Health Psychology, 18,* 63–71.

Lewis, M. A., Uhrig, J. D., Bann, C. M., Harris, J. L., Furberg, R. D., Coomes, C., & Kuhns, L. M. (2013). Tailored text messaging interventions for HIV adherence: A proof-of-concept study. *Health Psychology, 32,* 248–253.

Lewis, T. T., Everson-Rose, S. A., Karavolos, K., Janssen, I., Wesley, D., & Powell, L. H. (2009). Hostility is associated with visceral, but not with subcutaneous, fat in middle-aged African Amercian and White women. *Psychosomatic Medicine, 71,* 733–740.

Li, A. W., & Goldsmith, C. A. W. (2012). The effects of yoga on anxiety and stress. *Alternative Medicine Review, 17,* 21–35.

Li, J., Cowden, L. G., King, J. D., Briles, D. A., Schroeder, H. W., Stevens, A. B., . . . Go, R. C. (2007). Effects of chronic stress and interleukin-10 gene polymorphism on antibody response to tetanus vaccine in family caregivers of patients with Alzheimer's disease. *Psychosomatic Medicine, 69,* 551–559.

Li, J., Laursen, T. M., Precht, D. H., Olsen, J., & Mortensen, P. B. (2005). Hospitalization for mental illness among parents after the death of a child. *The New England Journal of Medicine, 352,* 1190–1196.

Li, L., Ji, G., Liang, L. J., Lin, C., Hsieh, J., Lan, C. W., & Xiao, Y. (2017). Efficacy of a multilevel intervention on the mental health of people living with HIV and their family members in rural China. *Health Psychology, 36,* 863–871.

Li, S. (2016, January 29). Barbie's bombshell: A new look. *The Los Angeles Times,* p. A1.

Li, Y., & Ferraro, K. F. (2005). Volunteering and depression in later life: Social benefit or selection processes? *Journal of Health and Social Behavior, 46,* 68–84.

Liberman, R. (1962). An analysis of the placebo phenomenon. *Journal of Chronic Diseases, 15,* 761–783.

Lichtenstein, E., & Cohen, S. (1990). Prospective analysis of two modes of unaided smoking cessation. *Health Education Research, 5,* 63–72.

Lichtenstein, E., Glasgow, R. E., Lando, H. A., Ossip-Klein, D. J., & Boles, S. M. (1996). Telephone counseling for smoking cessation: Rationales and meta-analytic review of evidence. *Health Education Research: Theory and Practice, 11,* 243–257.

Lichtenstein, E., Zhu, S. H., & Tedeschi, G. J. (2010). Smoking cessation quitlines: An underrecognized intervention success story. *American Psychologist, 65,* 252–261.

Lichtenstein, P., Holm, N. V., Verkasalo, P. K., Iliadou, A., Kaprio, J., Koskenvuo, M., . . . Hemminki, K. (2000). Environmental and heritable factors in the causation of cancer: Analyses of cohorts of twins from Sweden, Denmark, and Finland. *The New England Journal of Medicine, 343,* 78–85.

Lichtman, R. R., Taylor, S. E., Wood, J. V., Bluming, A. Z., Dosik, G. M., & Leibowitz, R. L. (1984). Relations with children after breast cancer: The mother–daughter relationship at risk. *Journal of Psychosocial Oncology, 2,* 1–19.

Lieberman, M. D., Jarcho, J. M., Berman, S., Naliboff, B. D., Suyenobu, B. Y., Mandelkern, M., & Mayer, E. A. (2004). The neural correlates of placebo effects: A disruption account. *NeuroImage, 22,* 447–455.

Lillis, J., Hayes, S. C., Bunting, K., & Masuda, A. (2009). Teaching acceptance and mindfulness to improve the lives of the obese: A preliminary test of a theoretical model. *Annals of Behavioral Medicine, 37,* 58–69.

Lin, K. Y., Hu, Y. T., Chang, K. J., Lin, H. F., & Tsauo, J. Y. (2011). Effects of yoga on psychological health, quality of life, and physical health of patients with cancer: A meta-analysis. *Evidence-Based Complementary and Alternative Medicine.*

Lindauer, R. T. L., van Meijel, E. P. M., Jaliuk, M., Olff, M., Carlier, I. V. E., & Gersons, B. P. R. (2006). Heart rate responsivity to script-driven imagery in posttraumatic stress disorder: Specificity of response and effects of psychotherapy. *Psychosomatic Medicine, 68,* 33–40.

Linde, K., Scholz, M., Ramirez, G., Clausius, N., Melchart, D., & Jonas, W. B. (1999). Impact of study quality on outcome in placebo-controlled trials of homeopathy. *Journal of Clinical Epidemiology, 52,* 631–636.

Linden, W., & Chambers, L. (1994). Clinical effectiveness of non-drug treatment for hypertension: A meta-analysis. *Annals of Behavioral Medicine, 16,* 35–45.

Lindsay, E. K., Young, S., Brown, K. W., Smyth, J. M., & Creswell, J. D. (2019). Mindfulness training reduces loneliness and increases social contact in a randomized controlled trial. *Proceedings of the National Academy of Sciences, 116,* 3488–3493.

Lindsay, M., & McCarthy, D. (1974). Caring for the brothers and sisters of a dying child. In T. Burton (Ed.), *Care of the child facing death* (pp. 189–206). Boston, MA: Routledge & Kegan Paul.

Linebaugh, K. (2012, June 11). Type 1 diabetes on rise among youth. *The Wall Street Journal,* p. A5.

Lingsweiler, V. M., Crowther, J. H., & Stephens, M. A. P. (1987). Emotional reactivity and eating in binge eating and obesity. *Journal of Behavioral Medicine, 10,* 287–300.

Link, B. G., Phelan, J. C., Miech, R., & Westin, E. L. (2008). The resources that matter: Fundamental social causes of health disparities and the challenge of intelligence. *Journal of Health and Social Behavior, 49,* 72–91.

Linke, S., Murray, E., Butler, C., & Wallace, P. (2007). Internet-based interactive health intervention for the promotion of sensible drinking: Patterns of use and potential impact on members of the general public. *Journal of Medical Internet Research, 9,* e10.

Linkins, R. W., & Comstock, G. W. (1990). Depressed mood and development of cancer. *American Journal of Epidemiology, 134,* 962–972.

Linton, S. J., & Buer, N. (1995). Working despite pain: Factors associated with work attendance versus dysfunction. *International Journal of Behavioral Medicine, 2,* 252–262.

Lipkus, I. M., Barefoot, J. C., Williams, R. B., & Siegler, I. C. (1994). Personality measures as predictors of smoking initiation and cessation in the UNC Alumni Heart Study. *Health Psychology, 13,* 149–155.

Lipkus, I. M., McBride, C. M., Pollak, K. I., Schwartz-Bloom, R. D., Tilson, E., & Bloom, P. N. (2004). A randomized trial comparing the effects of self-help materials and proactive telephone counseling on teen smoking cessation. *Health Psychology, 23,* 397–406.

Lipsitt, L. P. (2003). Crib death: A biobehavioral phenomenon? *Current Directions in Psychological Science, 12,* 164–170.

Lisspers, J., Sundin, Ö., Öhman, A., Hofman-Bang, C., Rydén, L., & Nygren, Å. (2005). Long-term effects of lifestyle behavior change in coronary artery disease: Effects on recurrent coronary events after percutaneous coronary intervention. *Health Psychology, 24,* 41–48.

Litcher-Kelly, L., Lam, Y., Broihier, J. A., Brand, D. L., Banker, S. V., Kotov, R., & Luft, B. J. (2014). Longitudinal study of the impact of psychological distress symptoms on new-onset upper gastrointestinal symptoms in world trade center responders. *Psychosomatic Medicine, 76,* 686–693.

Littlefield, C. H., Rodin, G. M., Murray, M. A., & Craven, J. L. (1990). Influence of functional impairment and social support on depressive symptoms in persons with diabetes. *Health Psychology, 9,* 737–749.

Littlewood, R. A., & Vanable, P. A. (2014). The relationship between CAM use and adherence to antiretroviral therapies among persons living with HIV. *Health Psychology, 33,* 660-667.

Littlewood, R. A., Vanable, P. A., Carey, M. P., & Blair, D. C. (2008). The association of benefit finding to psychosocial and health behavior adaptation among HIV+ men and women. *Journal of Behavioral Medicine, 31,* 145-155.

Liu, H., & Umberson, D. J. (2008). The times they are a changin': Marital status and health differentials from 1972 to 2003. *Journal of Health and Social Behavior, 49,* 239-253.

Liu, Y., & Tanaka, H. (2002). Overtime work, insufficient sleep, and risk of non-fatal acute myocardial infarction in Japanese men. *Occupational and Environmental Medicine, 59,* 447-451.

Loaring, J. M., Larkin, M., Shaw, R., & Flowers, P. (2015). Renegotiating sexual intimacy in the context of altered embodiment: The experiences of women with breast cancer and their male partners following mastectomy and reconstruction. *Health Psychology, 34,* 426-436.

Loder, N. (2017, September). Is there a doctor in my pocket? *The Economist,* 1843.

Logsdon, R. G., Gibbons, L. E., McCurry, S. M., & Teri, L. (2002). Assessing quality of life in older adults with cognitive impairment. *Psychosomatic Medicine, 64,* 510-519.

Lombardi, V. C., Ruscetti, F. W., Das Gupta, J., Pfost, M. A., Hagen, K. S., Peterson, D. L., . . . Mikovits, J. A. (2009). Detection of an infectious retrovirus, XMRV, in blood cells of patients with chronic fatigue syndrome. *Science, 326,* 585-589.

Longmire-Avital, B., Golub, S. A., & Parsons, J. T. (2010). Self-reevaluation as a critical component in sustained viral load change for HIV+ adults with alcohol problems. *Annals of Behavioral Medicine, 40,* 176-183.

Lopez, E. N., Drobes, D. J., Thompson, J. K., & Brandon, T. H. (2008). Effects of a body image challenge on smoking motivation among college females. *Health Psychology, 27,* S243-S251.

Lorig, K., Chastain, R. L., Ung, E., Shoor, S., & Holman, H. (1989). Development and evaluation of a scale to measure perceived self-efficacy in people with arthritis. *Arthritis and Rheumatism, 32,* 37-44.

Loucks, E. B., Almeida, N. D., Taylor, S. E., & Matthews, K. A. (2011). Childhood family psychosocial environment and coronary heart disease risk. *Psychosomatic Medicine, 73,* 563-571.

Lovallo, W. R., Al'Absi, M., Pincomb, G. A., Passey, R. B., Sung, B., & Wilson, M. F. (2000). Caffeine, extended stress, and blood pressure in borderline hypertensive men. *International Journal of Behavioral Medicine, 7,* 183-188.

Lovett, I., & Perez-Pena, R. (2015, October 6). Brown signs 'Right-to-Die' into law in California. *The New York Times,* p. A10.

Low, C. A., Bower, J. E., Kwan, L., & Seldon, J. (2008). Benefit finding in response to BRCA1/2 testing. *Annals of Behavioral Medicine, 35,* 61-69.

Low, C. A., Matthews, K. A., & Hall, M. (2013). Elevated C-reactive protein in adolescents: Roles of stress and coping. *Psychosomatic Medicine, 75,* 449-452.

Low, C. A., & Stanton, A. L. (2015). Activity disruption and depressive symptoms in women living with metastatic breast cancer. *Health Psychology, 34,* 89-92.

Low, C. A., Stanton, A. L., Bower, J. E., & Gyllenhammer, L. (2010). A randomized controlled trial of emotionally expressive writing for women with metastatic breast cancer. *Health Psychology, 29,* 460-466.

Low, C. A., Stanton, A. L., & Danoff-Burg, S. (2006). Expressive disclosure and benefit finding among breast cancer patients: Mechanisms for positive health effects. *Health Psychology, 25,* 181-189.

Low, C. A., Thurston, R. C., & Matthews, K. A. (2010). Psychosocial factors in the development of heart disease in women: Current research and future directions. *Psychosomatic Medicine, 72,* 842-854.

Löwe, B., Grafe, K., Kroenke, K., Zipfel, S., Quentier, A., Wild, B., . . . Herzog, W. (2003). Predictors of psychiatric comorbidity in medical outpatients. *Psychosomatic Medicine, 65,* 764-770.

Lowe, R., & Norman, P. (2017). Information processing in illness representation: Implications from an associative-learning framework. *Health Psychology, 36,* 280-290.

Lowe, S. R., Willis, M., & Rhodes, J. E. (2014). Health problems among low-income parents in the aftermath of Hurricane Katrina. *Health Psychology, 33,* 774-782.

Lozito, M. (2004). Chronic pain: The new workers' comp. *The Case Manager, 15,* 61-63.

Lu, Q., Zeltzer, L., & Tsao, J. (2013). Multiethnic differences in responses to laboratory pain stimuli among children. *Health Psychology, 32,* 905-914.

Lu, Q., Zheng, D., Young, L., Kagawa-Singer, M., & Loh, A. (2012). A pilot study of expressive writing intervention among Chinese-speaking breast cancer survivors. *Health Psychology, 31,* 548-551.

Lubitz, J., Cai, L., Kramarow, E., & Lentzner, H. (2003). Health, life expectancy, and health care spending among the elderly. *The New England Journal of Medicine, 349,* 1048-1055.

Luckow, A., Reifman, A., & McIntosh, D. N. (1998, August). *Gender differences in coping: A meta-analysis.* Poster session presented at the 106th annual convention of the American Psychological Association, San Francisco.

Ludescher, B., Leitlein, G., Schaefer, J. E., Vanhoeffen, S., Baar, S., Machann, J., . . . Eschweiler, G. W. (2009). Changes of body composition in bulimia nervosa: Increased visceral fat and adrenal gland size. *Psychosomatic Medicine, 71,* 93-97.

Luecken, L. J., Suarez, E., Kuhn, C., Barefoot, J., Blumenthal, J., Siegler, I., & Williams, R. B. (1997). Stress in employed women: Impact of marital status and children at home on neurohormone output and home strain. *Psychosomatic Medicine, 59,* 352-359.

Lumley, M. A., Shi, W., Wiholm, C., Slatcher, R. B., Sandmark, H., Wang, S., & Arnetz, B. B. (2014). The relationship of chronic and momentary work stress to cardiac reactivity in female managers: Feasibility of a smart phone-assisted assessment system. *Psychosomatic Medicine, 76,* 512-518.

Lundgren, T., Dahl, J., & Hayes, S. C. (2008). Evaluation of mediators of change in the treatment of epilepsy with acceptance and commitment therapy. *Journal of Behavioral Medicine, 31,* 225-235.

Lustman, P. J. (1988). Anxiety disorders in adults with diabetes mellitus. *Psychiatric Clinics of North America, 11,* 419-432.

Luszczynska, A., Sobczyk, A., & Abraham, C. (2007). Planning to lose weight: Randomized controlled trial of an implementation intention prompt to enhance weight reduction among overweight and obese women. *Health Psychology, 26,* 507-512.

Lutgendorf, S. K., & Andersen, B. L. (2015). Biobehavioral approaches to cancer progression and survival: Mechanisms and interventions. *American Psychologist, 70,* 186-197.

Lutgendorf, S. K., Anderson, B., Sorosky, J. I., Buller, R. E., & Lubaroff, D. M. (2000). Interleukin-6 and use of social support in gynecologic cancer patients. *International Journal of Behavioral Medicine, 7,* 127-142.

Lutgendorf, S. K., Antoni, M. H., Ironson, G., Starr, K., Costello, N., Zuckerman, M., . . . Schneiderman, N. (1998). Changes in cognitive coping skills and social support during cognitive behavioral stress management intervention and distress outcomes in symptomatic human immunodeficiency virus (HIV)-seropositive gay men. *Psychosomatic Medicine, 60,* 204-214.

Lutgendorf, S. K., Lamkin, D. M., Degeest, K., Anderson, B., Dao, M., McGinn, S., . . . Lubaroff, D. M. (2008). Depressed and anxious mood and T-cell cytokine expressing populations in ovarian cancer patients. *Brain, Behavior, and Immunity, 22,* 890-900.

Lutgendorf, S. K., & Sood, A. K. (2011). Biobehavioral factors and cancer progression: Physiological pathways and mechanisms. *Psychosomatic Medicine, 73,* 724-730.

Luyckx, K., Vanhalst, J., Seiffge-Krenke, I., & Wheets, I. (2010). A typology of coping with Type 1 diabetes in emerging adulthood: Associations with demographic, psychological, and clinical parameters. *Journal of Behavioral Medicine, 33,* 228-238.

Lynch, S., Ford, N., van Cutsem, G., Bygrave, H., Janssens, B., Decroo, T., . . . Goemaere, E. (2012). Getting HIV treatment to the most people. *Science, 337,* 298-300.

Lytle, L. A., Hearst, M. O., Fulkerson, J., Murray, D. M., Martinson, B., Klein, E., . . . Samuelson, A. (2011). Examining the relationships between family meal practices, family stressors, and the weight of youth in the family. *Annals of Behavioral Medicine, 41,* 353-362.

MacCoon, D. G., Imel, Z. E., Rosenkranz, M. A., Sheftel, J. G., Weng, H. Y., Sullivan, J. C., . . . Lutz, A. (2012). The validation of an active control intervention for Mindfulness Based Stress Reduction (MBSR). *Behaviour Research and Therapy, 50,* 3-12.

MacDorman, M. F., & Mathews, T. J. (2009). Behind international rankings of infant mortality: How the United States compares with Europe. *NCHS Data Brief, 23,* 1-8.

Maciejewski, P. K., Zhang, B., Block, S. D., & Prigerson, H. G. (2007). An empirical examination of the stage theory of grief. *Journal of the American Medical Association, 297,* 716-723.

Mackenbach, J. P., Stribu, I., Roskam, A. J. R., Schaap, M. M., Menvielle, G., Leinsalu, M., . . . European Union Working Group on Socioeconomic Inequalities in Health. (2008). Socioeconomic inequalities in health in 22 European countries. *The New England Journal of Medicine, 358,* 2468-2481.

Mackey, E. R., Struemph, K., Powell, P. W., Chen, R., Streisand, R., & Holmes, C. S. (2014). Maternal depressive symptoms and disease care status in youth with type 1 diabetes. *Health Psychology, 33,* 783-791.

Maddux, J. E., Roberts, M. C., Sledden, E. A., & Wright, L. (1986). Developmental issues in child health psychology. *American Psychologist, 41,* 25-34.

Madlensky, L., Natarajan, L., Flatt, S. W., Faerber, S., Newman, V. A., & Pierce, J. P. (2008). Timing of dietary change in response to a telephone counseling intervention: Evidence from the WHEL study. *Health Psychology, 27,* 539-547.

Madsen, M. V., Gøtzsche, P. C., & Hróbjartsson, A. (2009). Acupuncture treatment for pain: Systematic review of randomised clinical trials with acupuncture, placebo acupuncture, and no acupuncture groups. *British Medical Journal, 338,* a3115.

Maeland, J. G., & Havik, O. E. (1987). Psychological predictors for return to work after a myocardial infarction. *Journal of Psychosomatic Research, 31,* 471-481.

Maggi, S., Hertzman, C., & Vaillancourt, T. (2007). Changes in smoking behaviors from late childhood to adolescence: Insights from the Canadian National Longitudinal Survey of Children and Youth. *Health Psychology, 26,* 232-240.

Magill, M., & Ray, L. A. (2009). Cognitive-behavioral treatment with adult alcohol and illicit drug users: A meta-analysis of randomized controlled trials. *Journal of Studies on Alcohol and Drugs, 70,* 516-527.

Mahalik, J. R., Levine, C. R., McPherran Lombardi, C., Doyle Lynch, A., Markowitz, A. J., & Jaffee, S. R. (2013). Changes in health risk behaviors for males and females from early adolescence through early adulthood. *Health Psychology, 32,* 685-694.

Mahler, H. I. M., & Kulik, J. A. (1998). Effects of preparatory videotapes on self-efficacy beliefs and recovery from coronary bypass surgery. *Annals of Behavioral Medicine, 20,* 39-46.

Mahler, H. I. M., Kulik, J. A., Gerrard, M., & Gibbons, F. X. (2007). Long-term effects of appearance-based interventions on sun protection behaviors. *Health Psychology, 26,* 350-360.

Mahler, H. I. M., Kulick, J. A., Gibbons, F. X., Gerrard, M., & Harrell, J. (2003). Effects of appearance-based interventions on sun protection intentions and self-reported behaviors. *Health Psychology, 22,* 199-209.

Maisel, N. C., & Gable, S. L. (2009). The paradox of received social support: The importance of responsiveness. *Psychological Sciences, 20,* 928-932.

Majer, M., Welberg, L. A. M., Capuron, L., Miller, A. H., Pagnoni, G., & Reeves, W. C. (2008). Neuropsychological performance in persons with chronic fatigue syndrome: Results from a population-based study. *Psychosomatic Medicine, 70,* 829-836.

Major, B., Mendes, W. B., & Dovidio, J. F. (2013). Intergroup relations and health disparities: A social psychological perspective. *Health Psychology, 32,* 514-524.

Malik, V. S., Popkin, B. M., Bray, G. A., Després, J. P., Willett, W. C., & Hu, F. B. (2010). Sugar-sweetened beverages and risk of metabolic syndrome and type 2 diabetes. *Diabetes Care, 33,* 2477-2483.

Mallett, K., Price, J. H., Jurs, S. G., & Slenker, S. (1991). Relationships among burnout, death anxiety, and social support in hospice and critical care nurses. *Psychological Reports, 68,* 1347-1359.

Maloney, E. M., Boneva, R., Nater, U. M., & Reeves, W. C. (2009). Chronic fatigue syndrome and high allostatic load: Results from a population-based case-control study in Georgia. *Psychosomatic Medicine, 71,* 549-556.

Manber, R., Kuo, T. F., Cataldo, N., & Colrain, I. M. (2003). The effects of hormone replacement therapy on sleep-disordered breathing in postmenopausal women: A pilot study. *Journal of Sleep & Sleep Disorders Research, 26,* 163-168.

Mancuso, R. A., Dunkel-Schetter, C., Rini, C. M., Roesch, S. C., & Hobel, C. J. (2004). Maternal prenatal anxiety and corticitropin-releasing hormone associated with timing of delivery. *Psychosomatic Medicine, 66,* 762-769.

Mann, D. M., Ponieman, D., Leventhal, H., & Halm, E. A. (2009). Predictors of adherence to diabetes medications: The role of disease and medication beliefs. *Journal of Behavioral Medicine, 32,* 278-284.

Mann, T. (2001). Effects of future writing and optimism on health behaviors in HIV-infected women. *Annals of Behavioral Medicine, 23,* 26-33.

Mann, T., de Ridder, D., & Fujita, K. (2013). Self-regulation of health behavior: Social psychological approaches to goal setting and goal striving. *Health Psychology, 32,* 487-498.

Mann, T., Nolen-Hoeksema, S., Huang, K., Burgard, D., Wright, A., & Hanson, K. (1997). Are two interventions worse than none? Joint primary and secondary prevention of eating disorders in college females. *Health Psychology, 16,* 215-225.

Manne, S. L., Bakeman, R., Jacobsen, P. B., Gorfinkle, K., Bernstein, D., & Redd, W. H. (1992). Adult-child interaction during invasive medical procedures. *Health Psychology, 11,* 241-249.

Manne, S. L., Jacobsen, P. B., Gorfinkle, K., Gerstein, F., & Redd, W. H. (1993). Treatment adherence difficulties among children with cancer: The role of parenting style. *Journal of Pediatric Psychology, 18,* 47-62.

Manne, S. L., Markowitz, A., Winawer, S., Meropol, N. J., Haller, D., Rakowski, W., . . . Jandorf, L. (2002). Correlates of colorectal cancer screening compliance and stage of adoption among siblings of individuals with early onset colorectal cancer. *Health Psychology, 21,* 3-15.

Manne, S. L., Redd, W. H., Jacobsen, P. B., Gorfinkle, K., Schorr, O., & Rapkin, B. (1990). Behavioral intervention to reduce child and parent distress during venipuncture. *Journal of Consulting and Clinical Psychology, 58,* 565-572.

Manning, B. K., Catley, D., Harris, K. J., Mayo, M. S., & Ahluwalia, J. S. (2005). Stress and quitting among African American smokers. *Journal of Behavioral Medicine, 28,* 325-333.

Mantzari, E., Vogt, F., & Marteau, T. M. (2015). Financial incentives for increasing uptake of HPV vaccinations: A randomized controlled trial. *Health Psychology, 34,* 160-171.

Manuck, S. B., Phillips, J. E., Gianaros, P. J., Flory, J. D., & Muldoon, M. F. (2010). Subjective socioeconomic status and presence of the metabolic syndrome in midlife community volunteers. *Psychosomatic Medicine, 72,* 35-45.

Margolin, A., Avants, S. K., Warburton, L. A., Hawkins, K. A., & Shi, J. (2003). A randomized clinical trial of a manual-guided risk reduction intervention for HIV-positive injection drug users. *Health Psychology, 22,* 223-228.

Marin, T. J., Chen, E., Munch, J. A., & Miller, G. E. (2009). Double-exposure to acute stress and chronic family stress is associated with immune changes in children with asthma. *Psychosomatic Medicine, 71,* 378-384.

Marin, T. J., Martin, T. M., Blackwell, E., Stetler, C., & Miller, G. E. (2007). Differentiating the impact of episodic and chronic stressors on hypothalamic-pituitary-adrenocortical axis regulation in young women. *Health Psychology, 26,* 447-455.

Marks, M., Sliwinski, M., & Gordon, W. A. (1993). An examination of the needs of families with a brain injured child. *Neurological Rehabilitation, 3,* 1-12.

Marlatt, G. A. (1990). Cue exposure and relapse prevention in the treatment of addictive behaviors. *Addictive Behaviors, 15,* 395-399.

Marlatt, G. A., Baer, J. S., Kivlahan, D. R., Dimeff, L. A., Larimer, M. E., Quigley, L. A., . . . Williams, E. (1998). Screening and brief intervention for high-risk college student drinkers: Results from a 2-year follow-up assessment. *Journal of Consulting and Clinical Psychology, 66,* 604-615.

Marlatt, G. A., & George, W. H. (1988). Relapse prevention and the maintenance of optimal health. In S. Shumaker, E. Schron, & J. K. Ockene (Eds.), *The adoption and maintenance of behaviors for optimal health.* New York: Springer.

Marlatt, G. A., & Gordon, J. R. (1980). Determinants of relapse: Implications for the maintenance of behavior change. In P. O. Davidson & S. M. Davidson (Eds.), *Behavioral medicine: Changing health lifestyles.* New York: Brunner/Mazel.

Marrero, D., Mele, L., Doyle, T., Schwartz, F., Mather, K. J., Goldberg, R., . . . Knowler, W. C. (2018). Depressive symptoms, antidepressant medication use, and inflammatory markers in the diabetes prevention program. *Psychosomatic Medicine, 80,* 167-173.

Marsh, B. (2002, September 10). A primer on fat, some of it good for you. *New York Times,* p. D7.

Marshall, E. (1986). Involuntary smokers face health risks. *Science, 234,* 1066-1067.

Marsland, A. L., Petersen, K. L., Sathanoori, R., Muldoon, M. F., Neumann, S. A., Ryan, C., . . . Manuck, S. B. (2006). Interleukin-6 covaries inversely with cognitive performance among middle-aged community volunteers. *Psychosomatic Medicine, 68,* 895-903.

Marteau, T. M., Johnston, M., Baum, J. D., & Bloch, S. (1987). Goals of treatment in diabetes: A comparison of doctors and parents of children with diabetes. *Journal of Behavioral Medicine, 10,* 33-48.

Marteau, T. M., & Weinman, J. (2006). Self-regulation and the behavioural response to DNA risk information: A theoretical analysis and framework for future research. *Social Science & Medicine, 62,* 1360-1368.

Martens, E. J., Smith, O. R. F., & Denollet, J. (2007). Psychological symptom clusters, psychiatric comorbidity and poor self-reported health status following myocardial infarction. *Annals of Behavioral Medicine, 34,* 87-94.

Martin, J., Sheeran, P., Slade, P., Wright, A., & Dibble, T. (2009). Implementation intention formation reduces consultations for emergency contraception and pregnancy testing among teenage women. *Health Psychology, 28,* 762-769.

Martin, J. K., Tuch, S. A., & Roman, P. M. (2003). Problem drinking patterns among African Americans: The impacts of reports of discrimination, perceptions of prejudice, and "risky" coping strategies. *Journal of Health and Social Behavior, 44,* 408-425.

Martin, L. R., Friedman, H. S., Tucker, J. S., Tomlinson-Keasey, C., Criqui, M. H., & Schwartz, J. E. (2002). Life course perspective on childhood cheerfulness and its relations to mortality risk. *Personality and Social Psychology Bulletin, 28,* 1155-1165.

Martin, R., Davis, G. M., Baron, R. S., Suls, J., & Blanchard, E. B. (1994). Specificity in social support: Perceptions of helpful and unhelpful provider behaviors among irritable bowel syndrome, headache, and cancer patients. *Health Psychology, 13,* 432-439.

Martin, R., & Lemos, K. (2002). From heart attacks to melanoma: Do common sense models of somatization influence symptom interpretation for female victims? *Health Psychology, 21,* 25-32.

Martinez, I., Kershaw, T. S., Keene, D., Perez-Escamilla, R., Lewis, J. B., Tobin, J. N., & Ickovics, J. R. (2017). Acculturation and syndemic risk: Longitudinal evaluation of risk factors among pregnant Latina adolescents in New York City. *Annals of Behavioral Medicine, 52,* 42-52.

Martínez, M., Arantzamendi, M., Belar, A., Carrasco, J. M., Carvajal, A., Rullán, M., & Centeno, C. (2017). 'Dignity therapy', a promising intervention in palliative care: A comprehensive systematic literature review. *Palliative Medicine, 31,* 492-509.

Martinez, S. M., Ainsworth, B. E., & Elder, J. P. (2008). A review of physical activity measures used among US Latinos: Guidelines for developing culturally appropriate measures. *Annals of Behavioral Medicine, 36,* 195-207.

Martire, L. M., Lustig, A. P., Schulz, R., Miller, G. E., & Helgeson, V. S. (2004). Is it beneficial to involve a family member? A meta-analysis of psychosocial interventions for chronic illness. *Health Psychology, 23,* 599-611.

Martire, L. M., Schulz, R., Helgeson, V. S., Small, B. J., & Saghafi, E. M. (2010). Review and meta-analysis of couple-oriented interventions for chronic illness. *Annals of Behavioral Medicine, 40,* 325-342.

Martire, L. M., Stephens, M. A. P., Druley, J. A., & Wojno, W. C. (2002). Negative reactions to received spousal care: Predictors and consequences of miscarried support. *Health Psychology, 21,* 167-176.

Martire, L. M., Stephens, M. A. P., & Schulz, R. (2011). Independence centrality as a moderator of the effects of spousal support on patient well-being and physical functioning. *Health Psychology, 30,* 651-655.

Maselko, J., Kubzansky, L., Kawachi, I., Seeman, T., & Berkman, L. (2007). Religous service attendance and allostatic load among high-functioning elderly. *Psychosomatic Medicine, 69,* 464-472.

Masi, C. M., Chen, H. Y., Hawkley, L. C., & Cacioppo, J. T. (2011). A meta-analysis of interventions to reduce loneliness. *Personality and Social Psychology Review, 15,* 219-266.

Maslach, C. (1979). The burn-out syndrome and patient care. In C. Garfield (Ed.), *The emotional realities of life-threatening illness* (pp. 111-120). St. Louis, MO: Mosby.

Maslach, C. (2003). Job burnout: New directions in research and intervention. *Current Directions, 12,* 189-192.

Mason, A. E., Hecht, F. M., Daubenmier, J. J., Sbarra, D. A., Lin, J., Moran, P. J., . . . Epel, E. S. (2018). Weight loss maintenance and cellular aging in the supporting health through nutrition and exercise study. *Psychosomatic Medicine, 80,* 609-619.

Mason, H. R. C., Marks, G., Simoni, J. M., Ruiz, M. S., & Richardson, J. L. (1995). Culturally sanctioned secrets? Latino men's nondisclosure of HIV infection to family, friends, and lovers. *Health Psychology, 14,* 6-12.

Mason, J. W., Wang, S., Yehuda, R., Lubin, H., Johnson, D., Bremner, J. D., . . . Southwick, S. (2002). Marked lability in urinary cortisol levels in subgroups of combat veterans with posttraumatic stress disorder during an intensive exposure treatment program. *Psychosomatic Medicine, 64,* 238-246.

Master, S. L., Eisenberger, N. I., Taylor, S. E., Naliboff, B. D., Shirinyan, D., & Lieberman, M. D. (2009). A picture's worth: Partner photographs reduce experimentally induced pain. *Psychological Science, 20,* 1316-1318.

Masters, K. S., Ross, K. M., Hooker, S. A., & Wooldridge, J. L. (2018). A psychometric approach to theory-based behavior change intervention development: Example from the Colorado meaning-activity project. *Annals of Behavioral Medicine, 52,* 463-473.

Masters, K. S. (2018). Introduction to the special section on behavior change intervention development: theories, methods, and mechanisms. *Annals of Behavioral Medicine, 52,* 443-p445.

Masters, K. S., & Spielmans, G. I. (2007). Prayer and health: Review, meta-analysis, and research agenda. *Journal of Behavioral Medicine, 30,* 329-338.

Mata, J., Silva, M. N., Vieira, P. N., Carraca, E. V., Andrade, A. M., Coutinho, S. R., . . . Teixeira, P. J. (2009). Motivational "spill-over" during weight control: Increased self-determination and exercise intrinsic motivation predict eating self-regulation. *Health Psychology, 28,* 709-716.

Mathur, A., Jarrett, P., Broadbent, E., & Petrie, K. J. (2018). Open-label placebos for wound healing: A randomized controlled trial. *Annals of Behavioral Medicine, 52,* 902-908.

Matos, M., Bernardes, S. F., Goubert, L., & Beyers, W. (2017). Buffer or amplifier? Longitudinal effects of social support for functional autonomy/dependence on older adults' chronic pain experiences. *Health Psychology, 36,* 1195-1206.

Mattavelli, S., Avishai, A., Perugini, M., Richetin, J., & Sheeran, P. (2017). How can implicit and explicit attitudes both be changed? Testing two interventions to promote consumption of green vegetables. *Annals of Behavioral Medicine, 51,* 511-518.

Matthews, K. A., Boylan, J. M., Jakubowski, K. P., Cundiff, J. M., Lee, L., Pardini, D. A., & Jennings, J. R. (2017). Socioeconomic status and parenting during adolescence in relation to ideal cardiovascular health in Black and White men. *Health Psychology, 36,* 673-681.

Matthews, K. A., Gallo, L. C., & Taylor, S. E. (2010). Are psychosocial factors mediators of SES and health connections? A progress report and blueprint for the future. In N. Adler & J. Stewart (Eds.), *The biology of disadvantage: Socioeconomic status and health* (Vol. 1186, pp. 146-173). Malden, MA: Wiley-Blackwell.

Matthews, K. A., Gump, B. B., Block, D. R., & Allen, M. T. (1997). Does background stress heighten or dampen children's cardiovascular responses to acute stress? *Psychosomatic Medicine, 59,* 488-496.

Matthews, K. A., Gump, B. B., & Owens, J. F. (2001). Chronic stress influences cardiovascular and neuroendocrine responses during acute stress and recovery, especially in men. *Health Psychology, 20,* 403-410.

Matthews, K. A., Owens, J. F., Allen, M. T., & Stoney, C. M. (1992). Do cardiovascular responses to laboratory stress relate to ambulatory blood pressure levels? Yes, in some of the people, some of the time. *Psychosomatic Medicine, 54,* 686-697.

Matthews, K. A., Owens, J. F., Kuller, L. H., Sutton-Tyrrell, K., & Jansen-McWilliams, L. (1998). Are hostility and anxiety associated with carotid atherosclerosis in healthy postmenopausal women? *Psychosomatic Medicine, 60,* 633-638.

Matthews, K. A., Räikkönen, K., Gallo, L., & Kuller, L. H. (2008). Association between socioeconomic status and metabolic syndrome in women: Testing the reserve capacity model. *Health Psychology, 27,* 576-583.

Matthews, K. A., Salomon, K., Brady, S. S., & Allen, M. T. (2003). Cardiovascular reactivity to stress predicts future blood pressure in adolescence. *Psychosomatic Medicine, 65,* 410-415.

Matthews, K. A., Woodall, K. L., & Allen, M. T. (1993). Cardiovascular reactivity to stress predicts future blood pressure status. *Hypertension, 22,* 479-485.

Matthews, K. A., Woodall, K. L., Kenyon, K., & Jacob, T. (1996). Negative family environment as a predictor of boys' future status on measures of hostile attitudes, interview behavior, and anger expression. *Health Psychology, 15,* 30-37.

Mattson, M. P. (2004). Pathways towards and away from Alzheimer's disease. *Nature, 430,* 631-639.

Maugh, T. H. (2009, October 9). Virus is found in many people with chronic fatigue. *Los Angeles Times,* p. A18.

Mauksch, H. O. (1973). Ideology, interaction, and patient care in hospitals. *Social Science and Medicine, 7,* 817-830.

Mausbach, B. T., Bos, T., & Irwin, S. A. (2018). Mental health treatment dose and annual healthcare costs in patients with cancer and major depressive disorder. *Health Psychology, 37,* 1035-1040.

Mausbach, B. T., Chattillion, E., Roepke, S. K., Ziegler, M. G., Milic, M., von Känel, R., . . . Grant, I. (2012). A longitudinal analysis of the relations among stress, depressive symptoms, leisure satisfaction, and endothelial function in caregivers. *Health Psychology, 31,* 433-440.

Mausbach, B. T., Dimsdale, J. E., Ziegler, M. G., Mills, P. J., Ancoli-Israel, S., Patterson, T. L., & Grant, I. (2005). Depressive symptoms predict norepinephrine response to a psychological stressor task in Alzheimer's caregivers. *Psychosomatic Medicine, 67,* 638-642.

Mausbach, B. T., Patterson, T. L., Rabinowitz, Y. G., Grant, I., & Schulz, R. (2007). Depression and distress predict time to cardiovascular disease in dementia caregivers. *Health Psychology, 26,* 539-544.

Mausbach, B. T., Semple, S. J., Strathdee, S. A., Zians, J., & Patterson, T. L. (2007). Efficacy of a behavioral intervention for increasing safer sex behaviors in HIV-negative, heterosexual methamphetamine users: Results from the fast-lane study. *Annals of Behavioral Medicine, 34,* 263-274.

Mausbach, B. T., von Känel, R., Aschbacher, K., Roepke, S. K., Dimsdale, J. E., Ziegler, M. G., . . . Grant, I. (2007). Spousal caregivers of patients with Alzheimer's disease show longitudinal increases in plasma level of tissue-type plasminogen activator antigen. *Psychosomatic Medicine, 69,* 816-822.

Mayer-Davis, E. J., Lawrence, J. M., Dabelea, D., Divers, J., Isom, S., Dolan, L., . . . Pihoker, C. (2017). Incidence trends of type 1 and type 2 diabetes among youths, 2002-2012. *New England Journal of Medicine, 376,* 1419-1429.

Mayer, E. A., & Hsiao, E. Y. (2017). The gut and its microbiome as related to central nervous system functioning and psychological well-being: Introduction to the special issue of *Psychosomatic Medicine. Psychosomatic Medicine, 79,* 844-846.

May, M., McCarron, P., Stansfeld, S., Ben-Schlomo, Y., Gallacher, J., Yarnell, J., . . . Ebrahim, S. (2002). Does psychological distress predict the risk of ischemic stroke and transient ischemic attack? *Stroke, 33,* 7-12.

McAuley, E., Doerksen, S. E., Morris, K. S., Motl, R. W., Hu, L., Wójcicki, T. R., . . . Rosengren, K. R. (2008). Pathways from physical activity to quality of life in older women. *Annals of Behavioral Medicine, 36,* 13-20.

McAuley, E., White, S. M., Rogers, L. Q., Motl, R. W., & Courneya, K. S. (2010). Physical activity and fatigue in breast cancer and multiple sclerosis: Psychosocial mechanisms. *Psychosomatic Medicine, 72,* 88-96.

McBride, C. M., Pollack, K. I., Lyna, P., Lipkus, I. M., Samsa, G. P., & Bepler, G. (2001). Reasons for quitting smoking among low-income African American smokers. *Health Psychology, 20,* 334-340.

McCarroll, J. E., Ursano, R. J., Fullerton, C. S., Liu, X., & Lundy, A. (2002). Somatic symptoms in Gulf War mortuary workers. *Psychosomatic Medicine, 64,* 29-33.

McCaul, K. D., Monson, N., & Maki, R. H. (1992). Does distraction reduce pain-produced distress among college students? *Health Psychology, 11,* 210-217.

McClearn, G., Johansson, B., Berg, S., Pedersen, N., Ahern, F., Petrill, S. A., & Plomin, R. (1997). Substantial genetic influence on cognitive abilities in twins 80 or more years old. *Science, 276,* 1560-1563.

McClelland, L. E., & McCubbin, J. A. (2008). Social influence and pain response in women and men. *Journal of Behavioral Medicine, 31,* 413–420.

McConnell, A. R., Brown, C. M., Shoda, T. M., Stayton, L. E., & Martin, C. E. (2011). Friends with benefits: On the positive consequences of pet ownership. *Journal of Personality and Social Psychology, 101,* 1239–1252.

McCracken, L. M. (1991). Cognitive-behavioral treatment of rheumatoid arthritis: A preliminary review of efficacy and methodology. *Annals of Behavioral Medicine, 13,* 57–65.

McCracken, L. M., & Vowles, K. E. (2008). A prospective analysis of acceptance of pain and values-based action in patients with chronic pain. *Health Psychology, 27,* 215–220.

McCracken, L. M., & Vowles, K. E. (2014). Acceptance and commitment therapy and mindfulness for chronic pain: Model, process, and progress. *American Psychologist, 69,* 178–187.

McCrory, C., Dooley, C., Layte, R., & Kenny, R. A. (2015). The lasting legacy of childhood adversity for disease risk in later life. *Health Psychology, 34,* 687–696.

McCullough, M. E., Friedman, H. S., Enders, C. K., & Martin, L. R. (2009). Does devoutness delay death? Psychological investment in religion and its association with longevity in the Terman sample. *Journal of Personality and Social Psychology, 97,* 866–882.

McDonagh, A., Friedman, M., McHugo, G., Ford, J., Sengupta, A., Mueser, K., . . . Descamps, M. (2005). Randomized trial of cognitive-behavioral therapy for chronic posttraumatic stress disorder in adult female survivors of childhood sexual abuse. *Journal of Consulting and Clinical Psychology, 73,* 515–524.

McDonough, P., Williams, D. R., House, J. S., & Duncan, G. J. (1999). Gender and the socioeconomic gradient in mortality. *Journal of Health and Social Behavior, 40,* 17–31.

McEachan, R., Taylor, N., Harrison, R., Lawton, R., Gardner, P., & Conner, M. (2016). Meta-analysis of the reasoned action approach (RAA) to understanding health behaviors. *Annals of Behavioral Medicine, 50,* 592–612.

McEwen, B. S. (1998). Protective and damaging effects of stress mediators. *The New England Journal of Medicine, 338,* 171–179.

McGarrity, L. A., & Huebner, D. M. (2014). Behavioral intentions to HIV test and subsequent testing: The moderating role of sociodemographic characteristics. *Health Psychology, 33,* 396–400.

McGinty, H. L., Small, B. J., Laronga, C., & Jacobsen, P. B. (2016). Predictors and patterns of fear of cancer recurrence in breast cancer survivors. *Health Psychology, 35,* 1–9.

McGonagle, K. A., & Kessler, R. C. (1990). Chronic stress, acute stress, and depressive symptoms. *American Journal of Community Psychology, 18,* 681–706.

McGrady, A., Conran, P., Dickey, D., Garman, D., Farris, E., & Schumann-Brzezinski, C. (1992). The effects of biofeedback-assisted relaxation on cell-mediated immunity, cortisol, and white blood cell count in healthy adult subjects. *Journal of Behavioral Medicine, 15,* 343–354.

McGuire, L., Heffner, K., Glaser, R., Needleman, B., Malarkey, W., Dickinson, S., . . . Kiecolt-Glaser, J. K. (2006). Pain and wound healing in surgical patients. *Annals of Behavioral Medicine, 31,* 165–172.

McIntosh, D. N., Poulin, M. J., Silver, R. C., & Holman, E. A. (2011). The distinct roles of spirituality and religiosity in physical and mental health after collective trauma: A national longitudinal study of responses to the 9/11 attacks. *Journal of Behavioral Medicine, 34,* 497–507.

McKay, B. (2011, September 19). U.N. to address spread of chronic diseases. *The Wall Street Journal,* p. A13.

McKay, H. G., Seeley, J. R., King, D., Glasgow, R. E., & Eakin, E. G. (2001). The diabetes network Internet-based physical activity intervention. *Diabetes Care, 24,* 1328–1334.

McKenna, M. C., Zevon, M. A., Corn, B., & Rounds, J. (1999). Psychological factors and the development of breast cancer: A meta-analysis. *Health Psychology, 18,* 520–531.

McKnight, P. E., Afram, A., Kashdan, T. B., Kasle, S., & Zautra, A. (2010). Coping self-efficacy as a mediator between catastrophizing and physical functioning: Treatment target selection in an osteoarthritis sample. *Journal of Behavioral Medicine, 33,* 239–249.

McNally, R. J. (2012). Are we winning the war against posttraumatic stress disorder? *Science, 336,* 872–874.

McVea, K. L. S. P. (2006). Evidence for clinical smoking cessation for adolescents. *Health Psychology, 25,* 558–562.

Means-Christensen, A. J., Arnau, R. C., Tonidandel, A. M., Bramson, R., & Meagher, M. W. (2005). An efficient method of identifying major depression and panic disorder in primary care. *Journal of Behavioral Medicine, 28,* 565–572.

Meara, E., White, C., & Cutler, D. M. (2004). Trends in medical spending by age, 1963–2000. *Health Affairs, 23,* 176–183.

Mechanic, D. (1972). Social psychologic factors affecting the presentation of bodily complaints. *The New England Journal of Medicine, 286,* 1132–1139.

Mechanic, D. (1975). The organization of medical practice and practice orientation among physicians in prepaid and nonprepaid primary care settings. *Medical Care, 13,* 189–204.

Meert, K. L., Eggly, S., Kavanaugh, K., Berg, R. A., Wessel, D. L., Newth, C. J. L., & Park, C. L. (2015). Meaning making during parent-physician bereavement meetings at a child's death. *Health Psychology, 34,* 453–461.

Meechan, G., Collins, J., & Petrie, K. J. (2003). The relationship of symptoms and psychological factors to delay in seeking medical care for breast symptoms. *Preventive Medicine, 36,* 374–378.

Meichenbaum, D. H., & Jaremko, M. E. (Eds.). (1983). *Stress reduction and prevention.* New York: Plenum.

Melamed, B. G., & Brenner, G. F. (1990). Social support and chronic medical stress: An interaction-based approach. *Journal of Social and Clinical Psychology, 9,* 104–117.

Melamed, B. G., & Siegel, L. (1975). Reduction of anxiety in children facing hospitalization and surgery by use of filmed modeling. *Journal of Consulting and Clinical Psychology, 43,* 511–521.

Melzack, R. (1983). *Pain measurement and assessment.* New York: Raven Press.

Melzack, R., & Wall, P. D. (1982). *The challenge of pain.* New York: Basic Books.

Menaghan, E., Kowaleski-Jones, L., & Mott, F. (1997). The intergenerational costs of parental social stressors: Academic and social difficulties in early adolescence for children of young mothers. *Journal of Health and Social Behavior, 38,* 72–86.

Mendes de Leon, C. F. (1992). Anger and impatience/irritability in patients of low socioeconomic status with acute coronary heart disease. *Journal of Behavioral Medicine, 15,* 273–284.

Mendes de Leon, C. F., Kop, W. J., de Swart, H. B., Bar, F. W., & Appels, A. P. W. M. (1996). Psychosocial characteristics and recurrent events after percutaneous transluminal coronary angioplasty. *American Journal of Cardiology, 77,* 252–255.

Menning, C. L. (2006). Nonresident fathers' involvement and adolescents' smoking. *Journal of Health and Social Behavior, 47,* 32–46.

Menon, U., Belue, R., Wahab, S., Rugen, K., Kinney, A. Y., Maramaldi, P., . . . Szalacha, L. A. (2011). A randomized trial comparing the effect of two phone-based interventions on colorectal cancer screening adherence. *Annals of Behavioral Medicine, 42,* 294–303.

Mercado, A. C., Carroll, L. J., Cassidy, J. D., & Cote, P. (2000). Coping with neck and low back pain in the general population. *Health Psychology, 19,* 333–338.

Mercken, L., Steglich, C., Sinclair, P., Holliday, J., & Moore, L. (2012). A longitudinal social network analysis of peer influence, peer selection, and smoking behavior among adolescents in British schools. *Health Psychology, 31,* 450–459.

Mermelstein, R., Cohen, S., Lichtenstein, E., Baer, J. S., & Kamarck, T. (1986). Social support and smoking cessation and maintenance. *Journal of Consulting and Clinical Psychology, 54,* 447–453.

Merritt, M. M., Bennett, G. G., Williams, R. B., Sollers, J. J., III, & Thayer, J. F. (2004). Low educational attainment, John Henryism and cardiovascular reactivity to and recovery from personally relevant stress. *Psychosomatic Medicine, 66,* 49–55.

Mertens, M. C., Roukema, J. A., Scholtes, V. P. W., & De Vries, J. (2010). Trait anxiety predicts unsuccessful surgery in gallstone disease. *Psychosomatic Medicine, 72,* 198–205.

Merz, E. L., Fox, R. S., & Malcarne, V. L. (2014). Expressive writing interventions in cancer patients: A systematic review. *Health Psychology Review, 8,* 339–361.

Messina, C. R., Lane, D. S., Glanz, K., West, D. S., Taylor, V., Frishman, W., & Powell, L. (2004). Relationship of social support and social burden to repeated breast cancer screening in the women's health initiative. *Health Psychology, 23,* 582–594.

Mestel, R. (2012, June 5). Life expectancy gap narrows between blacks, whites. *Los Angeles Times.* Retrieved July 5, 2012, from http://articles.latimes.com/2012/jun/05/science/la-sci-life-expectancy-gap-20120606

Meyer, M. H., & Pavalko, E. K. (1996). Family, work, and access to health insurance among mature women. *Journal of Health and Social Behavior, 37,* 311–325.

Meyerowitz, B. E. (1983). Postmastectomy coping strategies and quality of life. *Health Psychology, 2,* 117–132.

Meyerowitz, B. E., & Hart, S. (1993, April). *Women and cancer: Have assumptions about women limited our research agenda?* Paper presented at the Women's Psychological and Physical Health Conference, Lawrence, KS.

Mezick, E. J., Matthews, K. A., Hall, M., Kamarck, T. W., Strollo, P. J., Buysse, D. J., . . . Reis, S. E. (2010). Low life purpose and high hostility are related to an attenuated decline in nocturnal blood pressure. *Health Psychology, 29,* 196–204.

Mezick, E. J., Matthews, K. A., Hall, M., Strollo, P. J., Buysse, D. J., Kamarck, T.W., . . . Reis, S. E. (2008). Influence of race and socioeconomic status on sleep: Pittsburgh sleep SCORE project. *Psychosomatic Medicine, 70,* 410–416.

Michael, Y. L., Carlson, N. E., Chlebowski, R. T., Aickin, M., Weihs, K. L., Ockene, J. K., . . . Ritenbaugh, C. (2009). Influence of stressors on breast cancer incidence in the women's health initiative. *Health Psychology, 28,* 137–146.

Michaud, D. S., Liu, S., Giovannucci, E., Willett, W. C., Colditz, G. A., & Fuchs, C. S. (2002). Dietary sugar, glycemic load, and pancreatic cancer risk in a prospective study. *Journal of the National Cancer Institute, 94,* 1293–1300.

Michela, J. L. (1987). Interpersonal and individual impacts of a husband's heart attack. In A. Baum & J. E. Singer (Eds.), *Handbook of psychology and health* (Vol. 5, pp. 255–301). Hillsdale, NJ: Erlbaum.

Michels, N., Sioen, I., Boone, L., Braet, C., Vanaelst, B., Huybrechts, I., & De Henauw, S. (2015). Longitudinal association between child stress and lifestyle. *Health Psychology, 34,* 40–50.

Michie, S., Carey, R. N., Johnston, M., Rothman, A. J., De Bruin, M., Kelly, M. P., & Connell, L. E. (2017). From theory-inspired to theory-based interventions: A protocol for developing and testing a methodology for linking behaviour change techniques to theoretical mechanisms of action. *Annals of Behavioral Medicine, 52,* 501–512.

Midei, A. J., & Matthews, K. A. (2009). Social relationships and negative emotional traits are associated with central adiposity and arterial stiffness in healthy adolescents. *Health Psychology, 28,* 347–353.

Midei, A. J., Matthews, K. A., Chang, Y. F., & Bromberger, J. T. (2013). Childhood physical abuse is associated with incident metabolic syndrome in mid-life women. *Health Psychology, 32,* 121–127.

Migneault, J. P., Dedier, J. J., Wright, J. A., Heeren, T., Campbell, M. K., Morisky, D. E., . . . Friedman, R. H. (2012). A culturally adapted telecommunication system to improve physical activity, diet quality, and medication adherence among hypertensive African-Americans: A randomized controlled trial. *Annals of Behavioral Medicine, 43,* 62–73.

Millar, B. M. (2017). Clocking self-regulation: Why time of day matters for health psychology. *Health Psychology Review, 11,* 345–357.

Miller, G. E., & Blackwell, E. (2006). Turning up the heat: Inflammation as a mechanism linking chronic stress, depression, and heart disease. *Current Directions in Psychological Science, 15,* 269–272.

Miller, G. E., & Chen, E. (2007). Unfavorable socioeconomic conditions in early life presage expression of proinflammatory phenotype in adolescence. *Psychosomatic Medicine, 69,* 402–409.

Miller, G. E., & Chen, E. (2010). Harsh family climate in early life presages the emergence of a proinflammatory phenotype in adolescence. *Psychological Science, 21,* 848–856.

Miller, G. E., Chen, E., & Parker, K. J. (2011). Psychological stress in childhood and susceptibility to the chronic diseases of aging: Moving toward a model of behavioral and biological mechanisms. *Psychological Bulletin, 137,* 959–997.

Miller, G. E., Chen, E., & Zhou, E. S. (2007). If it goes up, must it come down? Chronic stress and the hypothalamic-pituitary-adrenocortical axis in humans. *Psychological Bulletin, 133,* 25–45.

Miller, G. E., & Cohen, S. (2001). Psychological interventions and the immune system: A meta-analytic review and critique. *Health Psychology, 20,* 47–63.

Miller, G. E., Cohen, S., & Herbert, T. B. (1999). Pathways linking major depression and immunity in ambulatory female patients. *Psychosomatic Medicine, 61,* 850–860.

Miller, G. E., Cohen, S., & Ritchey, A. K. (2002). Chronic psychological stress and the regulation of pro-inflammatory cytokines: A glucocorticoid-resistance model. *Health Psychology, 21,* 531–541.

Miller, G. E., Lachman, M. E., Chen, E., Gruenewald, T. L., Karlamangla, A.S., & Seeman, T. E. (2011). Pathways to resilience: Maternal nurturance as a buffer against the effects of childhood poverty on metabolic syndrome at midlife. *Psychological Science, 22,* 1591–1599.

Miller, G. E., Rohleder, N., & Cole, S. W. (2009). Chronic interpersonal stress predicts activation of pro- and anti-inflammatory signaling pathways 6 months later. *Psychosomatic Medicine, 71,* 57–62.

Miller, M., Mangano, C. C., Beach, V., Kop, W. J., & Vogel, R. A. (2010). Divergent effects of joyful and anxiety-provoking music on endothelial vasoreactivity. *Psychosomatic Medicine, 72,* 354–356.

Miller, N. E. (1989). Placebo factors in types of treatment: Views of a psychologist. In M. Shepherd & N. Sartorius (Eds.), *Non-specific aspects of treatment* (pp. 39–56). Lewiston, NY: Hans Huber.

Miller, S. L., & Maner, J. K. (2012). Overperceiving disease cues: The basic cognition of the behavioral immune system. *Journal of Personality and Social Psychology, 102,* 1198–1213.

Miller, W. R., & Rose, G. S. (2009). Toward a theory of motivational interviewing. *American Psychologist, 64,* 527–537.

Mills, P. J., Meck, J. V., Waters, W. W., D'Aunno, D., & Ziegler, M. G. (2001). Peripheral leukocyte subpopulations and catecholamine levels in astronauts as a function of mission duration. *Psychosomatic Medicine, 63,* 886–890.

Milne, H. M., Wallman, K. E., Gordon, S., & Courneya, K. S. (2008). Impact of a combined resistance and aerobic exercise program on motivational variables in breast cancer survivors: A randomized controlled trial. *Annals of Behavioral Medicine, 36,* 158–166.

Milne, S., Orbell, S., & Sheeran, P. (2002). Combining motivational and volitional interventions to promote exercise participation: Protection motivation theory and implementation intentions. *British Journal of Health Psychology, 7,* 163–184.

Milne, S., Sheeran, P., & Orbell, S. (2000). Prediction and intervention in health-related behavior: A meta-analytic review of Protection Motivation Theory. *Journal of Applied Social Psychology, 30,* 106–143.

Milton, A. C., & Mullan, B. A. (2012). An application of the theory of planned behavior—a randomized controlled food safety pilot intervention for young adults. *Health Psychology, 31,* 250–259.

Minassian, A., Geyer, M. A., Baker, D. G., Nievergelt, C. M., O'Connor, D. T., & Risbrough, V. B., for the Marine Resiliency Study Team. (2014). Heart rate variability characteristics in a large group of active-duty marines and relationship to posttraumatic stress. *Psychosomatic Medicine, 76,* 292–301.

Miniño, A. M. (2010). Mortality among teenagers aged 12–19 years: United States, 1999–2006. *NCHS Data Brief, 37,* 1–8.

Minkler, M., Fuller-Thomson, E., & Guralnik, J. M. (2006). Gradient of disability across the socioeconomic spectrum in the United States. *The New England Journal of Medicine, 355,* 695–702.

Mintzer, J. E., Rubert, M. P., Loewenstein, D., Gamez, E., Millor, A., Quinteros, R., . . . Eisdorfer, C. (1992). Daughters caregiving for Hispanic and non-Hispanic Alzheimer patients: Does ethnicity make a difference? *Community Mental Health Journal, 28,* 293–303.

Mitchell, J. E., Agras, S., & Wonderlich, S. (2007). Treatment of bulimia nervosa: Where are we and where are we going? *International Journal of Eating Disorders, 40,* 95–101.

Mitchell, J. E., Laine, D. E., Morley, J. E., & Levine, A. S. (1986). Naloxone but not CCK-8 may attenuate binge-eating behavior in patients with the bulimia syndrome. *Biological Psychiatry, 21,* 1399–1406.

Mitrani, V. B., McCabe, B. E., Burns, M. J., & Feaster, D. J. (2012). Family mechanisms of structural ecosystems therapy for HIV-seropositive women in drug recovery. *Health Psychology, 31,* 591–600.

Mittag, W., & Schwarzer, R. (1993). Interaction of employment status and self-efficacy on alcohol consumption: A two-wave study on stressful life transitions. *Psychology and Health, 8,* 77–87.

Mittermaier, C., Dejaco, C., Waldhoer, T., Oefferlbauer-Ernst, A., Miehsler, W., Beier, M., . . . Moser, G. (2004). Impact of depressive mood on relapse in patients with inflammatory bowel disease: A prospective 18-month follow-up study. *Psychosomatic Medicine, 66,* 79–84.

Mohr, D., Bedantham, K., Neylan, T., Metzler, T. J., Best, S., & Marmar, C. R. (2003). The mediating effects of sleep in the relationship between traumatic stress and health symptoms in urban police officers. *Psychosomatic Medicine, 65,* 485–489.

Mohr, D., Hart, S. L., & Goldberg, A. (2003). Effects of treatment for depression on fatigue in multiple sclerosis. *Psychosomatic Medicine, 65,* 542–547.

Mohr, D. C., Siddique, J., Ho, J., Duffecy, J., Jin, L., & Fokuo, J. K. (2010). Interest in behavioral and psychological treatments delivered face-to-face, by telephone, and by Internet. *Annals of Behavioral Medicine, 40,* 89–98.

Mokdad, A. H., Marks, J. S., Stroup, D. F., & Gerberding, J. L. (2004). Actual cause of death in the United States, 2000. *Journal of the American Medical Society, 291,* 1238–1245.

Moller, J., Hallqvist, J., Diderichsen, F., Theorell, T., Reuterwall, C., & Ahlbom, A. (1999). Do episodes of anger trigger myocardial infarction? A case-crossover analysis in the Stockholm Heart Epidemiology Program (SHEEP). *Psychosomatic Medicine, 61,* 842–849.

Molloy, G. J., Noone, C., Caldwell, D., Welton, N. J., & Newell, J. (2018). Network meta-analysis in health psychology and behavioural medicine: A primer. *Health Psychology Review, 12,* 254–270.

Molloy, G. J., Perkins-Porras, L., Strike, P. C., & Steptoe, A. (2008). Type D personality and cortisol in survivors of acute coronary syndrome. *Psychosomatic Medicine, 70,* 863–868.

Molloy, G. J., Randall, G., Wikman, A., Perkins-Porras, L., Messerli-Bürgy, N., & Steptoe, A. (2012). Type D personality, self-efficacy, and medication adherence following an acute coronary syndrome. *Psychosomatic Medicine, 74,* 100–106.

Molton, I. R., & Terrill, A. L. (2014). Overview of persistent pain in older adults. *American Psychologist, 69,* 197–208.

Monaghan, M., Herbert, L. J., Wang, J., Holmes, C., Cogen, F., & Streisand, R. (2015). Mealtime behavior and diabetes-specific parent functioning in young children with type 1 diabetes. *Health Psychology, 34,* 794–780.

Moncrieft, A. E., Llabre, M. M., McCalla, J. R., Gutt, M., Mendez, A. J., Gellman, M. D., . . . Schneiderman, N. (2016). Effects of a multicomponent life-style intervention on weight, glycemic control, depressive symptoms, and renal function in low-income, minority patients with type 2 diabetes: Results of the community approach to lifestyle modification for diabetes randomized controlled trial. *Psychosomatic Medicine, 78,* 851–860.

Monson, C. M., Schnurr, P. P., Resnick, P. A., Friedman, M. J., Young-Xu, Y., & Stevens, S. P. (2006). Cognitive processing therapy for veterans with military-related posttraumatic stress disorder. *Journal of Consulting and Clinical Psychology, 74,* 898–907.

Montano, D. E., & Taplin, S. H. (1991). A test of an expanded theory of reasoned action to predict mammography participation. *Social Science and Medicine, 32,* 733–741.

Monteleone, P., Luisi, M., Colurcio, B., Casarosa, E., Ioime, R., Genazzani, A. R., & Maj, M. (2001). Plasma levels of neuroactive steroids are increased in untreated women with anorexia nervosa or bulimia nervosa. *Psychosomatic Medicine, 63,* 62–68.

Montgomery, G. H., & Bovbjerg, D. H. (2004). Presurgery distress and specific response expectancies predict postsurgery outcomes in surgery patients confronting breast cancer. *Health Psychology, 23,* 381–387.

Montgomery, G. H., Kangas, M., David, D., Hallquist, M. N., Green, S., Bovbjerg, D. H., & Schnur, J. B. (2009). Fatigue during breast cancer radiotherapy: An initial randomized study of cognitive–behavioral therapy plus hypnosis. *Health Psychology, 28,* 317–322.

Moody, L., McCormick, K., & Williams, A. (1990). Disease and symptom severity, functional status, and quality of life in chronic bronchitis and emphysema (CBE). *Journal of Behavioral Medicine, 13,* 297–306.

Moons, W. G., Eisenberger, N. I., & Taylor, S. E. (2010). Anger and fear responses to stress have different biological profiles. *Brain, Behavior, and Immunity, 24,* 215–219.

Moos, R. H. (1988). Life stressors and coping resources influence health and well-being. *Psychological Assessment, 4,* 133–158.

Moos, R. H., Brennan, P. L., & Moos, B. S. (1991). Short-term processes of remission and nonremission among later-life problem drinkers. *Alcoholism: Clinical and Experimental Review, 15,* 948–955.

Moos, R. H., & Schaefer, J. A. (1987). Evaluating health care work settings: A holistic conceptual framework. *Psychology and Health, 1,* 97–122.

Mora, P. A., Halm, E., Leventhal, H., & Ceric, F. (2007). Elucidating the relationship between negative affectivity and symptoms: The role of illness-specific affective responses. *Annals of Behavioral Medicine, 34,* 77–86.

Morell, V. (1993). Huntington's gene finally found. *Science, 260,* 28–30.

Morens, D. M., Folkers, G. K., & Fauci, A. S. (2004). The challenge of emerging and re-emerging infectious diseases. *Nature, 430,* 242–249.

Morgan, D. L. (1985). Nurses' perceptions of mental confusion in the elderly: Influence of resident and setting characteristics. *Journal of Health and Social Behavior, 26,* 102–112.

Morin, C. M., Rodrigue, S., & Ivers, H. (2003). Role of stress, arousal, and coping skills in primary insomnia. *Psychosomatic Medicine, 65,* 259–267.

Morozink, J. A., Friedman, E. M., Coe, C. L., & Ryff, C. D. (2010). Socio-economic and psychosocial predictors of interleukin-6 in the MIDUS national sample. *Health Psychology, 29,* 626–635.

Morrell, H. E. R., Song, A. V., & Halpern-Felsher, B. L. (2010). Predicting adolescent perceptions of the risks and benefits of cigarette smoking: A longitudinal investigation. *Health Psychology, 29,* 610–617.

Morris, P. L. P., & Raphael, B. (1987). Depressive disorder associated with physical illness: The impact of stroke. *General Hospital Psychiatry, 9,* 324–330.

Morrongiello, B. A., Corbett, M., & Bellissimo, A. (2008). "Do as I say, not as I do": Family influences on children's safety and risk behaviors. *Health Psychology, 27,* 498–503.

Morrongiello, B. A., Sandomierski, M., Zdzieborski, D., & McCollam, H. (2012). A randomized controlled trial evaluating the impact of the Supervising for Home Safety Program on parent appraisals of injury risk and need to actively supervise. *Health Psychology, 31,* 601–611.

Morrongiello, B. A., Schwebel, D. C., Bell, M., Stewart, J., & Davis, A. L. (2012). An evaluation of The Great Escape: Can an interactive computer game improve young children's fire safety knowledge and behaviors? *Health Psychology, 31,* 496–502.

Morton, G. J., Cummings, D. E., Baskin, D. G., Barsh, G. S., & Schwartz, M. W. (2006). Central nervous system control of food intake and body weight. *Nature, 443,* 289–295.

Moser, D. K., & Dracup, K. (2004). Role of spousal anxiety and depression in patients' psychosocial recovery after a cardiac event. *Psychosomatic Medicine, 66,* 527–532.

Moser, D. K., McKinley, S., Riegel, B., Doering, L. V., Meischke, H., Pelter, M., . . . Dracup, K. (2011). Relationship of persistent symptoms of anxiety to morbidity and mortality outcomes in patients with coronary heart disease. *Psychosomatic Medicine, 73,* 803–809.

Moses, H. (Producer). (1984, February 18). Helen. In *60 Minutes.* New York: CBS.

Moskowitz, J. T. (2003). Positive affect predicts lower risk of AIDS mortality. *Psychosomatic Medicine, 65,* 620–626.

Moss-Morris, R., & Spence, M. (2006). To "lump" or to "split" the functional somatic syndromes: Can infectious and emotional risk factors differentiate between the onset of chronic fatigue syndrome and irritable bowel syndrome? *Psychosomatic Medicine, 68,* 463–469.

Motivala, S. J., Hurwitz, B. E., Llabre, M. M., Klimas, N. G., Fletcher, M. A., Antoni, M. H., . . . Schneiderman, N. (2003). Psychological distress is associated with decreased memory and helper T-cell and B-cell counts in pre-AIDS HIV seropositive men and women but only in those with low viral load. *Psychosomatic Medicine, 65,* 627–635.

Motivala, S. J., Tomiyama, A. J., Ziegler, M., Khandrika, S., & Irwin, M. R. (2009). Nocturnal levels of ghrelin and leptin and sleep in chronic insomnia. *Psychoneuroendocrinology, 34,* 540–545.

Motl, R. W., & Snook, E. M. (2008). Physical activity, self-efficacy, and quality of life in multiple sclerosis. *Annals of Behavioral Medicine, 35,* 111–115.

Mõttus, R., Johnson, W., Murray, C., Wolf, M. S., Starr, J. M., & Deary, I. J. (2014). Towards understanding the links between health literacy and physical health. *Health Psychology, 33,* 164–173.

Mõttus, R., Luciano, M., Starr, J. M., Pollard, M. C., & Deary, I. J. (2013). Personality traits and inflammation in men and women in their early 70s: The Lothian Birth Cohort 1936 Study of Healthy Aging. *Psychosomatic Medicine, 75,* 11–19.

Mugavero, M. J., Raper, J. L., Reif, S., Whetten, K., Leserman, J., Thielman, N. M., & Pence, B. W. (2009). Overload: Impact of incident stressful events on antiretroviral medication adherence and virologic failure in a longitudinal, multisite human immunodeficiency virus cohort study. *Psychosomatic Medicine, 71,* 920–926.

Muhonen, T., & Torkelson, E. (2003). The demand-control-support model and health among women and men in similar occupations. *Journal of Behavioral Medicine, 26,* 601–613.

Mukherjee, S. (2017, April 3). The algorithm will see you now: When it comes to diagnosis, will A.I. replace M.D.? *The New Yorker,* pp. 46–53.

Mullen, B., & Smyth, J. M. (2004). Immigrant suicide rates as a function of ethnophaulisms: Hate speech predicts death. *Psychosomatic Medicine, 66,* 343–348.

Mullen, B., & Suls, J. (1982). The effectiveness of attention and rejection as coping styles: A meta-analysis of temporal differences. *Journal of Psychosomatic Research, 26,* 43–49.

Müller, F., Tuinman, M. A., Stephenson, E., Smink, A., DeLongis, A., & Hagedoorn, M. (2018). Associations of daily partner responses with fatigue interference and relationship satisfaction in colorectal cancer patients. *Health Psychology, 37,* 1015–1024.

Mulvaney, S. A., Rothman, R. L., Dietrich, M. S., Wallston, K. A., Grove, E., Elasy, T. A., & Johnson, K. B. (2012). Using mobile phones to measure adolescent diabetes adherence. *Health Psychology, 31,* 43–50.

Mund, M., & Mitte, K. (2012). The costs of repression: A meta-analysis on the relation between repressive coping and somatic diseases. *Health Psychology, 31,* 640–649.

Murphy, L., & Dockray, S. (2018). The consideration of future consequences and health behaviour: A meta-analysis. *Health Psychology Review, 12,* 357–381.

Murphy, M. L. M., Slavich, G. M., Chen, E., & Miller, G. E. (2015). Targeted rejection predicts decreased anti-inflammatory gene expression and increased symptom severity in youth with asthma. *Psychological Science, 26,* 111–121.

Murphy, S. L., Xu, J., & Kochanek, K. D. (2012). Deaths: Preliminary data for 2010. *National Vital Statistics Reports* (NCHS)*, 60,* 1–51.

Murphy, S. L., Xu, J. Q., Kochanek, K. D., & Arias, E. (2018). Mortality in the United States, 2017. *NCHS Data Brief, 328.* Retrieved March 26, 2019, from https://www.cdc.gov/nchs/data/databriefs/db328-h.pdf

Murray, D. M., Davis-Hearn, M., Goldman, A. I., Pirie, P., & Luepker, R. V. (1988). Four- and five-year follow-up results from four seventh-grade smoking prevention strategies. *Journal of Behavioral Medicine, 11,* 395–406.

Musick, M. A., House, J. S., & Williams, D. R. (2004). Attendance at religious services and mortality in a national sample. *Journal of Health and Social Behavior, 45,* 198–213.

Mutterperl, J. A., & Sanderson, C. A. (2002). Mind over matter: Internalization of the thinness norm as a moderator of responsiveness to norm misperception education in college women. *Health Psychology, 21,* 519–523.

Myers, H. F. (2009). Ethnicity and socio-economic status-related stresses in context: An integrative review and conceptual model. *Journal of Behavioral Medicine, 32,* 9–19.

Myers, M. M. (1996). Enduring effects of infant feeding experiences on adult blood pressure. *Psychosomatic Medicine, 58,* 612–621.

Myint, P. K., Luben, R. N., Surtees, P. G., Wainwright, N. W. J., Welch, A. A., Bingham, S. A., . . . Khaw, K. T. (2007). Self-reported mental health-related quality of life and mortality in men and women in the European perspective investigation into cancer (EPIC-Norfolk): A prospective population study. *Psychosomatic Medicine, 69,* 410–414.

Naar-King, S., Wright, K., Parsons, J. T., Frey, M., Templin, T., & Ondersma, S. (2006). Transtheoretical model and condom use in HIV-positive youths. *Health Psychology, 25,* 648–652.

Nahum-Shani, I., Smith, S. N., Spring, B. J., Collins, L. M., Witkiewitz, K., Tewari, A., & Murphy, S. A. (2017). Just-in-time adaptive interventions (JITAIs) in mobile health: Key components and design principles for ongoing health behavior support. *Annals of Behavioral Medicine, 52,* 446–462.

Naliboff, B. D., Mayer, M., Fass, R., Fitzgerald, L. Z., Chang, L., Bolus, R., & Mayer, E. A. (2004). The effect of life stress on symptoms of heartburn. *Psychosomatic Medicine, 66,* 426–434.

Napolitano, M. A., Fotheringham, M., Tate, D., Sciamanna, C., Leslie, E., Owen, N., . . . Marcus, B. (2003). Evaluation of an Internet-based physical activity intervention: A preliminary investigation. *Annals of Behavioral Medicine, 25,* 92–99.

Napolitano, M. A., Papandonatos, G. D., Lewis, B. A., Whiteley, J. A., Williams, D. M., King, A. C., . . . Marcus, B. H. (2008). Mediators of physical activity behavior change: A multivariate approach. *Health Psychology, 28,* 409–418.

Nash, J. M., Williams, D. M., Nicholson, R., & Trask, P. C. (2006). The contribution of pain-related anxiety to disability from headache. *Journal of Behavioral Medicine, 29,* 61–67.

Nater, U. M., Lin, J. M., Maloney, E. M., Jones, J. F., Tian, H., Boneva, R. S., . . . Heim, C. (2009). Psychiatric comorbidity in persons with chronic fatigue syndrome identified from the Georgia population. *Psychosomatic Medicine, 71,* 557–565.

National Academy of Medicine. (2002). *Unequal treatment: Confronting racial and ethnic disparities in health care.* Washington, DC: National Academic Press.

National Academy of Medicine. (2009). *Informing the future: Critical issues in health* (5th ed.). Washington, DC: The National Academies Press.

National Academy of Medicine. (2010). *Dietary reference intakes for calcium and vitamin D.* Retrieved March 28, 2013, from http://www.iom.edu/Reports/2010/Dietary-Reference-Intakes-for-Calcium-and-Vitamin-D.aspx

National Academy of Medicine. (2011a). *Clinical preventive services for women: Closing the gaps.* Report Brief. Washington, DC: The National Academies Press.

National Academy of Medicine. (2011b). *Informing the future: Critical issues in health* (6th ed.). Washington, DC: The National Academies Press.

National Academy of Medicine. (2011, March). *The health of lesbian, gay, bisexual, and transgender people: Building a foundation for better understanding.* Report Brief. Washington, DC: The National Academies Press.

National Academy of Medicine. (2011, October). *Essential health benefits: Balancing coverage and cost.* Report Brief. Washington, DC: The National Academies Press.

National Academy of Medicine. (2011c). *Relieving pain in America: A blueprint for transforming prevention, care, education, and research.* Washington, DC: The National Academies Press.

National Academy of Medicine. (2012, April). *For the public's health: Investing in a healthier future.* Report Brief. Washington, DC: The National Academies Press.

National Academy of Medicine. (2012, July). *The mental health and substance use workforce for older adults: In whose hands?* Report Brief. Washington, DC: The National Academies Press.

National Academy of Medicine. (2013, January). *U.S. health in international perspective: Shorter lives, poorer health* (pp. 1–4). Report Brief. Washington, DC: National Academy of Sciences.

National Academy of Medicine. (2013a, May). *Educating the student body: Taking physical activity and physical education to school.* Report Brief. Washington, DC: National Academy of Sciences.

National Academy of Medicine. (2013b, May). *Sodium intake in populations: Assessment of evidence.* Report Brief. Washington, DC: National Academy of Sciences.

National Academy of Medicine. (2013, October). *Sports-related concussions in youth: Improving the science, changing the culture* (pp. 1–4). Report Brief. Washington, DC: National Academy of Sciences.

National Cancer Institute. (2005). *Cancer health disparities: Fact sheet.* Retrieved March 1, 2007, from http://www.cancer.gov/cancertopics/factsheet/cancerhealthdisparities

National Cancer Institute. (2016). *Office of cancer survivorship.* Retrieved March 4, 2016, from http://cancer.control.cancer.gov/ocs/statistics/statistics.html.

National Cancer Institute (2018, October). *Cancer in children and adolescents.* Retrieved May 8, 2019, from https://www.cancer.gov/types/childhood-cancers/child-adolescent-cancers-fact-sheet

National Cancer Institute. (2019, March). *Cancer disparities.* Retrieved May 30, 2019, from https://www.cancer.gov/about-cancer/understanding/disparities

National Center for Complementary and Alternative Medicine. (2009). *Ayurvedic medicine: An introduction.* Retrieved March 26, 2013, from http://nccam.nih.gov/health/ayurveda/introduction.htm

National Center for Complementary and Alternative Medicine. (2010). *Meditation: An introduction.* Retrieved October 22, 2012, from http://nccam.nih.gov/health/meditation/overview.htm

National Center for Complementary and Alternative Medicine. (2012). *NCAAM facts-at-a-glance and mission.* Retrieved October 22, 2012, from http://nccam.nih.gov/about/ataglance

National Center for Complementary and Integrative Health. (2016). *Meditation: In depth.* Retrieved February 20, 2016, from https://nccih.nih.gov

National Center for Health Statistics. (2009). *Health, United States, 2008 with special feature on the health of young adults.* Retrieved September 29, 2009, from http://www.cdc.gov/nchs/data/hus/hus08.pdf

National Center for Complementary and Integrative Health. (2018). *National survey reveals increased use of yoga, meditation, and chiropractic care among U.S. adults.* Retrieved April 9, 2019, from https://nccih.nih.gov/research/results/spotlight/NHIS2017-Adult-Survey

National Center for Health Statistics. (2010, June). *Prevalence of obesity among children and adolescents: United States, trends 1963–1965 through 2007–2008.* Retrieved March 16, 2012, from http://www.cdc.gov/nchs/data/hestat/obesity_child_07_08/obesity_child_07_08.pdf

National Center for Health Statistics. (2011). *Health, United States, 2011: With special feature on socioeconomic status and health.* Retrieved April 5, 2013, from http://www.cdc.gov/nchs/data/hus/hus11.pdf#030

National Center for Health Statistics. (2017). *Table 79. Prescription drug use in the past 30 days, by sex, race, and Hispanic origin, and age: United States, selected years 1988–1994 through 2011–2014.* Retrieved April 24, 2019, from https://www.cdc.gov/nchs/data/hus/2017/079.pdf

National Center for Health Statistics. (2018, November). *Mortality in the United States, 2017.* Retrieved April 9, 2019, from https://www.cdc.gov/nchs/data/databriefs/db328-h.pdf

National Committee for Quality Assurance. (2001). *Health plan report card.* Retrieved from http://www.ncqa.org/index.asp

National Health Expenditures. (2017, April). *Fact sheet.* Retrieved March 12, 2019, from https://www.cms.gov/research-statistics-data-and-systems/statistics-trends-and-reports/nationalhealthexpenddata/nhe-fact-sheet.html

National Heart, Lung, and Blood Institute. (2010a). *What is cholesterol?* Retrieved June 6, 2010, from http://nhlbi.nih.gov/health/dci/Disease/Atherosclerosis/Atherosclerosis_WhatIs.html

National Heart, Lung, and Blood Institute. (2010b). *What are the signs and symptoms of atrial fibrillation?* Retrieved June 6, 2010, from http://nhlbi.nih.gov/health/dci/images/atrial_fib_stroke.jpg

National Heart, Lung, and Blood Institute. (2011). *What is asthma?* Retrieved May 12, 2012, from http://www.nhlbi.nih.gov/health/health-topics/topics/asthma

National Institutes of Health. (n.d.). *Body mass index table 1.* Retrieved April 8, 2019, from https://www.nhlbi.nih.gov/health/educational/lose_wt/BMI/bmi_tbl.htm

National Institutes of Health. (2017, March 22). *COPD National Action Plan.* Retrieved March 13, 2019, from https://www.nhlbi.nih.gov/sites/default/files/media/docs/COPD National Action Plan 508_0.pdf

National Institutes of Health. (2018a). *Cancer of the lung and bronchus-Cancer stat facts.* Retrieved March 30, 2019, from https://seer.cancer.gov/statfacts/html/lungb.html

National Institutes of Health. (2018b). *Vitamins and minerals.* Retrieved April 8, 2019, from https://nccih.nih.gov/health/vitamins

National Institute of Environmental Health Sciences. (2018). *Autoimmune diseases.* Retrieved March 26, 2019, from https://www.niehs.nih.gov/health/topics/conditions/autoimmune/index.cfm

National Highway Traffic Safety Administration. (2012). *Traffic safety facts 2010 data: Alcohol-impaired driving.* Retrieved May 3, 2012, from http://www-nrd.nhtsa.dot.gov/Pubs/811606.pdf

National Hospice and Palliative Care Organization. (2007). *Keys to quality care.* Retrieved June 13, 2007, from http://www.nhpco.org/i4a/pages/index.cfm?pageid53303

National Hospice and Palliative Care Organization. (2011). *NHPCO facts and figures: Hospice care in America.* Retrieved September 25, 2012, from http://www.nhpco.org/files/public/statistics_research/2011_facts_figures.pdf

National Hospice and Palliative Care Organization. (2015, September). *NHPCO's facts and figures: Hospice care in America.* Retrieved May 6, 2016, from http://www.nhpco.org/

National Institute of Neurological Disorders and Stroke. (2006). *Brain basics: Understanding sleep.* Retrieved April 25, 2007, from http://www.ninds.nih.gov/disorders/brain_basics/understanding_sleep.htm#sleep_disorders

National Institute of Neurological Disorders and Stroke. (2007). *Pain: Hope through research.* Retrieved April 14, 2007, from http://www.ninds.nih.gov/disorders/chronic_pain/detail_chronic_pain.htm

National Institute on Alcohol Abuse and Alcoholism. (2000a). *Alcohol alert: New advances in alcoholism treatment.* Retrieved from www.niaaa.nih.gov

National Institute on Alcohol Abuse and Alcoholism. (2000b). *10th special report to the U.S. Congress on alcohol and health.* Retrieved from http://silk.nih.gov/silk/niaaa1/publication/10report/10-order.htm

National Institute on Alcohol Abuse and Alcoholism. (2000c). *Estimated economic costs of alcohol abuse in the United States, 1992 and 1998.* Retrieved January 13, 2011, from http://www.niaaa.nih.gov/Resources/QuickFacts/EconomicData/Pages/cost8.aspx

National Institute on Alcohol Abuse and Alcoholism. (2009). *A snapshot of annual high-risk college drinking consequences.* Retrieved October 5, 2009, from http://www.collegedrinkingprevention.gov/StatsSummaries/snapshot.aspx

National Institute on Alcohol Abuse and Alcoholism. (2015, December). *College drinking.* Retrieved on February 28, 2016, from http://www.niaaa.nih.gov

National Institute on Diabetes and Digestive and Kidney Disorders. (1999). *Diabetes control and complications trial.* (National Institutes of Health Publication No. 97-3874). Retrieved from http://www.niddk.nih.gov/health/diabetes/pubs/dcct1/dcct.htm

National Institute on Diabetes and Digestive and Kidney Disorders. (2007). *Kidney disease of diabetes. USRDS 2007 Annual Report Data.* Retrieved from http://niddk.nih.gov/kudiseases/pubs/kdd

National Institute on Drug Abuse. (2011). *DrugFacts: Treatment statistics.* Retrieved March 6, 2013, from http://www.drugabuse.gov/publications/drugfacts/treatment-statistics

National Institutes of Health. (2006). NIH State-of-the-Science Conference statement on multivitamin/mineral supplements and chronic disease prevention. *Annals of Internal Medicine, 145,* 364-371.

National Multiple Sclerosis Society. (2016). *Multiple sclerosis FAQs.* Retrieved January 21, 2016, from nationalmssociety.org

National Research Council, & National Academy of Medicine. (2013). U.S. health in international perspective: Shorter lives, poorer health. *Consensus Report.* Washington, DC: National Academies Press

National Research Council. (2013). US health in international perspective: Shorter lives, poorer health. In *Panel on understanding cross-national health differences among high-income countries. Committee on Population, Division of Behavioral and Social Sciences and Education, and Board on Population Health and Public Health Practice.* Washington, DC: National Academies Press.

National Vital Statistics Reports. (2018, July 26). *Deaths: Final data for 2016.* Retrieved May 10, 2019, from http://www.cdc.gov

Navarro, A. M. (1996). Cigarette smoking among adult Latinos: The California tobacco baseline survey. *Annals of Behavioral Medicine, 18,* 238-245.

Nealey-Moore, J. B., Smith, T. W., Uchino, B. N., Hawkins, M. W., & Olson-Cerny, C. (2007). Cardiovascular reactivity during positive and negative marital interactions. *Journal of Behavioral Medicine, 30,* 505-519.

Neiberg, R. H., Aickin, M., Grzywacz, J. G., Lang, W., Quandt, S. A., Bell, R. A., & Arcury, T. A. (2011). Occurrence and co-occurrence of types of complementary and alternative medicine use by age, gender, ethnicity, and education among adults in the United States: The 2002 National Health Interview Survey (NHIS). *The Journal of Alternative and Complementary Medicine, 17,* 363-370.

Nelson, C., Franks, S., Brose, A., Raven, P., Williamson, J., Shi, X., . . . Harrell, E. (2005). The influence of hostility and family history of cardiovascular disease on autonomic activation in response to controllable versus non-controllable stress, anger imagery induction, and relaxation imagery. *Journal of Behavioral Medicine, 28,* 213-221.

Nelson, L. M., Wallin, M. T., Marrie, R. A., Culpepper, W. J., Langer-Gould, A., Campbell, J., . . . United States Multiple Sclerosis Prevalence Workgroup. (2019). A new way to estimate neurologic disease prevalence in the United States: Illustrated with MS. *Neurology, 92,* 469-480.

Nelson, W. L. Suls, J., & Padgett, L. (2014). Understanding "ChemoBrain." A challenge and invitation to psychological scientists. *Observer, 12,* 2.

Nemeroff, C. B., Bremner, J. D., Foa, E. B., Mayberg, H. S., North, C. S., & Stein, M. B. (2006). Posttraumatic stress disorder: A state-of-the-science review. *Journal of Psychiatric Research, 40,* 1-21.

Neu, P., Schlattmann, P., Schilling, A., & Hartmann, A. (2004). Cerebrovascular reactivity in major depression: A pilot study. *Psychosomatic Medicine, 66,* 6-8.

Neumark-Sztainer, D., Wall, M. M., Story, M., & Perry, C. L. (2003). Correlates of unhealthy weight-control behaviors among adolescents: Implications for prevention programs. *Health Psychology, 22,* 88-98.

Newcomb, M. E., & Mustanski, B. (2014). Cognitive influences on sexual risk and risk appraisals in men who have sex with men. *Health Psychology, 33,* 690-698.

New York Presbyterian Hospital. (2007). *Chronic pain.* Retrieved May 16, 2007, from http://www.nyp.org/health/chronic-pain.html

*New York Times.* (2001, May 22). Diabetics reminded of heart risk, p. D8.

Newsom, J. T., Mahan, T. L., Rook, K. S., & Krause, N. (2008). Stable negative social exchange and health. *Health Psychology, 27,* 78-86.

Newsom, J. T., & Schulz, R. (1998). Caregiving from the recipient's perspective: Negative reactions to being helped. *Health Psychology, 17,* 172-181.

New York University Langone Medical Center. (2012). *Osteopathic manipulative treatment.* Retrieved on November 15, 2012, from http://www.med.nyu.edu/content?ChunkIID=37409

Ng, D. M., & Jeffery, R. W. (2003). Relationships between perceived stress and health behaviors in a sample of working adults. *Health Psychology, 22,* 638-642.

Ng, J. Y. Y., Ntoumanis, N., Thøgersen-Ntoumani, C., Deci, E. L., Ryan, R. M., Duda, J. L., & Williams, G. C. (2012). Self-determination theory applied to health contexts: A meta-analysis. *Psychological Science, 7,* 325-340.

Nicassio, P. M., Meyerowitz, B. E., & Kerns, R. D. (2004). The future of health psychology interventions. *Health Psychology, 23,* 132-137.

Nicholson, A., Fuhrer, R., & Marmot, M. (2005). Psychological distress as a predictor of CHD events in men: The effect of persistence and components of risk. *Psychosomatic Medicine, 67,* 522-530.

Nicholson, A., Rose, R., & Bobak, M. (2010). Associations between different dimensions of religious involvement and self-rated health in diverse European populations. *Health Psychology, 29,* 227-235.

Nielsen, N. R., & Grønbaek, M. (2006). Stress and breast cancer: A systematic update on the current knowledge. *Nature Clinical Practice Oncology, 3,* 612-620.

Nielsen, S. J., & Popkin, B. M. (2003). Patterns and trends in food portion sizes, 1977-1998. *Journal of the American Medical Association, 289,* 450-453.

Niemcryk, S. J., Jenkins, S. D., Rose, R. M., & Hurst, M. W. (1987). The prospective impact of psychosocial variables on rates of illness and injury in professional employees. *Journal of Occupational Medicine, 29,* 645-652.

Nikoloudakis, I. A., Crutzen, R., Rebar, A. L., Vandelanotte, C., Quester, P., Dry, M., . . . Short, C. E. (2018). Can you elaborate on that? Addressing participants' need for cognition in computer-tailored health behavior interventions. *Health Psychology Review, 12,* 437-452.

Nivison, M. E., & Endresen, I. M. (1993). An analysis of relationships among environmental noise, annoyance and sensitivity to noise, and the consequences for health and sleep. *Journal of Behavioral Medicine, 16,* 257-271.

Nobles, J., & Frankenberg, E. (2009). Mothers' community participation and child health. *Journal of Health and Social Behavior, 50,* 16-30.

Noel, M., Rabbitts, J. A., Fales, J., Chorney, J., & Palermo, T. M. (2017). The influence of pain memories on children's and adolescents' post-surgical pain experience: A longitudinal dyadic analysis. *Health Psychology, 36,* 987-995.

Nolen-Hoeksema, S., McBride, A., & Larson, J. (1997). Rumination and psychological distress among bereaved partners. *Journal of Personality and Social Psychology, 72,* 855-862.

Norman, C. D., Maley, O., Skinner, H. A., & Li, X. (2008). Using the Internet to assist smoking prevention and cessation in schools: A randomized, controlled trial. *Health Psychology, 27,* 799-810.

North, R. B., Kidd, D. H., Olin, J., Sieracki, J. M., Farrokhi, F., Petrucci, L., & Cutchis, P. N. (2005). Spinal cord stimulation for axial low back pain: A prospective, controlled trial comparing dual with single percutaneous electrodes. *SPINE, 30,* 1412-1418.

Northouse, L., Templin, T., & Mood, D. (2001). Couples' adjustment to breast disease during the first year following diagnosis. *Journal of Behavioral Medicine, 24,* 115-136.

Nouwen, A., Ford, T., Balan, A. T., Twisk, J., Ruggiero, L., & White, D. (2011). Longitudinal motivational predictors of dietary self-care and diabetes control in adults with newly diagnosed type 2 diabetes mellitus. *Health Psychology, 30,* 771-779.

Novacek, D. (2016). How to get in: Applying to psychology grad school. *Association of Psychological Science, 29,* 39-40.

Novak, M., Ahlgren, C., & Hammarstrom, A. (2007). Inequalities in smoking: Influence of social chain of risks from adolescence to young adulthood: A prospective population-based cohort study. *International Journal of Behavioral Medicine, 14,* 181-187.

Novak, M., Molnar, M. Z., Szeifert, L., Kovacs, A. Z., Vamos, E. P., Zoller, R., . . . Mucsi, I. (2010). Depressive symptoms and mortality in patients after kidney transplantation: A prospective prevalent cohort study. *Psychosomatic Medicine, 72,* 527-534.

Novak, S. P., & Clayton, R. R. (2001). The influence of school environment and self-regulation on transitions between stages of cigarette smoking: A multilevel analysis. *Health Psychology, 20,* 196-207.

Noyes, R., Hartz, A. J., Doebbeling, C. C., Malis, R. W., Happel, R. L., Werner, L. A., & Yagla, S. J. (2000). Illness fears in the general population. *Psychosomatic Medicine, 62,* 318-325.

Nudelman, G., & Shiloh, S. (2018). Connectionism and behavioral clusters: Differential patterns in predicting expectations to engage in health behaviors. *Annals of Behavioral Medicine, 52,* 890-901.

Nurses' Health Study. (2004). *History.* Retrieved August 1, 2004, from http://www.channing.harvard.edu/nhs/history/index.shtml

Nwankwo, T., Yoon, S. S., Burt, V., & Gu, Q. (2013). Hypertension among adults in the United States: National health and nutrition examination survey, 2011-2012. *NCHS Data Brief, 133,* 1-8.

Nylén, L., Melin, B., & Laflamme, L. (2007). Interference between work and outside-work demands relative to health: Unwinding possibilities among full-time and part-time employees. *International Journal of Behavioral Medicine, 14,* 229-236.

Nyklíček, I., Mommersteeg, P. M. C., Van Beugen, S., Ramakers, C., & Van Boxtel, G. J. (2013). Mindfulness-based stress reduction and physiological activity during acute stress: A randomized controlled trial. *Health Psychology, 32,* 1110-1113.

Obama, B. (2009, September). *Remarks by the President to a joint session of Congress on health care.* Speech presented at the U.S. Capitol, Capitol Hill, Washington, DC.

Oberlander, J. (2010). A vote for health care reform. *The New England Journal of Medicine, 362,* e44(1)-e44(3).

O'Brien, A., Fries, E., & Bowen, D. (2000). The effect of accuracy of perceptions of dietary-fat intake on perceived risk and intentions to change. *Journal of Behavioral Medicine, 23,* 465-473.

O'Carroll, R., Whittaker, J., Hamilton, B., Johnston, M., Sudlow, C., & Dennis, M. (2011). Predictors of adherence to secondary preventive medication in stroke patients. *Annals of Behavioral Medicine, 41,* 383-390.

Ockene, J. K., Emmons, K. M., Mermelstein, R. J., Perkins, K. A., Bonollo, D. S., Voorhees, C. C., & Hollis, J. F. (2000). Relapse and maintenance issues for smoking cessation. *Health Psychology, 19,* 17-31.

O'Connor, A. (2004, February 6). Study details 30-year increase in calorie consumption. *New York Times,* p. A19.

O'Connor, D. B., Conner, M., Jones, F., McMillan, B., & Ferguson, E. (2009). Exploring the benefits of conscientiousness: An investigation of the role of daily stressors and health benefits. *Annals of Behavioral Medicine, 37,* 184-196.

O'Connor, D. B., Jones, F., Ferguson, E., Conner, M., & McMillan, B. (2008). Effects of daily hassles and eating style on eating behavior. *Health Psychology, 27,* S20-S31.

O'Connor, P. J. (2006). Improving medication adherence: Challenges for physicians, payers, and policy makers. *Archives of Internal Medicine, 166,* 1802-1804.

O'Donnell, M. L., Creamer, M., Elliott, P., & Bryant, R. (2007). Tonic and phasic heart rate as predictors of posttraumatic stress disorder. *Psychosomatic Medicine, 69,* 256-261.

O'Donnell, M. L., Varker, T., Creamer, M., Fletcher, S., McFarlane, A. C., Silove, D., . . . Forbes, D. (2013). Exploration of delayed-onset posttraumatic stress disorder after severe injury. *Psychosomatic Medicine, 75,* 68-75.

Oenema, A., Brug, J., Dijkstra, A., de Weerdt, I., & de Vries, H. (2008). Efficacy and use of an Internet-delivered computer-tailored lifestyle intervention, targeting saturated fat intake, physical activity and smoking cessation: A randomized controlled trial. *Annals of Behavioral Medicine, 35,* 125-135.

Office of Disease Prevention and Health Promotion. (2016, November 16). *2016 United States report card on physical activity for children and youth released.* Retrieved April 1, 2019, from https://health.gov/news/blog-bayw/2016/11/2016-united-states-report-card-on-physical-activity-for-children-and-youth-released/

Ogden, C. L., Carroll, M. D., Kit, B. K., & Flegal, K. M. (2012). Prevalence of obesity in the United States, 2009-2010. *NCHS Data Brief, 82,* 1-8.

Ogden, C. L., Lamb, M. M., Carroll, M. D., & Flegal, K. M. (2010). Obesity and socioeconomic status in adults: United States, 2005-2008. *NCHS Data Brief, 50,* 1-8.

Ogden, J. (2003). Some problems with social cognition models: A pragmatic and conceptual analysis. *Health Psychology, 22,* 424-428.

Oh, H., & Taylor, A. H. (2014). Self-regulating smoking and snacking through physical activity. *Health Psychology, 33,* 349-359.

Ohira, T., Diez Rouz, A. V., Polak, J. F., Homma, S., Iso, H., & Wasserman, B.A. (2012). Associations of anger, anxiety, and depressive symptoms with carotid arterial wall thickness: The multi-ethnic study of atherosclerosis. *Psychosomatic Medicine, 74,* 517-525.

Okely, J. A., Weiss, A., & Gale, C. R. (2017). The interaction between stress and positive affect in predicting mortality. *Journal of Psychosomatic Research, 100,* 53-60.

O'Leary, A., Jemmott, L. S., & Jemmott, J. B. (2008). Mediation analysis of an effective sexual risk-reduction intervention for women: The importance of self-efficacy. *Health Psychology, 27,* S180-S184.

Oleck, J. (2001, April 23). Dieting: More fun with a buddy? *Business Week,* p. 16.

Olive, L. S., Telford, R. M., Byrne, D. G., Abhayaratna, W. P., & Telford, R. D. (2017). Symptoms of stress and depression effect percentage of body fat and insulin resistance in healthy youth: LOOK longitudinal study. *Health Psychology, 36,* 749-759.

Oliver, G., Wardle, J., & Gibson, E. L. (2000). Stress and food choice: A laboratory study. *Psychosomatic Medicine, 62,* 853-865.

Olshansky, S. J. (2015). The demographic transformation of America. *Daedalus, 144, 2,* 13-19.

Olson, E. A., Mullen, S. P., Raine, L. B., Kramer, A. F., Hillman, C. H., & McAuley, E. (2016). Integrated social and neurocognitive model of physical activity behavior in older adults with metabolic disease. *Annals of Behavioral Medicine, 51,* 272-281.

O'Malley, L., Adair, P., Burnside, G., Robinson, L., Coffey, M., & Pine, C. (2017). An evaluation of a storybook targeting parental attitudes, intention, and self-efficacy to change their child's oral health behavior. *Health Psychology, 36,* 152-159.

O'Malley, P. M., & Johnston, L. D. (2002). Epidemiology of alcohol and other drug use among American college students. *Journal of Studies on Alcohol, 14,* 23-39.

Ong, A. D., Bergeman, C. S., Bisconti, T. L., & Wallace, K. A. (2006). Psychological resilience, positive emotions, and successful adaptation to stress in later life. *Journal of Personality and Social Psychology, 91,* 730-749.

Orbell, S., & Kyriakaki, M. (2008). Temporal framing and persuasion to adopt preventive health behavior: Moderating effect of individual differences in consideration of future consequences on sunscreen use. *Health Psychology, 27,* 770-779.

Orbell, S., Lidierth, P., Henderson, C. J., Geeraert, N., Uller, C., Uskul, A. K., & Kyriakaki, M. (2009). Social-cognitive beliefs, alcohol, and tobacco use: A prospective community study of change following a ban on smoking in public places. *Health Psychology, 28,* 753-761.

Oregon Department of Human Services. (2011). *Oregon's Death with Dignity Act-2011.* Retrieved June 12, 2012, from http://public.health.oregon.gov/ProviderPartnerResources/EvaluationResearch/DeathwithDignityAct/Documents/year14.pdf

Oregon Health Authority Public Health Division. (2018). *Oregon Death with Dignity Act: 2018 data summary.* Retrieved May 10, 2019, from https://www.oregon.gov/oha/PH/PROVIDERPARTNERRESOURCES/EVAL-UATIONRESEARCH/DEATHWITHDIGNITYACT/Documents/year21.pdf

Organisation for Economic Co-operation and Development. (2007). *OECD factbook 2007–economic, environmental and social statistics: Quality of life: Health.* Retrieved April 16, 2007, from http://oberon.sourceoecd.org/vl=3821204/cl=12/nw=1/rpsv/factbook/11-01-04-g01.htm

Organisation for Economic Co-operation and Development. (2012). *OECD obesity update 2012.* Retrieved March 6, 2013, from http://www.oecd.org/health/49716427.pdf

Orleans, C. T. (2000). Promoting the maintenance of health behavior change: Recommendations for the next generation of research and practice. *Health Psychology, 19,* 76-83.

Orr, S. T., Reiter, J. P., Blazer, D. G., & James, S. A. (2007). Maternal prenatal pregnancy-related anxiety and spontaneous preterm birth in Baltimore, Maryland. *Psychosomatic Medicine, 69,* 566-570.

Oslin, D. W., Sayers, S., Ross, J., Kane, V., Have, T. T., Conigliaro, J., & Cornelius, J. (2003). Disease management for depression and at-risk drinking via telephone in an older population of veterans. *Psychosomatic Medicine, 65,* 931-937.

Osman, A., Barrios, F., Gutierrez, P., Kopper, B., Merrifield, T., & Grittmann, L. (2000). The pain and catastrophizing scale: Further psychometric evaluation with adult samples. *Journal of Behavioral Medicine, 23,* 351-365.

Osman, A., Breitenstein, J. L., Barrios, F. X., Gutierrez, P. M., & Kopper, B. A. (2002). The Fear of Pain Questionnaire-III: Further reliability and validity with nonclinical samples. *Journal of Behavioral Medicine, 25,* 155-173.

Ossola, P., Gerra, M. L., De Panfilis, C., Tonna, M., & Marchesi, C. (2018). Anxiety, depression, and cardiac outcomes after a first diagnosis of acute coronary syndrome. *Health Psychology, 37,* 1115-1122.

Osterman, M. J., & Martin, J. A. (2018). System timing and adequacy of prenatal care in the United States, 2016. *National Vital Statistics Report, 67*(3), 1-14.

O'Toole, M. S., Bovbjerg, D. H., Renna, M. E., Lekander, M., Mennin, D. S., & Zachariae, R. (2018). Effects of psychological interventions on systemic levels of inflammatory biomarkers in humans: A systematic review and meta-analysis. *Brain, Behavior, and Immunity, 74,* 68-78.

Owen, J. E., Klapow, J. C., Roth, D. L., & Tucker, D. C. (2004). Use of the Internet for information and support: Disclosure among persons with breast and prostate cancer. *Journal of Behavioral Medicine, 27,* 491-505.

Owens, J. F., Matthews, K. A., Wing, R. R., & Kuller, L. H. (1990). Physical activity and cardiovascular risk: A cross-sectional study of middle-aged premenopausal women. *Preventive Medicine, 19,* 147-157.

Oxlad, M., Stubberfield, J., Stuklis, R., Edwards, J., & Wade, T. D. (2006). Psychological risk factors for increased post-operative length of hospital stay following coronary artery bypass graft surgery. *Journal of Behavioral Medicine, 29,* 179-190.

Ozer, E. J., & Weiss, D. S. (2004). Who develops posttraumatic stress disorder? *Current Directions in Psychological Science, 13,* 169-172.

Özkan, S., Zale, E. L., Ring, D., & Vranceanu, A. M. (2017). Associations between pain catastrophizing and cognitive fusion in relation to pain and upper extremity function among hand and upper extremity surgery patients. *Annals of Behavioral Medicine, 51,* 547-554.

Pachankis, J. E., Rendina, H. J., Restar, A., Ventuneac, A., Grov, C., & Parsons, J. T. (2015). A minority stress-emotion regulation model of sexual compulsivity among highly sexually active gay and bisexual men. *Health Psychology, 34,* 829-840.

Pai, M., & Carr, D. (2010). Do personality traits moderate the effect of late-life spousal loss on psychological distress? *Journal of Health and Social Behavior, 51,* 183-199.

Painter, J. E., Borba, C. P. C., Hynes, M., Mays, D., & Glanz, K. (2008). The use of theory in health behavior research from 2000 to 2005: A systematic review. *Annals of Behavioral Medicine, 35,* 358-362.

Pakenham, K. I., & Cox, S. (2012). Test of a model of the effects of parental illness on youth and family functioning. *Health Psychology, 31,* 580-590.

Palermo, T. M., Valrie, C. R., & Karlson C. W. (2014). Family and parent influences on pediatric chronic pain: A developmental perspective. *American Psychologist, 69,* 142-152.

Palesh, O., Scheiber, C., Kesler, S., Gevirtz, R., Heckler, C., Guido, J. J., . . . Mustian, K. (2019). Secondary outcomes of a behavioral sleep intervention: A randomized clinical trial. *Health Psychology, 38,* 196-205.

Palit, S., Kerr, K. L., Kuhn, B. L., Terry, E. L., DelVentura, J. L., Bartley, E. J., & Rhudy, J. L. (2013). Exploring pain processing differences in Native Americans. *Health Psychology, 32,* 1127-1136.

Palmero, T. M., Valrie, C. R., & Karlson, C. W. (2014). Family and parent influences on pediatric chronic pain: A developmental perspective. *American Psychologist, 69,* 142-152.

Pampel, F. C. (2001). Cigarette diffusion and sex differences in smoking. *Journal of Health and Social Behavior, 42,* 388-404.

Pampel, F. C., & Rogers, R. G. (2004). Socioeconomic status, smoking, and health: A test of competing theories of cumulative advantage. *Journal of Health and Social Behavior, 45,* 306-321.

Pan, M. H., Chiou, Y. S., Tsai, M. L., & Ho, C. T. (2011). Anti-inflammatory activity of traditional Chinese medicinal herbs. *Journal of Traditional and Complementary Medicine, 1,* 8-24.

Pandya, C., McHugh, M., & Batalova, J. (2011). *Limited English proficient individuals in the United States: Number, share, growth, and linguistic diversity.* Washington, DC: Migration Policy Institute.

Papandonatos, G. D., Williams, D. M., Jennings, E. G., Napolitano, M. A., Bock, B. C., Dunsiger, S., & Marcus, B. H. (2012). Mediators of physical activity behavior change: Findings from a 12-month randomized controlled trial. *Health Psychology, 31,* 512-520.

Paquet, C., Dubé, L., Gauvin, L., Kestens, Y., & Daniel, M. (2010). Sense of mastery and metabolic risk: Moderating role of the local fast-food environment. *Psychosomatic Medicine, 72,* 324-331.

Pardine, P., & Napoli, A. (1983). Physiological reactivity and recent life-stress experience. *Journal of Consulting and Clinical Psychology, 51,* 467-469.

Park, C. L., & Gaffey, A. E. (2007). Relationships between psychosocial factors and health behavior change in cancer survivors: An integrative review. *Annals of Behavioral Medicine, 34,* 115-134.

Park, C. L., Wortmann, J. H., & Edmondson, D. (2011). Religious struggle as a predictor of subsequent mental and physical well-being in advanced heart failure patients. *Journal of Behavioral Medicine, 34,* 426-436.

Park, D. C. (2007). Eating disorders: A call to arms. *American Psychologist, 62,* 158.

Park, M., Cherry, D., & Decker, S. L. (2011). Nurse practitioners, certified nurse midwives, and physician assistants in physician offices. *NCHS Data Brief, 69,* 1-8.

Park, S., Thøgersen-Ntoumani, C., Veldhuijzen van Zanten, J. J., & Ntoumanis, N. (2017). The role of physical activity and sedentary behavior in predicting daily pain and fatigue in older adults: A diary study. *Annals of Behavioral Medicine, 52,* 19-28.

Parker, J. C., Frank, R. G., Beck, N. C., Smarr, K. L., Buescher, K. L., Phillips, L. R., . . . Walker, S. E. (1988). Pain management in rheumatoid arthritis patients: A cognitive-behavioral approach. *Arthritis and Rheumatism, 31,* 593-601.

Parkinson's Foundation. (2018, July 10). *New study shows 1.2 million people in the United States estimated to be living with Parkinson's disease by 2030.* Retrieved March 12, 2019, from https://www.parkinson.org/about-us/Press-Room/Press-Releases/New-Study-Shows-Over-1-Million-People-in-the-United-States-Estimated-to-be-Living-with-Parkinsons-Disease-by-2030?_ga=2.172485155.1282953647.1552424688-2018650434.1552424688&_gac=1.89529833.1552425354.Cj0KCQjwsZ3kBRCnARIsAIuAV_RbL9PTLlh7Ydt21n-iEqkbkifxKMfP0ilNHd1Vg4fJthBso2qmq4aAoaDEALw_wcB

Parmelee, P. A., Scicolone, M. A., Cox, B. S., DeCaro, J. A., Keefe, F. J., & Smith, D. M. (2018). Global versus momentary osteoarthritis pain and emotional distress: Emotional intelligence as moderator. *Annals of Behavioral Medicine, 52*(8), 713-723.

Parrish, B. P., Zautra, A. J., & Davis, M. C. (2008). The role of positive and negative interpersonal events on daily fatigue in women with fibromyalgia, rheumatoid arthritis, and osteoarthritis. *Health Psychology, 27,* 694-702.

Parsons, J. T., Rosof, E., & Mustanski, B. (2008). The temporal relationship between alcohol consumption and HIV-medication adherence: A multilevel model of direct and moderating effects. *Health Psychology, 27,* 628-637.

Pascoe, M. C., Thompson, D. R., & Ski, C. F. (2017). Yoga, mindfulness-based stress reduction and stress-related physiological measures: A meta-analysis. *Psychoneuroendocrinology, 86,* 152-168.

Patel, J. S., Berntson, J., Polanka, B. M., & Stewart, J. C. (2018). Cardiovascular risk factors as differential predictors of incident atypical and typical major depressive disorder in US adults. *Psychosomatic Medicine, 80,* 508-514.

Patterson, F., Malone, S. K., Lozano, A., Grandner, M. A., & Hanlon, A. L. (2016). Smoking, screen-based sedentary behavior, and diet associated with habitual sleep duration and chronotype: Data from the UK Biobank. *Annals of Behavioral Medicine, 50,* 715-726.

Patterson, T. L., Sallis, J. F., Nader, P. R., Rupp, J. W., McKenzie, T. L., Roppe, B., & Bartok, P. W. (1988). Direct observation of physical activity and dietary behaviors in a structured environment: Effects of a family-based health promotion program. *Journal of Behavioral Medicine, 11,* 447-458.

Patton, G. C., Coffey, C., Cappa, C., Currie, D., Riley, L., Gore, F., . . . Ferguson, J. (2012). Health of the world's adolescents: A synthesis of internationally comparable data. *Lancet, 379,* 1665-1675.

Pavalko, E. K., Elder, G. H., Jr., & Clipp, E. C. (1993). Worklives and longevity: Insights from a life course perspective. *Journal of Health and Social Behavior, 34,* 363-380.

Pavalko, E. K., & Woodbury, S. (2000). Social roles as process: Caregiving careers and women's health. *Journal of Health and Social Behavior, 41,* 91-105.

PDQ® Screening and Prevention Editorial Board. (2019). *PDQ cancer prevention overview.* Bethesda, MD: National Cancer Institute. Retrieved June 25, 2019, from https://www.cancer.gov/about-cancer/causes-prevention/hp-prevention-overview-pdq.

Pear, R. (2015). Data on health law shows largest drop in uninsured in 4 decades, the U.S. says. *The New York Times.*

Pearlin, L. I., & Schooler, C. (1978). The structure of coping. *Journal of Health and Social Behavior, 19,* 2-21.

Pedersen, S. S., Herrmann-Lingen, C., de Jonge, P., & Scherer, M. (2010). Type D personality is a predictor of poor emotional quality of life in primary care heart failure patients independent of depressive symptoms and New York Heart Association functional class. *Journal of Behavioral Medicine, 33,* 72-80.

Pegram, S. E., Lumley, M. A., Jasinski, M. J., & Burns, J. W. (2016). Psychological trauma exposure and pain-related outcomes among people with chronic low back pain: Moderated mediation by thought suppression and social constraints. *Annals of Behavioral Medicine, 51,* 316–320

Peeters, A., Barendregt, J. J., Willekens, F., Mackenbach, J. P., Mamun, A. A., & Bonneux, L. (2003). Obesity in adulthood and its consequences for life expectancy: A life-table analysis. *Annals of Internal Medicine, 138,* 24–32.

Peirce, R. S., Frone, M. R., Russell, M., & Cooper, M. L. (1994). Relationship of financial strain and psychosocial resources to alcohol use and abuse: The mediating role of negative affect and drinking motives. *Journal of Health and Social Behavior, 35,* 291–308.

Pellowski, J. A., Kalichman, S. C., Matthews, K. A., & Adler, N. (2013). A pandemic of the poor: Social disadvantage and the U.S. HIV epidemic. *American Psychologist, 68,* 197–209.

Peltzer, K. (2010). Leisure time physical activity and sedentary behavior and substance use among in-school adolescents in eight African countries. *International Journal of Behavioral Medicine, 17,* 271–278.

Pennebaker, J. W. (1980). Perceptual and environmental determinants of coughing. *Basic and Applied Social Psychology, 1,* 83–91.

Pennebaker, J. W. (1983). Accuracy of symptom perception. In A. Baum, S. E. Taylor, & J. Singer (Eds.), *Handbook of psychology and health* (Vol. 4, pp. 189–218). Hillsdale, NJ: Erlbaum.

Pennebaker, J. W. (1997). Writing about emotional experiences as a therapeutic process. *Psychological Science, 8,* 162–166.

Pennebaker, J. W., & Beall, S. (1986). Confronting a traumatic event: Toward an understanding of inhibition and disease. *Journal of Abnormal Psychology, 95,* 274–281.

Pennebaker, J. W., Kiecolt-Glaser, J., & Glaser, R. (1988). Disclosure of traumas and immune function: Health implications for psychotherapy. *Journal of Consulting and Clinical Psychology, 56,* 239–245.

Pennebaker, J. W., & Smyth, J. M. (2016). *Opening up by writing it down, third edition: How expressive writing improves health and eases emotional pain.* New York: Guilford.

Penninx, B. W. J. H., van Tilburg, T., Boeke, A. J. P., Deeg, D. J. H., Kriegsman, D. M. W., & van Eijk, J. T. M. (1998). Effects of social support and personal coping resources on depressive symptoms: Different for various chronic diseases? *Health Psychology, 17,* 551–558.

Pereira, D. B., Antoni, M. H., Danielson, A., Simon, T. Efantis-Potter, J., Carver, C. S., . . . O'Sullivan, M. J. (2003). Life stress and cervical squamous intraepithelial lesions in women with human papillomavirus and human immunodeficiency virus. *Psychosomatic Medicine, 65,* 427–434.

Perez, M. A., Skinner, E. C., & Meyerowitz, B. E. (2002). Sexuality and intimacy following radical prostatectomy: Patient and partner. *Health Psychology, 21,* 288–293.

Perkins, K. A. (1985). The synergistic effect of smoking and serum cholesterol on coronary heart disease. *Health Psychology, 4,* 337–360.

Perkins-Porras, L., Whitehead, D. L., Strike, P. C., & Steptoe, A. (2008). Causal beliefs, cardiac denial and pre-hospital delays following the onset of acute coronary syndromes. *Journal of Behavioral Medicine, 31,* 498–505.

Perlman, D. M., Salomons, T. V., Davidson, R. J., & Lutz, A. (2010). Differential effects on pain intensity and unpleasantness of two meditation practices. *Emotion, 10,* 65–71.

Perna, F. M., & McDowell, S. L. (1995). Role of psychological stress in cortisol recovery from exhaustive exercise among elite athletes. *International Journal of Behavioral Medicine, 2,* 13–26.

Persky, I., Spring, B., Vander Wal, J. S., Pagoto, S., & Hedeker, D. (2005). Adherence across behavioral domains in treatment promoting smoking cessation plus weight control. *Health Psychology, 24,* 153–160.

Pesonen, A., Räikkönen, K., Paavonen, E. J., Heinonen, K., Komsi, N., Lahti, J., . . . Strandberg, T. (2009). Sleep duration and regularity are associated with behavioral problems in 8-year-old children. *International Journal of Behavioral Medicine, 17,* 298–305.

Petersen, K. L., Marsland, A. L., Flory, J., Votruba-Drzal, E., Muldoon, M.F., & Manuck, S. B. (2008). Community socioeconomic status is associated with circulating interleukin-6 and c-reactive protein. *Psychosomatic Medicine, 70,* 646–652.

Peterson, M. S., Lawman, H. G., Wilson, D. K., Fairchild, A., & Van Horn, M. L. (2013). The association of self-efficacy and parent social support on physical activity in male and female adolescents. *Health Psychology, 32,* 666–674.

Petrie, K. J., Booth, R. J., Pennebaker, J. W., Davison, K. P., & Thomas, M. G. (1995). Disclosure of trauma and immune response to a hepatitis B vaccination program. *Journal of Consulting and Clinical Psychology, 63,* 787–792.

Petrie, K. J., Buick, D. L., Weinman, J., & Booth, R. J. (1999). Positive effects of illness reported by myocardial infarction and breast cancer patients. *Journal of Psychosomatic Research, 47,* 537–543.

Petrie, K. J., Fontanilla, I., Thomas, M. G., Booth, R. J., & Pennebaker, J. W. (2004). Effect of written emotional expression on immune function in patients with human immunodeficiency virus infection: A randomized trial. *Psychosomatic Medicine, 66,* 272–275.

Petrie, K. J., MacKrill, K., Derksen, C., & Dalbeth, N. (2018). An illness by any other name: The effect of renaming gout on illness and treatment perceptions. *Health Psychology, 37,* 37–41.

Petrie, K. J., Myrtveit, S. M., Partridge, A. H., Stephens, M., & Stanton, A. L. (2015). The relationship between the belief in a genetic cause for breast cancer and bilateral mastectomy. *Health Psychology, 34,* 473–476.

Petrie, K. J., & Weinman, J. (2012). Patients' perceptions of their illness: The dynamo of volition in health care. *Current Directions in Psychological Science, 21,* 60–65.

Petrova, D., Garcia-Retamero, R., Catena, A., Cokely, E., Heredia Carrasco, A., Arrebola Moreno, A., & Ramírez Hernández, J. A. (2016). Numeracy predicts risk of pre-hospital decision delay: A retrospective study of acute coronary syndrome survival. *Annals of Behavioral Medicine, 51,* 292–306.

Petrovic, P., Kalso, E., Peterson, K. M., & Ingvar, M. (2002). Placebo and opioid analgesia–imaging a shared neuronal network. *Science, 295,* 1737–1740.

Peyrot, M., McMurry, J. F., Jr., & Kruger, D. F. (1999). A biopsychosocial model of glycemic control in diabetes: Stress, coping and regimen adherence. *Journal of Health and Social Behavior, 40,* 141–158.

Pfeifer, J. E., & Brigham, J. C. (Eds.). (1996). Psychological perspectives on euthanasia. *Journal of Social Issues, 52* (entire issue).

Philips, H. C. (1983). Assessment of chronic headache behavior. In R. Meizack (Ed.), *Pain measurement and assessment* (pp. 97–104). New York: Raven Press.

Phillips, A. C., Batty, G. D., Gale, C. R., Deary, I. J., Osborn, D., MacIntyre, K., & Carroll, D. (2009). Generalized anxiety disorder, major depressive disorder, and their comorbidity as predictors of all-cause and cardiovascular mortality: The Vietnam experience study. *Psychosomatic Medicine, 71,* 395–403.

Phillips, A. C., Carroll, D., Ring, C., Sweeting, H., & West, P. (2005). Life events and acute cardiovascular reactions to mental stress: A cohort study. *Psychosomatic Medicine, 67,* 384–392.

Phillips, K. M., Antoni, M. H., Lechner, S. C., Blomberg, B. B., Llabre, M. M., Avisar, E., . . . Carver, C. S. (2008). Stress management intervention reduces serum cortisol and increases relaxation during treatment for nonmetastatic breast cancer. *Psychosomatic Medicine, 70,* 1044–1049.

Phillips, L. A., & Gardner, B. (2016). Habitual exercise instigation (vs. execution) predicts healthy adults' exercise frequency. *Health Psychology, 35,* 69–77.

Phipps, S., & Steele, R. (2002). Repressive adaptive style in children with chronic illness. *Psychosomatic Medicine, 64,* 34–42.

Phipps, S., Steele, R. G., Hall, K., & Leigh, L. (2001). Repressive adaptation in children with cancer: A replication and extension. *Health Psychology, 20,* 445-451.

Piasecki, T. M. (2006). Relapse to smoking. *Clinical Psychology Review, 26,* 196-215.

Picardi, A., Battisti, F., Tarsitani, L., Baldassari, M., Copertaro, A., Mocchegiani, E., & Biondi, M. (2007). Attachment security and immunity in healthy women. *Psychosomatic Medicine, 69,* 40-46.

Pichon, L. C., Arredondo, E. M., Roesch, S., Sallis, J. F., Ayala, G. X., & Elder, J. P. (2007). The relation of acculturation to Latina's perceived neighborhood safety and physical activity: A structural equation analysis. *Annals of Behavioral Medicine, 34,* 295-303.

Pickering, T. G., Devereux, R. B., James, G. D., Gerin, W., Landsbergis, P., Schnall, P. L., & Schwartz, J. E. (1996). Environmental influences on blood pressure and the role of job strain. *Journal of Hypertension, 14* (Suppl.), S179-S185.

Pickett, M. (1993). Cultural awareness in the context of terminal illness. *Cancer Nursing, 16,* 102-106.

Pieper, S., & Brosschot, J. F. (2005). Prolonged stress-related cardiovascular activation: Is there any? *Annals of Behavioral Medicine, 30,* 91-103.

Pieper, S., Brosschot, J. F., van der Leeden, R., & Thayer, J. F. (2007). Cardiac effects of momentary assessed worry episodes and stressful events. *Psychosomatic Medicine, 69,* 901-909.

Pieper, S., Brosschot, J. F., van der Leeden, R., & Thayer, J. F. (2010). Prolonged cardiac effects of momentary assessed stressful events and worry episodes. *Psychosomatic Medicine, 72,* 570-577.

Pietras, S. A., & Goodman, E. (2013). Socioeconomic status gradients in inflammation in adolescence. *Psychosomatic Medicine, 75,* 442-448.

Pietromonaco, P. R., & Collins, N. L. (2017). Interpersonal mechanisms linking close relationships to health. *American Psychologist, 72,* 531-542

Pietrzak, R. H., Goldstein, R. B., Southwick, S. M., & Grant, B. F. (2011). Medical comorbidity of full and partial Posttraumatic Stress Disorder in US adults: Results from wave 2 of the National Epidemiologic Survey on Alcohol and Related Conditions. *Psychosomatic Medicine, 73,* 697-707.

Pignone, M. P., Gaynes, B. N., Rushton, J. L., Burchell, C. M., Orleans, C. T., Mulrow, C. D., & Lohr, K. N. (2002). Screening for depression in adults: A summary of the evidence for the U.S. preventive services task force. *Annals of Internal Medicine, 136,* 765-776.

Pike, J., Smith, T., Hauger, R., Nicassio, P., Patterson, T., McClintock, J., . . . Irwin, M. R. (1997). Chronic life stress alters sympathetic, neuroendocrine, and immune responsivity to an acute psychological stressor in humans. *Psychosomatic Medicine, 59,* 447-457.

Pike, K. M., & Rodin, J. (1991). Mothers, daughters, and disordered eating. *Journal of Abnormal Psychology, 100,* 1-7.

Piliavin, J. A., & Siegl, E. (2007). Health benefits of volunteering in the Wisconsin longitudinal study. *Journal of Health and Social Behavior, 48,* 450-464.

Pilutti, L. A., Greenlee, T. A., Motl, R. W., Nickrent, M. S. & Petruzzello, S. J. (2013). Effects of exercise training on fatigue in multiple sclerosis: A meta-analysis. *Psychosomatic Medicine, 75,* 575-580.

Piper, M. E., Cook, J. W., Schlam, T. R., Jorenby, D. E., Smith, S. S., Collins, L. M., . . . Baker, T. B. (2018). A randomized controlled trial of an optimized smoking treatment delivered in primary care. *Annals of Behavioral Medicine, 52,* 854-864.

Piper, M. E., Kenford, S., Fiore, M. C., & Baker, T. B. (2012). Smoking cessation and quality of life: Changes in life satisfaction over 3 years following a quit attempt. *Annals of Behavioral Medicine, 43,* 262-270.

Pinheiro, M. B., Morosoli, J. J., Ferreira, M. L., Madrid-Valero, J. J., Refshauge, K., Ferreira, P. H., & Ordoñana, J. R. (2018). Genetic and environmental contributions to sleep quality and low back pain: A population-based twin study. *Psychosomatic Medicine, 80,* 263-270.

Pinto, B. M., Papandonatos, G. D., & Goldstein, M. G. (2013). A randomized trial to promote physical activity among breast cancer patients. *Health Psychology, 32,* 616-626.

Pischke, C. R., Scherwitz, L., Weidner, G., & Ornish, D. (2008). Long-term effects of lifestyle changes on well-being and cardiac variables among coronary heart disease patients. *Health Psychology, 27,* 584-592.

Polanka, B. M., Berntson, J., Vrany, E. A., & Stewart, J. C. (2018). Are cardiovascular risk factors stronger predictors of incident cardiovascular disease in US adults with versus without a history of clinical depression? *Annals of Behavioral Medicine, 52,* 1036-1045.

Polk, D. E., Cohen, S., Doyle, W. J., Skoner, D. P., & Kirschbaum, C. (2005). State and trait affect as predictors of salivary cortisol in healthy adults. *Psychoneuroendocrinology, 30,* 261-272.

Poole, L., Ronaldson, A., Kidd, T., Leigh, E., Jahangiri, M., & Steptoe, A. (2016). Pre-operative cognitive functioning and inflammatory and neuroendocrine responses to cardiac surgery. *Annals of Behavioral Medicine, 50,* 545-553.

Posadzki, P., & Ernst, E. (2011). Guided imagery for musculoskeletal pain: A systematic review. *Clinical Journal of Pain, 27,* 648-653.

Posadzki, P., Lewandowski, W., Terry, R., Ernst, E., & Stearns, A. (2012). Guided imagery for non-musculoskeletal pain: A systematic review of randomized clinical trials. *Journal of Pain and Symptom Management, 44,* 95-104.

Poulin, M. J. (2014). Volunteering predicts health among those who value others: Two national studies. *Health Psychology, 33,* 120-129.

Powell, D. J., McMinn, D., & Allan, J. L. (2017). Does real time variability in inhibitory control drive snacking behavior? An intensive longitudinal study. *Health Psychology, 36*(4), 356-364.

Powell, L. H., Appelhans, B. M., Ventrelle, J., Karavolos, K., March, M. L., Ong, J. C., . . . Kazlauskaite, R. (2018). Development of a lifestyle intervention for the metabolic syndrome: Discovery through proof-of-concept. *Health Psychology, 37,* 929-939.

Powell, L. H., Shahabi, L., & Thoresen, C. E. (2003). Religion and spirituality: Linkages to physical health. *American Psychologist, 58,* 36-52.

Power, E., Van Jaarsveld, C. H. M., McCaffery, K., Miles, A., Atkin, W., & Wardle, J. (2008). Understanding intentions and action in colorectal cancer screening. *Annals of Behavioral Medicine, 35,* 285-294.

Power, M., Bullinger, M., Harper, A., & the World Health Organization Quality of Life Group. (1999). The World Health Organization WHO-QOL-100: Tests of the universality of quality of life in 15 different cultural groups worldwide. *Health Psychology, 18,* 495-505.

Pratt, L. A., & Brody, D. J. (2010). Depression and smoking in the U.S. household population aged 20 and over, 2005-2008. *NCHS Data Brief, 34,* 1-8.

Presseau, J., Tait, R. I., Johnston, D. W., Francis, J. J., & Sniehotta, F. F. (2013). Goal conflict and goal facilitation as predictors of daily accelerometer-assessed physical activity. *Health Psychology, 32,* 1179-1187.

Pressman, E., & Orr, W. C. (Eds.). (1997). *Understanding sleep: The evolution and treatment of sleep disorders.* Washington, DC: American Psychological Association.

Pressman, S. D., & Cohen, S. (2007). Use of social words in autobiographies and longevity. *Psychosomatic Medicine, 69,* 262-269.

Pressman, S. D., & Cohen, S. (2011). Positive emotion word use and longevity in famous deceased psychologists. *Health Psychology, 31,* 297-305.

Pressman, S. D., Cohen, S., Miller, G. E., Barkin, A., Rabin, B. S., & Treanor, J. J. (2005). Loneliness, social network size, and immune response to influenza vaccination in college freshmen. *Health Psychology, 24,* 297-306.

Pressman, S. D., Matthews, K. A., Cohen, S., Martire, L. M., Scheier, M., Baum, A., & Schulz, R. (2009). Association of enjoyable leisure activities with psychological and physical well-being. *Psychosomatic Medicine, 71,* 725-732.

Prestwich, A., Conner, M. T., Lawton, R. J., Ward, J. K., Ayres, K., & McEachan, R. R. C. (2012). Randomized controlled trial of collaborative implementation intentions targeting working adults' physical activity. *Health Psychology, 31,* 486–495.

Prestwich, A., Perugini, M., & Hurling, R. (2010). Can implementation intentions and text messages promote brisk walking? A randomized trial. *Health Psychology, 29,* 40–49.

Pribicevic, M., Pollard, H., Bonello, R., & de Luca, K. (2010). A systematic review of manipulative therapy for the treatment of shoulder pain. *Journal of Manipulative and Physiological Therapeutics, 33,* 679–689.

Prinstein, M. J., & La Greca, A. M. (2009). Childhood depressive symptoms and adolescent cigarette use: A six-year longitudinal study controlling for peer relations correlates. *Health Psychology, 28,* 283–291.

Prochaska, J. J., & Sallis, J. F. (2004). A randomized controlled trial of single versus multiple health behavior change: Promoting physical activity and nutrition among adolescents. *Health Psychology, 23,* 314–318.

Prochaska, J. O. (1994). Strong and weak principles for progressing from precontemplation to action on the basis of 12 problem behaviors. *Health Psychology, 13,* 47–51.

Prochaska, J. O., DiClemente, C. C., & Norcross, J. C. (1992). In search of how people change: Applications to addictive behaviors. *American Psychologist, 47,* 1102–1114.

Protogerou, C., Johnson, B. T., & Hagger, M. S. (2018). An integrated model of condom use in Sub-Saharan African youth: A meta-analysis. *Health Psychology, 37,* 586–602.

Pruessner, J. C., Hellhammer, D. H., & Kirschbaum, C. (1999). Burnout, perceived stress, and cortisol responses to awakening. *Psychosomatic Medicine, 61,* 197–204.

Pruessner, M., Hellhammer, D. H., Pruessner, J. C., & Lupien, S. J. (2003). Self-reported depressive symptoms and stress levels in healthy young men: Associations with the cortisol response to awakening. *Psychosomatic Medicine, 65,* 92–99.

Puig, J., Englund, M. M., Simpson, J. A., & Collins, A. W. (2013). Predicting adult physical illness from infant attachment: A prospective longitudinal study. *Health Psychology, 32,* 409–417.

Pulkki-Råback, L., Elovainio, M., Kivimäki, M., Raitakari, O. T., & Keltikangas-Järvinen, L. (2005). Temperament in childhood predicts body mass in adulthood: The cardiovascular risk in young Finns study. *Health Psychology, 24,* 307–315.

Puterman, E., Adler, N., Matthews, K. A., & Epel, E. (2012). Financial strain and impaired fasting glucose: The moderating role of physical activity in the Coronary Artery Risk Development in Young Adults study. *Psychosomatic Medicine, 74,* 187–192.

Puterman, E., Prather, A. A., Epel, E. S., Loharuka, S., Adler, N. E., Laraia, B., & Tomiyama, A. J. (2016). Exercise mitigates cumulative associations between stress and BMI in girls age 10 to 19. *Health Psychology, 35,* 191–194.

Puustinen, P. J., Koponen, H., Kautiainen, H., Mäntyselkä, P., & Vanhala, M. (2011). Psychological distress predicts the development of the metabolic syndrome: A prospective population-based study. *Psychosomatic Medicine, 73,* 158–165.

Quadagno, J. (2004). Why the United States has no national health insurance: Stakeholder mobilization against the welfare state, 1945–1996. *Journal of Health and Social Behavior, 45* (extra issue), 25–44.

Quartana, P. J., Bounds, S., Yoon, K. L., Goodin, B. R., & Burns, J. W. (2010). Anger suppression predicts pain, emotional, and cardiovascular responses to the cold pressor. *Annals of Behavioral Medicine, 39,* 211–221.

Quartana, P. J., Burns, J. W., & Lofland, K. R. (2007). Attentional strategy moderates effects of pain catastrophizing on symptom-specific physiological response in chronic low back pain patients. *Journal of Behavioral Medicine, 30,* 221–231.

Quinlan, K. B., & McCaul, K. D. (2000). Matched and mismatched interventions with young adult smokers: Testing a stage theory. *Health Psychology, 19,* 165–171.

Quinn, J. M., Pascoe, A., Wood, W., & Neal, D. T. (2010). Can't control yourself? Monitor those bad habits. *Personality and Social Psychology Bulletin, 36,* 499–511.

Quon, E. C., & McGrath, J. J. (2014). Subjective socioeconomic status and adolescent health: A meta-analysis. *Health Psychology, 33,* 433–447.

Rabin, C. (2011). Review of health behaviors and their correlates among young adult cancer survivors. *Journal of Behavioral Medicine, 34,* 41–52.

Rabin, C., Ward, S., Leventhal, H., & Schmitz, M. (2001). Explaining retrospective reports of symptoms in patients undergoing chemotherapy: Anxiety, initial symptom experience and posttreatment symptoms. *Health Psychology, 20,* 91–98.

Rabin, R. C. (2012, October 22). Curbing the enthusiasm on daily multivitamins. *New York Times.* Retrieved October 24, 2012, from http://well.blogs.nytimes.com/2012/10/22/curbing-the-enthusiasm-on-daily-multivitamins

Rabius, V., McAlister, A. L., Geiger, A., Huang, P., & Todd, R. (2004). Telephone counseling increases cessation rates among young adult smokers. *Health Psychology, 23,* 539–541.

Rabkin, J. G., McElhiney, M., Ferrando, S. J., Van Gorp, W., & Lin, S. H. (2004). Predictors of employment of men with HIV/AIDS: A longitudinal study. *Psychosomatic Medicine, 66,* 72–78.

Rachman, S. J., & Phillips, C. (1978). *Psychology and medicine.* Baltimore, MD: Penguin.

Raeburn, P., Forster, D., Foust, D., & Brady, D. (2002, October 21). Why we're so fat. *Business Week,* pp. 112–114.

Räikkönen, K., Matthews, K. A., Flory, J. D., Owens, J. F., & Gump, B. B. (1999). Effects of optimism, pessimism, and trait anxiety on ambulatory blood pressure and mood during everyday life. *Journal of Personality and Social Psychology, 76,* 104–113.

Rakoff, V. (1983). Multiple determinants of family dynamics in anorexia nervosa. In P. L. Darby, P. E. Garfinkel, D. M. Garner, & D. V. Coscina (Eds.), *Anorexia nervosa: Recent developments in research* (pp. 29–40). New York: Liss.

Ramirez-Maestre, C., Lopez-Martinez, A. E., & Zarazaga, R. E. (2004). Personality characteristics as differential variables of the pain experience. *Journal of Behavioral Medicine, 27,* 147–165.

Randall, G., Molloy, G. J., & Steptoe, A. (2009). The impact of an acute cardiac event on the partners of patients: A systematic review. *Health Psychology Review, 3,* 1–84.

Rapoff, M. A., & Christophersen, E. R. (1982). Improving compliance in pediatric practice. *Pediatric Clinics of North America, 29,* 339–357.

Raposa, E. B., Hammen, C. L., Brennan, P. A., O'Callaghan, F., & Najman, J. M. (2014). Early adversity and health outcomes in young adulthood: The role of ongoing stress. *Health Psychology, 33,* 410–418.

Rasmussen, H. N., Scheier, M. F., & Greenhouse, J. B. (2009). Optimism and physical health: A meta-analytic review. *Annals of Behavioral Medicine, 42,* 239–256.

Rassart, J., Luyckx, K., Berg, C. A., Bijttebier, P., Moons, P., & Weets, I. (2015). Psychosocial functioning and glycemic control in emerging adults with Type 1 diabetes: A 5-year follow-up study. *Health Psychology, 34,* 1058–1065.

Rauma, P., Koivumaa-Honkanen, H., Williams, L. J., Tuppurainen, M. T., Kroger, H. P., & Honkanen, R. J. (2014). Life satisfaction and bone mineral density among postmenopausal women: Cross-sectional and longitudinal associations. *Psychosomatic Medicine, 76,* 709–715.

Raven, B. H., Freeman, H. E., & Haley, R. W. (1982). Social science perspectives in hospital infection control. In A. W. Johnson, O. Grusky, & B. Raven (Eds.), *Contemporary health services: Social science perspectives* (pp. 139–176). Boston, MA: Auburn House.

Read, J. P., Wardell, J. D., Vermont, L. N., Colder, C. R., Ouimette, P., & White, J. (2013). Transition and change: Prospective effects of posttraumatic stress on smoking trajectories in the first year of college. *Health Psychology, 32,* 757–767.

Reddy, S. (2017, February 14). No drugs for your back pain. *The Wall Street Journal,* p. A11.

Reddy, K. S., Shah, B., Varghese, C., & Ramadoss, A. (2005). Responding to the threat of chronic diseases in India. *The Lancet, 366,* 1744–1749.

Redelmeier, D., & Ross, L. (2018, November). The objectivity illusion in medical practice. *Association for Psychological Science, 31,* 5–7.

Redman, S., Webb, G. R., Hennrikus, D. J., Gordon, J. J., & Sanson-Fisher, R. W. (1991). The effects of gender on diagnosis of psychological disturbance. *Journal of Behavioral Medicine, 14,* 527–540.

Redwine, L., Dang, J., Hall, M., & Irwin, M. (2003). Disordered sleep, nocturnal cytokines, and immunity in alcoholics. *Psychosomatic Medicine, 65,* 75–85.

Reed, G. M. (1989). *Stress, coping, and psychological adaptation in a sample of gay and bisexual men with AIDS.* Unpublished doctoral dissertation, University of California, Los Angeles.

Reed, G. M., Kemeny, M. E., Taylor, S. E., & Visscher, B. R. (1999). Negative HIV-specific expectancies and AIDS-related bereavement as predictors of symptom onset in asymptomatic HIV-positive gay men. *Health Psychology, 18,* 354–363.

Reed, G. M., Kemeny, M. E., Taylor, S. E., Wang, H. Y. J., & Visscher, B. R. (1994). Realistic acceptance as a predictor of decreased survival time in gay men with AIDS. *Health Psychology, 13,* 299–307.

Reger, G. M., Holloway, K. M., Candy, C., Rothbaum, B. O., Difede, J., Rizzo, A. A., & Gahm, G. A. (2011). Effectiveness of virtual reality exposure therapy for active duty soldiers in a military mental health clinic. *Journal of Traumatic Stress, 24,* 93–96.

Reid, A. E., Taber, J. M., Ferrer, R. A., Biesecker, B. B., Lewis, K. L., Biesecker, L. G., & Klein, W. M. P. (2018). Associations of perceived norms with intentions to learn genomic sequencing results: Roles for attitudes and ambivalence. *Health Psychology, 37*(6), 553–561.

Reitman, V. (2003, March 24). Healing sound of a word: "Sorry." *Los Angeles Times,* pp. F1, F8.

Reitman, V. (2004, June 28). Ill effects of cutting back on medications. *Los Angeles Times,* p. F2.

Rendina, H. J., Gamarel, K. E., Pachankis, J. E., Ventuneac, A., Grov, C., & Parsons, J. T. (2016). Extending the minority stress model to incorporate HIV-positive gay and bisexual men's experiences: A longitudinal examination of mental health and sexual risk behavior. *Annals of Behavioral Medicine, 51,* 147–158.

Repetti, R. L. (1989). Effects of daily workload on subsequent behavior during marital interactions: The role of social withdrawal and spouse support. *Journal of Personality and Social Psychology, 57,* 651–659.

Repetti, R. L. (1993b). Short-term effects of occupational stressors on daily mood and health complaints. *Health Psychology, 12,* 125–131.

Repetti, R. L., & Pollina, S. L. (1994). *The effects of daily social and academic failure experiences on school-age children's subsequent interactions with parents.* Unpublished manuscript, University of California, Los Angeles.

Repetti, R. L., Taylor, S. E., & Seeman, T. E. (2002). Risky families: Family social environments and the mental and physical health of offspring. *Psychological Bulletin, 128,* 330–336.

Repetti, R. L., Wang, S. W., & Saxbe, D. E. (2011). Adult health in the context of everyday family life. *Annals of Behavioral Medicine, 42,* 285–293.

Repetto, M. J., & Petitto, J. M. (2008). Psychopharmacology in HIV-infected patients. *Psychosomatic Medicine, 70,* 585–592.

Repetto, P. B., Caldwell, C. H., & Zimmerman, M. A. (2005). A longitudinal study of the relationship between depressive symptoms and cigarette use among African American adolescents. *Health Psychology, 24,* 209–219.

Resnick, B., Orwig, D., Yu-Yahiro, J., Hawkes, W., Shardell, M., Hebel, J. R., . . . Magaziner, J. (2007). Testing the effectiveness of the exercise plus program in older women post-hip fracture. *Annals of Behavioral Medicine, 34,* 67–76.

Resnicow, K., Davis, R., Zhang, N., Konkel, J., Strecher, V. J., Shaikh, A. R., . . . Wiese, C. (2008). Tailoring a fruit and vegetable intervention on novel motivational constructs: Results of a randomized study. *Annals of Behavioral Medicine, 35,* 159–169.

Resnicow, K., DiIorio, C., Soet, J. E., Borrelli, B., Hecht, J., & Ernst, D. (2002). Motivational interviewing in health promotion: It sounds like something is changing. *Health Psychology, 21,* 444–451.

Resnicow, K., Reddy, S. P., James, S., Gabebodeen Omardien, R., Kambaran, N. S., Langner, R. G., . . . Nichols, T. (2008). Comparison of two school-based smoking prevention programs among South African high school students: Results of a randomized trial. *Annals of Behavioral Medicine, 36,* 231–243.

Resolve: The National Fertility Association. (2013). *What are my chances of success with an IVF?* Retrieved January 21, 2016, from http://www.resolve.org

Reyes, E. A. (2013, November 22). U.S. attitudes on end of life show a change. *The New York Times,* pp. AA1–AA2.

Reyes del Paso, G. A., Garrido, S., Pulgar, Á., Martín-Vázquez, M., & Duschek, S. (2010). Aberrances in autonomic cardiovascular regulation in fibromyalgia syndrome and their relevance for clinical pain reports. *Psychosomatic Medicine, 72,* 462–470.

Reynolds, D. V. (1969). Surgery in the rat during electrical analgesia induced by focal brain stimulation. *Science, 164,* 444–445.

Reynolds, J. S., & Perrin, N. A. (2004). Mismatches in social support and psychological adjustment to breast cancer. *Health Psychology, 23,* 425–430.

Reynolds, K. A., & Helgeson, V. S. (2011). Children with diabetes compared to peers: Depressed? Distressed? A meta-analytic review. *Annals of Behavioral Medicine, 42,* 29–41.

Reynolds, N., Mrug, S., Wolfe, K., Schwebel, D., & Wallander, J. (2016). Spiritual coping, psychosocial adjustment, and physical health in youth with chronic illness: A meta-analytic review. *Health Psychology Review, 10*(2), 226–243.

Rhee, H., Holditch-Davis, D., & Miles, M. S. (2005). Patterns of physical symptoms and relationships with psychosocial factors in adolescents. *Psychosomatic Medicine, 67,* 1006–1012.

Rhodes, R. E., Blanchard, C. M., Benoit, C., Levy-Milne, R., Naylor, P., Symons, Downs, D., & Warburton, D. E. R. (2014). Social cognitive correlates of physical activity across 12 months in cohort samples of couples without children, expecting their first child, and expecting their second child. *Health Psychology, 33,* 792–802.

Rhodes, R. E., Naylor, P. J., & McKay, H. A. (2010). Pilot study of a family physical activity planning intervention among parents and their children. *Journal of Behavioral Medicine, 33,* 91–100.

Rhodes, R. E., Plotnikoff, R. C., & Courneya, K. S. (2008). Predicting the physical activity intention-behavior profiles of adopters and maintainers using three social cognition models. *Annals of Behavioral Medicine, 36,* 244–252.

Rice, E. L., & Klein, W. M. (2019). Interactions among perceived norms and attitudes about health-related behaviors in US adolescents. *Health Psychology, 38,* 268–275.

Richardson, L. (2004, January 9). Obesity blamed as disability rates soar for those under 60. *Los Angeles Times,* p. A22.

Rief, W., Hessel, A., & Braehler, E. (2001). Somatization symptoms and hypochondriacal features in the general population. *Psychosomatic Medicine, 63,* 595–602.

Rietschlin, J. (1998). Voluntary association membership and psychological distress. *Journal of Health and Social Behavior, 39*, 348–355.

Riley, K. E., & Kalichman, S. (2015). Mindfulness-based stress reduction for people living with HIV/AIDS: Preliminary review of intervention trial methodologies and findings. *Health Psychology Review, 9*(2), 224–243.

Riley, W.T. (2017). Behavioral and social sciences at the National Institutes of Health: Adoption of research findings in health research and practice as a scientific priority. *Translational Behavioral Medicine, 7*(2), 380–384.

Rimes, K. A., Salkovskis, P. M., Jones, L., & Lucassen, A. M. (2006). Applying a cognitive–behavioral model of health anxiety in a cancer genetics service. *Health Psychology, 25*, 171–180.

Rini, C., Dunkel-Schetter, C., Wadhwa, P., & Sandman, C. (1999). Psychological adaptation and birth outcomes: The role of personal resources, stress, and socio-cultural context in pregnancy. *Health Psychology, 18*, 333–345.

Rini, C., Manne, S., DuHamel, K., Austin, J., Ostroff, J., Boulad, F., . . . Redd, W. H. (2008). Social support from family and friends as a buffer of low social support among mothers of critically ill children: A multi-level modeling approach. *Health Psychology, 27*, 593–603.

Rios, R., & Zautra, A. J. (2011). Socioeconomic disparities in pain: The role of economic hardship and daily financial worry. *Health Psychology, 30*, 58–66.

Ritz, T., & Steptoe, A. (2000). Emotion and pulmonary function in asthma: Reactivity in the field and relationship with laboratory induction of emotion. *Psychosomatic Medicine, 62*, 808–815.

Rizzo, A. A., Difede, J., Rothbaum, B. O., Johnston, S., McLay, R. N., Reger, G., & Pair, J. (2009). VR PTSD exposure therapy results with active duty OIF/OEF combatants. *Studies in Health Technology and Informatics, 142*, 277–282.

Robinson, H., Norton, S., Jarrett, P., & Broadbent, E. (2017). The effects of psychological interventions on wound healing: A systematic review of randomized trials. *British Journal of Health Psychology, 22*, 805–835.

Robbins, C. A., & Martin, S. S. (1993). Gender, styles of deviance, and drinking problems. *Journal of Health and Social Behavior, 34*, 302–321.

Roberts, M. C., & Turner, D. S. (1984). Preventing death and injury in childhood: A synthesis of child safety seat efforts. *Health Education Quarterly, 11*, 181–193.

Roberts, M. E., Gibbons, F. X., Gerrard, M., & Alert, M. D. (2011). Optimism and adolescent perception of skin cancer risk. *Health Psychology, 30*, 810–813.

Robinson, E., Fleming, A., & Higgs, S. (2014). Prompting healthier eating: Testing the use of health and social norm based messages. *Health Psychology, 33*, 1057–1064.

Robinson, H., Jarrett, P., Vedhara, K., & Broadbent, E. (2017). The effects of expressive writing before or after punch biopsy on wound healing. *Brain, Behavior, and Immunity, 61*, 217–227.

Robinson, H., Ravikulan, A., Nater, U. M., Skoluda, N., Jarrett, P., & Broadbent, E. (2017). The role of social closeness during tape stripping to facilitate skin barrier recovery: Preliminary findings. *Health Psychology, 36*(7), 619–629.

Robles, T. F. (2007). Stress, social support, and delayed skin barrier recovery. *Psychosomatic Medicine, 69*, 807–815.

Robles, T. F. (2014). Marital quality and health: Implications for marriage in the 21st century. *Current Directions in Psychological Science, 23*, 427–432.

Robles, T. F., Brooks, K. P., & Pressman, S. D. (2009). Trait positive affect buffers the effects of acute stress on skin barrier recovery. *Health Psychology, 28*, 373–378.

Robles, T. F., Glaser, R., & Kiecolt-Glaser, J. K. (2005). Out of balance: A new look at chronic stress, depression, and immunity. *Current Directions in Psychological Science, 14*, 111–115.

Rodgers, A., Corbett, T., Bramley, D., Riddell, T., Wills, M., Lin, R. B., & Jones, M. (2005). Do u smoke after txt? Results of a randomized trial of smoking cessation using mobile phone text messaging. *Tobacco Control, 14*, 255–261.

Rodin, J., & McAvay, G. (1992). Determinants of change in perceived health in a longitudinal study of older adults. *Journal of Gerontology, 47*, P373–P384.

Rodin, J., & Plante, T. (1989). The psychological effects of exercise. In R. S. Williams & A. Wellece (Eds.), *Biological effects of physical activity* (pp. 127–137). Champaign, IL: Human Kinetics.

Rodrigues, A. M., O'Brien, N., French, D. P., Glidewell, L., & Sniehotta, F. F. (2015). The question-behavior effect: Genuine effect or spurious phenomenon? A systematic review of randomized controlled trials with meta-analysis. *Health Psychology, 34*, 61–78.

Rodriguez, C. J., Gwathmey, T. M., Jin, Z., Schwartz, J., Beech, B. M., Sacco, R. L., . . . Homma, S. (2016). Perceived discrimination and nocturnal blood pressure dipping among Hispanics: The influence of social support and race. *Psychosomatic Medicine, 78*, 841–850.

Rodriguez, F. S., Schroeter, M. L., Arélin, K., Witte, A. V., Baber, R., Burkhardt, R., . . . Riedel-Heller, S. G. (2018). APOE e4-genotype and lifestyle interaction on cognitive performance: Results of the LIFE-Adult-study. *Health Psychology, 37*, 194–205.

Roepke, S. K., Chattillion, E. A., von Känel, R., Allison, M., Ziegler, M. G., Dimsdale, J. E., . . . Grant, I. (2011). Carotid plaque in Alzheimer caregivers and the role of sympathoadrenal arousal. *Psychosomatic Medicine, 73*, 206–213.

Roepke, S. K., & Grant, I. (2011). Toward a more complete understanding of the effects of personal mastery on cardiometabolic health. *Health Psychology, 30*, 615–632.

Roest, A. M., Heideveld, A., Martens, E. J., de Jonge, P., & Denollet, J. (2014). Symptom dimensions of anxiety following myocardial infarction: Associations with depressive symptoms and prognosis. *Health Psychology, 33*, 1468–1476.

Roest, A. M., Martens, E. J., Denollet, J., & de Jonge, P. (2010). Prognostic association of anxiety post myocardial infarction with mortality and new cardiac events: A meta-analysis. *Psychosomatic Medicine, 72*, 563–569.

Rogers, R. W. (1975). A protection motivation theory of fear appeals and attitude change. *The Journal of Psychology, 91*, 93–114.

Rohan, J. M., Rausch, J. R., Pendley, J. S., Delamater, A. M., Dolan, L., Reeves, G., & Drotar, D. (2014). Identification and prediction of group-based glycemic control trajectories during the transition to adolescence. *Health Psychology, 33*, 1143–1152.

Rohleder, N. (2014). Stimulation of systemic low-grade inflammation by psychosocial stress. *Psychosomatic Medicine, 76*, 181–189.

Roitt, I., Brostoff, J., & Male, D. (1998). *Immunology* (5th ed.). London, England: Mosby International.

Rollman, B. L. & Huffman, J. C. (2013). Treating anxiety in the presence of medical comorbidity: calmly moving forward. *Psychosomatic Medicine, 75*, 710–712.

Roman, M. J., Shanker, B. A., Davis, A., Lockshin, M. D., Sammaritano, L., Simantov, R., . . . Salmon, J. E. (2003). Prevalence and correlates of accelerated atherosclerosis in systematic lupus erythematosus. *The New England Journal of Medicine, 349*, 2399–2406.

Rook, K. S., & Charles, S. T. (2017). Close social ties and health in later life: Strengths and vulnerabilities. *American Psychologist, 72*(6), 567–577.

Romero, C., Friedman, L. C., Kalidas, M., Elledge, R., Chang, J., & Liscum, K. R. (2006). Self-forgiveness, spirituality, and psychological adjustment in women with breast cancer. *Journal of Behavioral Medicine, 29*, 29–36.

Rooks-Peck, C. R., Adegbite, A. H., Wichser, M. E., Ramshaw, R., Mullins, M. M., Higa, D., . . . The Prevention Research Synthesis Project, Division of HIV/AIDS Prevention, Centers for Disease Control and Prevention. (2018). Mental health and retention in HIV care: A systematic review and meta-analysis. *Health Psychology, 37,* 574-585.

Rosenfield, S. (1992). The costs of sharing: Wives' employment and husbands' mental health. *Journal of Health and Social Behavior, 33,* 213-225.

Rosenstock, I. M. (1966). Why people use health services. *Milbank Memorial Fund Quarterly, 44,* 94ff.

Rosenstock, I. M. (1974). Historical origins of the health belief model. *Health Education Monographs, 2,* 328-335.

Ross, C. E., & Mirowsky, J. (1988). Child care and emotional adjustment to wives' employment. *Journal of Health and Social Behavior, 29,* 127-138.

Ross, C. E., & Mirowsky, J. (2001). Neighborhood disadvantages, disorder, and health. *Journal of Health and Social Behavior, 42,* 258-276.

Rossy, L. A., Buckelew, S. P., Dorr, N., Hagglund, K. J., Thayer, J. F., McIntosh, M. J., . . . Johnson, J. C. (1999). A meta-analysis of fibromyalgia treatment interventions. *Annals of Behavioral Medicine, 21,* 180-191.

Roth, B., & Robbins, D. (2004). Mindfulness-based stress reduction and health-related quality of life: Findings from a bilingual inner-city patient population. *Psychosomatic Medicine, 66,* 113-123.

Rothbaum, B. O., Kearns, M. C., Price, M., Malcoun, E., Davis, M., Ressler, K. J., . . . Houry, D. (2012). Early intervention may prevent the development of posttraumatic stress disorder: A randomized pilot civilian study with modified prolonged exposure. *Biological Psychiatry, 72,* 957-863.

Rotheram-Borus, M. J., Murphy, D. A., Reid, H. M., & Coleman, C. L. (1996). Correlates of emotional distress among HIV+ youths: Health status, stress, and personal resources. *Annals of Behavioral Medicine, 18,* 16-23.

Rothman, A. J. (2000). Toward a theory-based analysis of behavioral maintenance. *Health Psychology, 19,* 64-69.

Rothman, A. J., & Salovey, P. (1997). Shaping perceptions to motivate healthy behavior: The role of message framing. *Psychological Bulletin, 121,* 3-19.

Rottenberg, J., Yaroslavsky, I., Carney, R. M., Freedland, K. E., George, C. J., Baji, I., & Kovacs, M. (2014). The association between major depressive disorder in childhood and risk factors for cardiovascular disease in adolescence. *Psychosomatic Medicine, 76,* 122-127.

Rottman, B. M., Marcum, Z. A., Thorpe, C. T., & Gellad, W. F. (2017). Medication adherence as a learning process: Insights from cognitive psychology. *Health Psychology Review, 11,* 17-32.

Rottmann, N., Hansen, D. G., Larsen, P. V., Nicolaisen, A., Flyger, H., Johansen, C., & Hagedoorn, M. (2015). Dyadic coping within couples dealing with breast cancer: A longitudinal, population-based study. *Health Psychology, 34,* 486-495.

Rowe, M. M. (1999). Teaching health-care providers coping: Results of a two-year study. *Journal of Behavioral Medicine, 22,* 511-527.

Roy, B., Diez-Roux, A. V., Seeman, T., Ranjit, N., Shea, S., & Cushman, M. (2010). Association of optimism and pessimism with inflammation and hemostasis in the multi-ethnic study of artherosclerosis (MESA). *Psychosomatic Medicine, 72,* 134-140.

Rozanski, A. (2005). Integrating psychological approaches into the behavioral management of cardiac patients. *Psychosomatic Medicine, 67,* S67-S73.

Ruben, M. A., Blanch-Hartigan, D., & Shipherd, J. C. (2018). To know another's pain: A meta-analysis of caregivers' and healthcare providers' pain assessment accuracy. *Annals of Behavioral Medicine, 52,* 662-685.

Rubin, G. J., Cleare, A., & Hotopf, M. (2004). Psychological factors in post-operative fatigue. *Psychosomatic Medicine, 66,* 959-964.

Ruble, D. N. (1972). Premenstrual symptoms: A reinterpretation. *Science, 197,* 291-292.

Ruby, M. B., Dunn, E. W., Perrino, A., Gillis, R., & Viel, S. (2011). The invisible benefits of exercise. *Health Psychology, 30,* 67-74.

Ruissen, G. R., Rhodes, R. E., Crocker, P. R. E., & Beauchamp, M. R. (2018). Affective mental contrasting to enhance physical activity: A randomized controlled trial. *Health Psychology, 37,* 51-60.

Ruiz, J. M., & Brondolo, E. (2016). Introduction to the special issue Disparities in cardiovascular health: Examining the contributions of social and behavioral factors. *Health Psychology, 35,* 309-312.

Ruiz-Párraga, G. T., & López-Martínez, A. E. (2014). The contribution of posttraumatic stress symptoms to chronic pain adjustment. *Health Psychology, 33,* 958-967.

Rushing, B., Ritter, C., & Burton, R. P. D. (1992). Race differences in the effects of multiple roles on health: Longitudinal evidence from a national sample of older men. *Journal of Health and Social Behavior, 33,* 126-139.

Ruthig, J. C., & Chipperfield, J. G. (2007). Health incongruence in later life: Implications for subsequent well-being and health care. *Health Psychology, 26,* 753-761.

Rutledge, T., Linden, W., & Paul, D. (2000). Cardiovascular recovery from acute laboratory stress: Reliability and concurrent validity. *Psychosomatic Medicine, 62,* 648-654.

Rutledge, T., Linke, S. E., Krantz, D. S., Johnson, B. D., Bittner, V., Eastwood, J. A., . . . Merz, C. N. (2009). Comorbid depression and anxiety symptoms as predictors of cardiovascular events: Results from the NHLBI-sponsored women's ischemia syndrome evaluations (WISE) study. *Psychosomatic Medicine, 71,* 958-964.

Rutledge, T., Matthews, K., Lui, L. Y., Stone, K. L., & Cauley, J. A. (2003). Social networks and marital status predict mortality in older women: Prospective evidence from the Study of Osteoporotic Fractures (SOF). *Psychosomatic Medicine, 65,* 688-694.

Rutledge, T., Redwine, L. S., Linke, S. E., & Mills, P. J. (2013). A meta-analysis of mental health treatments and cardiac rehabilitation for improving clinical outcomes and depression among patients with coronary heart disease. *Psychosomatic Medicine, 75,* 335-349.

Rutledge, T., Reis, S. E., Olson, M., Owens, J., Kelsey, S. F., Pepine, C. J., . . . National Heart, Lung, and Blood Institute. (2004). Social networks are associated with lower mortality rates among women with suspected coronary disease: The national heart, lung, and blood institute-sponsored women's ischemia syndrome evaluation study. *Psychosomatic Medicine, 66,* 882-888.

Ryan, J., Zwerling, C., & Orav, E. J. (1992). Occupational risks associated with cigarette smoking: A prospective study. *American Journal of Public Health, 82,* 29-32.

Ryan, J. P., Sheu, L. K., Crtichley, H. D., & Gianaros, P. J. (2012). A neural circuitry linking insulin resistance to depressed mood. *Psychosomatic Medicine, 74,* 476-482.

Ryan, R. M., & Deci, E. L. (2000). Self-determination theory and the facilitation of intrinsic motivation, social development, and well-being. *American Psychologist, 55,* 68-78.

Ryff, C. D., Keyes, C. L. M., & Hughes, D. L. (2003). Status inequalities, perceived discrimination, and eudaimonic well-being: Do the challenges of minority life hone purpose and growth? *Journal of Health and Social Behavior, 44,* 275-291.

Saab, P. G., Llabre, M. M., Schneiderman, N., Hurwitz, B. E., McDonald, P. G., Evans, J., . . . Klein, B. (1997). Influence of ethnicity and gender on cardiovascular responses to active coping and inhibitory-passive coping challenges. *Psychosomatic Medicine, 59,* 434-446.

Sacco, W. P., Malone, J. I., Morrison, A. D., Friedman, A., & Wells, K. (2009). Effect of a brief, regular telephone intervention by paraprofessionals for type 2 diabetes. *Journal of Behavioral Medicine, 32,* 349-359.

Sacker, A., Head, J., & Bartley, M. (2008). Impact of coronary heart disease on health functioning in an aging population: Are there differences according to socioeconomic position? *Psychosomatic Medicine, 70,* 133-140.

Sadava, S. W., & Pak, A. W. (1994). Problem drinking and close relationships during the third decade of life. *Psychology of Addictive Behaviors, 8,* 251-258.

Safer, M. A., Tharps, Q. J., Jackson, T. C., & Leventhal, H. (1979). Determinants of three stages of delay in seeking care at a medical care clinic. *Medical Care, 17,* 11-29.

Safren, S. A., Blashill, A. J., Lee, J. S., O'Cleirigh, C., Tomassili, J., Biello, K. B., . . . Mayer, K. H. (2018). Condom-use self-efficacy as a mediator between syndemics and condomless sex in men who have sex with men (MSM). *Health Psychology, 37,* 820-827.

Safren, S. A., O'Cleirigh, C., Tan, J. Y., Raminani, S. R., Reilly, L. C., Otto, M. W., & Mayer, K. H. (2009). A randomized controlled trial of cognitive behavioral therapy for adherence and depression (CBT-AD) in HIV-infected individuals. *Health Psychology, 28,* 1-10.

Safren, S. A., O'Cleirigh, C. M., Skeer, M., Elsesser, S. A., & Mayer, K. H. (2013). Project enhance: A randomized controlled trial of an individualized HIV prevention intervention for HIV-infected men who have sex with men conducted in a primary care setting. *Health Psychology, 32,* 171-179.

Safren, S. A., Traeger, L., Skeer, M. R., O'Cleirigh, C., Meade, C. S., Covahey, C., & Mayer, K. H. (2010). Testing a social-cognitive model of HIV transmission risk behaviors in HIV-infected MSM with and without depression. *Health Psychology, 29,* 215-221.

Sagherian, M. J., Huedo-Medina, T. B., Pellowski, J. A., Eaton, L. A., & Johnson, B. T. (2016). Single-session behavioral interventions for sexual risk reduction: A meta-analysis. *Annals of Behavioral Medicine, 50,* 920-934.

Salamon, J. D., & Correa, M. (2013). Dopamine and food addiction: Lexicon badly needed. *Biological Psychiatry, 73,* 15-24.

Sallis, J. F., King, A. C., Sirard, J. R., & Albright, C. L. (2007). Perceived environmental predictors of physical activity over 6 months in adults: Activity counseling trial. *Health Psychology, 26,* 701-709.

Salmon, J., Owen, N., Crawford, D., Bauman, A., & Sallis, J. F. (2003). Physical activity and sedentary behavior: A population-based study of barriers, enjoyment, and preference. *Health Psychology, 22,* 178-188.

Salmon, P., Humphris, G. M., Ring, A., Davies, J. C., & Dowrick, C. F. (2007). Primary care consultations about medically unexplained symptoms: Patient presentations and doctor responses that influence the probability of somatic intervention. *Psychosomatic Medicine, 69,* 571-577.

Salomon, K., & Jagusztyn, N. E. (2008). Resting cardiovascular levels and reactivity to interpersonal incivility among Black, Latino/a, and White individuals: The moderating role of ethnic discrimination. *Health Psychology, 27,* 473-481.

Salzmann, S., Euteneuer, F., Laferton, J. A., Auer, C. J., Shedden-Mora, M. C., Schedlowski, M., . . . Rief, W. (2017). Effects of preoperative psychological interventions on catecholamine and cortisol levels after surgery in coronary artery bypass graft patients: The randomized controlled PSY-HEART trial. *Psychosomatic Medicine, 79,* 806-814.

Samuel-Hodge, C. D., Gizlice, Z., Cai, J., Brantley, P. J., Ard, J. D., & Svetkey, L. P. (2010). Family functioning and weight loss in a sample of African Americans and Whites. *Annals of Behavioral Medicine, 40,* 294-301.

Sanchez, L. M., & Turner, S. M. (2003). Practicing psychology in the era of managed care: Implications for practice and training. *American Psychologist, 58,* 116-129.

Sanderson, C. A., Darley, J. M., & Messinger, C. S. (2002). "I'm not as thin as you think I am": The development and consequences of feeling discrepant from the thinness norm. *Personality and Social Psychology Bulletin, 28,* 172-183.

Sandgren, A. K., & McCaul, K. D. (2003). Short-term effects of telephone therapy for breast cancer patients. *Health Psychology, 22,* 310-315.

Saphire-Bernstein, S., Way, B. M., Kim, H. S., Sherman, D. K., & Taylor, S. E. (2011). Oxytocin receptor gene (OXTR) is related to psychological resources. *Proceedings of the National Academy of Sciences, 108,* 15118-15122.

Sarason, I. G., Johnson, J. H., & Siegel, J. M. (1978). Assessing the impact of life changes: Development of the Life Experiences Survey. *Journal of Consulting and Clinical Psychology, 46,* 932-946.

Sarason, I. G., Sarason, B. R., Pierce, G. R., Shearin, E. N., & Sayers, M. H. (1991). A social learning approach to increasing blood donations. *Journal of Applied Social Psychology, 21,* 896-918.

Sareen, J., Cox, B. J., Stein, M. B., Afifi, T. O., Fleet, C., & Asmundson, G. J. G. (2007). Physical and mental comorbidity, disability, and suicidal behavior associated with posttraumatic stress disorder in a large community sample. *Psychosomatic Medicine, 69,* 242-248.

Sargent, J. D., & Heatherton, T. F. (2009). Comparison of trends for adolescent smoking and smoking in movies, 1990-2007. *Journal of the American Medical Association, 301,* 2211-2213.

Sarkar, U., Ali, S., & Whooley, M. A. (2009). Self-efficacy as a marker of cardiac function and predictor of heart failure hospitalization and mortality in patients with stable coronary heart disease: Findings from the heart and soul study. *Health Psychology, 28,* 166-173.

Sausen, K. P., Lovallo, W. R., Pincomb, G. A., & Wilson, M. F. (1992). Cardiovascular responses to occupational stress in male medical students: A paradigm for ambulatory monitoring studies. *Health Psychology, 11,* 55-60.

Savelieva, K., Pulkki-Råback, L., Jokela, M., Kubzansky, L. D., Elovainio, M., Mikkilä, V., . . . Keltikangas-Järvinen, L. (2017). Intergenerational transmission of socioeconomic position and ideal cardiovascular health: 32-year follow-up study. *Health Psychology, 36,* 270-279.

Saxbe, D. E., Margolin, G., Spies Shapiro, L., Ramos, M., Rodriguez, A., & Iturralde, E. (2014). Relative influences: Patterns of HPA axis concordance during triadic family interaction. *Health Psychology, 33,* 273-281.

Saxbe, D. E., Repetti, R. L., & Nishina, A. (2008). Marital satisfaction, recovery from work, and diurnal cortisone among men and women. *Health Psychology, 27,* 15-25.

Saxby, B. K., Harrington, F., McKeith, I. G., Wesnes, K., & Ford, G. A. (2003). Effects of hypertension in attention, memory and executive function in older adults. *Health Psychology, 22,* 587-591.

Sbarra, D. A. (2009). Marriage protects men from clinically meaningful elevations in C-reactive protein: Results from the national social life, health, and aging project (NSHAP). *Psychosomatic Medicine, 71,* 828-835.

Sbarra, D. A., Boals, A., Mason, A. E., Larson, G. M., & Mehl, M. R. (2013). Expressive writing can impede emotional recovery following marital separation. *Clinical Psychological Science, 1,* 120-134.

Sbarra, D. A., & Nietert, P. J. (2009). Divorce and death: Forty years of the Charleston heart study. *Psychological Science, 20,* 107-113.

Scanlan, J. M., Vitaliano, P. P., Zhang, J., Savage, M., & Ochs, H. D. (2001). Lymphocyte proliferation is associated with gender, caregiving, and psychosocial variables in older adults. *Journal of Behavioral Medicine, 24,* 537-559.

Schaa, K. L., Roter, D. L., Biesecker, B. B., Cooper, L. A., & Erby, L. H. (2015). Genetic counselors' implicit racial attitudes and their relationship to communication. *Health Psychology, 34,* 111-119.

Schaffer, J. A., Edmondson, D., Wasson, L. T., Falzon, L., Homma, K., Ezeokoli, N., & Davidson, K. W. (2014). Vitamin D supplementation for depressive symptoms: A systematic review and meta-analysis of randomized controlled trials. *Psychosomatic Medicine, 76,* 190-196.

Schechtman, K. B., Ory, M. G., & the FICSIT Group. (2001). The effects of exercise on the quality of life of frail older adults: A preplanned meta-analysis of the FICSIT trials. *Annals of Behavioral Medicine, 23,* 186-197.

Scheier, M. F., & Carver, C. S. (2018). Dispositional optimism and physical health: A long look back, a quick look forward. *American Psychologist, 73,* 1082-1094.

Scheier, M. F., Carver, C. S., & Bridges, M. W. (1994). Distinguishing optimism from neuroticism (and trait anxiety, self-mastery, and self-esteem): A reevaluation of the Life Orientation Test. *Journal of Personality and Social Psychology, 67,* 1063-1078.

Scheier, M. F., Weintraub, J. K., & Carver, C. S. (1986). Coping with stress: Divergent strategies of optimists and pessimists. *Journal of Personality and Social Psychology, 51,* 1257-1264.

Schernhammer, E. (2005). Taking their own lives—The high rate of physician suicide. *The New England Journal of Medicine, 352,* 2473-2476.

Scheufele, P. M. (2000). Effects of progressive relaxation and classical music on measurements of attention, relaxation, and stress responses. *Journal of Behavioral Medicine, 23,* 207-228.

Schins, A., Honig, A., Crijns, H., Baur, L., & Hamulyak, K. (2003). Increased coronary events in depressed cardiovascular patients: 5HT2A receptor as missing link? *Psychosomatic Medicine, 65,* 729-737.

Schirda, B., Nicholas, J. A., & Prakash, R. S. (2015). Examining trait mindfulness, emotion dysregulation, and quality of life in multiple sclerosis. *Health Psychology, 34,* 1107-1115.

Schlotz, W., Hellhammer, J., Schulz, P., & Stone, A. A. (2004). Perceived work overload and chronic worrying predict weekend-weekday differences in the cortisol awakening response. *Psychosomatic Medicine, 66,* 207-214.

Schnall, E., Wassertheil-Smoller, S., Swencionis, C., Zemon, V., Tinker, L., O'Sullivan, M. J., . . . Goodwin, M. (2010). The relationship between religion and cardiovascular outcomes and all-cause mortality in the women's health initiative observational study. *Psychology and Health, 25,* 249-263.

Schneider, M. S., Friend, R., Whitaker, P., & Wadhwa, N. K. (1991). Fluid noncompliance and symptomatology in end-stage renal disease: Cognitive and emotional variables. *Health Psychology, 10,* 209-215.

Schneider, S., Moyer, A., Knapp-Oliver, S., Sohl, S., Cannella, D., & Targhetta, V. (2010). Pre-intervention distress moderated the efficacy of psychosocial treatment for cancer patients: A meta-analysis. *Journal of Behavioral Medicine, 33,* 1-14.

Schnurr, P. P., Friedman, M. J., Engel, C. C., Foa, E. B., Shea, M. T., Chow, B. K., . . . Bernardy, N. (2007). Cognitive behavioral therapy for posttraumatic stress disorder in women: A randomized controlled trial. *Journal of the American Medical Association, 297,* 820-830.

Schoenthaler, A. M., Butler, M., Chaplin, W., Tobin, J., & Ogedegbe, G. (2016). Predictors of changes in medication adherence in Blacks with hypertension: Moving beyond cross-sectional data. *Annals of Behavioral Medicine, 50,* 642-652.

Schöllgen, I., Huxhold, O., Schüz, B., & Tesch-Römer, C. (2011). Resources for health: Differential effects of optimistic self-beliefs and social support according to socioeconomic status. *Health Psychology, 30,* 326-335.

Schreier, H. M., & Chen, E. (2012). Socioeconomic status and health of youth: A multilevel, multidomain approach to conceptualizing pathways. *Psychological Bulletin, 139,* 606-654.

Schreier, H. M. C., & Chen, E. (2010). Longitudinal relationships between family routines and biological profiles among youth with asthma. *Health Psychology, 29,* 82-90.

Schreier, H. M. C., Roy, L. B., Frimer, L. T., & Chen, E. (2014). Family chaos and adolescent inflammatory profiles: The moderating role of socioeconomic status. *Psychosomatic Medicine, 76,* 460-467.

Schrepf, A., Markon, K., & Lutgendorf, S. K. (2014). From childhood to trauma to elevated C-reactive protein in adulthood: The role of anxiety and emotional eating. *Psychosomatic Medicine, 76,* 327-336.

Schrimshaw, E. W. (2003). Relationship-specific unsupportive social interactions and depressive symptoms among women living with HIV/AIDS: Direct and moderating effects. *Journal of Behavioral Medicine, 26,* 297-313.

Schofield, P. E., Stockler, M. R., Zannino, D., Tebbutt, N. C., Price, T. J., Simes, R. J., . . . Jefford, M. (2016). Hope, optimism and survival in a randomised trial of chemotherapy for metastatic colorectal cancer. *Supportive Care in Cancer, 24,* 401-408.

Schulz, R., & Beach, S. R. (1999). Caregiving as a risk factor for mortality: The caregiver health effects study. *Journal of the American Medical Association, 282,* 2215-2219.

Schulz, R., Bookwala, J., Knapp, J. E., Scheier, M., & Williamson, G. (1996). Pessimism, age, and cancer mortality. *Psychology and Aging, 11,* 304-309.

Schulz, R., & Decker, S. (1985). Long-term adjustment to physical disability: The role of social support, perceived control, and self-blame. *Journal of Personality and Social Psychology, 48,* 1162-1172.

Schüz, B., Papadakis, T., & Ferguson, S. G. (2018). Situation-specific social norms as mediators of social influence on snacking. *Health Psychology, 37,* 153-159.

Schüz, N., Schüz, B., & Eid, M. (2013). When risk communication backfires: Randomized controlled trial on self-affirmation and reactance to personalized risk feedback in high-risk individuals. *Health Psychology, 32,* 561-570.

Schvey, N. A., Puhl, R. M., & Brownell, K. D. (2014). The stress of stigma: Exploring the effect of weight stigma on cortisol reactivity. *Psychosomatic Medicine, 76,* 156-162.

Schwebel, D. C., McClure, L. A., & Severson, J. (2014). Teaching children to cross streets safely: A randomized, controlled trial. *Health Psychology, 33,* 628-638.

Schwartz, M. B., & Brownell, K. D. (1995). Matching individuals to weight loss treatments: A survey of obesity experts. *Journal of Consulting and Clinical Psychology, 63,* 149-153.

Schwartz, M. D., Taylor, K. L., & Willard, K. S. (2003). Prospective association between distress and mammography utilization among women with a family history of breast cancer. *Journal of Behavioral Medicine, 26,* 105-117.

Scott-Sheldon, L. A. J., Fielder, R. L., & Carey, M. P. (2010). Sexual risk reduction interventions for patients attending sexually transmitted disease clinics in the United States: A meta-analytic review, 1986 to early 2009. *Annals of Behavioral Medicine, 40,* 191-204.

Scott-Sheldon, L. A. J., Kalichman, S. C., Carey, M. P., & Fielder, R. L. (2008). Stress management interventions for HIV+ adults: A meta-analysis of randomized controlled trials, 1989-2006. *Health Psychology, 27,* 129-139.

Scrimshaw, S. M., Engle, P. L., & Zambrana, R. E. (1983, August). *Prenatal anxiety and birth outcome in U.S. Latinas: Implications for psychosocial interventions.* Paper presented at the annual meeting of the American Psychological Association, Anaheim, CA.

Sears, S. R., & Stanton, A. L. (2001). Physician-assisted dying: Review of issues and roles for health psychologists. *Health Psychology, 20,* 302-310.

Seeman, M., Seeman, A. Z., & Budros, A. (1988). Powerlessness, work, and community: A longitudinal study of alienation and alcohol use. *Journal of Health and Social Behavior, 29,* 185-198.

Seeman, T. E., Berkman, L. F., Gulanski, B. I., Robbins, R. J., Greenspan, S. L., Charpentier, P. A., & Rowe, J. W. (1995). Self-esteem and neuroendocrine response to challenge: MacArthur studies of successful aging. *Journal of Psychosomatic Research, 39,* 69-84.

Seeman, T. E., Dubin, L. F., & Seeman, M. (2003). Religiosity/spirituality and health: A critical review of the evidence for biological pathways. *American Psychologist, 58,* 53-63.

Seeman, T. E., Singer, B., Horwitz, R., & McEwen, B. S. (1997). The price of adaptation—Allostatic load and its health consequences: MacArthur studies of successful aging. *Archives of Internal Medicine, 157,* 2259-2268.

Segan, C. J., Borland, R., & Greenwood, K. M. (2004). What is the right thing at the right time? Interactions between stages and processes of change among smokers who make a quit attempt. *Health Psychology, 23,* 86–93.

Segerstrom, S. C. (2001). Optimism, goal conflict, and stressor-related immune change. *Journal of Behavioral Medicine, 24,* 441–46*l*.

Segerstrom, S. C. (2006a). How does optimism suppress immunity? Evaluation of three affective pathways. *Health Psychology, 25,* 653–657.

Segerstrom, S. C. (2006b). Optimism and resources: Effects on each other and on health over 10 years. *Journal of Research in Personality, 41,* 772–786.

Segerstrom, S. C. (2010). Resources, stress, and immunity: An ecological perspective on human psychoneuroimmunology. *Annals of Behavioral Medicine, 40,* 114–125.

Segerstrom, S. C., Al-Attar, A., & Lutz, C. T. (2012). Psychosocial resources, aging, and natural killer cell terminal maturity. *Psychology and Aging, 27,* 892–902.

Segerstrom, S. C., Castañeda, J. O., & Spencer, T. E. (2003). Optimism effects on cellular immunity: Testing the affective and persistence models. *Personality and Individual Differences, 35,* 1615–1624.

Segerstrom, S. C., & Miller, G. E. (2004). Psychological stress and the human immune system: A meta-analytic study of 30 years of inquiry. *Psychological Bulletin, 130,* 601–630.

Segerstrom, S. C., & Sephton, S. E. (2010). Optimistic expectancies and cell-mediated immunity: The role of positive affect. *Psychological Science, 21,* 448–455.

Segerstrom, S. C., Taylor, S. E., Kemeny, M. E., & Fahey, J. L. (1998). Optimism is associated with mood, coping, and immune change in response to stress. *Journal of Personality and Social Psychology, 74,* 1646–1655.

Segerstrom, S. C., Taylor, S. E., Kemeny, M. E., Reed, G. M., & Visscher, B. R. (1996). Causal attributions predict rate of immune decline in HIV-seropositive gay men. *Health Psychology, 15,* 485–493.

Segrin, C., Badger, T. A., & Harrington, J. (2012). Interdependent psychological quality of life in dyads adjusting to prostate cancer. *Health Psychology, 31,* 70–79.

Seidman, D. F., Westmaas, J. L., Goldband, S., Rabius, V., Katkin, E. S., Pike, K. J., . . . Sloan, R. P. (2010). Randomized controlled trial of an interactive Internet smoking cessation program with long-term follow-up. *Annals of Behavioral Medicine, 39,* 48–60.

Selby, A., & Smith-Osborne, A. (2013). A systematic review of effectiveness of complementary and adjunct therapies and interventions involving equines. *Health Psychology, 32,* 418–432.

Selcuk, E., & Ong, A. D. (2013). Perceived partner responsiveness moderates the association between received emotional support and all-cause mortality. *Health Psychology, 32,* 231–235.

Self, C. A., & Rogers, R. W. (1990). Coping with threats to health: Effects of persuasive appeals on depressed, normal, and antisocial personalities. *Journal of Behavioral Medicine, 13,* 343–358.

Selye, H. (1956). *The stress of life.* New York: McGraw-Hill.

Selye, H. (1976). *Stress in health and disease.* Woburn, MA: Butterworth.

Seneff, M. G., Wagner, D. P., Wagner, R. P., Zimmerman, J. E., & Knaus, W. A. (1995). Hospital and 1-year survival of patients admitted to intensive care units with acute exacerbation of chronic obstructive pulmonary disease. *Journal of the American Medical Association, 274,* 1852–1857.

Sénémeaud, C., Georget, P., Guéguen, N., Callé, N., Plainfossé, C., Touati, C., & Mange, J. (2014). Labeling of previous donation to encourage subsequent donation among experienced blood donors. *Health Psychology, 33,* 656–659.

Sengupta, M., Bercovitz, A., & Harris-Kojetin, L. D. (2010). Prevalence and management of pain, by race and dementia among nursing home residents: United States, 2004. *NCHS Data Brief, 30,* 1–8.

Serbic, D., Pincus, T., Fife-Schaw, C., & Dawson, H. (2016). Diagnostic uncertainty, guilt, mood, and disability in back pain. *Health Psychology, 35,* 50–59.

Serido, J., Almeida, D. M., & Wethington, E. (2004). Chronic stress and daily hassles: Unique and interactive relationships with psychological distress. *Journal of Health and Social Behavior, 45,* 17–33.

Sevick, M. A., Stone, R. A., Zickmund, S., Wang, Y., Korytkowski, M., & Burke, L. E. (2010). Factors associated with probability of personal digital assistant-based dietary self-monitoring in those with type 2 diabetes. *Journal of Behavioral Medicine, 33,* 315–325.

SeyedAlinaghi, S., Jam, S., Foroughi, M., Imani, A., Mohraz, M., Djavid, G. E., & Black, D. S. (2012). Randomized controlled trial of mindfulness-based stress reduction delivered to human immunodeficiency virus-positive patients in Iran: Effects on CD4+ T lymphocyte count and medical and psychological symptoms. *Psychosomatic Medicine, 74,* 620–627.

Shadel, W. G., Martino, S. C., Setodji, C., Cervone, D., Witkiewitz, K., Beckjord, E. B., . . . Shih, R. (2011). Lapse-induced surges in craving influence relapse in adult smokers: An experimental investigation. *Health Psychology, 30,* 588–596.

Shadel, W. G., & Mermelstein, R. J. (1996). Individual differences in self-concept among smokers attempting to quit: Validation and predictive utility of measures of the smoker self-concept and abstainer self-concept. *Annals of Behavioral Medicine, 18,* 151–156.

Shadel, W. G., Niaura, R., & Abrams, D. B. (2004). Who am I? The role of self-conflict in adolescents' responses to cigarette advertising. *Journal of Behavioral Medicine, 27,* 463–475.

Shadish, W. R. (2010). Introduction: The perils of science in the world of policy and practice. *Health Psychology, 29,* 105–106.

Shaffer, V. A., Focella, E. S., Hathaway, A., Scherer, L. D., & Zikmund-Fisher, B. J. (2018). On the usefulness of narratives: An interdisciplinary review and theoretical model. *Annals of Behavioral Medicine, 52,* 429–442.

Shaffer, W. J., Duszynski, K. R., & Thomas, C. B. (1982). Family attitudes in youth as a possible precursor of cancer among physicians: A search for explanatory mechanisms. *Journal of Behavioral Medicine, 15,* 143–164.

Shankar, A., Hamer, M., McMunn, A., & Steptoe, A. (2013). Social isolation and loneliness: Relationships with cognitive function during 4 years of follow-up in the English Longitudinal Study of Ageing. *Psychosomatic Medicine, 75,* 161–170.

Shankar, A., McMunn, A., Banks, J., & Steptoe, A. (2011). Loneliness, social isolation, and behavioral and biological health indicators in older adults. *Health Psychology, 30,* 377–385.

Shapiro, A. K. (1960). A contribution to a history of the placebo effect. *Behavioral Science, 5,* 109–135.

Shapiro, A. K. (1964). Factors contributing to the placebo effect: Their implications for psychotherapy. *American Journal of Psychotherapy, 18,* 73–88.

Shapiro, D., Hui, K. K., Oakley, M. E., Pasic, J., & Jamner, L. D. (1997). Reduction in drug requirements for hypertension by means of a cognitive-behavioral intervention. *American Journal of Hypertension, 10,* 9–17.

Sharman, S. J., Garry, M., Jacobson, J. A., Loftus, E. F., & Ditto, P. H. (2008). False memories for end-of-life decisions. *Health Psychology, 27,* 291–296.

Sharpe, T. R., Smith, M. C., & Barbre, A. R. (1985). Medicine use among the rural elderly. *Journal of Health and Social Behavior, 26,* 113–127.

Sheeran, P., & Conner, M. (2017). Improving the translation of intentions into health actions: The role of motivational coherence. *Health Psychology, 36,* 1065–1073.

Sheeran, P., Gollwitzer, P. M., & Bargh, J. A. (2013). Nonconscious processes and health. *Health Psychology, 32,* 460–473.

Shelby, R. A., Somers, T. J., Keefe, F. J., Silva, S. G., McKee, D. C., She, L., . . . Johnson, P. (2009). Pain catastrophizing in patients with noncardiac chest pain: Relationships with pain, anxiety, and disability. *Psychosomatic Medicine, 71,* 861–868.

Shelton, J. L., & Levy, R. L. (1981). *Behavioral assignments and treatment compliance: A handbook of clinical strategies.* Champaign, IL: Research Press.

Shen, B. J., Eisenberg, S. A., Maeda, U., Farrell, K. A., Schwarz, E. R., Penedo, F. J., . . . Mallon, S. (2011). Depression and anxiety predict decline in physical health functioning in patients with heart failure. *Annals of Behavioral Medicine, 41,* 373–382.

Shen, B. J., & Maeda, U. (2018). Psychosocial predictors of self-reported medical adherence in patients with heart failure over 6 months: An examination of the influences of depression, self-efficacy, social support, and their changes. *Annals of Behavioral Medicine, 52,* 613–619.

Sherman, A. C., Pennington, J., Simonton, S., Latif, U., Arent, L., & Farley, H. (2008). Determinants of participation in cancer support groups: The role of health beliefs. *International Journal of Behavioral Medicine, 15,* 92–100.

Sherman, A. C., Plante, T. G., Simonton, S., Latif, U., & Anaissie, E. J. (2009). A prospective study of religious coping among patients undergoing autologous stem cell transplantation. *Journal of Behavioral Medicine, 32,* 118–128.

Sherman, D. K., Bunyan, D. P., Creswell, J. D., & Jaremka, L. M. (2009). Psychological vulnerability and stress: The effects of self-affirmation on sympathetic nervous system responses to naturalistic stressors. *Health Psychology, 28,* 554–562.

Sherman, D. K., & Cohen, G. L. (2006). The psychology of self-defense: Self-affirmation theory. In M. P. Zanna (Ed.), *Advances in experimental social psychology* (Vol. 38, pp. 183–242). San Diego, CA: Academic Press.

Sherman, J. J., LeResche, L., Hanson Huggins, K., Mancl, L. A., Sage, J. C., & Dworkin, S. F. (2004). The relationship of somatization and depression to experimental pain response in women with temporomandibular disorders. *Psychosomatic Medicine, 66,* 852–860.

Shiels, M. S., Chernyavskiy, P., Anderson, W. F., Best, A. F., Haozous, E. A., Hartge, P., . . . de Gonzalez, A. B. (2017). Trends in premature mortality in the USA by sex, race, and ethnicity from 1999 to 2014: An analysis of death certificate data. *The Lancet, 389,* 1043–1054.

Shiffman, S., Fischer, L. A., Paty, J. A., Gnys, M., Hickcox, M., & Kassel, J. D. (1994). Drinking and smoking: A field study of their association. *Annals of Behavioral Medicine, 16,* 203–209.

Shiffman, S., Hickcox, M., Paty, J. A., Gnys, M., Kassel, J. D., & Richards, T. J. (1996). Progression from a smoking lapse to relapse: Prediction from abstinence violation effects, nicotine dependence, and lapse characteristics. *Journal of Consulting and Clinical Psychology, 64,* 993–1002.

Shifren, K., Park, D. C., Bennett, J. M., & Morrell, R. W. (1999). Do cognitive processes predict mental health in individuals with rheumatoid arthritis? *Journal of Behavioral Medicine, 22,* 529–547.

Shiloh, S., Drori, E., Orr-Urtreger, A., & Friedman, E. (2009). Being "at-risk" for developing cancer: Cognitive representations and psychological outcomes. *Journal of Behavioral Medicine, 32,* 197–208.

Shiota, M. N., & Levenson, R. W. (2012). Turn down the volume or change the channel? Emotional effects of detached versus positive reappraisal. *Journal of Personality and Social Psychology, 103,* 416–429.

Shipley, B. A., Weiss, A., Der, G., Taylor, M. D., & Deary, I. J. (2007). Neuroticism, extraversion, and mortality in the UK health and lifestyle survey: A 21-year prospective cohort study. *Psychosomatic Medicine, 69,* 923–931.

Shirom, A., Toker, S., Alkaly, Y., Jacobson, O., & Balicer, R. (2011). Work-based predictors of mortality: A 20-year follow-up of healthy employees. *Health Psychology, 30,* 268–275.

Shively, C. A., Register, T. C., Adams, M. R., Golden, D. L., Willard, S. L., & Clarkson, T. B. (2008). Depressive behavior and coronary artery atherogenesis in adult female cynomolgus monkeys. *Psychosomatic Medicine, 70,* 637–645.

Shnabel, N., Purdie-Vaughns, V., Cook, J. E., Garcia, J., & Cohen, G. L. (2013). Demystifying values-affirmation interventions: Writing about social belonging is a key to buffering against identity threat. *Personality and Social Psychology Bulletin, 39,* 663–676.

Shomaker, L. B., Kelly, N. R., Pickworth, C. K., Cassidy, O. L., Radin, R. M., Shank, L. M., . . . Demidowich, A. P. (2016). A randomized controlled trial to prevent depression and ameliorate insulin resistance in adolescent girls at risk for type 2 diabetes. *Annals of Behavioral Medicine, 50,* 762–774.

Sidney, S., Friedman, G. D., & Siegelaub, A. B. (1987). Thinness and mortality. *American Journal of Public Health, 77,* 317–322.

Sieber, W. J., Rodin, J., Larson, L., Ortega, S., Cummings, N., Levy, S., . . . Herberman, R. (1992). Modulation of human natural killer cell activity by exposure to uncontrollable stress. *Brain, Behavior, and Immunity, 6,* 1–16.

Siegel, J. T., Navarro, M. A., Tan, C. N., & Hyde, M. K. (2014). Attitude-behavior consistency, the principle of compatibility, and organ donation: A classic innovation. *Health Psychology, 33,* 1084–1091.

Siegel, R. L., Miller, K. D., & Jemal, A. (2019). Cancer statistics, 2019. *CA Cancer Journal for Clinicians, 69,* 7–34.

Siegler, I. C., Costa, P. T., Brummett, B. H., Helms, M. J., Barefoot, J. C., Williams, R. B., . . . Rimer, B. K. (2003). Patterns of change in hostility from college to midlife in the UNC alumni heart study predict high-risk status. *Psychosomatic Medicine, 65,* 738–745.

Siegler, I. C., Peterson, B. L., Barefoot, J. C., & Williams, R. B. (1992). Hostility during late adolescence predicts coronary risk factors at mid-life. *American Journal of Epidemiology, 136,* 146–154.

Siegman, A. W., & Snow, S. C. (1997). The outward expression of anger, the inward experience of anger, and CVR: The role of vocal expression. *Journal of Behavioral Medicine, 20,* 29–46.

Siegman, A. W., Townsend, S. T., Civelek, A. C., & Blumenthal, R. S. (2000). Antagonistic behavior, dominance, hostility, and coronary heart disease. *Psychosomatic Medicine, 62,* 248–257.

Siegrist, J., Peter, R., Runge, A., Cremer, P., & Seidel, D. (1990). Low status control, high effort at work, and ischemic heart disease: Prospective evidence from blue-collar men. *Social Science and Medicine, 31,* 1127–1134.

Sieverding, M., Matterne, U., & Ciccarello, L. (2010). What role do social norms play in the context of men's cancer screening intentions and behavior? Application of an extended theory of planned behavior. *Health Psychology, 29,* 72–81.

Sikkema, K. J., Hansen, N. B., Ghebremichael, M., Kochman, A., Tarakeshwar, N., Meade, C. S., & Zhang, H. (2006). A randomized controlled trial of a coping group intervention for adults with HIV who are AIDS bereaved: Longitudinal effects on grief. *Health Psychology, 25,* 563–570.

Silver, E. J., Bauman, L. J., & Ireys, H. T. (1995). Relationships of self-esteem and efficacy to psychological distress in mothers of children with chronic physical illnesses. *Health Psychology, 14,* 333–340.

Silver, R. C., Holman, E. A., McIntosh, D. N., Poulin, M., & Gil-Rivas, V. (2002). Nationwide longitudinal study of psychological responses to September 11. *Journal of the American Medical Association, 288,* 1235–1244.

Simon, N. (2003). Can you hear me now? *Time.*

Simon, R. (2012, May 7). U.S. traffic deaths at record low; economy may be a factor. *The Los Angeles Times.* Retrieved August 8, 2012, from http://articles. latimes.com/2012/may/07/nation/la-na-nn-traffic-deaths-20120507

Simon, R. W. (1992). Parental role strains, salience of parental identity and gender differences in psychological distress. *Journal of Health and Social Behavior, 33,* 25–35.

Simon, R. W. (1998). Assessing sex differences in vulnerability among employed parents: The importance of marital status. *Journal of Health and Social Behavior, 39,* 38–54.

Simoni, J. M., Frick, P. A., & Huang, B. (2006). A longitudinal evaluation of a social support model of medication adherence among HIV-positive men and women on antiretroviral therapy. *Health Psychology, 25,* 74–81.

Simoni, J. M., & Ng, M. T. (2002). Abuse, health locus of control, and perceived health among HIV-positive women. *Health Psychology, 21,* 89–93.

Simons-Morton, B. G., Bingham, C. R., Falk, E. B., Li, K., Pradhan, A. K., Ouimet, M. C., & Shope, J. T. (2014). Experimental effects of injunctive norms on simulated risky driving among teenage males. *Health Psychology, 33,* 616–627.

Sin, N. L., Almeida, D. M., Crain, T. L., Kossek, E. E., Berkman, L. F., & Buxton, O. M. (2017). Bidirectional, temporal associations of sleep with positive events, affect, and stressors in daily life across a week. *Annals of Behavioral Medicine, 51,* 402–415.

Sin, N. L., Graham-Engeland, J. E., Ong, A. D., & Almeida, D. M. (2015). Affective reactivity to daily stressors is associated with elevated inflammation. *Health Psychology, 34,* 1154–1165.

Sin, N. L., Kumar, A. D., Gehi, A. K., & Whooley, M. A. (2016). Direction of association between depressive symptoms and lifestyle behaviors in patients with coronary heart disease: The Heart and Soul Study. *Annals of Behavioral Medicine, 50,* 523–532.

Sinha, R., & Jastreboff, A. M. (2013). Stress as a common risk factor for obesity and addiction. *Biological Psychiatry, 73,* 827–835.

Singer, B. H. (Ed.). (2000). *Future directions for behavioral and social sciences research at the National Institutes of Health.* Washington, DC: National Academy of Sciences Press.

Singh-Manoux, A., Richards, M., & Marmot, M. (2003). Leisure activities and cognitive function in middle age: Evidence from the Whitehall II study. *Journal of Epidemiology and Community Health, 57,* 907–913.

Sinha, R., Fisch, G., Teague, B., Tamborlane, W. V., Banyas, B., Allen, K., . . . Caprio, S. (2002). Prevalence of impaired glucose tolerance among children and adolescents with marked obesity. *The New England Journal of Medicine, 346,* 802–810.

Sirota, M., Round, T., Samaranayaka, S., & Kostopoulou, O. (2017). Expectations for antibiotics increase their prescribing: Causal evidence about localized impact. *Health Psychology, 36,* 402–409.

Skapinakis, P., Lewis, G., & Mavreas, V. (2004). Temporal relations between unexplained fatigue and depression: Longitudinal data from an international study in primary care. *Psychosomatic Medicine, 66,* 330–335.

Slatcher, R. B., & Robles, T. F. (2012). Preschoolers' everyday conflict at home and diurnal cortisol patterns. *Health Psychology, 31,* 834–838.

Slatcher, R. B., Selcuk, E., & Ong, A. D. (2015). Perceived partner responsiveness predicts diurnal cortisol profiles 10 years later. *Psychological Science, 26,* 972–982.

Slater, R., Cantarella, A., Gallella, S., Worley, A., Boyd, S., Meek, J., & Fitzgerald, M. (2006). Cortical pain responses in human infants. *Journal of Neuroscience, 26,* 3662–3666.

Sledjeski, E. M., Speisman, B., & Dierker, L. C. (2008). Does number of lifetime traumas explain the relationship between PTSD and chronic medical conditions? Answers from the national comorbidity survey-replication (NCS-R). *Journal of Behavioral Medicine, 31,* 341–349.

Slesnick, N., & Kang, M. J. (2008). The impact of an integrated treatment on HIV risk behavior among homeless youth: A randomized controlled trial. *Journal of Behavioral Medicine, 31,* 45–59.

Sloan, R. P., Schwarz, E., McKinley, P. S., Weinstein, M., Love, G., Ryff, C., . . . Seeman, T. (2017). Vagally-mediated heart rate variability and indices of well-being: Results of a nationally representative study. *Health Psychology, 36*(1), 73–81.

Slovinec, D., Monika, E., Pelletier, L. G., Reid, R. D., & Huta, V. (2014). The roles of self-efficacy and motivation in the prediction of short- and long-term adherence to exercise among patients with coronary heart disease. *Health Psychology, 33,* 1344–1353.

Smalec, J. L., & Klingle, R. S. (2000). Bulimia interventions via interpersonal influence: The role of threat and efficacy in persuading bulimics to seek help. *Journal of Behavioral Medicine, 23,* 37–57.

Smart Richman, L., Pek, J., Pascoe, E., & Bauer, D. J. (2010). The effects of perceived discrimination on ambulatory blood pressure and affective responses to interpersonal stress modeled over 24 hours. *Health Psychology, 29,* 403–411.

Smith, A. M., Loving, T. J., Crockett, E. E., & Campbell, L. (2009). What's closeness got to do with it? Men's and women's cortisol responses when providing and receiving support. *Psychosomatic Medicine, 71,* 843–851.

Smith, B. (2013). Disability, sport and men's narratives of health: A qualitative study. *Health Psychology, 32,* 110–119.

Smith, B. W., & Zautra, A. J. (2002). The role of personality in exposure and reactivity to interpersonal stress in relation to arthritis disease activity and negative effects in women. *Health Psychology, 21,* 81–88.

Smith, D. G., & Robbins, T. W. (2013). The neurobiological underpinnings of obesity and binge eating: A rationale for adopting the food addiction model. *Biological Psychiatry, 73,* 804–810.

Smith, J. A., Lumley, M. A., & Longo, D. J. (2002). Contrasting emotional approach coping with passive coping for chronic myofascial pain. *Annals of Behavioral Medicine, 24,* 326–335.

Smith, K. B., & Pukall, C. F. (2009). An evidence-based review of Yoga as a complementary intervention for patients with cancer. *Psycho-Oncology, 18,* 465–475.

Smith, P., Frank, J., Bondy, S., & Mustard, C. (2008). Do changes in job control predict differences in health status? Results from a longitudinal national survey of Canadians. *Psychosomatic Medicine,* 85–91.

Smith, T. W., & Baucom, B. R. W. (2017). Intimate relationships, individual adjustment, and coronary heart disease: Implications of overlapping associations in psychosocial risk. *American Psychologist, 72,* 578–589.

Smith, T. W., Eagle, D. E., & Proeschold-Bell, R. J. (2017). Prospective associations between depressive symptoms and the metabolic syndrome: The Spirited Life Study of Methodist pastors in North Carolina. *Annals of Behavioral Medicine, 51,* 610–619.

Smith, T. W., & Gallo, L. C. (1999). Hostility and cardiovascular reactivity during marital interaction. *Psychosomatic Medicine, 61,* 436–445.

Smith, T. W., & Ruiz, J. M. (2002). Psychosocial influences on the development and course of coronary heart disease: Current status and implications for research and practice. *Journal of Consulting and Clinical Psychology, 70,* 548–568.

Smith, T. W., Ruiz, J. M., & Uchino, B. N. (2000). Vigilance, active coping, and cardiovascular reactivity during social interaction in young men. *Health Psychology, 19,* 382–392.

Smith, T. W., Ruiz, J. M., & Uchino, B. N. (2004). Mental activation of supportive ties, hostility, and cardiovascular reactivity to laboratory stress in young men and women. *Health Psychology, 23,* 476–485.

Smith, T. W., Turner, C. W., Ford, M. H., Hunt, S. C., Barlow, G. K., Stults, B. M., & Williams, R. R. (1987). Blood pressure reactivity in adult male twins. *Health Psychology, 6,* 209–220.

Sneed, R. S., & Cohen, S. (2014). Negative social interactions and incident hypertension among older adults. *Health Psychology, 33,* 554–565.

Sneed, R. S., Cohen, S., Turner, R. B., & Doyle, W. J. (2012). Parenthood and host resistance to the common cold. *Psychosomatic Medicine, 74,* 567–573.

Sobel, H. (1981). Toward a behavioral thanatology in clinical care. In H. Sobel (Ed.), *Behavioral therapy in terminal care: A humanistic approach* (pp. 3–38). Cambridge, MA: Ballinger.

Sone, T., Nakaya, N., Ohmori, K., Shimazu, T., Higashiguchi, M., Kakizaki, M., . . . Tsuji, I. (2008). Sense of life worth (ikigai) and mortality in Japan: Ohsaki study. *Psychosomatic Medicine, 70,* 709–715.

Sonnenburg, J., & Sonnenburg, E. (2015). *The good gut.* New York: Penguin.

Sood, E. D., Pendley, J. S., Delamater, A. M., Rohan, J. M., Pulgaron, E. R., & Drotar, D. (2012). Mother–father informant discrepancies regarding diabetes management: Associations with diabetes-specific family conflict and glycemic control. *Health Psychology, 31,* 571–579.

Sorkin, D. H., Mavandadi, S., Rook, K. S., Biegler, K. A., Kilgore, D., Dow, E., & Ngo-Metzger, Q. (2014). Dyadic collaboration in shared health behavior change: The effects of a randomized trial to test a lifestyle intervention for high-risk Latinas. *Health Psychology, 33,* 566–575.

Spanos, S., Vartanian, L. R., Herman, C. P., & Polivy, J. (2014). Failure to report social influences on food intake: Lack of awareness or motivated denial? *Health Psychology, 33,* 1487–1494.

Sorkin, D., Rook, K. S., & Lu, J. L. (2002). Loneliness, lack of emotional support, lack of companionship, and the likelihood of having a heart condition in an elderly sample. *Annals of Behavioral Medicine, 24,* 290–298.

Speca, M., Carlson, L. E., Goodey, E., & Angen, M. (2000). A randomized, wait-list controlled clinical trial: The effect of a mindfulness meditation-based stress reduction program on mood and symptoms of stress in cancer outpatients. *Psychosomatic Medicine, 62,* 613–622.

Spina, M., Arndt, J., Landau, M. J., & Cameron, L. D. (2018). Enhancing health message framing with metaphor and cultural values: Impact on Latinas' cervical cancer screening. *Annals of Behavioral Medicine, 52,* 106–115.

Spinetta, J. J. (1974). The dying child's awareness of death: A review. *Psychological Bulletin, 81,* 256–260.

Spinetta, J. J. (1982). Behavioral and psychological research in childhood cancer: An overview. *Cancer, 50* (Suppl.), 1939–1943.

Spitzer, R. L., Yanovski, S., Wadden, T., Wing, R., Marcus, M. D., Stunkard, A., . . . Horne, R. L. (1993). Binge eating disorder: Its further validation in a multisite study. *International Journal of Eating Disorders, 13,* 137–153.

Springer, K. W., & Mouzon, D. M. (2011). "Macho men" and preventive health care: Implications for older men in different social classes. *Journal of Health and Social Behavior, 52,* 212–227.

Srinivasan, K., & Joseph, W. (2004). A study of lifetime prevalence of anxiety and depressive disorders in patients presenting with chest pain to emergency medicine. *General Hospital Psychiatry, 26,* 470–474.

Stadler, G., Oettingen, G., & Gollwitzer, P. M. (2010). Intervention effects of information and self-regulation on eating fruits and vegetables over two years. *Health Psychology, 29,* 274–283.

Stafford, L., Jackson, H. J., & Berk, M. (2008). Illness beliefs about heart disease and adherence to secondary prevention regimens. *Psychosomatic Medicine, 70,* 942–948.

Stagl, J. M., Antoni, M. H., Lechner, S. C., Bouchard, L. C., Blomberg, B. B., Gluck, S., & Charles, S. (2015). Randomized controlled trial of cognitive behavioral stress management in breast cancer: A brief report of effects on 5-year depressive symptoms. *Health Psychology, 34,* 175–180.

Stagl, J. M., Bouchard, L. C., Lechner, S. C., Blomberg, B. B., Gudenkauf, L. M., Jutagir, D. R., . . . Antoni, M. H. (2015). Long-term psychological benefits of cognitive–behavioral stress management for women with breast cancer: 11-year follow-up of a randomized controlled trial. *Cancer, 121,* 1873–1881.

Stall, R., & Biernacki, P. (1986). Spontaneous remission from the problematic use of substances: An inductive model derived from a comparative analysis of the alcohol, opiate, tobacco, and food/obesity literatures. *International Journal of the Addictions, 21,* 1–23.

Stampfer, M. J., Hu, F. B., Manson, J. E., Rimm, E. B., & Willett, W. C. (2000). Primary prevention of coronary heart disease in women through diet and lifestyle. *The New England Journal of Medicine, 343,* 16–22.

Stansfeld, S. A., Bosma, H., Hemingway, H., & Marmot, M. G. (1998). Psychosocial work characteristics and social support as predictors of SF-36 health functioning: The Whitehall II study. *Psychosomatic Medicine, 60,* 247–255.

Stansfeld, S. A., Fuhrer, R., Shipley, M. J., & Marmot, M. G. (2002). Psychological distress as a risk factor for coronary heart disease in the Whitehall II study. *International Journal of Epidemiology, 31,* 248–255.

Stanton, A. L. (1987). Determinants of adherence to medical regimens by hypertensive patients. *Journal of Behavioral Medicine, 10,* 377–394.

Stanton, A. L. (2010). Regulating emotions during stressful experiences: The adaptive utility of coping through emotional approach. In S. Folkman (Ed.), *Oxford handbook of stress, health and coping.* New York: Oxford University Press.

Stanton, A. L., Kirk, S. B., Cameron, C. L., & Danoff-Burg, S. (2000). Coping through emotional approach: Scale construction and validation. *Journal of Personality and Social Psychology, 78,* 1150–1169.

Stanton, A. L., & Low, C. A. (2012). Expressing emotions in stressful contexts: Benefits, moderators, and mechanisms. *Current Directions in Psychological Science, 21,* 124–128.

Stanton, A. L., Rowland, J. H., & Ganz, P. A. (2015). Life after diagnosis and treatment of cancer in adulthood: Contributions from psychosocial oncology research. *American Psychologist, 70,* 159–174.

Stanton, A. L., Wiley, J., Krull, J., Crespi, C. C., & Weihs, K. L. (2018). Cancer-related coping processes as predictors of depressive symptoms, trajectories, and episodes. *Journal of Consulting and Clinical Psychology, 86,* 820–830.

Starace, F., Massa, A., Amico, K. R., & Fisher, J. D. (2006). Adherence to antiretroviral therapy: An empirical test of the information-motivation-behavioral skills model. *Health Psychology, 25,* 153–162.

Starkman, M. N., Giordani, B., Berent, S., Schork, M. A., & Schteingart, D. E. (2001). Elevated cortisol levels in Cushing's disease are associated with cognitive decrements. *Psychosomatic Medicine, 63,* 985–993.

Starks, T. J., Grov, C., & Parsons, J. T. (2013). Sexual compulsivity and interpersonal functioning: Sexual relationship quality and sexual health in gay relationships. *Health Psychology, 32,* 1047–1056.

Starr, K. R., Antoni, M. H., Hurwitz, B. E., Rodriguez, M. S., Ironson, G., Fletcher, M. A., . . . Schneiderman, N. (1996). Patterns of immune, neuroen-docrine, and cardiovascular stress responses in asymptomatic HIV seropositive and seronegative men. *International Journal of Behavioral Medicine, 3,* 135–162.

Steele, C. (1988). The psychology of self-affirmation: Sustaining the integrity of the self. In L. Berkowitz (Ed.), *Advances in experimental social psychology* (Vol. 21, pp. 261–302). San Diego, CA: Academic Press.

Steele, C., & Josephs, R. A. (1990). Alcohol myopia: Its prized and dangerous effects. *American Psychologist, 45,* 921–933.

Steenland, K., Hu, S., & Walker, J. (2004). All-cause and cause-specific mortality by socioeconomic status among employed persons in 27 US states, 1984–1997. *American Journal of Public Health, 94,* 1037–1042.

Steffen, P. R., Smith, T. B., Larson, M., & Butler, L. (2006). Acculturation to western society as a risk factor for high blood pressure: A meta-analytic review. *Psychosomatic Medicine, 68,* 386–397.

Steginga, S. K., & Occhipinti, S. (2006). Dispositional optimism as a predictor of men's decision-related distress after localized prostate cancer. *Health Psychology, 25,* 135–143.

Stein, J. Y., Levin, Y., Lahav, Y., Uziel, O., Abumock, H., & Solomon, Z. (2018). Perceived social support, loneliness, and later life telomere length following wartime captivity. *Health Psychology, 37,* 1067–1076.

Stein, M. B., Belik, S. L., Jacobi, F., & Sareen, J. (2008). Impairment associated with sleep problems in the community: Relationship to physical and mental health comorbidity. *Psychosomatic Medicine, 70,* 913–919.

Stein, N., Folkman, S., Trabasso, T., & Richards, T. A. (1997). Appraisal and goal processes as predictors of psychological well-being in bereaved caregivers. *Journal of Personality and Social Psychology, 72,* 872–884.

Steinberg, D. M., Christy, J., Batch, B. C., Askew, S., Moore, R. H., Parker, P., & Bennett, G. G. (2017). Preventing weight gain improves sleep quality among black women: Results from a RCT. *Annals of Behavioral Medicine, 51,* 555–566.

Steinbrook, R. (2006). Imposing personal responsibility for health. *The New England Journal of Medicine, 355,* 753–756.

Stephan, Y., Sutin, A. R., Bayard, S., Križan, Z., & Terracciano, A. (2018). Personality and sleep quality: Evidence from four prospective studies. *Health Psychology, 37,* 271–281.

Stephens, M. A. P., Druley, J. A., & Zautra, A. J. (2002). Older adults' recovery from surgery for osteoarthritis of the knee: Psychological resources and constraints as predictors of outcomes. *Health Psychology, 21,* 377–383.

Stephens, M. A. P., Franks, M. M., Rook, K. S., Iida, M., Hemphill, R. C., & Salem, J. K. (2013). Spouses' attempts to regulate day-to-day dietary adherence among patients with type 2 diabetes. *Health Psychology, 32,* 1029–1037.

Steptoe, A., Brydon, L., & Kunz-Ebrecht, S. (2005). Changes in financial strain over three years, ambulatory blood pressure, and cortisol responses to awakening. *Psychosomatic Medicine, 67,* 281–287.

Steptoe, A., Demakakos, P., de Oliveira, C., & Wardle, J. (2012). Distinctive biological correlates of positive psychological well-being in older men and women. *Psychosomatic Medicine, 74,* 501–508.

Steptoe, A., Doherty, S., Kerry, S., Rink, E., & Hilton, S. (2000). Sociodemographic and psychological predictors of changes in dietary fat consumption in adults with high blood cholesterol following counseling in primary care. *Health Psychology, 19,* 411–419.

Steptoe, A., Kerry, S., Rink, E., & Hilton, S. (2001). The impact of behavioral counseling on stage of change in fat intake, physical activity, and cigarette smoking in adults at increased risk of coronary heart disease. *American Journal of Public Health, 91,* 265–269.

Steptoe, A., & Marmot, M. (2003). Burden of psychosocial adversity and vulnerability in middle age: Associations with biobehavioral risk factors and quality of life. *Psychosomatic Medicine, 65,* 1029–1037.

Steptoe, A., Perkins-Porras, L., Rink, E., Hilton, S., & Cappuccio, F. P. (2004). Psychological and social predictors of changes in fruit and vegetable consumption over 12 months following behavioral and nutrition education counseling. *Health Psychology, 23,* 574–581.

Steptoe, A., Roy, M. P., & Evans, O. (1996). Psychosocial influences on ambulatory blood pressure over working and non-working days. *Journal of Psychophysiology, 10,* 218–227.

Steptoe, A., Siegrist, J., Kirschbaum, C., & Marmot, M. (2004). Effort-reward imbalance, overcommitment, and measures of cortisol and blood pressure over the working day. *Psychosomatic Medicine, 66,* 323–329.

Stetler, C. A., & Miller, G. E. (2008). Social integration of daily activities and cortisol secretion: A laboratory based manipulation. *Journal of Behavioral Medicine, 31,* 249–257.

Stevens, V., Peterson, R., & Maruta, T. (1988). Changes in perception of illness and psychosocial adjustment. *The Clinical Journal of Pain, 4,* 249–256.

Stewart, A. L., King, A. C., Killen, J. D., & Ritter, P. L. (1995). Does smoking cessation improve health-related quality-of-life? *Annals of Behavioral Medicine, 17,* 331–338.

Stewart, D. E., Abbey, S. E., Shnek, Z. M., Irvine, J., & Grace, S. L. (2004). Gender differences in health information needs and decisional preferences in patients recovering from an acute ischemic coronary event. *Psychosomatic Medicine, 66,* 42–48.

Stewart, J. C., Fitzgerald, G. J., & Kamarck, T. W. (2010). Hostility now, depression later? Longitudinal associations among emotional risk factors for coronary artery disease. *Annals of Behavioral Medicine, 39,* 258–266.

Stewart, J. C., Perkins, A. J., & Callahan, C. M. (2014). Effect of collaborative care for depression on risk of cardiovascular events: Data from the IMPACT randomized controlled trial. *Psychosomatic Medicine, 76,* 29–37.

Stewart-Williams, S. (2004). The placebo puzzle: Putting together the pieces. *Health Psychology, 23,* 198–206.

Stice, E., Durant, S., Rohde, P., & Shaw, H. (2014). Effects of a prototype internet dissonance-based eating disorder prevention program at 1- and 2-year follow-up. *Health Psychology, 33,* 1558–1567.

Stice, E., Presnell, K., & Spangler, D. (2002). Risk factors for binge eating onset in adolescent girls: A 2-year prospective investigation. *Health Psychology, 21,* 131–138.

Stice, E., Yokum, S., & Burger, K. S. (2013). Elevated reward region responsivity predicts future substance use onset but not overweight/obesity onset. *Biological Psychiatry, 73,* 869–876.

Stilley, C. S., Bender, C. M., Dunbar-Jacob, J., Sereika, S., & Ryan, C. M. (2010). The impact of cognitive function on medication management: Three studies. *Health Psychology, 29,* 50–55.

Stock, M. L., Gibbons, F. X., Peterson, L., & Gerrard, M. (2013). The effects of racial discrimination on the HIV-risk cognitions and behaviors of Black adolescents and young adults. *Health Psychology, 32,* 543–550.

Stommel, M., Kurtz, M. E., Kurtz, J. C., Given, C. W., & Given, B. A. (2004). A longitudinal analysis of the course of depressive symptomatology in geriatric patients with cancer of the breast, colon, lung, or prostate. *Health Psychology, 23,* 564–573.

Stoney, C. M., Owens, J. F., Guzick, D. S., & Matthews, K. A. (1997). A natural experiment on the effects of ovarian hormones on cardiovascular risk factors and stress reactivity: Bilateral salpingo oophorectomy versus hysterectomy only. *Health Psychology, 16,* 349–358.

Stotts, A. L., DiClemente, C. C., Carbonari, J. P., & Mullen, P. D. (2000). Postpartum return to smoking: Staging a "suspended" behavior. *Health Psychology, 19,* 324–332.

Strachan, E. D., Bennett, W. R. M., Russo, J., & Roy-Byrne, P. P. (2007). Disclosure of HIV status and sexual orientation independently predicts increased absolute CD4 cell counts over time for psychiatric patients. *Psychosomatic Medicine, 69,* 74–80.

Strating, M. M. H., van Schuur, W. H., & Suurmeijer, T. P. B. M. (2006). Contribution of partner support in self-management of rheumatoid arthritis patients. An application of the theory of planned behavior. *Journal of Behavioral Medicine, 29,* 51–60.

Straus, R. (1988). Interdisciplinary biobehavioral research on alcohol problems: A concept whose time has come. *Drugs and Society, 2,* 33–48.

Streisand, B. (2006, October 9). Treating war's toll on the mind. *U.S. News & World Report,* pp. 55–62.

Strickhouser, J. E., Zell, E., & Krizan, Z. (2017). Does personality predict health and well-being? A metasynthesis. *Health Psychology, 36,* 797–810.

Striegel, R. H., Bedrosian, R., Wang, C., & Schwartz, S. (2012). Why men should be included in research on binge eating: Results from a comparison of psychosocial impairment in men and women. *International Journal of Eating Disorders, 45,* 233–240.

Striegel-Moore, R. H., & Bulik, C. M. (2007). Risk factors for eating disorders. *American Psychologist, 62,* 181–198.

Strigo, I. A., Simmons, A. N., Matthews, S. C., Craig, A. D., & Paulus, M. P. (2008). Increased affective bias revealed using experimental graded heat stimuli in young depressed adults: Evidence of "emotional allodynia." *Psychosomatic Medicine, 70,* 338–344.

Strike, P. C., Magid, K., Brydon, L., Edwards, S., McEwan, J. R., & Steptoe, A. (2004). Exaggerated platelet and hemodynamic reactivity to mental stress in men with coronary artery disease. *Psychosomatic Medicine, 66,* 492–500.

Strike, P. C., & Steptoe, A. (2005). Behavioral and emotional triggers of acute coronary syndromes: A systematic review and critique. *Psychosomatic Medicine, 67,* 179-186.

Stroebe, M., Gergen, M. M., Gergen, K. J., & Stroebe, W. (1992). Broken hearts or broken bonds: Love and death in historical perspective. *American Psychologist, 47,* 1205-1212.

Stroebe, W., & Stroebe, M. S. (1987). *Bereavement and health: The psychological and physical consequences of partner loss.* New York: Cambridge University Press.

Strong, K., Mathers, C., Leeder, S., & Beaglehole, R. (2005). Preventing chronic diseases: How many lives can we save? *Lancet, 366,* 1578-1582.

Strube, M. J., Smith, J. A., Rothbaum, R., & Sotelo, A. (1991). Measurement of health care attitudes in cystic fibrosis patients and their parents. *Journal of Applied Social Psychology, 21,* 397-408.

Stuber, K. J., & Smith, D. L. (2008). Chiropractic treatment of pregnancy-related low back pain: A systematic review of the evidence. *Journal of Manipulative Physiological Therapy, 31,* 447-454.

Stunkard, A. J. (1979). Behavioral medicine and beyond: The example of obesity. In O. F. Pomerleau & J. P. Brady (Eds.), *Behavioral medicine: Theory and practice* (pp. 279-298). Baltimore, MD: Williams & Wilkins.

Sturgeon, J. A., Carriere, J. S., Kao, M. C. J., Rico, T., Darnall, B. D., & Mackey, S. C. (2016). Social disruption mediates the relationship between perceived injustice and anger in chronic pain: A collaborative health outcomes information registry study. *Annals of Behavioral Medicine, 50,* 802-812.

Su, D., & Li, L. (2011). Trends in the use of complementary and alternative medicine in the United States: 2002-2007. *Journal of Health Care for the Poor and Underserved, 22,* 295-309.

Suarez, E. C. (2004). C-reactive protein is associated with psychological risk factors of cardiovascular disease in apparently healthy adults. *Psychosomatic Medicine, 66,* 684-691.

Substance Abuse and Mental Health Services Administration (SAMHSA). (2015). *Results from the 2015 national survey on drug use and health (NSDUH): Detailed tables. Table 5.6A—substance use disorder in past year among persons aged 18 or older, by demographic characteristics: Numbers in thousands, 2014 and 2015.* Retrieved January 18, 2017, from https://www.samhsa.gov/data/sites/default/files/NSDUH-DetTabs-2015/NSDUH-DetTabs-2015/NSDUH-DetTabs-2015.htm#tab5-6a.

Suendermann, O., Ehlers, A., Boellinghaus, I., Gamer, M., & Glucksman, E. (2010). Early heart rate responses to standardized trauma-related pictures predict posttraumatic stress disorder: A prospective study. *Psychosomatic Medicine, 72,* 301-308.

Suls, J., & Bunde, J. (2005). Anger, anxiety, and depression as risk factors for cardiovascular disease: The problems and implications of overlapping affective dispositions. *Psychological Bulletin, 131,* 260-300.

Suls, J., & Fletcher, B. (1985). The relative efficacy of avoidant and nonavoidant coping strategies: A meta-analysis. *Health Psychology, 4,* 249-288.

Suls, J., & Wan, C. K. (1993). The relationship between trait hostility and cardiovascular reactivity: A quantitative review and analysis. *Psychophysiology, 30,* 1-12.

Sundin, J., Öhman, L., & Simrén, M. (2017). Understanding the gut microbiota in inflammatory and functional gastrointestinal diseases. *Psychosomatic Medicine, 79,* 857-867.

Surwit, R. S., & Schneider, M. S. (1993). Role of stress in the etiology and treatment of diabetes mellitus. *Psychosomatic Medicine, 55,* 380-393.

Surwit, R. S., & Williams, P. G. (1996). Animal models provide insight into psychosomatic factors in diabetes. *Psychosomatic Medicine, 58,* 582-589.

Sussman, S., Sun, P., & Dent, C. W. (2006). A meta-analysis of teen cigarette smoking cessation. *Health Psychology, 25,* 549-557.

Sutin, A. R., Ferrucci, L., Zonderman, A. B., & Terracciano, A. (2011). Personality and obesity across the adult life span. *Journal of Personality and Social Psychology, 101,* 579-592.

Sutin, A. R., Zonderman, A. B., Uda, M., Deiana, B., Taub, D. D., Longo, D. L., & Terracciano, A. (2013). Personality traits and leptin. *Psychosomatic Medicine, 75,* 505-509.

Suzuki, N. (2004). Complementary and alternative medicine: A Japanese perspective. *Evidence-based Complementary and Alternative Medicine, 1,* 113-118.

Swaim, R. C., Oetting, E. R., & Casas, J. M. (1996). Cigarette use among migrant and nonmigrant Mexican American youth: A socialization latent-variable model. *Health Psychology, 15,* 269-281.

Sweeney, A. M., & Moyer, A. (2015). Self-affirmation and responses to health messages: A meta-analysis on intentions and behavior. *Health Psychology, 34,* 149-159.

Sweet, S. N., Martin Ginis, K. A., & Tamasone J. R. (2013). Investigating intermediary variables in the physical activity and quality of life relationship in persons with spinal cord injury. *Health Psychology, 32,* 877-885.

Sweet, S. N., Tulloch, H., Fortier, M. S., Pipe, A. L., & Reid, R. D. (2011). Patterns of motivation and ongoing exercise activity in cardiac rehabilitation settings: A 24-month exploration from the TEACH study. *Annals of Behavioral Medicine, 42,* 55-63.

Swencionis, C., Wylie-Rosett, J., Lent, M. R., Ginsberg, M., Cimino, C., Wassertheil-Smoller, S., Caban, A., & Segal-Isaacson, C. J. (2013). Weight change, psychological well-being, and vitality in adults participating in a cognitive–behavioral weight loss program. *Health Psychology, 32,* 439-446.

Swindle, R. E., Jr., & Moos, R. H. (1992). Life domains in stressors, coping, and adjustment. In W. B. Walsh, R. Price, & K. B. Crak (Eds.), *Person environment psychology: Models and perspectives* (pp. 1-33). New York: Erlbaum.

Szapocznik, J. (1995). Research on disclosure of HIV status: Cultural evolution finds an ally in science. *Health Psychology, 14,* 4-5.

Szrek, H., & Bundorf, M. K. (2014). Enrollment in prescription drug insurance: The interaction of numeracy and choice set size. *Health Psychology, 33,* 340-348.

Taber, D. R., Chriqui, J. F., Perna, F. M., Powell, L. M., & Chaloupka, F. J. (2012). Weight status among adolescents in states that govern competitive food nutrition content. *Pediatrics, 130,* 437-444.

Taber, J. M., Klein, W. M., Suls, J. M., & Ferrer, R. A. (2016). Lay awareness of the relationship between age and cancer risk. *Annals of Behavioral Medicine, 51,* 214-225.

Tamres, L., Janicki, D., & Helgeson, V. S. (2002). Sex differences in coping behavior: A meta-analytic review. *Personality and Social Psychology Review, 6,* 2-30.

Taub, E., Uswatte, G., King, D. K., Morris, D., Crago, J. E., & Chatterjec, A. (2006). A placebo-controlled trial of constraint-induced movement therapy for upper extremity after stroke. *Stroke, 37,* 1045-1049.

Taubes, G. (1993). Claim of higher risk for women smokers attacked. *Science, 262,* 1375.

Tavernise, S. (2015, October 28). Death rate study finds long U.S. decline stalled. *The New York Times,* p. A15.

Tavernise, S. (2015, November 13). Socioeconomic divide in smoking rates. *The New York Times,* p. A23.

Tavernise, S. (2016, February 13). Life spans of the rich leave the poor behind. *The New York Times,* p. A11.

Taylor, C. B., Bandura, A., Ewart, C. K., Miller, N. H., & DeBusk, R. F. (1985). Exercise testing to enhance wives' confidence in their husbands' cardiac capability soon after clinically uncomplicated acute myocardial infarction. *American Journal of Cardiology, 55,* 635-638.

Taylor, M. D., Whiteman, M. C., Fowkes, G. R., Lee, A. J., Allerhand, M., & Deary, I. J. (2009). Five factor model personality traits and all-cause mortality in the Edinburgh artery study cohort. *Psychosomatic Medicine, 71*, 631–641.

Taylor, M. J., Vlaev, I., Maltby, J., Brown, G. D. A., & Wood, A. M. (2015). Improving social norms interventions: Rank-framing increases excessive alcohol drinkers' information-seeking. *Health Psychology, 34*, 1200–1203.

Taylor, R. (2004). Causation of type 2 diabetes—The Gordian Knot unravels. *The New England Journal of Medicine, 350*, 639–641.

Taylor, R. R., Jason, L. A., & Jahn, S. C. (2003). Chronic fatigue and sociodemographic characteristics as predictors of psychiatric disorders in a community-based sample. *Psychosomatic Medicine, 65*, 896–901.

Taylor, S. E. (1983). Adjustment to threatening events: A theory of cognitive adaptation. *American Psychologist, 41*, 1161–1173.

Taylor, S. E. (1989). *Positive illusions: Creative self-deception and the healthy mind.* New York: Basic Books.

Taylor, S. E. (2002). *The tending instinct: How nurturing is essential to who we are and how we live.* New York: Holt.

Taylor, S. E. (2003). *Health psychology* (5th ed.). New York: McGraw-Hill.

Taylor, S. E. (2011). Social support: A review. In H. S. Friedman (Ed.), *Oxford handbook of health psychology.* New York: Oxford University Press.

Taylor, S. E., & Aspinwall, L. G. (1990). Psychological aspects of chronic illness. In G. R. VandenBos & P. T. Costa, Jr. (Eds.), *Psychological aspects of serious illness.* Washington, DC: American Psychological Association.

Taylor, S. E., & Broffman, J. I. (2011). Psychosocial resources: Functions, origins, and links to mental and physical health. In J. M. Olson and M. P. Zanna (Eds.), *Advances in experimental social psychology* (pp. 1–57). New York: Academic Press.

Taylor, S. E., Eisenberger, N. I., Saxbe, D., Lehman, B. J., & Lieberman, M. D. (2006). Neural responses to emotional stimuli are associated with childhood family stress. *Biological Psychiatry, 60*, 296–301.

Taylor, S. E., Falke, R. L., Shoptaw, S. J., & Lichtman, R. R. (1986). Social support, support groups, and the cancer patient. *Journal of Consulting and Clinical Psychology, 54*, 608–615.

Taylor, S. E., Helgeson, V. S., Reed, G. M., & Skokan, L. A. (1991). Self-generated feelings of control and adjustment to physical illness. *Journal of Social Issues, 47*, 91–109.

Taylor, S. E., Kemeny, M. E., Reed, G. M., Bower, J. E., & Gruenewald, T. L. (2000). Psychological resources, positive illusions, and health. *American Psychologist, 55*, 99–109.

Taylor, S. E., Klein, L. C., Lewis, B. P., Gruenewald, T. L., Gurung, R. A. R., & Updegraff, J. A. (2000). Biobehavioral responses to stress in females: Tend-and-befriend, not fight-or-flight. *Psychological Review, 107*, 411–429.

Taylor, S. E., Lichtman, R. R., & Wood, J. V. (1984). Attributions, beliefs about control, and adjustment to breast cancer. *Journal of Personality and Social Psychology, 46*, 489–502.

Taylor, S. E., & Stanton, A. (2007). Coping resources, coping processes, and mental health. *Annual Review of Clinical Psychology, 3*, 129–153.

Tegethoff, M., Greene, N., Olsen, J., Meyer, A. H., & Meinlschmidt, G. (2010). Maternal psychosocial adversity during pregnancy is associated with length of gestation and offspring size at birth: Evidence from a population-based cohort study. *Psychosomatic Medicine, 72*, 419–426.

Teguo, M. T., Simo-Tabue, N., Stoykova, R., Meillon, C., Cogne, M., Amiéva, H., & Dartigues, J. F. (2016). Feelings of loneliness and living alone as predictors of mortality in the elderly: The PAQUID study. *Psychosomatic Medicine, 78*, 904–909.

Teh, C. F., Zasylavsky, A. M., Reynolds, C. F., & Cleary, P. D. (2010). Effect of depression treatment on chronic pain outcomes. *Psychosomatic Medicine, 72*, 61–67.

Teixeira, P. J., Going, S. B., Houtkooper, L. B., Cussler, E. C., Martin, C. J., Metcalfe, L. L., . . . Lohman, T. G. (2002). Weight loss readiness in middle-aged women: Psychosocial predictors of success for behavioral weight reduction. *Journal of Behavioral Medicine, 25*, 499–523.

Telch, C. F., & Agras, W. S. (1996). Do emotional states influence binge eating in the obese? *International Journal of Eating Disorders, 20*, 271–279.

Temoshok, L. R., Wald, R. L., Synowski, S., & Garzino-Demo, A. (2008). Coping as a multisystem construct associated with pathways mediating HIV-relevant immune function and disease progression. *Psychosomatic Medicine, 70*, 555–561.

ten Brummelhuis, L. L., & Bakker, A. B. (2012). A resource perspective on the work-home interface: The work-home resources model. *American Psychologist, 67*, 545–556.

Tennen, H., Affleck, G., & Zautra, A. (2006). Depression history and coping with chronic pain: A daily process analysis. *Health Psychology, 25*, 370–379.

Teno, J. M., Fisher, E. S., Hamel, M. B., Coppola, K., & Dawson, N. V. (2002). Medical care inconsistent with patients' treatment goals: Association with 1-year medicare resource use and survival. *Journal of the American Geriatrics Society, 50*, 496–500.

Teno, J. M., Gozalo, P., Trivedi, A. N., Bunker, J., Lima, J., Ogarek, J., & Mor, V. (2018). Site of death, place of care, and health care transitions among US Medicare beneficiaries, 2000–2015. *Journal of the American Medical Association, 320*, 264–271.

Terracciano, A., Löckenhoff, C. E., Zonderman, A. B., Ferrucci, L., & Costa, P. T. (2008). Personality predictors of longevity: Activity, emotional stability, and conscientiousness. *Psychosomatic Medicine, 70*, 621–627.

Terracciano, A., Strait, J., Scuteri, A., Meirelles, O., Sutin, A. R., Tarasov, K., & Schlessinger, D. (2014). Personality traits and circadian blood pressure patterns: A 7-year prospective study. *Psychosomatic Medicine, 76*, 237–243.

Tesson, S., Butow, P. N., Sholler, G. F., Sharpe, L., Kovacs, A. H., & Kasparian, N. A. (2019). Psychological interventions for people affected by childhood-onset heart disease: A systematic review. *Health Psychology, 38*, 151–161.

Teunissen, H. A., Spijkerman, R., Larsen, H., Kremer, K. A., Kuntsche, E., Gibbons, F. X., . . . Engels, R. C. (2012). Stereotypic information about drinkers and students' observed alcohol intake: An experimental study on prototype-behavior relations in males and females in a naturalistic drinking context. *Drug and Alcohol Dependence, 125*, 301–306.

Thaler, R., & Sunstein, C. (2009). *Nudge: Improving decisions about health, wealth, and happiness.* New York: Penguin Books.

*The Economist.* (2015, May 30). Health care: *Bedside manners*, p. 65.

*The Economist.* (2015, June 20). Displaying braille: *Reading lessons*, p. 79.

*The Economist.* (2015, November 28). *Stopping splurging*, p. 67–68.

*The Economist.* (2016, March 5). *Schools and hard knocks*, p. 14.

*The Economist.* (2016, March 5). Concussion: *Bang to rights*, p. 73.

*The Economist.* (2017, August 26). *Health care: The right treatment*, pp. 10–12.

*The Economist.* (2017, August 26). *Primary health care: Diagnosing doctors*, pp. 50–52.

*The Economist.* (2018, April 28). *An affordable necessity*, pp. 3–12.

*The Economist.* (2018, July 28). *Debauchery and public finances: The taxes of sin*, p. 44.

*The Economist.* (2018, July 28). *The price of vice: "Sin" taxes—eg, on tobacco—are less efficient than they look*, p. 45.

*The Economist.* (2018, November 24). *Tobacco companies: Here comes the government*, p. 58.

The Lancet. (2015, June 8). Global, regional, and national incidence, prevalence, and years lived with disability for 301 acute and chronic diseases and injuries in 188 countries, 1990–2013: A systematic analysis for the Global burden of Disease Study 2013. *The Lancet, 386*, 743–800.

*The New York Times.* (2014, September 9). *Passing on risk for diabetes*, p.D4.

Theorell, T., Blomkvist, V., Lindh, G., & Evengard, B. (1999). Critical life events, infections, and symptoms during the year preceding chronic fatigue syndrome (CFS): An examination of CFS patients and subjects with a nonspecific life crisis. *Psychosomatic Medicine, 61,* 304-310.

Thoits, P. A. (1994). Stressors and problem-solving: The individual as psychological activist. *Journal of Health and Social Behavior, 35,* 143-159.

Thomas, J. M., Ursell, A., Robinson, E. L., Aveyard, P., Jebb, S. A., Herman, C. P., & Higgs, S. (2017). Using a descriptive social norm to increase vegetable selection in workplace restaurant settings. *Health Psychology, 36,* 1026-1033.

Thomas, K. S., Nelesen, R. A., & Dimsdale, J. E. (2004). Relationships between hostility, anger expression, and blood pressure dipping in an ethnically diverse sample. *Psychosomatic Medicine, 66,* 298-304.

Thomas, M. R., Wara, D., Saxton, K., Truskier, M., Chesney, M. A., & Boyce, W. T. (2013). Family adversity and automatic reactivity association with immune change in HIV-affected school children. *Psychosomatic Medicine, 75,* 557-565.

Thompson, S. C. (1981). Will it hurt less if I can control it? A complex answer to a simple question. *Psychological Bulletin, 90,* 89-101.

Thompson, S. C., Cheek, P. R., & Graham, M. A. (1988). The other side of perceived control: Disadvantages and negative effects. In S. Spacapan & S. Oskamp (Eds.), *The social psychology of health: The Claremont Applied Social Psychology Conference* (Vol. 2, pp. 69-94). Beverly Hills, CA: Sage.

Thompson, S. C., Nanni, C., & Schwankovsky, L. (1990). Patient-oriented interventions to improve communication in a medical office visit. *Health Psychology, 9,* 390-404.

Thompson, S. C., Sobolew-Shubin, A., Graham, M. A., & Janigian, A. S. (1989). Psychosocial adjustment following a stroke. *Social Science and Medicine, 28,* 239-247.

Thompson, S. C., & Spacapan, S. (1991). Perceptions of control in vulnerable populations. *Journal of Social Issues, 47,* 1-22.

Thompson, T., Rodebaugh, T. L., Pérez, M., Schootman, M., & Jeffe, D. B. (2013). Perceived social support change in patients with early stage breast cancer and controls. *Health Psychology, 32,* 886-895.

Thornton, B., Gibbons, F. X., & Gerrard, M. (2002). Risk perception and prototype perception: Independent processes predicting risk behaviors. *Personality and Social Psychology Bulletin, 28,* 986-999

Thornton, C. M., Kerr, J., Conway, T. L., Saelens, B. E., Sallis, J. F., Ahn, D. K., ... King, A. C. (2016). Physical activity in older adults: An ecological approach. *Annals of Behavioral Medicine, 51,* 159-169.

Thornton, L. M., Andersen, B. L., & Blakely, W. P. (2010). The pain, depression, and fatigue symptom cluster in advanced breast cancer: Covariation with the hypothalamic-pituitary-adrenal axis and the sympathetic nervous system. *Health Psychology, 29,* 333-337.

Thornton, L. M., Andersen, B. L., Schuler, T. A., & Carson, W. E. (2009). A psychological intervention reduces inflammatory markers by alleviating depressive symptoms: Secondary analysis of a randomized contolled trial. *Psychosomatic Medicine, 71,* 715-724.

Thurston, R. C., Chang, Y., Barinas-Mitchell, E., von Känel, R., Jennings, J. R., Santoro, N., ... Matthews, K. A. (2017). Child abuse and neglect and subclinical cardiovascular disease among midlife women. *Psychosomatic Medicine, 79,* 441-449.

Thurston, R. C., Sherwood, A., Matthews, K. A., & Blumenthal, J. A. (2011). Household responsibilities, income, and ambulatory blood pressure among working men and women. *Psychosomatic Medicine, 73,* 200-205.

Timberlake, D. S., Haberstick, B. C., Lessem, J. M., Smolen, A., Ehringer, M., Hewitt, J. K., & Hopfer, C. (2006). An association between the DAT1 polymorphism and smoking behavior in young adults from the National Longitudinal Study of Adolescent Health. *Health Psychology, 25,* 190-197.

Timko, C., Stovel, K. W., Moos, R. H., & Miller, J. J., III. (1992). A longitudinal study of risk and resistance factors among children with juvenile rheumatic disease. *Journal of Clinical Child Psychology, 21,* 132-142.

Timman, R., Roos, R., Maat-Kievit, A., & Tibben, A. (2004). Adverse effects of predictive testing for Huntington disease underestimated: Long-term effects 7-10 years after the test. *Health Psychology, 23,* 189-197.

Tindle, H., Belnap, B. H., Houck, P. R., Mazumdar, S., Scheier, M. F., Matthews, K. A., ... Rollman, B. L. (2012). Optimism, response to treatment of depression, and rehospitalization after coronary artery bypass graft surgery. *Psychosomatic Medicine, 74,* 200-207.

Tobin, E. T., Kane, H. S., Saleh, D. J., Naar-King, S., Poowuttikul, P., Secord, Elizabeth, Pierantoni, & Slatcher, R. B. (2015). Naturalistically observed conflict and youth asthma symptoms. *Health Psychology, 34,* 622-631.

Tobin, J. J., & Friedman, J. (1983). Spirits, shamans, and nightmare death: Survivor stress in a Hmong refugee. *American Journal of Orthopsychiatry, 53,* 439-448.

Toker, S., Melamed, S., Berliner, S., Zeltser, D., & Shapira, I. (2012). Burnout and risk of coronary heart disease: A prospective study of 8838 employees. *Psychosomatic Medicine, 74,* 840-847.

Tombor, I., Shahab, L., Herbec, A., Neale, J., Michie, S., & West, R. (2015). Smoker identity and its potential role in young adults' smoking behavior: A meta-ethnography. *Health Psychology, 34,* 992-1003.

Tomenson, B., McBeth, J., Chew-Graham, C. A., MacFarlane, G., Davies, I., Jackson, J., ... Creed, F. H. (2012). Somatization and health anxiety as predictors of health care use. *Psychosomatic Medicine, 74,* 656-664.

Tomiyama, A. J., Epel, E. S., McClatchey, T. M., Poelke, G., Kemeny, M. E., McCoy, S. K., & Daubenmier, J. (2014). Associations of weight stigma with cortisol and oxidative stress independent of adiposity. *Health Psychology, 33,* 862-867.

Tomiyama, A. J., Mann, T., Vinas, D., Hunger, J. M., DeJager, J., & Taylor, S. E. (2010). Low calorie dieting increases cortisol. *Psychosomatic Medicine, 72,* 357-364.

Toobert, D. J., Strycker, L. A., Barrera, M., Osuna, D., King, D. K., & Glasgow, R. E. (2011). Outcomes from a multiple risk factor diabetes self-management trial for Latinas: ¡Viva Bien! *Annals of Behavioral Medicine, 41,* 310-323.

Topol, E. (2015). *The patient will see you now: The future of medicine is in your hands.* New York: Basic Books.

Torres, J. M., Deardorff, J., Gunier, R. B., Harley, K. G., Alkon, A., Kogut, K., & Eskenazi, B. (2018). Worry about deportation and cardiovascular disease risk factors among adult women: The center for the health assessment of mothers and children of Salinas study. *Annals of Behavioral Medicine, 52,* 186-193.

Toups, M. S. P., Myers, A. K., Wisniewski, S. R., Kurian, B., Morris, D. W., Rush, A. J., Fava, M., & Trivedi, M. H. (2013). Relationship between obesity and depression: Characteristics and treatment outcomes with antidepressant medication. *Psychosomatic Medicine, 75,* 863-872.

Tran, V., Wiebe, D. J., Fortenberry, K. T., Butler, J. M., & Berg, C. A. (2011). Benefit finding, affective reactions to diabetes stress, and diabetes management among early adolescents. *Health Psychology, 30,* 212-219.

Travagin, G., Margola, D., & Revenson, T. A. (2015). How effective are expressive writing interventions for adolescents? A meta-analytic review. *Clinical Psychology Review, 36,* 42-55.

Troisi, A., Di Lorenzo, G., Alcini, S., Nanni, C., Di Pasquale, C., & Siracusano, A. (2006). Body dissatisfaction in women with eating disorders: Relationship to early separation anxiety and insecure attachment. *Psychosomatic Medicine, 68,* 449-453.

Troxel, W. M., Matthews, K. A., Bromberger, J. T., & Sutton-Tyrrell, K. (2003). Chronic stress burden, discrimination, and subclinical carotid artery disease in African American and Caucasian women. *Health Psychology, 22,* 300-309.

Trudel-Fitzgerald, C., Tworoger, S. S., Poole, E. M., Zhang, X., Giovannucci, E. L., Meyerhardt, J. A., & Kubzansky, L. D. (2018). Psychological symptoms and subsequent healthy lifestyle after a colorectal cancer diagnosis. *Health Psychology, 37*(3), 207-217.

Trumbetta, S. L., Seltzer, B. K., Gottesman, I. I., & McIntyre, K. M. (2010). Mortality predictors in a 60-year follow up of adolescent males: Exploring delinquency, socioeconomic status, IQ, high school drop-out status, and personality. *Psychosomatic Medicine, 72,* 46-52.

Tsenkova, V., Pudrovska, T., & Karlamangla, A. (2014). Childhood socioeconomic disadvantage and prediabetes and diabetes in later life: A study of biopsychosocial pathways. *Psychosomatic Medicine, 76,* 622-628.

Tsenkova, V. K., Karlamangla, A. S., & Ryff, C. D. (2016). Parental history of diabetes, positive affect, and diabetes risk in adults: Findings from MIDUS. *Annals of Behavioral Medicine, 50,* 836-843.

Tucker, J. S., Elliott, M. N., Wenzel, S. L., & Hambarsoomian, K. (2007). Relationship commitment and its implications for unprotected sex among impoverished women living in shelters and low-income housing in Los Angeles county. *Health Psychology, 26,* 644-649.

Tucker, J. S., Orlando, M., Burnam, M. A., Sherbourne, C. D., Kung, F. Y., & Gifford, A. L. (2004). Psychosocial mediators of antiretroviral nonadherence in HIV-positive adults with substance use and mental health problems. *Health Psychology, 23,* 363-370.

Tugade, M. M., & Fredrickson, B. L. (2004). Resilient individuals use positive emotions to bounce back from negative emotional experiences. *Journal of Personality and Social Psychology, 86,* 320-333.

Tully, P. J., Baumeister, H., Martin, S., Atlantis, E., Jenkins, A., Januszewski, A., . . . Wittert, G. A. (2016). Elucidating the biological mechanisms linking depressive symptoms with type 2 diabetes in men: The longitudinal effects of inflammation, microvascular dysfunction, and testosterone. *Psychosomatic Medicine, 78,* 221-232.

Tuomilehto, J., Lindstrom, J., Eriksson, J. G., Valle, T. T., Hamalainen, H., Ilanne-Parikka, P., . . . Finnish Diabetes Prevention Study Group. (2001). Prevention of Type 2 diabetes mellitus by changes in lifestyle among subjects with impaired glucose tolerance. *The New England Journal of Medicine, 344,* 1343-1350.

Turiano, N. A., Chapman, B. P., Gruenwald, T. L., & Mroczek, D. K. (2015). Personality and the leading behavioral contributors of mortality. *Health Psychology, 34,* 51-60.

Turk, D. C., & Feldman, C. S. (1992a). Facilitating the use of noninvasive pain management strategies with the terminally ill. In D. C. Turk & C. S. Feldman (Eds.), *Non-invasive approaches to pain management in the terminally ill* (pp. 1-25). New York: Haworth Press.

Turk, D. C., & Feldman, C. S. (1992b). Noninvasive approaches to pain control in terminal illness: The contribution of psychological variables. In D. C. Turk & C. S. Feldman (Eds.), *Non-invasive approaches to pain management in the terminally ill* (pp. 193-214). New York: Haworth Press.

Turk, D. C., & Fernandez, E. (1990). On the putative uniqueness of cancer pain: Do psychological principles apply? *Behavioural Research and Therapy, 28,* 1-13.

Turk, D. C., Kerns, R. D., & Rosenberg, R. (1992). Effects of marital interaction on chronic pain and disability: Examining the downside of social support. *Rehabilitation Psychology, 37,* 259-274.

Turk, D. C., & Meichenbaum, D. (1991). Adherence to self-care regimens: The patient's perspective. In R. H. Rozensky, J. J. Sweet, & S. M. Tovian (Eds.), *Handbook of clinical psychology in medical settings* (pp. 249-266). New York: Plenum.

Turk, D. C., & Rudy, T. E. (1991). Neglected topics in the treatment of chronic pain patients—Relapse, noncompliance, and adherence enhancement. *Pain, 44,* 5-28.

Turk, D. C., Wack, J. T., & Kerns, R. D. (1995). An empirical examination of the "pain-behavior" construct. *Journal of Behavioral Medicine, 8,* 119-130.

Turner, J. C., Keller, A., Wu, H., Zimmerman, M., Zhang, J., & Barnes, L. E. (2018). Utilization of primary care among college students with mental health disorders. *Health Psychology, 37,* 385-393

Turner, L. R., & Mermelstein, R. J. (2005). Psychosocial characteristics associated with sun protection practices among parents of young children. *Journal of Behavioral Medicine, 28,* 77-90.

Turner, R. J., & Avison, W. R. (1992). Innovations in the measurement of life stress: Crisis theory and the significance of event resolution. *Journal of Health and Social Behavior, 33,* 36-50.

Turner, R. J., & Avison, W. R. (2003). Status variations in stress exposure: Implications for the interpretation of research on race, socioeconomic status, and gender. *Journal of Health and Social Behavior, 44,* 488-505.

Turner, R. J., & Noh, S. (1988). Physical disability and depression: A longitudinal analysis. *Journal of Health and Social Behavior, 29,* 23-37.

Turner-Cobb, J. M., Gore-Felton, C., Marouf, F., Koopman, C., Kim, P., Israelski, D., & Spiegel, D. (2002). Coping, social support, and attachment style as psychosocial correlates of adjustment in men and women with HIV/AIDS. *Journal of Behavioral Medicine, 25,* 337-353.

Turner-Cobb, J. M., Sephton, S. E., Koopman, C., Blake-Mortimer, J., & Spiegel, D. (2000). Social support and salivary cortisol in women with metastatic breast cancer. *Psychosomatic Medicine, 62,* 337-345.

Turner-Stokes, L., Erkeller-Yuksel, F., Miles, A., Pincus, T., Shipley, M., & Pearce, S. (2003). Outpatient cognitive behavioral pain management programs: A randomized comparison of a group-based multidisciplinary versus an individual therapy model. *Archives of Physical Medicine and Rehabilitation, 84,* 781-788.

Turnwald, B. P., Jurafsky, D., Conner, A., & Crum, A. J. (2017). Reading between the menu lines: Are restaurants' descriptions of "healthy" foods unappealing? *Health Psychology, 36,* 1034-1037.

Turrisi, R., Hillhouse, J., Gebert, C., & Grimes, J. (1999). Examination of cognitive variables relevant to sunscreen use. *Journal of Behavioral Medicine, 22,* 493-509.

Tyson, M., Covey, J., & Rosenthal, H. E. S. (2014). Theory of planned behavior interventions for reducing heterosexual risk behaviors: A meta-analysis. *Health Psychology, 33,* 1454-1467.

Uchino, B. N., Bosch, J. A., Smith, T. W., Carlisle, M., Birmingham, W., Bowen, K. S., & O'Hartaigh, B. (2013). Relationships and cardiovascular risk: Perceived spousal ambivalence in specific relationship contexts and its links to inflammation. *Health Psychology, 32,* 1067-1075.

Uchino, B. N., Cawthon, R. M., Smith, T. W., Light, K. C., McKenzie, J., Carlisle, . . .Bowen, K. (2012). Social relationships and health: Is feeling positive, negative, or both (ambivalent) about your social ties related to telomeres? *Health Psychology, 31,* 789-796.

Uchino, B. N., Trettevik, R., Kent de Grey, R. G., Cronan, S., Hogan, J., & Baucom, B. R. W. (2018). Social support, social integration, and inflammatory cytokines: A meta-analysis. *Health Psychology, 37,* 462-471.

Uchino, B. N., & Way, B. M. (2017). Integrative pathways linking close family ties to health: A neurochemical perspective. *American Psychologist, 72,* 590-600.

Ueda, H., Howson, J. M., Esposito, L., Heward, J., Snook, H., Chamberlain, G., . . . Gough, S. C. (2003). Association of the T-cell regulatory gene CTLA-4 with susceptibility to autoimmune disease. *Nature, 423,* 506-511.

Umberson, D. (1987). Family status and health behaviors: Social control as a dimension of social integration. *Journal of Health and Social Behavior, 28,* 306-319.

Umberson, D., & Montez, J. K. (2010). Social relationships and health: A flashpoint for health policy. *Journal of Health and Social Behavior, 51,* S54-S66.

Umberson, D., Wortman, C. B., & Kessler, R. C. (1992). Widowhood and depression: Explaining long-term gender differences in vulnerability. *Journal of Health and Social Behavior, 33,* 10–24.

UNAIDS. (2010). *2010 report on the global AIDS epidemic.* Retrieved March 26, 2012, from www.unaids.org/globalreport/global_report.htm.

UNAIDS. (2014, July). *UNAIDS report shows that 19 million of the 35 million people living with HIV today do not know that they have the virus.* Retrieved May 25, 2016, from http://www.unaids.org/

UNAIDS. (2018). *UNAIDS data 2018.* Retrieved May 29, 2019, from https://www.unaids.org/sites/default/files/media_asset/unaids-data-2018_en.pdf

Unger, J. B., Hamilton, J. E., & Sussman, S. (2004). A family member's job loss as a risk factor for smoking among adolescents. *Health Psychology, 23,* 308–313.

United Nations, Department of Economic and Social Affairs, Population Division. (2011). *World population prospects: The 2010 revision.* Retrieved March 28, 2012, from http://esa.un.org/wpp/excel-data/population.htm

Updegraff, J. A., Brick, C., Emanuel, A. S., Mintzer, R. E., & Sherman, D. K. (2015). Message framing for health: Moderation by perceived susceptibility and motivational orientation in a diverse sample of Americans. *Health Psychology, 34,* 20–29.

Updegraff, J. A., Taylor, S. E., Kemeny, M. E., & Wyatt, G. E. (2002). Positive and negative effects of HIV infection in women with low socioeconomic resources. *Personality and Social Psychology Bulletin, 28,* 382–394.

U.S. Burden of Disease Collaborators. (2013). The state of US health, 1990–2010: Burden of diseases, injuries, and risk factors. *JAMA, 310,* 591–606.

U.S. Bureau of Labor Statistics (May, 2014) *Women in the labor Force: A databook.* Report 1049.

U.S. Census Bureau. (2011). *Income, poverty, and health insurance coverage in the United States: 2010.* Retrieved March 29, 2012, from http://www.census.gov/prod/2011pubs/p60-239.pdf

U.S. Census Bureau. (2012). *Persons living alone by sex and age.* Retrieved September 11, 2012, from http://www.census.gov/compendia/statab/2012/tables/12s0072.pdf

U.S. Census Bureau. (2019, June). *U.S. and world population clock.* Retrieved June 26, 2019, from https://www.census.gov/popclock/

U.S. Department of Agriculture. (2007). *Electronic outlook report from the economic research service: Tobacco outlook.* Retrieved March 20, 2012, from http://usda.mannlib.cornell.edu/usda/ers/TBS//2000s/2007/TBS-10-24-2007.pdf

U.S. Department of Commerce. (2009). Current population reports: Consumer income. Income, Poverty, and Health Insurance Coverage in the United States: 2008, 20–25.

U.S. Department of Health and Human Services. (2014). The health consequences of smoking–50 years of progress: A report of the Surgeon General.

U.S. Department of Health and Human Services. (2018). *Physical activity guidelines for Americans* (2nd ed.). Washington, DC: U.S. Department of Health and Human Services. Retrieved April 1, 2019, from https://health.gov/paguidelines/second-edition/pdf/Physical_Activity_Guidelines_2nd_edition.pdf

U.S. Department of Health & Human Services. (2019, March 21). *Female infertility.* Retrieved March 26, 2019, from https://www.hhs.gov/opa/reproductive-health/fact-sheets/female-infertility/index.html

U.S. Department of Health, Education, and Welfare and U.S. Public Health Service. (1964). *Smoking and health: Report of the advisory committee to the surgeon general of the Public Health Service* (Publication No. PHS-1103). Washington, DC: U.S. Government Printing Office.

U.S. Department of Labor. (2012). *Occupational Outlook Handbook*, 2012–13 Edition, *Physical Therapists.* Retrieved June 5, 2012, from http://www.bls.gov/ooh/healthcare/physical-therapists.htm

U.S. Food and Drug Administration. (2019). *How tobacco can harm your lungs.* Retrieved April 8, 2019, from https://www.fda.gov/tobacco-products/health-information/keep-your-air-clear-how-tobacco-can-harm-your-lungs

U.S. Preventive Services Task Force. (2009). Screening for breast cancer: U.S. preventive services task force recommendation statement. *Annals of Internal Medicine, 151,* 716–726.

Uysal, A., & Lu, Q. (2011). Is self-concealment associated with acute and chronic pain? *Health Psychology, 30,* 606–614.

Vahtera, J., Kivimäki, M., Väänänen, A., Linna, A., Pentti, J., Helenius, H., & Elovainio, M. (2006). Sex differences in health effects of family death or illness: Are women more vulnerable than men? *Psychosomatic Medicine, 68,* 283–291.

Valet, M., Gündel, H., Sprenger, T., Sorg, C., Mühlau, M., Zimmer, C., . . . Tölle, T. R. (2009). Patients with pain disorder show gray-matter loss in pain-processing structures: A voxel-based morphometric study. *Psychosomatic Medicine, 71,* 49–56.

Valkanova, V., & Ebmeier, K. P. (2013). Vascular risk factors and depression in later life: A systematic review and meta-analysis. *Biological Psychiatry, 73,* 406–413.

Vallance, J. K. H., Courneya, K. S., Plotnikoff, R. C., & Mackey, J. R. (2008). Analyzing theoretical mechanisms of physical activity behavior change in breast cancer survivors: Results from the activity promotion (ACTION) trial. *Annals of Behavioral Medicine, 35,* 150–158.

Vamos, E. P., Mucsi, I., Keszei, A., Kopp, M. S., & Novak, M. (2009). Comorbid depression is associated with increased healthcare utilization and lost productivity in persons with diabetes: A large nationally representative Hungarian population survey. *Psychosomatic Medicine, 71,* 501–507.

Van den Berg, J. F., Miedema, H. M. E., Tulen, J. H. M., Neven, A. K., Hofman, A., Witteman, J. C. M., & Tiemeier, H. (2008). Long sleep duration is associated with serum cholesterol in the elderly: The Rotterdamn study. *Psychosomatic Medicine, 70,* 1005–1011.

van den Boom, W., Stolte, I. G., Rogggen, A., Sandfort, T., Prins, M., & Davidovich, U. (2015). Is anyone around me using condoms? Site-specific condom-use norms and their potential impact on condomless sex across various gay venues and websites in the Netherlands. *Health Psychology, 34,* 857–864.

VanderDrift, L. E., Agnew, C. R., Harvey, S. M., & Warren, J. T. (2013). Whose intentions predict? Power over condom use within heterosexual dyads. *Health Psychology, 32,* 1038–1046.

Van den Putte, B., Yzer, M., Willemsen, M. C., & de Bruijn, G. J. (2009). The effects of smoking self-identity and quitting self-identity on attempts to quit smoking. *Health Psychology, 28,* 535–544.

Van der Laan, L. N., Papies, E. K., Hooge, I. T. C., & Smeets, P. A. M. (2017). Goal-directed visual attention drives health goal priming: An eye-tracking experiment. *Health Psychology, 36,* 82–90.

Van der Ploeg, H. P., Streppel, K. R. M., van der Beek, A. J., van der Woude, L. H. V., van Harten, W. H., & van Mechelen, W. (2008). Underlying mechanisms of improving physical activity behavior after rehabilitation. *International Journal of Behavioral Medicine, 15,* 101–108.

Van der Velde, F. W., & Van der Pligt, J. (1991). AIDS-related health behavior: Coping, protection, motivation, and previous behavior. *Journal of Behavioral Medicine, 14,* 429–452.

Van der Zwaluw, C. S., Scholte, R. H. J., Vermulst, A. A., Buitelaar, J. K., Verkes, R. J., & Engels, R. C. M. E. (2008). Parental problem drinking, parenting, and adolescent alcohol use. *Journal of Behavioral Medicine, 31,* 189–200.

Van Dijk, S., van den Beukel, T., Dekker, F. W., le Cessie, S., Kaptein, A. A., Honig, A., . . . Verduijn, M. (2012). Short-term versus long-term effects of depressive symptoms on mortality in patients on dialysis. *Psychosomatic Medicine, 74,* 854–860.

Vangeepuram, N., Galvez, M. P., Teitelbaum, S. L., Brenner, B., & Wolff, M. S. (2012). The association between parental perception of neighborhood safety and asthma diagnosis in ethnic minority urban children. *Journal of Urban Health, 89,* 758–768.

Van Gils, A., Janssens, K. A. M., & Rosmalen, J. G. M. (2014). Family disruption increases functional somatic symptoms in late adolescence: The TRAILS study. *Health Psychology, 33,* 1354–1361.

Van Jaarsveld, C. H. M., Fidler, J. A., Simon, A. E., & Wardle, J. (2007). Persistent impact of pubertal timing on trends in smoking, food choice, activity, and stress in adolescents. *Psychosomatic Medicine, 96,* 798–806.

Van Kessel, K., Moss-Morris, R., Willoughby, E., Chalder, T., Johnson, M. H., & Robinson, E. (2008). A randomized controlled trial of cognitive behavior therapy for multiple sclerosis fatigue. *Psychosomatic Medicine, 70,* 205–213.

Van Koningsbruggen, G. M., Das, E., & Roskos-Ewoldsen, D. R. (2009). How self-affirmation reduces defensive processing of threatening health information: Evidence at the implicit level. *Health Psychology, 28,* 563–568.

Van Lankveld, W., Naring, G., van der Staak, C., van't Pad Bosch, P., & van de Putte, L. (1993). Stress caused by rheumatoid arthritis: Relation among subjective stressors of the disease, disease status, and well-being. *Journal of Behavioral Medicine, 16,* 309–322.

Van Liew, J. R., Christensen, A. J., Howren, M. B., Hynds Karnell, L., & Funk, G. F. (2014). Fear of recurrence impacts health-related quality of life and continued tobacco use in head and neck cancer survivors. *Health Psychology, 33,* 373–381.

Vannucci, A., Shomaker, L. B., Field, S. E., Sbrocco, T., Stephens, M., Kozlosky, M., Reynolds, J. C., Yanovski, J. A., & Tanofsky-Kraff, M. (2014). History of weight control attempts among adolescent girls with loss of control eating. *Health Psychology, 33,* 419–423.

Van Reedt Dortland, A. K. B., Giltay, E. J., van Veen, T., Zitman, F. G., & Penninx, B. W. J. J. (2013). Longitudinal relationship of depressive and anxiety symptoms with dyslipidemia and abdominal obesity. *Psychosomatic Medicine, 75,* 83–89.

Van Rijn, I, Wegman, J., Aarts, E., de Graaf, C., & Smeets, P. A. M. (2017). Health interest modulates brain reward responses to a perceived low-caloric beverage in females. *Health Psychology, 36,* 65–72.

Van Rood, Y. R., Bogaards, M., Goulmy, E., & van Houwelingen, H. C. (1993). The effects of stress and relaxation on the in vitro immune response in man: A meta-analytic study. *Journal of Behavioral Medicine, 16,* 163–182.

Van Ryn, M., & Fu, S. S. (2003). Paved with good intensions: Do public health and human service providers contribute to racial/ethnic disparities in health? *American Journal of Public Health, 93,* 248–255.

Van Stralen, M. M., De Vries, H., Bolman, C., Mudde, A. N., & Lechner, L. (2010). Exploring the efficacy and moderators of two computer-tailored physical activity interventions for older adults: A randomized controlled trial. *Annals of Behavioral Medicine, 39,* 139–150.

Van YPeren, N. W., Buunk, B. P., & Schaufelli, W. B. (1992). Communal orientation and the burnout syndrome among nurses. *Journal of Applied Social Psychology, 22,* 173–189.

van Zon, S. K., Reijneveld, S. A., van der Most, P. J., Swertz, M. A., Bültmann, U., & Snieder, H. (2018). The interaction of genetic predisposition and socioeconomic position with type 2 diabetes mellitus: Cross-sectional and longitudinal analyses from the Lifelines Cohort and Biobank Study. *Psychosomatic Medicine, 80,* 252–262.

Van Zundert, R. M. P., Ferguson, S. G., Shiffman, S., & Engels, R. C. M. (2010). Dynamic effects of self-efficacy on smoking lapses and relapse among adolescents. *Health Psychology, 29,* 246–254.

Varni, J. W., Burwinkle, T. M., Rapoff, M. A., Kamps, J. L., & Olson, N. (2004). The PedsQL in pediatric asthma: Reliability and validity of the Pediatric Quality of Life Inventory Generic Core Scales and Asthma Module. *Journal of Behavioral Medicine, 27,* 297–318.

Vedhara, K., Brant, E., Adamopoulos, E., Byrne-Davis, L., Mackintosh, B., Hoppitt, L., . . . Pennebaker, J. W. (2010). A preliminary investigation into whether attentional bias influences mood outcomes following emotional disclosure. *International Journal of Behavioral Medicine, 17,* 195–206.

Veehof, M. M., Trompetter, H. R., Bohlmeijer, E. T., & Schreurs, K. M. G. (2016). Acceptance- and mindfulness-based interventions for the treatment of chronic pain: A meta-analytic review. *Cognitive Behaviour Therapy, 45,* 5–31.

Veitch, J., Timperio, A., Crawford, D., Abbott, G., Giles-Corti, B., & Salmon, J. (2011). Is the neighbourhood environment associated with sedentary behaviour outside of school hours among children? *Annals of Behavioral Medicine, 41,* 333–341.

Vendrig, A. (1999). Prognostic factors and treatment-related changes associated with return to working: The multimodal treatment of chronic back pain. *Journal of Behavioral Medicine, 22,* 217–232.

Verbrugge, L. M. (1983). Multiple roles and physical health of women and men. *Journal of Health and Social Behavior, 24,* 16–30.

Verbrugge, L. M. (1995). Women, men, and osteoarthritis. *Arthritis Care and Research, 8,* 212–220.

Vila, G., Porche, L., & Mouren-Simeoni, M. (1999). An 18-month longitudinal study of posttraumatic disorders in children who were taken hostage in their school. *Psychosomatic Medicine, 61,* 746–754.

Villarosa, L. (2002, September 23). As Black men move into middle age, dangers rise. *New York Times,* pp. E1, E8.

Visotsky, H. M., Hamburg, D. A., Goss, M. E., & Lebovitz, B. Z. (1961). Coping behavior under extreme stress. *Archives of General Psychiatry, 5,* 423–428.

Vitaliano, P. P., Maiuro, R. D., Russo, J., Katon, W., DeWolfe, D., & Hall, G. (1990). Coping profiles associated with psychiatric, physical health, work, and family problems. *Health Psychology, 9,* 348–376.

Vitaliano, P. P., Scanlan, J. M., Zhang, J., Savage, M. V., Hirsch, I. B., & Siegler, I. C. (2002). A path model of chronic stress, the metabolic syndrome, and coronary heart disease. *Psychosomatic Medicine, 64,* 418–435.

Vitality Compass. Retrieved February 20, 2013, from http://apps.bluezones.com/vitality

Vittinghoff, E., Shlipak, M. G., Varosy, P. D., Furberg, C. D., Ireland, C. C., Khan, S. S., . . . Heart and Estrogen/progestin Replacement Study Research Group. (2003). Risk factors and secondary prevention in women with heart disease: The Heart and Estrogen/Progestin Replacement Study. *Annals of Internal Medicine, 138,* 81–89.

Vogt, F., Hall, S., Hankins, M., & Marteau, T. M. (2009). Evaluating three theory-based interventions to increase physicians recommendations of smoking cessation services. *Health Psychology, 28,* 174–182.

Volkow, N. D., Wang, G., Tomasi, D., & Baler, R. D. (2013). The addictive dimensionality of obesity. *Biological Psychiatry, 73,* 811–818.

Von Dawans, B., Fischbacher, U., Kirschbaum, C., Fehr, E., & Heinrichs, M. (2012). The social dimension of stress reactivity: Acute stress increases prosocial behavior in humans. *Psychological Science, 23,* 651–660.

Von Känel, R., Bellingrath, S., & Kudielka, B. M. (2009). Overcommitment but not effort–reward imbalance relates to stress-induced coagulation changes in teachers. *Annals of Behavioral Medicine, 37,* 20–28.

Von Korff, M., Katon, W., Lin, E. H. B., Simon, G., Ludman, E., Ciechanowski, P., . . . Bush, T. (2005). Potentially modifiable factors associated with disability among people with diabetes. *Psychosomatic Medicine, 67,* 233–240.

Vos, J., & Vitali, D. (2018). The effects of psychological meaning-centered therapies on quality of life and psychological stress: A meta-analysis. *Palliative & Supportive Care, 16,* 608–632.

Vos, P. J., Garssen, B., Visser, A. P., Duivenvoorden, H. J., & de Haes, C. J. M. (2004). Early stage breast cancer: Explaining level of psychosocial adjustment using structural equation modeling. *Journal of Behavioral Medicine, 27,* 557-580.

Voss, U., Kolling, T., & Heidenreich, T. (2006). Role of monitoring and blunting coping styles in primary insomnia. *Psychosomatic Medicine, 68,* 110-115.

Vowles, K. E., McCracken, L. M., & Eccleston, C. (2008). Patient functioning and catastrophizing in chronic pain: The mediating effects of acceptance. *Health Psychology, 27,* S136-S143.

Vowles, K. E., Zvolensky, M. J., Gross, R. T., & Sperry, J. A. (2004). Pain-related anxiety in the prediction of chronic low-back pain distress. *Journal of Behavioral Medicine, 27,* 77-89.

Wachholtz, A. B., & Pargament, K. I. (2008). Migraines and meditation: does spirituality matter? *Journal of Behavioral Medicine, 31,* 351-366.

Wade, T. D., Bulik, C. M., Sullivan, P. F., Neale, M. C., & Kendler, K. S. (2000). The relation between risk factors for binge eating and bulimia nervosa: A population-based female twin study. *Health Psychology, 19,* 115-123.

Wager, T. D., Rilling, J. K., Smith, E. E., Sokolik, A., Casey, K. L., Davidson, R. J., . . . Cohen, J. D. (2004). Placebo-induced changes in fMRI in the anticipation and experience of pain. *Science, 303,* 1162-1167.

Waggoner, C. D., & LeLieuvre, R. B. (1981). A method to increase compliance to exercise regimens in rheumatoid arthritis patients. *Journal of Behavioral Medicine, 4,* 191-202.

Wagner, H. S., Ahlstrom, B., Redden, J. P., Vickers, Z., & Mann, T. (2014). The myth of comfort food. *Health Psychology, 33,* 1552-1557.

Wagner, H. S., Howland, M., & Mann, T. (2015). Effects of subtle and explicit health messages on food choice. *Health Psychology, 34,* 79-82.

Wainstock, T., Lerner-Geva, L., Glasser, S., Shoham-Vardi, I., & Anteby, E. Y. (2013). Prenatal stress and risk of spontaneous abortion. *Psychosomatic Medicine, 75,* 228-235.

Waldstein, S. R., Burns, H. O., Toth, M. J., & Poehlman, E. T. (1999). Cardiovascular reactivity and central adiposity in older African Americans. *Health Psychology, 18,* 221-228.

Waldstein, S. R., Jennings, J. R., Ryan, C. M., Muldoon, M. F., Shapiro, A. P., Polefrone, J. M., . . . Manuck, S. B. (1996). Hypertension and neuropsychological performance in men: Interactive effects of age. *Health Psychology, 15,* 102-109.

Walker, H. A., & Chen, E. (2010). The impact of family asthma management on biology: A longitudinal investigation of youth with asthma. *Journal of Behavioral Medicine, 33,* 326-334.

Walker, L. S., Smith, C. A., Garber, J., & Claar, R. L. (2005). Testing a model of pain appraisal and coping in children with chronic abdominal pain. *Health Psychology, 24,* 364-374.

*Wall Street Journal.* (2005, August 9). Fatalities rise after repeal of helmet laws, p. D6.

*Wall Street Journal.* (2016, February 18). Economics and populists don't mix, p. A2.

Waller, J., McCaffery, K. J., Forrest, S., & Wardle, J. (2004). Human papillomavirus and cervical cancer: Issues for biobehavioral and psychosocial research. *Annals of Behavioral Medicine, 27,* 68-79.

Wallston, B. S., Alagna, S. W., DeVellis, B. M., & DeVellis, R. F. (1983). Social support and physical health. *Health Psychology, 2,* 367-391.

Walsh, J. L., Senn, T. E., Scott-Sheldon, L. A. J., Vanable, P. A., & Carey, M. P. (2011). Predicting condom use using the Information-Motivation-Behavioral Skills (IMB) model: A multivariate latent growth curve analysis. *Annals of Behavioral Medicine, 42,* 235-244.

Wang, A. W. T., Chang, C. S., Chen, S. T., Chen, D. R., Fan, F., Carver, C. S., & Hsu, W. Y. (2017). Buffering and direct effect of posttraumatic growth in predicting distress following cancer. *Health Psychology, 36,* 549-559.

Wang, F., DesMeules, M., Luo, W., Dai, S., Lagace, C., & Morrison, H. (2011). Leisure-time physical activity and marital status in relation to depression between men and women: A prospective study. *Health Psychology, 30,* 204-211.

Wang, H. L., Kroenke, K., Wu, J., Tu, W., Theobald, D., & Rawl, S. M. (2012). Predictors of cancer-related pain improvement over time. *Psychosomatic Medicine, 74,* 642-647.

Ward, A., & Mann, T. (2000). Don't mind if I do: Disinhibited eating under cognitive load. *Journal of Personality and Social Psychology, 78,* 753-763.

Ward, B. W., & Schiller, J. S. (2011). Prevalence of complex activity limitations among racial/ethnic groups and Hispanic subgroups of adults: United States, 2003-2009. *NCHS Data Brief, 73,* 1-8.

Ward, S., Donovan, H., Gunnarsdottier, S., Serlin, R. C., Shapiro, G. R., & Hughes, S. (2008). A randomized trial of a representational intervention to decrease cancer pain (RIDcancerPAIN). *Health Psychology, 27,* 59-67.

Wardle, J., Robb, K. A., Johnson, F., Griffith, J., Brunner, E., Power, C., & Tovee, M. (2004). Socioeconomic variation in attitudes to eating and weight in female adolescents. *Health Psychology, 23,* 275-282.

Wardle, J., Williamson, S., McCaffery, K., Sutton, S., Taylor, T., Edwards, R., & Atkin, W. (2003). Increasing attendance at colorectal cancer screening: Testing the efficacy of a mailed, psychoeducational intervention in a community sample of older adults. *Health Psychology, 22,* 99-105.

Ware, J. E., Jr. (1994). Norm-based interpretation. *Medical Outcomes Trust Bulletin, 2,* 3.

Ware, J. E., Jr., Davies-Avery, A., & Stewart, A. L. (1978). The measurement and meaning of patient satisfaction: A review of the literature. *Health and Medical Care Services Review, 1,* 1-15.

Warner, M., Chen, L. H., Makuc, D. M., Anderson, R. N., & Miniño, A. M. (2011). Drug poisoning deaths in the United States, 1980-2008. *NCHS Data Brief, 81,* 1-8.

Warziski, M. T., Sereika, S. M., Styn, M. A., Music, E., & Burke, L. E. (2008). Changes in self-efficacy and dietary adherence: The impact on weight loss in the PREFER study. *Journal of Behavioral Medicine, 31,* 81-92.

Watson, D., & Clark, L. A. (1984). Negative affectivity: The disposition to experience aversive emotional states. *Psychological Bulletin, 96,* 465-490.

Watson, D., & Pennebaker, J. W. (1989). Health complaints, stress, and distress: Exploring the central role of negative affectivity. *Psychological Review, 96,* 234-264.

Watts, K. J., Meiser, B., Wakefield, C. E., Barratt, A. L., Howard, K., Cheah, B. C., Mann, G. J., & Patel, M. I. (2014). Online prostate cancer screening decision aid for men at-risk: A randomized trial. *Health Psychology, 33,* 986-997.

Weaver, J. (2018, July 16). More people search for health online. *NBC News.* Retrieved from https://www.nbcnews.com/

Weaver, K. E., Llabre, M. M., Durán, R. E., Antoni, M. H., Ironson, G., Penedo, F., & Schneiderman, N. (2005). A stress coping model of medication adherence and viral load in HIV-positive men and women on highly active antiretroviral therapy (HAART). *Health Psychology, 24,* 385-392.

Webb, M. S., Simmons, V. N., & Brandon, T. H. (2005). Tailored interventions for motivating smoking cessation: Using placebo tailoring to examine the influence of expectancies and personalization. *Health Psychology, 24,* 179-188.

Webb, M. S., Vanable, P. A., Carey, M. P., & Blair, D. C. (2007). Cigarette smoking among HIV+ men and women: Examining health, substance use, and psychological correlates across the smoking spectrum. *Journal of Behavioral Medicine, 30,* 371-383.

Webb, T. L., & Sheeran, P. (2006). Does changing behavioral intentions engender behavior change? A meta-analysis of the experimental evidence. *Psychological Bulletin, 132,* 249-268.

Weber-Hamann, B., Hentschel, F., Kniest, A., Deuschle, M., Colla, M., Lederbogen, F., & Heuser, I. (2002). Hypercortisolemic depression is associated with increased intra-abdominal fat. *Psychosomatic Medicine, 64,* 274-277.

WebMD. (2014, December). *Type 1 diabetes on the rise in children.* Retrieved May 25, 2016, from http://www.webmd.com/

WebMD. (2015). *Lupus overview.* Retrieved January 21, 2016, from http://www.webmd.com/lupus/arthritis-lupus

Wechsler, H., Lee, J. E., Kuo, M., Seibring, M., Nelson, T. F., & Lee, H. (2002). Trends in college binge drinking during a period of increased prevention efforts. *Journal of American College Health, 50,* 203-217.

Wechsler, H., Seibring, M., Liu, I. C., & Ahl, M. (2004). Colleges respond to student binge drinking: Reducing student demand or limiting access. *Journal of American College Health, 52,* 159-168.

Wegman, H. L., & Stetler, C. (2009). A meta-analytic review of the effects of childhood abuse on medical outcomes in adulthood. *Psychosomatic Medicine, 71,* 805-812.

Weidner, G., Boughal, T., Connor, S. L., Pieper, C., & Mendell, N. R. (1997). Relationship of job strain to standard coronary risk factors and psychological characteristics in women and men of the family heart study. *Health Psychology, 16,* 239-247.

Weidner, G., Rice, T., Knox, S. S., Ellison, C., Province, M. A., Rao, D. C., & Higgins, M. W. (2000). Familial resemblance for hostility: The National Heart, Lung, and Blood Institute Family Heart Study. *Psychosomatic Medicine, 62,* 197-204.

Weihs, K. L., Enright, T. M., & Simmens, S. J. (2008). Close relationships and emotional processing predict decreased mortality in women with breast cancer: Preliminary evidence. *Psychosomatic Medicine, 70,* 117-124.

Weinhardt, L. S., Carey, M. P., Carey, K. B., Maisto, S. A., & Gordon, C. M. (2001). The relation of alcohol use to sexual HIV risk behavior among adults with a severe and persistent mental illness. *Journal of Consulting and Clinical Psychology, 69,* 77-84.

Weinhardt, L. S., Carey, M. P., Johnson, B. T., & Bickman, N. L. (1999). Effects of HIV counseling and testing on sexual risk behavior: A meta-analytic review of published research, 1985-1997. *American Journal of Public Health, 89,* 1397-1405.

Weintraub, A. (2004, January 26). "I can't sleep." *Business Week,* pp. 67-70, 72, 74.

Weir, H. K., Anderson, R. N., Coleman King, S. M., Soman, A., Thompson, T. D., Hong, Y., . . . Leadbetter, S. (2016). Heart disease and cancer deaths—Trends and projections in the United States, 1969-2020. *Preventing Chronic Disease, 13,* E157.

Weisman, A. D. (1972). *On death and dying.* New York: Behavioral Publications.

Weisman, A. D. (1977). The psychiatrist and the inexorable. In H. Feifel (Ed.), *New meanings of death* (pp. 107-122). New York: McGraw-Hill.

Weisman, C. S., & Teitelbaum, M. A. (1985). Physician gender and the physician–patient relationship: Recent evidence and relevant questions. *Social Sciences and Medicine, 20,* 1119-1127.

Weiss, A., Gale, C. R., Batty, D., & Deary, I. J. (2009). Emotionally stable, intelligent men live longer: The Vietnam experience study cohort. *Psychosomatic Medicine, 71,* 385-394.

Weller, J. A., Shackleford, C., Dieckmann, N., & Slovic, P. (2013). Possession attachment predicts cell phone use while driving. *Health Psychology, 32,* 379-387.

Wen, C. K. F., Liao, Y., Maher, J. P., Huh, J., Belcher, B. R., Dzubur, E., & Dunton, G. F. (2018). Relationships among affective states, physical activity, and sedentary behavior in children: Moderation by perceived stress. *Health Psychology, 37,* 904-914.

Wenninger, K., Weiss, C., Wahn, U., & Staab, D. (2003). Body image in cystic fibrosis—Development of a brief diagnostic scale. *Journal of Behavioral Medicine, 26,* 81-94.

Werthmann, J., Jansen, A., Vreugdenhil, A. C. E., Nederkoorn, C., Schyns, G., & Roefs, A. (2015). Food through the child's eye: An eye-tracking study on attentional bias for food in healthy-weight children and children with obesity. *Health Psychology, 34,* 1123-1132.

Whalen, C. K., Jamner, L. D., Henker, B., & Delfino, R. J. (2001). Smoking and moods in adolescents with depressive and aggressive dispositions: Evidence from surveys and electronic diaries. *Health Psychology, 20,* 99-111.

Whetten, K., Reif, S., Whetten, R., & Murphy-McMillan, L. K. (2008). Trauma, mental health, distrust, and stigma among HIV-positive persons: Implications for effective care. *Psychosomatic Medicine, 70,* 531-538.

Whisman, M. A., & Kwon, P. (1993). Life stress and dysphoria: The role of self-esteem and hopelessness. *Journal of Personality and Social Psychology, 65,* 1054-1060.

Whisman, M. A., Li, A., Sbarra, D. A., & Raison, C. L. (2014). Marital quality and diabetes: Results from the Health and Retirement study. *Health Psychology, 33,* 832-840.

Whisman, M. A., & Uebelacker, L. A. (2011). A longitudinal investigation of marital adjustment as a risk factor for metabolic syndrome. *Health Psychology, 31,* 80-86.

Whitbeck, L. B., Hoyt, D. R., McMorris, B. J., Chen, X., & Stubben, J. D. (2001). Perceived discrimination and early substance abuse among American Indian children. *Journal of Health and Social Behavior, 42,* 405-424.

Whitbeck, L. B., McMorris, B. J., Hoyt, D. R., Stubben, J. D., & LaFromboise, T. (2002). Perceived discrimination, traditional practices, and depressive symptoms among American Indians in the upper Midwest. *Journal of Health and Social Behavior, 43,* 400-418.

White, L. P., & Tursky, B. (1982). Where are we? Where are we going? In L. White & B. Tursky (Eds.), *Clinical biofeedback: Efficacy and mechanisms* (pp. 438-448). New York: Guilford Press.

Wichstrom, L. (1994). Predictors of Norwegian adolescents' sunbathing and use of sunscreen. *Health Psychology, 13,* 412-420.

Wichstrom, L., von Soest, T., & Kvalem, I. L. (2013). Predictors of growth and decline in leisure time physical activity from adolescence to adulthood. *Health Psychology, 32,* 775-784.

Wickrama, K., O'Neal, C. W., Lee, T. K., & Wickrama, T. (2015). Early socioeconomic adversity, youth positive development, and young adults' cardiometabolic disease risk. *Health Psychology, 34,* 905-914.

Widman, L., Noar, S. M., Choukas-Bradley, S., & Francis, D. B. (2014). Adolescent sexual health communication and condom use: A meta-analysis. *Health Psychology, 33,* 1113-1124.

Widows, M., Jacobsen, P., Booth-Jones, M., & Fields, K. K. (2005). Predictors of posttraumatic growth following bone marrow transplantation for cancer. *Health Psychology, 24,* 266-273.

Widows, M., Jacobsen, P., & Fields, K. (2000). Relation of psychological vulnerability factors to posttraumatic stress disorder symptomatology in bone marrow transplant recipients. *Psychosomatic Medicine, 62,* 873-882.

Wiest, M., Schüz, B., Webster, N., & Wurm, S. (2011). Subjective well-being and mortality revisited: Differential effects of cognitive and emotional facets of well-being on mortality. *Health Psychology, 30,* 728-735.

Wijngaards-Meij, L., Stroebe, M., Schut, H., Stroebe, W., van den Bout, J., van der Heijden, P., et al. (2005). Couples at risk following the death of their child: Predictors of grief versus depression. *Journal of Consulting and Clinical Psychology, 73,* 617-623.

Wilbert-Lampen, U., Leistner, D., Greven, S., Pohl, T., Sper, S., Völker, C., . . . Steinbeck, G. (2008). Cardiovascular events during world cup soccer. *The New England Journal of Medicine, 358,* 475-483.

Wilcox, S., Evenson, K. R., Aragaki, A., Wassertheil-Smoller, S., Mouton, C. P., & Loevinger, B. L. (2003). The effects of widowhood on physical and mental health, health behaviors, and health outcomes: The women's health initiative. *Health Psychology, 22,* 513–522.

Wild, B., Heider, D., Maatouk, I., Slaets, J., König, H., Niehoff, D., Saum, K., Brenner, H., Söllner, W., & Herzog, W. (2014). Significance and costs of complex biopsychosocial health care needs in elderly people: Results of a population-based study. *Psychosomatic Medicine, 76,* 497–502.

Wilfley, D. E., Tibbs, T. L., Van Buren, D. J., Reach, K. P., Walker, M. S., & Epstein, L. H. (2007). Lifestyle interventions in the treatment of childhood overweight: A meta-analytic review of randomized controlled trials. *Health Psychology, 26,* 521–532.

Willenbring, M. L., Levine, A. S., & Morley, J. E. (1986). Stress induced eating and food preference in humans: A pilot study. *International Journal of Eating Disorders, 5,* 855–864.

Williams, D. R. (2002). Racial/ethnic variations in women's health: The social embeddedness of health. *American Journal of Public Health, 92,* 588–597.

Williams, D. R. (2003). The health of men: Structured inequalities and opportunities. *American Journal of Public Health, 93,* 724–731.

Williams, D. R., & Mohammed, S. A. (2009). Discrimination and racial disparities in health: Evidence and needed research. *Journal of Behavioral Medicine, 32,* 20–47.

Williams, D. R., Priest, N., & Anderson, N. B. (2016). Understanding associations among race, socioeconomic status, and health: Patterns and prospects. *Health Psychology, 35,* 407–411.

Williams, G. C., Gagne, M., Ryan, R. M., & Deci, E. L. (2002). Supporting autonomy to motivate smoking cessation: A test of self-determination theory. *Health Psychology, 21,* 40–50.

Williams, G. C., Lynch, M., & Glasgow, R. E. (2007). Computer-assisted intervention improves patient-centered diabetes care by increasing autonomy support. *Health Psychology, 26,* 728–734.

Williams, G. C., McGregor, H. A., Sharp, D., Kouides, R. W., Levesque, C. S., Ryan, R. M., & Deci, E. L. (2006). A self-determination multiple risk intervention trial to improve smokers health. *Journal of General Internal Medicine, 21,* 1288–1294.

Williams, L., O'Carroll, R. E., & O'Connor, R. C. (2008). Type D personality and cardiac output in response to stress. *Psychology and Health, 24,* 489–500.

Williams, R. B. (1984). An untrusting heart. *The Sciences, 24,* 31–36.

Williams, S., & Kohout, J. L. (1999). Psychologists in medical schools in 1997. *American Psychologist, 54,* 272–276.

Williams, S. A., Kasil, S. V., Heiat, A., Abramson, J. L., Krumholtz, H. M., & Vaccarino, V. (2002). Depression and risk of heart failure among the elderly: A prospective community-based study. *Psychosomatic Medicine, 64,* 6–12.

Williams, S. C., Schmaltz, S. P., Morton, D. J., Koss, R. G., & Loeb, J. M. (2005). Quality of care in U.S. hospitals as reflected by standardized measures, 2002–2004. *The New England Journal of Medicine, 353,* 255–264.

Williamson, G. M., Walters, A. S., & Shaffer, D. R. (2002). Caregiver models of self and others, coping, and depression: Predictors of depression in children with chronic pain. *Health Psychology, 21,* 405–410.

Willmott, L., Harris, P., Gellaitry, G., Cooper, V., & Horne, R. (2011). The effects of expressive writing following first myocardial infarction: A randomized controlled trial. *Health Psychology, 30,* 642–650.

Wills, T. A. (1984). Supportive functions of interpersonal relationships. In S. Cohen & L. Syme (Eds.), *Social support and health* (pp. 61–82). New York: Academic Press.

Wills, T. A., Bantum, E. O., Pokhrel, P., Maddock, J. E., Ainette, M. G., Morehouse, E., & Fenster, B. (2013). A dual-process model of early

substance use: Tests in two diverse populations of adolescents. *Health Psychology, 32,* 533–542.

Wills, T. A., Gibbons, F. X., Sargent, J. D., Gerrard, M., Lee, H. R., & Dal Cin, S. (2010). Good self-control moderates the effect of mass media on adolescent tobacco and alcohol use: Tests with studies of children and adolescents. *Health Psychology, 29,* 539–549.

Wills, T. A., Sandy, J. M., & Yaeger, A. M. (2002). Stress and smoking in adolescence: A test of directional hypotheses. *Health Psychology, 21,* 122–130.

Wills, T. A., & Vaughan, R. (1989). Social support and substance use in early adolescence. *Journal of Behavioral Medicine, 12,* 321–340.

Wilson, R. (1963). The social structure of a general hospital. *Annals of the American Academy of Political and Social Science, 346,* 67–76.

Wilson, P. A., Stadler, G., Boone, M. R., & Bolger, N. (2014). Fluctuations in depression and well-being are associated with sexual risk episodes among HIV-positive men. *Health Psychology, 33,* 681–685.

Wilson, R. S., Beck, T. L., Bienias, J. L., & Bennett, D. A. (2007). Terminal cognitive decline: Accelerated loss of cognition in the last years of life. *Psychosomatic Medicine, 69,* 131–137.

Wilson, T. E., Weedon, J., Cohen, M. H., Golub, E. T., Milam, J., Young, M. A., . . . Fredrickson, B. L. (2017). Positive affect and its association with viral control among women with HIV infection. *Health Psychology, 36,* 91–100.

Winett, R. A., Wagner, J. L., Moore, J. F., Walker, W. B., Hite, L. A., Leahy, M., . . . Lombard, D. (1991). An experimental evaluation of a prototype public access nutrition information system for supermarkets. *Health Psychology, 10,* 75–78.

Wing, R. R. (2000). Cross-cutting themes in maintenance of behavior change. *Health Psychology, 19,* 84–88.

Wing, R. R., Blair, E., Marcus, M., Epstein, L. H., & Harvey, J. (1994). Year-long weight loss treatment for obese patients with type II diabetes: Does including an intermittent very-low-calorie diet improve outcome? *American Journal of Medicine, 97,* 354–362.

Wing, R. R., Epstein, L. H., Nowalk, M. P., Scott, N., Koeske, R., & Hagg, S. (1986). Does self-monitoring of blood glucose levels improve dietary competence for obese patients with Type II diabetes? *American Journal of Medicine, 81,* 830–836.

Wing, R. R., Matthews, K. A., Kuller, L. H., Meilahn, E. N., & Plantinga, P. L. (1991). Weight gain at the time of menopause. *Archives of Internal Medicine, 151,* 97–102.

Winning, A., McCormick, M. C., Glymour, M. M., Gilsanz, P., & Kubzansky, L. D. (2018). Childhood psychological distress and healthy cardiovascular lifestyle 17–35 years later: The potential role of mental health in primordial prevention. *Annals of Behavioral Medicine, 52,* 621–632.

Winslow, R. (2016, January 28). Cancer centers urge vaccinations for HPV. *Wall Street Journal,* p. A3.

Wirtz, P. H., Ehlert, U., Emini, L., Rüdisüli, K., Groessbauer, S., Gaab, J., . . . von Känel, R. (2006). Anticipatory cognitive stress appraisal and the acute procoagulant stress response in men. *Psychosomatic Medicine, 68,* 851–858.

Wirtz, P. H., von Känel, R., Schnorpfeil, P., Ehlert, U., Frey, K., & Fischer, J. E. (2003). Reduced glucocorticoid sensitivity of monocyte interleukin-6 production in male industrial employees who are vitally exhausted. *Psychosomatic Medicine, 65,* 672–678.

Wise, R. (2013). Dual roles of dopamine in food and drug seeking: The drive-reward paradox. *Biological Psychiatry, 73,* 819–826.

Wisniewski, L., Epstein, L., Marcus, M. D., & Kaye, W. (1997). Differences in salivary habituation to palatable foods in bulimia nervosa patients and controls. *Psychosomatic Medicine, 59,* 427–433.

Witkiewitz, K., & Marlatt, G. A. (2004). Relapse prevention for alcohol and drug problems: That was Zen, this is Tao. *American Psychologist, 59,* 224–235.

Wolf, L. D., & Davis, M. C. (2014). Loneliness, daily pain, and perceptions of interpersonal events in adults with fibromyalgia. *Health Psychology, 33,* 929–937.

Wolf, S. L., Thompson, P. A., Winstein, C. J., Miller, J. P., Blanton, S, R., Nichols-Larsen, D. S., . . . Sawaki, L. (2010). The EXCITE stroke trial: Comparing early and delayed constraint-induced movement therapy. *Stroke, 41,* 2309–2315.

Wolf, T., Tsenkova, V., Ryff, C. D., Davidson, R. J., & Willette, A. A. (2018). Neural, hormonal, and cognitive correlates of metabolic dysfunction and emotional reactivity. *Psychosomatic Medicine, 80,* 452–459.

Wolff, B., Burns, J. W., Quartana, P. J., Lofland, K., Bruehl, S., & Chung, O. Y. (2008). Pain catastrophizing, physiological indexes, and chronic pain severity: Tests of mediation and moderation models. *Journal of Behavioral Medicine, 31,* 105–114.

Wolff, N. J., Darlington, A. E., Hunfeld, J. A. M., Verhulst, F. C., Jaddoe, V. W. V., Moll, H. A., . . . Tiemeier, H. (2009). The association of parent behaviors, chronic pain, and psychological problems with venipuncture distress in infants: The generation R study. *Health Psychology, 28,* 605–613.

Womack, V. Y., De Chavez, P. J., Albrecht, S. S., Durant, N., Loucks, E. B., Puterman, E., . . . Carnethon, M. R. (2016). A longitudinal relationship between depressive symptoms and development of metabolic syndrome: The coronary artery risk development in young adults (CARDIA) study. *Psychosomatic Medicine, 78,* 867–873.

Wong, M., & Kaloupek, D. G. (1986). Coping with dental treatment: The potential impact of situational demands. *Journal of Behavioral Medicine, 9,* 579–598.

Wong, M. D., Shapiro, M. F., Boscardin, W. J., & Ettner, S. L. (2002). Contribution of major diseases to disparities in mortality. *The New England Journal of Medicine, 347,* 1585–1592.

Woodall, K. L., & Matthews, K. A. (1993). Changes in and stability of hostile characteristics: Results from a 4-year longitudinal study of children. *Journal of Personality and Social Psychology, 64,* 491–499.

*The World Factbook 2009.* Washington, DC: Central Intelligence Agency, 2009. Retrieved July 2, 2012, from https://www.cia.gov/library/publications/the-world-factbook/index.html

World Health Organization. (1948). *Constitution of the World Health Organization.* Geneva, Switzerland: World Health Organization Basic Documents.

World Health Organization. (2008, May). *World health statistics, 2008.* Retrieved August 23, 2012, from http://www.who.int/whosis/whostat/EN_WHS08_Full.pdf

World Health Organization. (2010). *Diabetes programme.* Retrieved July 22, 2010, from http://www.who.int/diabetes/actionnow/en/mapdiabprev.pdf

World Health Organization. (2011, March). *Obesity and overweight.* Retrieved April 24, 2012, from http://www.who.int/mediacentre/factsheets/fs311/en

World Health Organization. (2015). *Hepatitis C.* Retrieved January 21, 2016, from http://www.who.int

World Health Organization. (2015, November). *Number of women living with HIV.* Retrieved May 25, 2016, from http://www.who.int

World Health Organization. (2016a). *Global health estimates 2016.* Geneva: Author.

World Health Organization. (2016b). *Headache disorders.* Retrieved April 30, 2019, from https://www.who.int/news-room/fact-sheets/detail/headache-disorders

World Health Organization. (2017, August 31). *Asthma: Key facts.* Retrieved March 11, 2019, from https://www.who.int/en/news-room/fact-sheets/detail/asthma

World Health Organization. (2017, October). *Tenfold increase in childhood and adolescent obesity in four decades: New study by Imperial College London and WHO.* Retrieved June 4, 2019, from https://www.who.int

World Health Organization. (2018a). *Global status report on alcohol and health 2018.* Retrieved April 8, 2019, from https://apps.who.int/iris/bitstream/handle/10665/274603/9789241565639-eng.pdf

World Health Organization. (2018b). *Life expectancy and healthy life expectancy data by WHO region.* Retrieved from http://apps.who.int/gho/data/view.main.SDG2016LEXREGv?lang=en

World Health Organization. (2018, February 16). *Obesity and overweight.* Retrieved April 8, 2019, from https://www.who.int/news-room/fact-sheets/detail/obesity-and-overweight

World Health Organization. (2018, May). *The top 10 causes of death.* Retrieved March 11, 2019, from https://www.who.int/news-room/fact-sheets/detail/the-top-10-causes-of-death

World Health Organization. (2018, November 12). *Projections of mortality and causes of death, 2016 to 2060.* Retrieved March 11, 2019, from https://www.who.int/healthinfo/global_burden_disease/projections/en/

World Health Organization. (2018, December 7). *Road traffic injuries: Key facts.* Retrieved April 1, 2019, from https://www.who.int/news-room/fact-sheets/detail/road-traffic-injuries

World Health Organization. (2019a). *HIV.* Retrieved May 29, 2019, from https://www.who.int/hiv/en/

World Health Organization. (2019b). *The top 10 causes of death.* Retrieved May 29, 2019, from https://www.who.int/news-room/fact-sheets/detail/the-top-10-causes-of-death

World Health Organization. (2019c). *Life expectancy.* Retrieved May 7, 2019, from https://www.who.int/gho/mortality_burden_disease/life_tables/situation_trends_text/en/

World Health Organization. (2019d). *HIV.* Retrieved May 29, 2019, from https://www.who.int/hiv/en/

World Health Organization. (2019, May 29). *Tobacco.* Retrieved April 8, 2019, from https://www.who.int/news-room/fact-sheets/detail/tobacco

Worobey, M., Watts, T. D., McKay, R. A., Suchard, M. A., Granade, T., Teuwen, D. E., . . . Jaffe, H. W. (2016). 1970s and 'Patient 0'HIV-1 genomes illuminate early HIV/AIDS history in North America. *Nature, 539,* 98–101.

Worthington, E. L., Witvliet, C. V. O., Pietrini, P., & Miller, A. J. (2007). Forgiveness, health, and well-being: A review of evidence for emotional versus decisional forgiveness, dispositional forgivingness, and reduced unforgiving. *Journal of Behavioral Medicine, 30,* 291–302.

Wroe, A. L. (2001). Intentional and unintentional nonadherence: A study of decision making. *Journal of Behavioral Medicine, 25,* 355–372.

Wrosch, C., Miller, G. E., & Schulz, R. (2009). Cortisol secretion and functional disabilities in old age: Importance of using adaptive control strategies. *Psychosomatic Medicine, 71,* 996–1003.

Wrulich, M., Brunner, M., Stadler, G., Schalke, D., Keller, U., & Martin, R. (2014). Forty years on: Childhood intelligence predicts health in middle adulthood. *Health Psychology, 33,* 292–296.

Wu, S., Fisher-Hoch, S. P., Reininger, B. M., & McCormick, J. B. (2018). Association between fruit and vegetable intake and symptoms of mental health conditions in Mexican Americans. *Health Psychology, 37,* 1059–1066.

Wu, T., Treiber, F. A., & Snieder, H. (2013). Genetic influence on blood pressure and underlying hemodynamics measured at rest and during stress. *Psychosomatic Medicine, 75,* 404–412.

Wu, Y., Rausch, J., Rohan, J. M., Hood, K. K., Pendley, J. S., Delamater, A., & Drotar, D. (2014). Autonomy support and responsibility-sharing predict blood glucose monitoring frequency among youth with diabetes. *Health Psychology, 33,* 1224–1231.

Wulsin, L. R., Vaillant, G. E., & Wells, V. E. (1999). A systematic review of the mortality of depression. *Psychosomatic Medicine, 61,* 6–17.

Wyatt, G. E., Gomez, C. A., Hamilton, A. B., Valencia-Garcia, D., Gant, L. M., & Graham, C. E. (2013). The intersection of gender and ethnicity in

HIV risk, interventions, and prevention: New frontiers for psychology. *American Psychologist, 68,* 247–260.

Wynder, E. L., Kajitani, T., Kuno, I. J., Lucas, J. C., Jr., DePalo, A., & Farrow, J. (1963). A comparison of survival rates between American and Japanese patients with breast cancer. *Surgery, Gynecology, Obstetrics, 117,* 196–200.

Wysocki, T., Green, L., & Huxtable, K. (1989). Blood glucose monitoring by diabetic adolescents: Compliance and metabolic control. *Health Psychology, 8,* 267–284.

Wyszynski, C. M., Bricker, J. B., & Comstock, B. A. (2011). Parental smoking cessation and child daily smoking: A 9-year longitudinal study of mediation by child cognitions about smoking. *Health Psychology, 30,* 171–176.

Xian, H., Scherrer, J. F., Franz, C. E., McCaffery, J., Stein, P. K., Lyons, M. J., . . . Kremen, W. S. (2010). Genetic vulnerability and phenotypic expression of depression and risk for ischemic heart disease in the Vietnam Era Twin Study of Aging. *Psychosomatic Medicine, 72,* 370–375.

Xu, J., Kochanek, K. D., Murphy, S. L., & Arias, E. (2014). Mortality in the United States, 2012. *NCHS Data Brief, 168,* 1–7.

Xu, J., Murphy, S. L., Kochanek, K. D., Bastian, B., & Arias, E. (2018). Deaths: Final data for 2016. *National Vital Statistics Report, 67*(5), 1–76.

Xu, J., & Roberts, R. E. (2010). The power of positive emotions: It's a matter of life or death—Subjective well-being and longevity over 28 years in a general population. *Health Psychology, 29,* 9–19.

Xu, W., Qiu, C., Gatz, M., Pedersen, N. L., Johansson, B., & Fratiglioni, L. (2009). Mid- and late-life diabetes in relation to the risk of dementia: A population-based twin study. *Diabetes, 58,* 71–77.

Xu, X., Bao, H., Strait, K. M., Edmondson, D. E., Davidson, K. W., Beltrame, J. F., . . . Krumholz, H. M. (2017). Perceived stress after acute myocardial infarction: A comparison between young and middle-aged women versus men. *Psychosomatic Medicine, 79,* 50–58.

Yali, A. M., & Revenson, T. A. (2004). How changes in population demographics will impact health psychology: Incorporating a broader notion of cultural competence into the field. *Health Psychology, 23,* 147–155.

Yamada, T. (2008). In search of new ideas for global health. *New England Journal of Medicine, 358,* 1324–1325.

Yamada, Y., Izawa, H., Ichihara, S., Takatsu, F., Ishihara, H., Hirayama, H., . . . Yokata, M. (2002). Prediction of the risk of myocardial infarction from polymorphisms in candidate genes. *The New England Journal of Medicine, 347,* 1916–1923.

Ybema, J. F., Kuijer, R. G., Buunk, B. P., DeJong, G. M., & Sanderman, R. (2001). Depression and perceptions of inequity among couples facing cancer. *Personality and Social Psychology Bulletin, 27,* 3–13.

Yi, J. P., Yi, J. C., Vitaliano, P. P., & Weinger, K. (2008). How does anger coping style affect glycemic control in diabetes patients? *International Journal of Behavioral Medicine, 15,* 167–172.

Yong, H., Borland, R., Thrasher, J. F., Thompson, M. E., Nagelhout, G. E., Fong, G. T., & Cummings, K. M. (2014). Mediational pathways of the impact of cigarette warning labels on quit attempts. *Health Psychology, 33,* 1410–1420.

Yong, H. H., & Borland, R. (2008). Functional beliefs about smoking and quitting activity among adult smokers in four countries: Findings from the international tobacco control four-country survey. *Health Psychology, 27,* S216–S223.

Yoon, S. S., Burt, V., Louis, T., & Carroll, M. D. (2012). Hypertension among adults in the United States, 2009–2010. *NCHS Data Brief, 107,* 1–8.

Young, D. R., He, X., Genkinger, J., Sapun, M., Mabry, I., & Jehn, M. (2004). Health status among urban African American women: Associations among well-being, perceived stress, and demographic factors. *Journal of Behavioral Medicine, 27,* 63–76.

Zajacova, A., & Burgard, S. A. (2010). Body weight and health from early to mid-adulthood: A longitudinal analysis. *Journal of Health and Social Behavior, 51,* 92–107.

Zajdel, M., Helgeson, V. S., Seltman, H. J., Korytkowski, M. T., & Hausmann, L. R. M. (2018). Daily communal coping in couples with type 2 diabetes: Links to mood and self-care. *Annals of Behavioral Medicine, 52,* 228–238.

Zakowski, S. G., Hall, M. H., Klein, L. C., & Baum, A. (2001). Appraised control, coping, and stress in a community sample: A test of the goodness-of-fit hypothesis. *Annals of Behavioral Medicine, 23,* 158–165.

Zastowny, T. R., Kirschenbaum, D. S., & Meng, A. L. (1986). Coping skills training for children: Effects on distress before, during, and after hospitalization for surgery. *Health Psychology, 5,* 231–247.

Zautra, A. J. (2009). Resilience: One part recovery, two parts sustainability. *Journal of Personality, 77,* 1935–1943.

Zautra, A. J., Fasman, R., Davis, M. C., & Craig, A. D. (2010). The effects of slow breathing on affective responses to pain stimuli: An experimental study. *Pain, 149,* 12–18.

Zautra, A. J., Fasman, R., Reich, J. W., Harakas, P., Johnson, L. M., Olmsted, M. E., & Davis, M. C. (2005). Fibromyalgia: Evidence for deficits in positive affect regulation. *Psychosomatic Medicine, 67,* 147–155.

Zautra, A. J., Hall, J. S., & Murray, K. E. (2008). Resilience: A new integrative approach to health and mental health research. *Health Psychology Review, 2,* 41–64.

Zautra, A. J., & Manne, S. L. (1992). Coping with rheumatoid arthritis: A review of a decade of research. *Annals of Behavioral Medicine, 14,* 31–39.

Zautra, A. J., Okun, M. A., Roth, S. H., & Emmanual, J. (1989). Life stress and lymphocyte alterations among patients with rheumatoid arthritis. *Health Psychology, 8,* 1–14.

Zautra, A. J., & Smith, B. W. (2001). Depression and reactivity to stress in older women with rheumatoid arthritis and osteoarthritis. *Psychosomatic Medicine, 63,* 687–696.

Zawadzki, M. J., Graham, J. E., & Gerin, W. (2013). Rumination and anxiety mediate the effect of loneliness on depressed mood and sleep quality in college students. *Health Psychology, 32,* 212–222.

Zelinski, E. M., Crimmins, E., Reynolds, S., & Seeman, T. (1998). Do medical conditions affect cognition in older adults? *Health Psychology, 17,* 504–512.

Zernicke, K. A., Campbell, T. S., Speca, M., McCabe-Ruff, K., Flowers, S., & Carlson, L. E. (2014). A randomized wait-list controlled trial of feasibility and efficacy of an online mindfulness-based cancer recovery program: The eTherapy for cancer applying mindfullness trial. *Psychosomatic Medicine, 76,* 257–267.

Zhang, J., Kahana, B., Kahana, E., Hu, B., & Pozuelo, L. (2009). Joint modeling of longitudinal changes in depressive symptoms and mortality in a sample of community-dwelling elderly people. *Psychosomatic Medicine, 71,* 704–714.

Zhao, J., Bremner, J. D., Goldberg, J., Quyyumi, A. A., & Vaccarino, V. (2013). Monoamine oxidase a genotype, childhood trauma, and subclinical atherosclerosis: A twin study. *Psychosomatic Medicine, 75,* 471–477.

Zheng, Z. J., Croft, J. B., Labarthe, D., Williams, J. E., & Mensah, G. A. (2001). Racial disparity in coronary heart disease mortality in the United States: Has the gap narrowed? *Circulation 2001, 104,* 787.

Zhu, C. (2010). Science-based health care. *Science, 327,* 1429.

Zhu, L., Ranchor, A. V., Helgeson, V. S., van der Lee, M., Garssen, B., Stewart, R. E., . . . Schroevers, M. J. (2018). Benefit finding trajectories in cancer patients receiving psychological care: Predictors and relations to depressive and anxiety symptoms. *British Journal of Health Psychology, 23,* 238–252.

Ziadni, M. S., Carty, J. N., Doherty, H. K., Porcerelli, J. H., Rapport, L. J., Schubiner, H., & Lumley, M. A. (2018). A life-stress, emotional awareness, and expression interview for primary care patients with medically unexplained symptoms: A randomized controlled trial. *Health Psychology, 37,* 282–290.

Ziegelstein, R. C., Kim, S. Y., Kao, D., Fauerbach, J. A., Thombs, B. D., McCann, U., . . . Bush, D. E. (2005). Can doctors and nurses recognize depression in patients hospitalized with an acute myocardial infarction in the absence of formal screening? *Psychosomatic Medicine, 67,* 393–397.

Zillman, D., de Wied, M., King-Jablonski, C., & Jenzowsky, S. (1996). Drama-induced affect and pain sensitivity. *Psychosomatic Medicine, 58,* 333–341.

Zimbardo, P. G. (1969). The human choice: Individuation, reason, and order versus deindividuation, impulse, and chaos. In W. J. Arnold & D. Levine (Eds.), *Nebraska symposium on motivation.* Lincoln: University of Nebraska Press.

Zimmer, C. (2001). Do chronic diseases have an infectious root? *Science, 293,* 1974–1977.

Zimmerman, R. (2005, March 15). Nonconventional therapies gain broader acceptance. *Wall Street Journal,* p. 24.

Zimmermann, T., Heinrichs, N., & Baucom, D. H. (2007). "Does one size fit all?" Moderators in psychosocial interventions for breast cancer patients: A meta-analysis. *Annals of Behavioral Medicine, 34,* 225–239.

Zisook, S., Shuchter, S. R., Irwin, M., Darko, D. F., Sledge, P., & Resovsky, K. (1994). Bereavement, depression, and immune function. *Psychiatry Research, 52,* 1–10.

Zoccola, P. M., Dickerson, S. S., & Lam, S. (2009). Rumination predicts longer sleep onset latency after an acute psychosocial stressor. *Psychosomatic Medicine, 71,* 771–775.

Zoccola, P. M., Figueroa, W. S., Rabideau, E. M., Woody, A., & Benencia, F. (2014). Differential effects of poststressor rumination and distraction on cortisol and C-reactive protein. *Health Psychology, 33,* 1606–1609.

Trompetter, H. R., 155
Troop, N., 99
Trouillet, R., 47
Troxel, W. M., 273, 275
Trudel-Fitzgerald, C., 292, 314
Trumbetta, S. L., 329
Truskier, M., 299
Tsai, M. L., 197
Tsao, J., 212
Tsauo, J. Y., 200
Tschann, J. M., 43, 126
Tseng, M., 139, 298
Tsenkova, V. K., 292, 294
Tsuji, I., 150
Tu, W., 314
Tucker, D. C., 317
Tucker, J. S., 148–149, 308
Tugade, M. M., 150
Tuinman, M. A., 314
Tulen, J. H. M., 80
Tulloch, H., 280
Tully, P. J., 292
Tuomilehto, J., 293
Tuomisto, M., 142
Tuppurainen, M. T., 233
Turiano, N. A., 148
Turk, D. C., 187, 212–213,
    218–219, 226
Turkheimer, E., 89
Turner, D. S., 72
Turner, E., 299
Turner, J. C., 174
Turner, L. R., 76
Turner, N., 154
Turner, R. A., 131
Turner, R. B., 131, 142
Turner, R. J., 133, 138, 235
Turner, S. L., 320
Turner-Cobb, J. M., 161, 309
Turnwald, B. P., 78
Turrisi, R., 76
Tursky, B., 222
Tuschen-Caffier, B., 99
Tweed, R. G., 267
Tworoger, S. S., 314
Tyrrell, D. A. J., 299
Tyson, M., 50
Tzourio, C., 19

## U

Ubel, P. A., 49
Uchino, B. N., 132, 151, 159, 161–163,
    277, 282
Uda, M., 88
Uddin, S., 180
Uebelacker, L. A., 292
Ueda, H., 299
Ulbricht, C. M., 211
Uller, C., 115
Umberson, D., 161, 162, 267, 330
Umberson, D. J., 162
Ung, E., 246

Updegraff, J. A., 48, 123, 305
Urban, M. A., 305
Urcuyo, K. R., 310
Urry, H. L., 80, 237
Ursano, R. J., 132
Ursell, A., 78
Uskul, A. K., 115
Uswatte, G., 289
Uutela, A., 150
Uysal, A., 117
Uziel, O., 159

## V

Väänänen, A., 267
Vaccarino, V., 31
Vago, D. R., 155, 200
Vahtera, J., 80, 139, 141, 267
Vaillancourt, T., 110
Vaillant, G. E., 199, 235
Valach, L., 51
Valdimarsdottir, H. B., 58, 313
Valencia-Garcia, D., 305
Valet, M., 212
Valkanova, V., 330
Vallance, J. K. H., 316
Valle, T. T., 293
Valrie, C. R., 211
Valverde, R. H., 247, 264
Vamos, E. P., 174
Vanable, P. A., 304, 305, 307, 308
Vanaelst, B., 142
Van Beugen, S., 155, 200
Van Boxtel, G. J., 155, 200
Van Buren, D. J., 97
van Cutsem, G., 303
Vandelanotte, C., 43, 79
van den Berg, J. F., 80
Vandenberg, R. J., 70
van den Boom, W., 308
van den Bout, J., 267
Van den Putte, B., 111
van de Putte, L., 318
van der Beek, A. J., 238
VanderDrift, L. E., 307
van der Heijden, P., 267
Van der Heijden, P. G. M., 245
Van der Laan, L. N., 79
van der Lee, M., 315
van der Leeden, R., 126, 174
Vandermorris, S., 69
van der Most, P. J., 292
Van der Ploeg, H. P., 238
Van Der Pol, W. J., 27
van der Staak, C., 318
van der Voort, P. H., 11
Vander Wal, J. S., 59
Vander Weg, M. W., 57
van der Woude, L. H. V., 238
Van der Zwaluw, C. S., 101
van Doornen, L. J., 239
van Dulmen, M. H. M., 155
Vangeepuram, N., 24

van Gils, A., 239
Van Gorp, W., 309
Vanhala, M., 275
Vanhalst, J., 320
van Harten, W. H., 238
Vanhoeffen, S., 99
Van Horn, L., 77
Van Horn, M. L., 69
van Houwelingen, H. C., 223
Van Jaarsveld, C. H. M., 85
Van Kessel, K., 58–59, 246
van Koningsbruggen, G. M., 52, 156
VanLanduyt, L. M., 68
Van Lankveld, W., 318
Van Lieshout, R. J., 196
Van Liew, J. R., 315
Van Loey, N., E. E., 245
van Mechelen, W., 238
van Meijel, E. P. M., 132
Vannatta, K., 264
Vannucci, A., 85
Van Os, J., 126
Van Reedt Dortland, A. K. B., 91
Van Rijn, I., 78
Van Rood, Y. R., 223
Van Ryn, M., 183
van Schuur, W. H., 318
Van Son, M. J. M., 245
van Sonderen, E., 278
Van Stralen, M. M., 70
van Straten, A., 64
van't Pad Bosch, P., 318
van Veen, T., 91
van Veldhuisen, D. J., 278
Van Wasshenova, E., 48
Van YPeren, N. W., 193
van Zon, S. K., 292
Van Zundert, R. M. P., 114
Varker, T., 132
Varosy, P. D., 275
Vartanian, L. R., 91, 94
Vaughan, R., 160
Vavak, C. R., 276
Vedhara, K., 156
Veehof, M. M., 155
Veitch, J., 89
Vela-Bueno, A., 80
Veldhuijzen van Zanten, J. J., 47
Velicer, W., 335
Velicer, W. F., 59
Vella, L., 235
Vena, J. E., 107
Vendrig, A., 225
Ventrelle, J., 271
Ventuneac, A., 307
Verbrugge, L. M., 142, 268, 318
ver Halen, N. B., 138
Verhulst, F. C., 196
Verkes, R. J., 101
Vermont, L. N., 108
Vermulst, A. A., 101
Vermunt, J. K., 300
Vesper, J. M., 278

## A

AA (AlcoholicsAnonymous), 104
abstinence violation effect, 57, 113-114
ACA (Patient Protection and Affordable Care Act), 325
acceptance, as stage of dying, 261
acceptance and commitment therapy (ACT), 155, 224-225, 247
accidents, 71-73, 107, 253
acquired immune deficiency syndrome (AIDS). *See* HIV/AIDS
ACT (acceptance and commitment therapy), 155, 224-225, 247
ACTH (adrenocorticotropic hormone), 19, 125
action stage, 60
acupuncture, 199, 225
acute disorders, 7
acute illness, model of, 171
acute pain
    defined, 217
    recurrent, 217
    *vs.* chronic pain, 217-218
acute stress paradigm, 131, 160-161
addiction, 101, 220
A-delta fibers, 215
ADH (antidiuretic hormone), 19
adherence, 186, 187, 189, 238, 293, 308-309, 320. *See also* health behavior change
adolescents
    and alcoholism/problem drinking, 106-107
    death in, 254
    and diabetes, 320-321
    and diet, 77
    health behaviors in, 45
    and health-compromising behaviors, 84
    and HIV/AIDS, 306
    and smoking, 110-111, 113
adoption studies, 30
adrenal glands, 19, 20
adrenocorticotropic hormone (ACTH), 19, 125
aerobic exercise, 68
African Americans. *See also* race
    hypertension among, 284-285
aftereffects of stress, 130
aging. *See* older adults
AIDS. *See* HIV/AIDS
alarm phase of stress, 122
AlcoholEdu, 106
Alcoholics Anonymous (AA), 104
alcoholism/problem drinking, 54, 100-107
    extent of, 100-101
    interventions for, 102-104
    origins of, 101-102
allergies, 24, 35

allostatic load, 127-128
Alzheimer's disease, 19, 235
amenorrhea, 29
American Psychological Association (APA), 7
amygdala, 16
anatomical barriers, 33
anger, 275, 276, 284
    as stage of dying, 261
angina pectoris, 22
anorexia nervosa, 98-99
antabuse, 54
antibiotics, 35
antibodies, 34
anticipatory grief, 261, 263
antidiuretic hormone (ADH), 19
antigens, 34
antimicrobial substances, 33
antiretroviral therapy (ART), 303-304, 308
anxiety, 92, 174, 205, 234, 261
appendicitis, 26
appraisal delay, 176
approach (confrontative, vigilant) coping style, 150-153, 278
arrhythmia, 22
ART (antiretroviral therapy), 303-304, 308
arthritis, 317-319
artificial intelligence, 186
aspirin, 288
assertiveness training, 56
assisted death, 257, 258, 259
asthma, 24, 35
atherosclerosis, 22, 272. *See also* coronary heart disease (CHD)
at-risk people, 41
    interventions with, 45-46
attentional retraining, 94, 112
attitude theories, criticisms of, 50-51
autoimmune disorders, 36
    defined, 299
    multiple sclerosis, 18
    rheumatoid arthritis, 317-318
    Type 1 diabetes, 20
automobile accidents, 72, 73, 254
avoidant (minimizing) coping style, 150-153
avoidant/passive coping, 313
ayurvedic medicine, 197

## B

baby talk, 183
bacterial infections, 24
Barbie doll, 97
bargaining, 261
bargaining, as stage of dying, 261
behavioral assignments, 55-56
behavioral delay, 176

behavioral immunization, 326
behavior change. *See* health behavior change
beliefs, about chronic health disorders, 237-238
benefit finding, 301
bereavement, 265-268
Berlin Wall, 103
bile, 25
bilirubin, 27
binge eating disorder, 100
biofeedback, 222
biological transmission, 32
biomedical model, 5
biopsychosocial model, 160-161
    advantages of, 5-6
    clinical implications of, 6
    defined, 5
    nightmare deaths, case of, 6
blood, 20, 22-23
blood pressure, 22
BMI (body mass index), 86, 87
body image, 235-236
body mass index (BMI), 86, 87
body systems, 15-36
    cardiovascular system, 20-23
    digestive system, 25-27
    endocrine system, 19-20
    immune system, 31-36
    nervous system, 15-19
    renal system, 27-28
    reproductive system, 28-30
    respiratory system, 23-25
bolus, 25
Bonica, John, 225
brain, 15-17, 155, 212-213, 215-216
    and gut communication, 27
    health behavior change and, 52-53
breast cancer, 73, 74
Brief COPE, 151
bronchial pneumonia, 25
bronchitis, 24
buffering hypothesis, 161
bulimia, 99-100
burnout, 192, 193

## C

CABG (coronary artery bypass graft) surgery, 279
CAM. *See* complementary and alternative medicine (CAM)
cancer, 310-317
    in children, 253
    hard to study, 311
    interventions for, 314-316
    and placebo effect, 204

creative nonadherence, 187–188
CRH (corticotrophin-releasing hormone), 125
CSN (Combat Stress Now), 157
cue elimination, 58
cultural differences, 47, 212, 266.
    *See also* ethnicity; race
curative care, 262
CVD. *See* cardiovascular disease (CVD)
cyclic illness, 171
cystic fibrosis (CF), 248
cysts, 29
cytokines, 297

## D

daily hassles, 134–136
death/dying, 251–268
    in adolescents, 254
    alternatives to hospitalization, 264–265
    assisted, 257, 258, 259
    and bereavement, 265–268
    causes of, 7, 8, 11, 41, 252–254
    in children, 252–254, 264, 267–268
    in infancy and childhood, 252–254
    life expectancy, 255, 256
    in middle age, 255
    and nontraditional treatment, 260
    and older adults, 255
    physician-assisted, 257–259
    psychological issues in, 257–260, 262–264
    stages of, 260–262
    in young adulthood, 254–255
death education, 268
delay behavior, 175–177, 279
demand-control-support model, 140
dementia, 18–19
denial, 233–234, 260
depersonalization, 183
depression
    and alcoholism/problem drinking, 102
    and cancer, 313, 314
    and chronic health disorders, 234–235
    and coronary heart disease, 277–278, 281
    defined, 234
    and diabetes, 294
    HIV/AIDS and, 304
    and hypertension, 284
    and immune system, 299–300
    and obesity, 91
    and pain, 219
    and smoking, 108
    as stage of dying, 261
    and stress eating, 92
    and use of health care services, 174
detoxification, 102
diabetes, 19–20, 25, 290–294, 319–321
    health implications of, 292
    psychosocial factors in development, 282–283
diarrhea, 26
diet, 76–79
    balanced, USDA recommendations for, 76
    and complementary and alternative
        medicine, 198

and coronary heart disease, 280
and hypertension, 286
and obesity, 86, 89
dietary supplements, 198
dieting, 91–92, 93
dietitians, 241
digestive system, 25–27
direct effects hypothesis, 161
direct transmission, 31
disclosure, 304–305, 309
discriminative stimulus, 52
distraction, 223
doctors. *See* health care services
double-blind experiment, 206
drug abuse. *See* substance abuse
drugs. *See* medication
drunk driving, 107
duodenum, 25
dysbiosis, 27
dysentery, 26

## E

eating disorders, 97–100
education. *See* community-based
        interventions
elderly people. *See* older adults
emotional support, 159
emotion-focused coping, 153
emotions, 43
employment. *See* workplace
endocrine system, 19–20
endogenous opioid peptides, 216
endometrial cancer, 29
endometriosis, 29
epidemiology, 11
epilepsy, 17–18, 240
epinephrine, 17, 19, 125
estrogen, 28, 274–275
ethnicity
    and health behaviors, 47
    and health promotion, 329
    and patient–provider communication, 183
etiology, 3
euthanasia, 257
evidence-based medicine, 10, 335
exercise, 68–71, 247
    aerobic, 68
    benefits of, 68–69
    and coronary heart disease, 280
    determinants of, 69
    interventions, 70–71
    and obesity, 89, 95
    settings, 70
    and stress, 125
exhaustion phase of stress, 122
experiments, 10, 206
expressive writing, 155–156, 246, 316

## F

Facebook, 164
family. *See* family-based interventions;
        social support

family-based interventions, 61–62
    for cancer, 316
    for chronic health disorders, 246–248
    for coronary heart disease, 282
    for diet, 78
    for eating disorders, 98
    for obesity, 95
    for pain, 226
fear appeals, 48
feces, 26
fertilization, 28–29
fibroids, 29
fibromyalgia, 239
fight-or-flight response, 121
*Final Exit* (Humphry), 257
forebrain, 16
Freud, Sigmund, 5
functional somatic syndromes, 239
future challenges, 325–338
    chronic health disorders, 331–332
    and cost containment, 334
    and evidence-based medicine, 335
    health disparities, 328–330
    health promotion, 326–330
    international health, 335–337
    progress, 325–326
    research, 332–333

## G

gastroenteritis, 26
gastroesophageal reflux disease
        (GERD), 26
gate-control theory of pain, 214–216
gender
    and caregiving, 243
    and chronic health disorders, 243–244
    and health promotion, 329–330
    and hostility, 276
    and hypertension, 284
    and life expectancy, 255, 256
    and patient–provider communication, 183
    and stress, 138, 142, 330
    and use of health care services,
        172–173, 174
general adaptation syndrome, 121–122
genetic counseling, 18, 31
genetics, 30–31
    and alcoholism/problem drinking, 101
    and eating disorders, 98, 99
    genetic counseling, 18, 31
    and hypertension, 284
    and obesity, 89
GERD (gastroesophageal reflux disease), 26
gestation, 28–29
ghrelin, 89, 100
glomerular nephritis, 28
gonadotropic hormones, 19, 28
Greece, ancient, 4
grief, 266–267
guided imagery, 200–201, 225
gut-brain connection, 27
gynecologic cancer, 29

# H

hassles, 134–135
headache, 214
health, defined, 3
health behavior change. *See also* interventions
  affective aspects of, 48
  and brain, 52–53
  cognitive-behavioral approaches to.
    *See* cognitive-behavioral therapy (CBT)
  future challenges, 326–330
  health practitioner as effective
    agent of, 190
  and implementation intentions, 52
  and older adults, 326–327
  social engineering approaches, 61
  social support and, 58
  stages of change model, 59–61, 70, 308
  venues for, 61–64
health behaviors, 41–64. *See also* health
    behavior change
  in adolescents, 45
  attitude change and, 47–49
  change, affective aspects of, 48
  defined, 41
  factors in, 42–43
  and health habits, 41–42
  information-motivation-behavioral skills
    model, 190
  instability of, 43
  intervening with at-risk people, 45–46
  and negative affectivity, 145–146
  and older adults, 46–47
  overview, 41
  poor, modifying, barriers to, 43
  and race/ethnicity, 47
  self-regulation and, 51
  and socialization, 43–44, 173
  and stress, 123
health belief model, 49–50, 173
health care services, 168–177, 180–206
  access to, 42–43, 253, 325, 328, 331
  complementary and alternative medicine.
    *See* complementary and alternative
      medicine (CAM)
  delivery system structure, 180–181
  evidence-based medicine, 10, 335
  expansion of, 8
  future challenges, 331, 333–334
  and health promotion, 328
  hospitals, 190–194
  misuse of, 174–177
  and obesity, 88
  and patient consumerism, 180, 331
  patient–provider communication,
    182–190, 331
  and placebo effect, 203–206
  provider burnout, 192, 193
  providers, types of, 180
  and smoking, 115
  spending on, 328, 336
  and stress, 126
  and symptoms, 169–172, 176, 177, 185

and terminal illness, 262
  use of, 172–173
  as venues for behavior change, 61
health-compromising behaviors, 84–116
  alcoholism/problem drinking, 100–107
  characteristics of, 84–85
  eating disorders, 97–100
  marijuana use, 85
  obesity. *See* obesity
health disparities, 328–330
health habits, 41–42. *See also* health
    behavior change
health illiteracy, 185
health locus of control, 42
health maintenance organizations (HMOs),
    180–182, 191
health-promoting behaviors, 68–81
  accident prevention, 71–73
  and cancer, 316
  diet, 76–79
  exercise. *See* exercise
  rest/renewal/savoring, 81
  screenings, 73–75
  sleep, 79–81
  sun safety practices, 75–76
  vaccinations, 73
health promotions, 41, 326–330.
    *See also* health behavior change
  mass media campaigns and, 63
  and older adults, 46–47
health psychologists
  medical acceptance of, 9
  role of, 192
health psychology
  careers in, 12, 337–338
  defined, 3–4
  development, need for, 3–4
  need for, 6–9
  research. *See* research
heart, 21, 280
heart attack. *See* myocardial infarction (MI)
hedonic eating, 77
"Helen," 32
*Helicobacter pylori*, 26, 311
hepatitis, 26–27
high blood pressure. *See* hypertension
hindbrain, 15–16
hippocampus, 16
Hispanic Americans. *See* race
histamine, 33
historical overviews
  HIV/AIDS, 302–303
  mind-body relationship, 4–5
  placebo effect, 203–204
  research on stress, 121–124
  smoking, 108–109
HIV/AIDS, 302–310
  carriers for, 32
  coping with, 152, 309
  history of, 302–303
  interventions for, 304, 305–309
  progression of, 303, 309–310
  psychosocial impact of, 304–305

HMOs (health maintenance organizations),
    180–182, 191
Hodgkin's disease, 35
holistic medicine, 197
home care, 265
homeopathy, 197–198
homicide, 254
hormones, 19, 28, 274–275
hormone therapy (HT), 30
hospice, 264
hospice care, 264–265, 334
hospitalization, 190–194
  of children, 194–196
  goals of, 191–192
  impact on patient, 192–194
  interventions for, 194
  structure of, 191–192
  and terminal illness, 262
hostility, 275–277, 278
HPA (hypothalamic–pituitary adrenal)
    system, 125, 126
HPV (human papillomavirus), 73
HT (hormone therapy), 30
humoral immunity, 34
Huntington's disease, 18
hyperlipidemia, 25
hypertension, 22, 28, 283–287
  among African Americans,
    284–285
  assessment of, 283
  causes of, 283–284
  stress and, 284
  white coat, 285
hypnosis, 200, 225
hypochondriacs, 169
hypothalamic–pituitary adrenal (HPA)
    system, 125, 126
hypothalamus, 16, 19
hysterical contagion, 175

# I

illness delay, 176
illness representations, 170–172
IMB (information-motivation-behavioral)
    skills model, 190
immune system, 31–36, 125, 126,
    297–302
immunity, 33–34
implementation intentions, 52, 70, 95, 112
inattentiveness, 183
indirect transmission, 32
infant mortality rate, 252
infections, 32–33
inflammation, 25, 300
inflammatory response, 33–34, 36
  and complementary and alternative
    medicine, 197
  and coping, 163
  and coronary heart disease, 277, 278
  and stress, 126
influenza, 24, 32
informational support, 159